W9-BKB-232

Musculoskeletal Imaging

A Teaching File

Musculoskeletal Imaging
A Teaching File

Second Edition

Felix S. Chew, M.D., ED.M., M.B.A.
Professor and Vice-Chairman for Radiology Informatics
Section Head of Musculoskeletal Radiology
University of Washington, Seattle, Washington

Clinical Professor of Radiology
Wake Forest University School of Medicine
Winston-Salem, North Carolina

and

Catherine C. Roberts, M.D.
Associate Professor of Radiology
Associate Dean, Mayo School of Health Sciences Mayo Clinic
Phoenix, Arizona

With contributions from:

Anand P. Lalaji, M.D.
The Radiology Group of Stephens County
Toccoa, Georgia

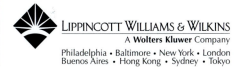
LIPPINCOTT WILLIAMS & WILKINS
A Wolters Kluwer Company
Philadelphia • Baltimore • New York • London
Buenos Aires • Hong Kong • Sydney • Tokyo

Acquisitions Editor: Lisa McAllister
Managing Editor: Kerry Barrett
Production Editor: Dave Murphy
Manufacturing Manager: Ben Rivera
Marketing Manager: Angela Panetta
Design Manager: Doug Smock
Compositor: TechBooks
Printer: RR Donnelley

Copyright © 2006 Text and Illustrations by Felix S. Chew, M.D.
Copyright © 2006 Design and Publication Rights by Lippincott Williams & Wilkins

© 2006 by LIPPINCOTT WILLIAMS & WILKINS
530 Walnut Street
Philadelphia, PA 19106 USA
LWW.com

All rights reserved. This book is protected by copyright. No part of this book may be reproduced in any form or by any means, including photocopying, or utilized by any information storage and retrieval system without written permission from the copyright owner, except for brief quotations embodied in critical articles and reviews. Materials appearing in this book prepared by individuals as part of their official duties as U.S. government employees are not covered by the above-mentioned copyright.

Printed in China

Library of Congress Cataloging-in-Publication Data

Chew, Felix S.
   Musculoskeletal imaging : a teaching file / Felix S. Chew and Catherine C. Roberts, with contributions from Anand P. Lalaji.– 2nd ed.
       p. ; cm.
   Includes bibliographical references and index.
   ISBN-13: 978-0-7817-5754-6
   ISBN-10: 0-7817-5754-1 (alk. paper)
   1. Musculoskeletal system—Imaging.   2. Musculoskeletal system—Diseases—Diagnosis.   I. Roberts, Catherine C.   II. Lalaji, Anand P.   III. Title.
       [DNLM: 1. Musculoskeletal Diseases—radiography—Case Reports.   2. Diagnostic Imaging—Case Reports.   WE 141 C529m 2006]
   RC925.7.C47 2006
   616.7′0754–dc22

                                                                        2005024857

Care has been taken to confirm the accuracy of the information presented and to describe generally accepted practices. However, the authors, editors, and publisher are not responsible for errors or omissions or for any consequences from application of the information in this book and make no warranty, expressed or implied, with respect to the currency, completeness, or accuracy of the contents of the publication. Application of this information in a particular situation remains the professional responsibility of the practitioner.

The authors, editors, and publisher have exerted every effort to ensure that drug selection and dosage set forth in this text are in accordance with current recommendations and practice at the time of publication. However, in view of ongoing research, changes in government regulations, and the constant flow of information relating to drug therapy and drug reactions, the reader is urged to check the package insert for each drug for any change in indications and dosage and for added warnings and precautions. This is particularly important when the recommended agent is a new or infrequently employed drug.

Some drugs and medical devices presented in this publication have Food and Drug Administration (FDA) clearance for limited use in restricted research settings. It is the esponsibility of the health care provider to ascertain the FDA status of each drug or device planned for use in their clinical practice.

To purchase additional copies of this book, call our customer service department at (800) 638-3030 or fax orders to (301) 824-7390. International customers should call (301) 714-2324.

Visit Lippincott Williams & Wilkins on the Internet: at LWW.com. Lippincott Williams & Wilkins customer service representatives are available from 8:30 am to 6 pm, EST.

10 9 8 7 6

RRS1001

We dedicate this work to our families.

CONTENTS

CHAPTER 3 SPINE

CHAPTER 4 PELVIS

CHAPTER 5 PROXIMAL FEMUR AND THIGH

CHAPTER 6 KNEE

CHAPTER 7 LOWER LEG

CHAPTER 8 ANKLE AND FOOT

Contributors to the First Edition:

Felix S. Chew, M.D.
Seattle, Washington

Susan G. Leffler, M.D.
Richmond, Virginia

Catherine Maldjian, M.D.
West Caldwell, New Jersey

Michael E. Mulligan, M.D.
Baltimore, Maryland

Donald J. Flemming, M.D.
Frederick, Maryland

PUBLISHER'S FOREWORD

Teaching Files are one of the hallmarks of education in radiology. There has long been a need for a comprehensive series of books, using the Teaching File format, that would provide the kind of personal consultation with the experts normally found only in the setting of a teaching hospital. Lippincott Williams & Wilkins is proud to have created such a series; our goal is to provide the resident and practicing radiologist with a useful resource that answers this need.

Actual cases have been culled from extensive teaching files in major medical centers. The discussions presented mimic those performed on a daily basis between residents and faculty members in all radiology departments.

The format of this series is designed so that each case can be studied as an unknown, if desired. A consistent format is used to present each case. A brief clinical history is given, followed by several images. Then, relevant findings, differential diagnosis, and final diagnosis are given, followed by a discussion of the case. The authors thereby guide the reader through the interpretation of each case.

We hope that this series will become a valuable and trusted teaching tool for radiologists at any stage of training or practice, and that it will also be a benefit to clinicians whose patients undergo these imaging studies.

The Publisher

Are you in need of a quick reference book on the subject of musculoskeletal imaging? Are you preparing to take the American Board of Radiology examination? Would you like to have in your possession an easy way to refresh or periodically assess your skills in musculoskeletal imaging? Do you require a simple method of testing your competence in musculoskeletal imaging? Would you like something portable that you could do at home or at the office or while on the road?

Well, look no further. You have in your hands all that you require: the second edition of *Musculoskeletal Imaging: A Teaching File*. As they say, it is new and improved, updated and authoritative, and all that you need for upgrading your skills and maintaining your competence in MSK imaging.

Each page or two contains a separate case with images, and each of the eight chapters contains up to 60 or more cases devoted to a single anatomic region of the skeleton; for example Chapter 1 is entitled Hand and Wrist. The selected cases cover the entire spectrum of disease encountered in this region: arthritis, trauma, infection, tumor, and metabolic and congenital diseases. It is hard to imagine that you would encounter a topic on the oral Board examination about MSK that wasn't covered in this text. The pertinent imaging findings are discussed, a germane differential diagnosis is presented, and each case is concluded with a brief review of the pertinent pathophysiology and etiology of the disease—all-in-all a remarkably concise and informative one- or two-page format highlighting the principal features of both the imaging and clinical characteristics of each case.

How you use this book is up to you. You can read it like any other text at your own pace, cover to cover, and be infinitely more informed about MSK radiology. Or you can go at it until the wee hours of the morning, as in cramming for the Board examination. You could look up cases as you encounter them in your practice to substantiate your diagnoses or to make certain you include the most likely alternative diagnoses. Or you might want to test yourself by reviewing the images and coming up with an answer before reading the accompanying text to see if you noted the important findings and made the correct diagnosis. Nothing to fear by doing so; after all, you keep your own score. It is like having your very own private self-assessment module.

This book's unique format is adaptable to many purposes, so the choice is yours.

Even if you have a previous edition of this book, you should seriously consider the purchase of this new edition. Advances in musculoskeletal imaging have occurred at a rapid pace, and you certainly want to keep abreast of new developments. This new edition will aid in this endeavor. Older, less relevant cases have been removed and replaced with new and better examples. The book has been expanded to include more timely cases illustrating up-to-date imaging technologies, particularly multidetector-row CT and MRI, so essential to today's musculoskeletal imaging.

Drs. Chew and Roberts are to be commended for maintaining the same high-quality standards in the selection and presentation of their material in this second edition of *Musculoskeletal Imaging: A Teaching File* as had been brought to bear in the first edition. I know from experience that this was not an easy task.

It is now up to you to read, mark, and inwardly digest the fruits of these authors' labor. I am certain that this will prove to be both refreshing and informative. Enjoy!

Lee F. Rogers, M.D.
Professor of Radiology
University of Arizona
Tucson, Arizona

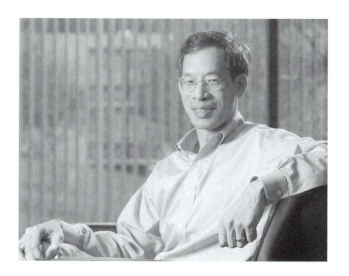 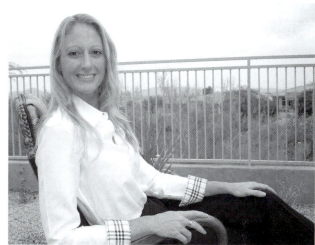

This book of teaching file cases is intended to duplicate the learning experience of sitting at the viewbox with an expert skeletal radiologist and master teacher. Unlike a comprehensive textbook organized according to pathophysiology, this book is organized by anatomic regions. It provides a broad variety of cases, each intended to teach the nuances of image-based diagnostic reasoning. The cases encompass all imaging modalities, including radiography, CT, MR imaging, nuclear imaging, and sonography, as well as all categories of disease, including trauma, tumors, joint disease, endocrine and metabolic bone disease, infections, congenital and developmental conditions, and musculoskeletal manifestations of systemic disease. The cases are presented as unknowns in a consistent format. Each begins with a brief clinical history and one or more radiologic images. A description of the relevant findings, the diagnosis, and comments regarding the case follow, with emphasis on image-based diagnostic reasoning. The discussions reflect those that typically occur between radiologic consultant and clinician or between a faculty member and radiology trainee. An extensive subject index and lists of diagnoses organized by pathophysiology and anatomic region make the material accessible for use as a reference or as an atlas.

Case selection is not intended to parallel ones daily clinical experience at the viewbox, nor to provide an exhaustive subject review. Rather, the cases make specific teaching points, raise clinically relevant issues, satisfy intellectual curiosity, and reflect the particular interests of the authors. By including a number of companion cases, we hope to give the reader an appreciation of the range of radiologic variety in specific diseases. Although the teaching file is organized by anatomic region, in some cases of systemic or polyostotic disease, companion images from other regions are included for convenience. Many diagnoses are represented by more than one case. Some discussions range well beyond the analysis of imaging features and differential diagnosis to include the pathophysiology underlying the images, as well as clinical and management considerations.

FELIX S. CHEW, M.D.
CATHERINE C. ROBERTS, M.D.

ACKNOWLEDGMENTS

Preparation of the first edition of *Musculoskeletal Imaging: A Teaching File*, was begun at Massachusetts General Hospital (MGH), during the time that Susan G. Leffler, M.D., and I were members of the Division of Bone and Joint Radiology. With the help of Catherine Maldjian, M.D., who was on the faculty at Temple University at the time and subsequently at New York University Medical Center, the book was completed while I was Section Head of Musculoskeletal Radiology at Wake Forest. Drs. Leffler and Maldjian have since left academic radiology for private practices, where they are both doing superb work. Contributions to the first edition were also made by Michael E. Mulligan, M.D., and Donald J. Flemming, M.D. The preponderance of the case material for the first edition was drawn from MGH, and most of the remaining material was drawn from the personal teaching collections of the authors. I acknowledge the gracious help of my former MGH colleagues, Drs. Daniel I. Rosenthal, Susan V. Kattapuram, and William E. Palmer, for providing me with or guiding me to interesting cases.

For the second edition of this book, some new cases and illustrations were added, while a few were deleted, and the remainder were updated. Much of the new material was developed by Anand P. Lalaji, M.D., from cases at Wake Forest University School of Medicine. I am also grateful to my former Wake Forest colleagues, Drs. Carol A. Boles, Leon Lenchik, and Lee F. Rogers, for bringing many interesting cases to my attention. Some additional material was developed at the University of Washington with the help of Dr. Michael L. Richardson. I also wish to thank the many residents and fellows whose comments helped shape the final product.

FELIX S. CHEW, M.D.

It was a pleasure and an honor to be involved with revising the 'purple book.' I memorized the first edition of this book when I was studying for the Oral Radiology Boards. Felix Chew is a dedicated teacher and is the best mentor I could have imagined. His mentoring has changed the course of my career and I am forever indebted to him.

My Mayo Clinic colleagues, Drs. Patrick T. Liu, Ethan M. Braunstein, F. Spencer Chivers and William W. Daniel, helped identify cases for inclusion in this second edition. My most sincere thanks go to my family who support my work wholeheartedly.

CATHERINE C. ROBERTS, M.D.

ABBREVIATIONS AND ACRONYMS

ACL — anterior cruciate ligament
AIDS — acquired immunodeficiency syndrome
ANA — antinuclear antibodies
AP — anteroposterior
C1, C2, etc. — first cervical vertebra (atlas), second cervical vertebra (axis), etc.
CMC joint — carpometacarpal joint
CPPD — calcium pyrophosphate dihydrate
CT — computed tomography
DDH — developmental dysplasia of the hip
DIP joint — distal interphalangeal joint
DISH — diffuse idiopathic skeletal hyperostosis
DISI — dorsal intercalated segment instability (dorsiflexion instability)
DPA — dual photon absorptiometry
DXA — dual x-ray absorptiometry
FS — fat suppression
FSE — fast spin-echo
GRE — gradient-recalled echo
HIV — human immunodeficiency virus
HLA — human lymphocyte antigens
HU — Hounsfield unit (unit of x-ray attenuation on a CT scan)
IM rod — intramedullary rod
IP joint — interphalangeal joint
IR — inversion recovery
K-wire — Kirschner wire
L1, L2, etc. — first lumbar vertebra, second lumbar vertebra, etc.
LCL — lateral collateral ligament
MCL — medial collateral ligament
MCP joint — metacarpophalangeal joint

MDP — methylene diphosphonate
MFH — malignant fibrous histiocytoma
MR imaging — magnetic resonance imaging
MRI — magnetic resonance imaging
MTP joint — metatarsophalangeal joint
ORIF — open reduction internal fixation
PA — posteroanterior
PCL — posterior cruciate ligament
PD — proton density
PIP joint — proximal interphalangeal joint
PMNs — polymorphonuclear leukocytes
PVNS — pigmented villonodular synovitis
QCT — quantitative computed tomography
RF — rheumatoid factor
S1, S2, etc. — first sacral vertebra, second sacral vertebra, etc.
SCFE — slipped capital femoral epiphysis
SI joint — sacroiliac joint
SLE — systemic lupus erythematosus
STIR — short tau inversion recovery
T1, T2, etc. — first thoracic vertebra, second thoracic vertebra, etc.
Tc-99m — technetium-99m
TFCC — triangular fibrocartilage complex
THA — total hip arthroplasty
THR — total hip replacement
TKA — total knee arthroplasty
TKR — total knee replacement
TMT joint — tarsometatarsal joint
VISI — volar intercalated segment instability (volar flexion instability)
WBC — white blood cells

FIGURE CREDITS

Figures 1–24 and 3–27 from Chew FS. Radiologic manifestations in the musculoskeletal system of miscellaneous endocrine disorders. Radiol Clin North Am 1991;29(1):135–147.

Figures 2–32A and 2–32B from Chew FS, Schulze ES, Mattia AR. Osteomyelitis. AJR AM J Roentgenol 1994; 162:942.

Figures 2–51A, 2–51B, and 2–51C from Chew FS, Huang-Hellinger F. Brown tumor. AJR AM J Roentgenol 1993;160:752.

Figures 3–14A and 3–14B from Chew FS, Pena CS, Keel SB. Cervical spine osteoblastoma. AJR AM J Roentgenol 1998;171:1244.

Figures 5–38A, 5–38B, and 5–38D from Ramsdell MG, Chew FS, Keel SB. Myxoid liposarcoma of the thigh. AJR AM J Roentgenol 1998;170:1242.

Figures 6–45A and 6–45C from Chew FS, Ramsdell MG, Keel SB. Metallosis after total knee replacement. AJR Am J Roentegnol 1998;170:1556.

Figures 7–19A, 7–19B, 7–19C, and 7–19D from Chew FS, al-Sinan AA. Periosteal osteosarcoma of the tibia. AJR Am J Roentgenol 1977;169:1034.

Figures 7–31A and 7–31B from Spillane RM, Whitman GJ, Chew FS. Peroneal nerve ganglion cyst. AJR Am J Roentgenol 1996;166:682.

CHAPTER ONE
HAND AND WRIST

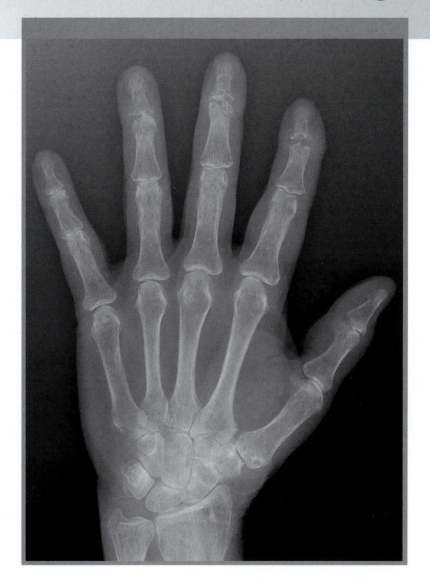

CASE 1-1

Clinical History: 37-year-old man.

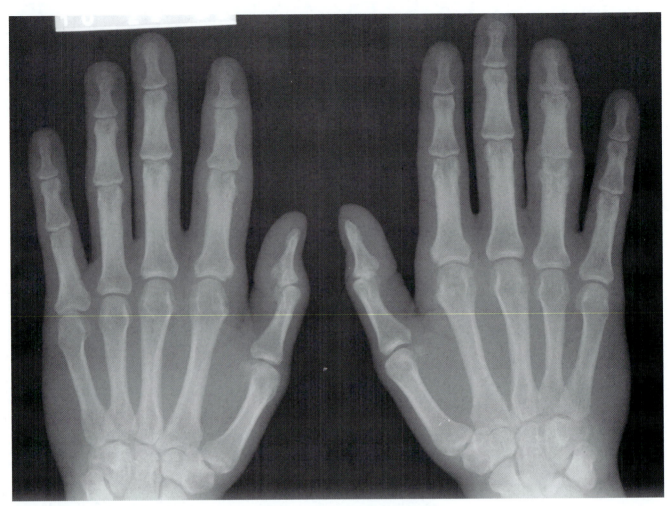

Figure 1-1

Findings: Posteroanterior (PA) radiographs of both hands. On the left side, sausage-digit soft tissue swelling involves the entire index finger. The other fingers are normal. There is a single erosion at the metacarpophalangeal (MCP) joint of the index finger at the radial aspect of the proximal phalanx, and fluffy periostitis is present adjacent to the proximal interphalangeal (PIP) and distal interphalangeal (DIP) joints. Overall bone mineralization is preserved, and there is no abnormality of alignment or narrowing of the cartilage spaces. On the right side, the ring finger shows sausage-digit soft tissue swelling. There are erosions at the PIP and DIP joints, and periostitis.

Differential Diagnosis: Psoriatic arthritis, erosive osteoarthritis, rheumatoid arthritis, gout.

Diagnosis: Psoriatic arthritis.

Discussion: Sausage-digit soft tissue swelling is characteristic of diffuse inflammation, raising the possibility of cellulitis and underlying osteomyelitis as well as one of the seronegative spondyloarthropathies such as psoriatic arthritis. This pattern of swelling, reflecting involvement of the tendons and ligaments as well as the joint capsules, is different from the fusiform soft tissue swelling that is characteristic of effusion or synovial joint inflammation. The presence of erosions, as well as the fluffy periostitis, is pathognomonic for an inflammatory process. In this case, the periostitis is more evident when the cortex and shapes of the abnormal bones are compared with that of their normal neighbors. The distribution of involvement—a single, entire digit, with normal adjacent digits—is characteristic of psoriatic arthritis. Psoriatic arthritis is more prevalent in HIV-positive patients [1]. Early changes of psoriatic arthritis may precede or follow dermatologic manifestations of psoriasis, sometimes by many years. Although many patients have relatively indolent arthritic changes, some patients may have a very aggressive, deforming, and disabling arthritis for which early, aggressive treatment is indicated [2].

CASE 1-2

Clinical History: 55-year-old man with rash.

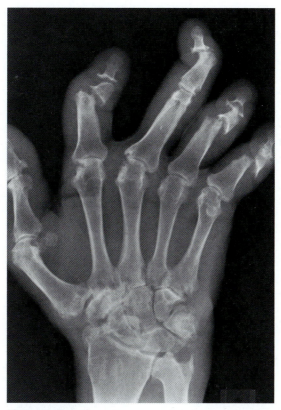

Figure 1-2

Findings: PA radiograph of the right hand. Polyarticular arthritis is distributed through the entire hand and wrist. The DIP and PIP joints of all the fingers are severely involved, with erosions of the articular ends of the bones resulting in complete loss of cartilage and subarticular bone. Several joints have pencil-in-cup deformities. There is pancompartmental involvement of the wrist, with erosions and mature periosteal new bone. The periosteal bone is best seen at the ulnar styloid processes. The contralateral hand has a similar appearance.

Differential Diagnosis: Psoriatic arthritis, erosive osteoarthritis, rheumatoid arthritis, gout.

Diagnosis: Psoriatic arthritis, arthritis mutilans appearance.

Discussion: Psoriasis is a common, genetically predisposed skin disease characterized by dry, pink, scaly, nonpruritic lesions. Psoriatic arthritis is an inflammatory arthropathy associated with psoriasis and characterized by the absence of rheumatoid factor [3]. As many as 5% of patients with psoriasis has an associated arthritis. Psoriatic arthritis has five patterns of clinical presentation:

1. Asymmetric oligoarthritis, seen in more than 50% of cases.

2. Polyarthritis with predominantly DIP involvement, of which the classic presentation is seen in 5% to 19% of cases.
3. Symmetric seronegative polyarthritis simulating rheumatoid arthritis, seen in up to 25% of cases.
4. Sacroiliitis and spondylitis resembling ankylosing spondylitis, seen in 20% to 40% of cases.
5. Arthritis mutilans with resorption of phalanges, seen in 5% of cases.

Individual patients may progress from one clinical pattern to another. The dominant radiologic features in this case—erosions and periostitis—are those of inflammatory arthritis [4]. The features of degenerative joint disease—osteophytes, subchondral sclerosis, and asymmetric joint space loss—are conspicuously absent. The preservation of normal bone mineralization mitigates against rheumatoid arthritis, in which profound osteoporosis is an invariable feature in chronic, severe disease. The greater severity of interphalangeal (IP) joint involvement, compared with carpal and MCP joint involvement, favors psoriatic arthritis over rheumatoid arthritis. The complete erosions of the articular ends of the phalanges and the involvement of the DIP joints are characteristic of the arthritis mutilans pattern of peripheral psoriatic arthritis.

Clinical History: 55-year-old woman with stiff hands.

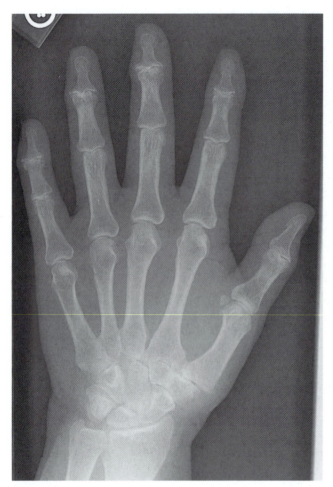

Figure 1-3   A

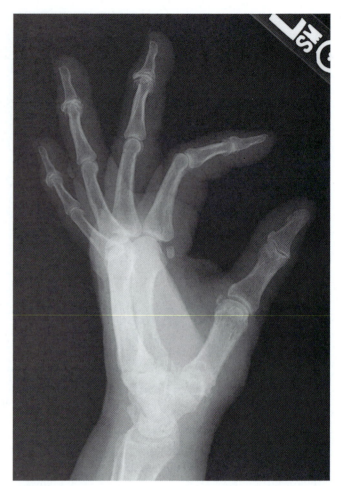

Figure 1-3   B

Findings: PA (**A**) and lateral (**B**) radiographs of the left hand. Arthritic changes involve the PIP and DIP joints of the fingers, and the IP, MCP, and basal joints of the thumb. These changes are characterized by bony hypertrophy, with large osteophytes and subchondral sclerosis. The cartilage spaces are narrowed asymmetrically. Mineralization of the hand is normal. Soft tissue swelling is not prominent, and there are no erosions.

Differential Diagnosis: Osteoarthritis, pyrophosphate arthropathy.

Diagnosis: Primary osteoarthritis.

Discussion: The presence of hypertrophic degenerative changes at the basal joint of the thumb (first carpometacarpal joint and scaphoid-trapezium-trapezoid joints) is generally seen only in primary osteoarthritis. Involvement of the PIP and DIP joints is also characteristic. Soft tissue swelling, juxtaarticular osteoporosis, erosions, and ankylosis should be absent, unless inflammatory changes are also present. Osteoarthritis is the most common form of polyarticular arthritis. Its prevalence increases with age, so that it is nearly ubiquitous in patients older than 65. In addition to the hand, other common sites of osteoarthritis include the hip, the knee, the first metatarsophalangeal joint, and the synovial joints of the cervical and lumbar spine. The early morphologic abnormality in osteoarthritis is fibrillation of the surface of the articular cartilage, reflecting disruption of the molecular structure of the cartilage. Progressive mechanical erosion of the cartilage, thinning of the cartilage, and formation of fissures will eventually expose the subchondral bone. An adaptive response of osteophyte formation and subchondral sclerosis, combined with asymmetric cartilage space narrowing, results in the characteristic radiographic appearance [5]. In pyrophosphate arthropathy, involvement of the MCP and radial-carpal joints is more typical.

Clinical History: 58-year-old woman with arthritis.

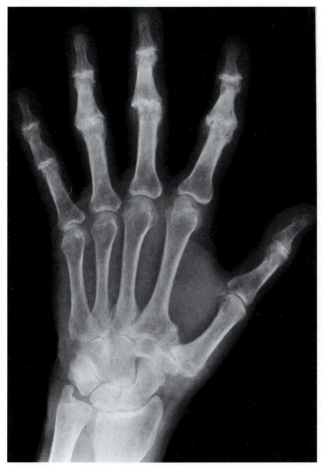

Figure 1-4 A

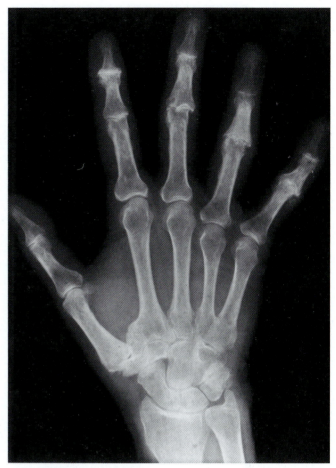

Figure 1-4 B

Findings: (A, B). PA radiographs of both hands. There is polyarticular disease with asymmetric joint space narrowing, osteophytes, and subchondral sclerosis. The predominant sites of involvement are the IP joints and the basal joints of the thumb, with sparing of the MCP and radiocarpal joints. A seagull appearance is present at the PIP joints of the middle, ring, and little fingers. Bone mineralization is normal.

Differential Diagnosis: Osteoarthritis, erosive osteoarthritis, psoriatic arthritis, pyrophosphate arthropathy.

Diagnosis: Erosive osteoarthritis.

Discussion: The presence of osteophytes and subchondral sclerosis indicates a degenerative form of arthritis. The particular distribution of involvement is characteristic of osteoarthritis (IP joints, basal joint of the thumb). Although joint degeneration always has some component of synovial inflammation because of the presence of joint debris and cartilage breakdown products, when the inflammation has erosive changes that dominate the clinical presentation, the condition may be called erosive osteoarthritis [6]. Radiographs show the degenerative features and distribution of primary osteoarthritis, but the acute synovitis causes inflammatory erosions, uniform joint space narrowing, and sometimes ankylosis. A characteristic "gull-wing" appearance may be seen on PA radiographs at the IP joints of the fingers, corresponding to central erosions and bony hypertrophy [7]. The typical patient is a postmenopausal woman (female-to-male ratio of about 12:1). The inflammation usually subsides within a few months to a couple of years, leaving the residual degenerative changes. Although psoriatic arthritis may have a similar distribution, the presence of subchondral sclerosis and osteophytes eliminates psoriatic arthritis as a diagnostic consideration.

CASE 1-5

Clinical History: 81-year-old woman presents with progressive index finger swelling.

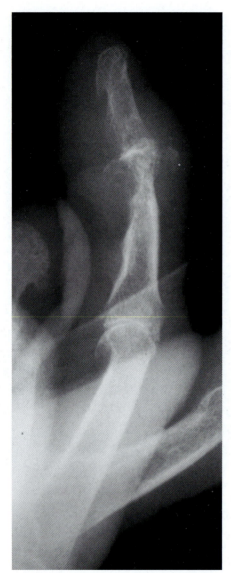

Figure 1-5   A

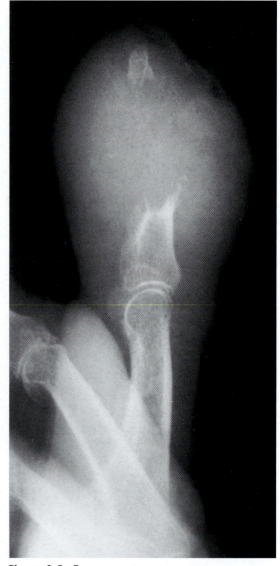

Figure 1-5   B

Findings: (A) Lateral radiograph of the DIP joint of the index finger demonstrates marked soft tissue swelling. The joint space is obliterated, and there is osteolysis and ossific debris at the margins. (B) Lateral radiograph of the DIP joint taken 3 months later demonstrates progressive soft tissue swelling, with complete destruction of the normal osseous architecture on both sides of the joint. Debris is again noted in the surrounding soft tissues.

Differential Diagnosis: None.

Diagnosis: Septic arthritis.

Discussion: Joint effusion is the first radiographic sign of a joint infection, but it is a nonspecific finding. Hyperemia associated with the inflammatory change leads to juxtaarticular osteoporosis, and destruction of cartilage by enzymes elaborated by inflammatory cells results in decreasing joint space. Erosions of bone with osteolysis and fragmentation may follow, with osteomyelitis from contiguous spread. Joint destruction caused by pyogenic infection may progress rapidly over only a few days. Risk factors for developing septic arthritis include advanced age (80 years or older), diabetes mellitus, rheumatoid arthritis, joint surgery or joint replacement, and skin infection [8]. Septic arthritis may also occur as a postoperative complication. The most common organism recovered from a septic joint is *Staphylococcus aureus* [9]. The most commonly infected joint is the knee.

Clinical History: 50-year-old immunocompromised man with deformed, tender, swollen thumb.

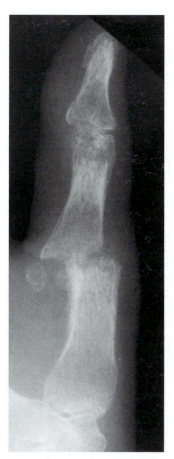
Figure 1-6   A

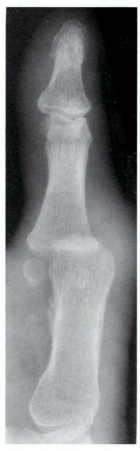
Figure 1-6   B

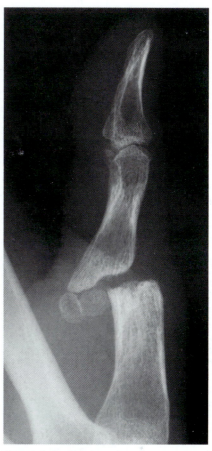
Figure 1-6   C

Findings: (A) Lateral radiograph demonstrates soft tissue swelling and erosion of the articular surfaces of the first MCP joint. The surfaces of the erosions have indistinct margins. Volar subluxation is present. (B) Oblique radiograph taken 2 months after presentation demonstrates increased reactive bone at the articular erosions and metadiaphyseal periostitis. (C) Lateral radiograph taken 9 months after initial presentation, following treatment, demonstrates smooth, amputated, well-corticated margins with resolved periostitis.

Differential Diagnosis: Osteomyelitis, septic arthritis, tuberculous arthritis, psoriatic arthritis.

Diagnosis: Tuberculous arthritis.

Discussion: The images in this case document a slowly destructive arthritis of a single joint that healed without ankylosis. Tuberculous arthritis may be caused by direct extension from tuberculous osteomyelitis of initial seeding of the synovium, generally from a pre-existing focus of infection of the lung. The overgrowth of granulation tissue from the synovium extends into the joint, destroying both the articular cartilage as well as the subchondral bone. There is virtually no reactive bone formation. Although fibrous ankylosis may result, bony ankylosis ordinarily does not. The process may be protracted and evolve with only mild symptoms occurring over a period of months. Tuberculous arthritis is an unusual form of extrapulmonary tuberculosis, appearing in no more than 1% of patients with tuberculosis. Both *Mycobacterium tuberculosis* as well as atypical mycobacteria may be the infective agents. Often seen in association with Human Immunodeficiency Virus (HIV) infection, patients with tuberculous arthritis who are not infected with HIV are usually adults between 30 and 60 years of age. Predisposing factors for joint involvement include joint trauma, systemic disease such as diabetes mellitus, intravenous drug abuse, intra-articular corticosteroid injection, and HIV infection. HIV specifically eliminates the tissue macrophages and CD4 lymphocytes that provide immunity against tuberculosis; therefore, it is not surprising that tuberculosis, one of the more virulent of opportunistic infections, appears fairly early in HIV disease and is becoming much more common [10]. A large proportion of patients who are infected with tuberculosis will also be seropositive for HIV, and patients with tuberculosis are more likely to have extrapulmonary involvement if they are seropositive for HIV [11].

Clinical History: 63-year-old woman with chronic cough.

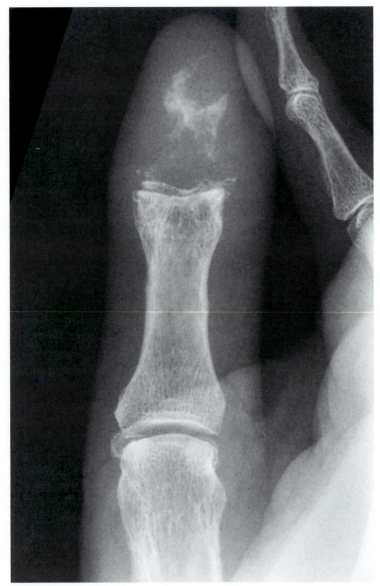

Figure 1-7

Findings: Detail of thumb reveals mixed lytic and permeative destruction of the distal phalanx with associated soft tissue swelling. The joint space is preserved.

Differential Diagnosis: Infection, trauma, squamous cell carcinoma, metastases, melanoma.

Diagnosis: Lytic metastasis (lung carcinoma).

Discussion: The radiographic appearance is that of an aggressive bone-destroying lesion. Differential diagnostic considerations might include infection, but one might expect an infection to spread into the joint space and involve the adjacent bone. Metastases to the hands and feet, particularly the digits, are uncommon. Location in the distal phalanx of a digit, or in a subungual location, is rare [12] and is associated with a poor prognosis. Phalangeal metastasescommonly display inflammatory symptoms that may mimic an acute infection [13]. They may also present as onycholysis (detachment of a nail plate from its distal and lateral attachments) [14]. The most common responsible primary sites are lung, kidney, and breast, and in 44% of patients with subungual metastases, this was the presenting symptom [15]. The most common primary malignant lesions of the distal phalanges are epidermoid carcinoma and malignant melanoma. External cortical erosions radiographically characterize primary nail bed lesions, whereas metastatic lesions tend to show extensive permeated destruction [16].

Clinical History: 35-year-old man with aching pain and exquisite tenderness at the tip of his thumb. There is no history of trauma.

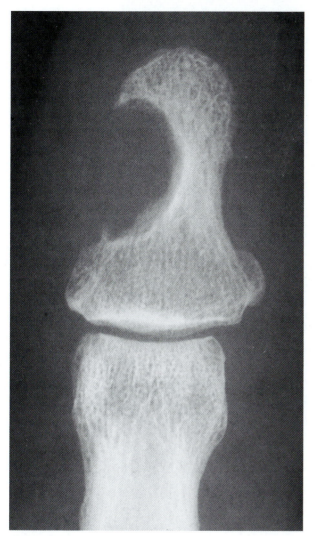

Figure 1-8 A

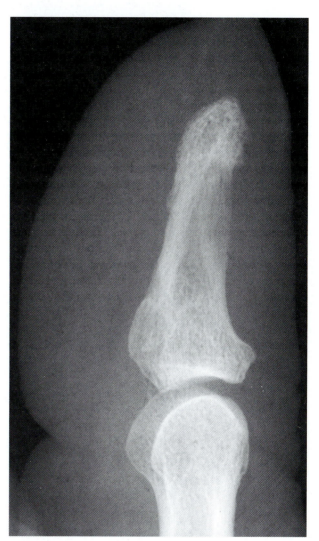

Figure 1-8 B

Findings: (A) PA radiograph of the thumb demonstrates a well-defined eccentric lesion with sclerotic borders replacing more than 50% of the midsubstance of the terminal phalanx, beneath the nail bed. (B) Lateral view shows the bony abnormality is a shallow, well-marginated erosion on the dorsal aspect of the distal phalanx, with associated soft tissue swelling in the nail bed.

Differential Diagnosis: Glomus tumor, epidermoid inclusion cyst, foreign body granuloma, enchondroma, sarcoidosis.

Diagnosis: Glomus tumor.

Discussion: Locating the lesion in the soft tissues of the nail bed rather than as an intramedullary bone lesion is key to approaching the diagnosis. Although the differential diagnosis would include foreign body granuloma, epidermoid inclusion cyst, enchondroma, and sarcoidosis, the clinical presentation suggests the correct diagnosis. Glomus tumors are hamartomas that arise from the neuromyoarterial glomus, a normal, specialized vascular anastomotic complex surrounded by nerve elements [17]. Located in diverse internal organs and in the dermis and superficial subcutaneous tissues in the extremities, particularly around the fingertips, the neuromyoarterial glomus functions in the regulation of body temperature. Glomus tumors are typically small, soft tissue lesions that are highly vascular. In the fingers, most are located in the subungual region, with the remaining located in the pulp [18]. Radiographically, they produce shallow erosions in adjacent bone. Direct demonstration by magnetic resonance imaging (MRI) has been described, and multiple lesions may occur [19]. Intraosseous glomus tumors are rare. Complete surgical excision is curative.

Clinical History: 43-year-old construction worker with chronically swollen finger.

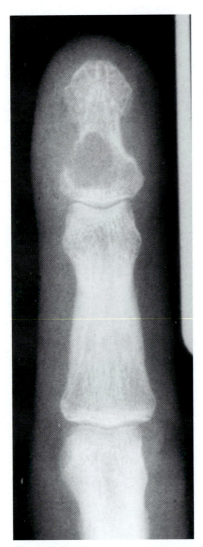
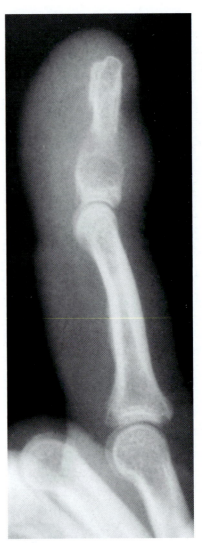

Figure 1-9 A   **Figure 1-9 B**

Findings: (A) PA radiograph of the finger shows a round lucent lesion in the distal phalanx with a well-defined sclerotic margin. The lesion is slightly eccentric in location. (B) Lateral radiograph shows a subungual soft tissue mass raising the nail bed and eroding the dorsal surface of the cortex of the distal phalanx.

Differential Diagnosis: Glomus tumor, epidermoid inclusion cyst, foreign body granuloma, enchondroma, sarcoidosis.

Diagnosis: Epidermoid inclusion cyst.

Discussion: Bone cysts lined with epidermis are uncommon and are found only in the skull and the distal phalanges. Epidermoid inclusion cysts are posttraumatic lesions that result from penetrating trauma in which dermoid elements are implanted into the bone [20,21]. Growth of these elements results in a slowly enlarging cyst filled with desquamated keratin flakes, sebaceous material, and foreign-body reactive tissue and debris. Nearly all lesions involving the phalanges are reported to be in the hand. In the majority of cases, a definite history of trauma to the affected finger exists. The typical injury is a fairly severe crushing wound to the fingertip. Men are affected more frequently than women by a 2:1 ratio. The episode of trauma may have occurred decades before presentation, often when the patient was a child or young adult. Epidermoid inclusion cysts present clinically with swelling, often with associated redness and tenderness. They may occasionally be asymptomatic. The classic radiologic appearance is a clear-cut, lucent, rounded lesion with a sclerotic rim, causing destruction and expansion of the phalanx. Sometimes a retained foreign body, implanted at the time of trauma, will be visible [22]. Treatment is surgical excision or curettage; amputation is generally not required.

CASE 1-10

Clinical History: 38-year-old woman with abnormal chest radiograph.

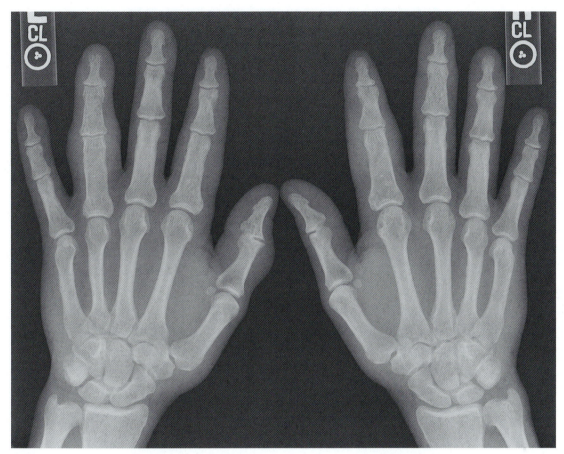

Figure 1-10

Findings: PA radiograph of both hands shows asymmetric soft tissue swelling, involving the index and ring fingers on the left, and the index and middle fingers on the right. The bones of these fingers show bone loss characterized by cortical thinning, small punched-out erosions, and endosteal scalloping. A lace-like appearance is best seen in the middle phalanx of the right middle finger.

Differential Diagnosis: Sarcoidosis, hemangiomatosis, enchondromatosis, tophaceous gout.

Diagnosis: Sarcoidosis.

Discussion: Sarcoidosis may involve the joints in about 10% of cases, but sarcoidosis most often causes transient migratory polyarticular arthralgias without radiographic findings. A chronic granulomatous arthritis develops in only a few patients, leading to chronic noncaseating granulomatous inflammation of the synovium. Granulomas within or adjacent to the bone may result in punched-out cortical erosions or central lytic lesions with nonaggressive features within the medullary cavity. The process appears not to provoke reactive bone, and the remaining portions of cortex and trabeculae become reinforced and thickened. The middle and distal phalanges of the fingers are the typical sites of involvement. The characteristic appearance caused by the presence of multiple granulomatous lesions has been described as lace-like, latticework, or honeycomb. The most common radiographic appearance in bone is lace-like or honeycomb involvement of the hands or feet. Cyst-like lesions in bone are, in fact, bone that has been replaced by solid sarcoid granulomas, and are not actually cysts. Soft tissue involvement by sarcoid may occur in one-third of patients. The hand, bone, muscle, tendon, cutaneous or subcutaneous tissue, or synovium may be involved [23,24]. The natural history of sarcoid bone lesions is variable, ranging from rare cases of recovery to gradual progression and eventual auto-amputation. Treatment with systemic corticosteroids may result in improvement or stabilization of bone lesions, but bone usually does not return to normal.

Radiologic appearances consist of cyst-like lesions, a lace-like pattern, or extensive bone destruction. Asymmetric soft tissue swelling may be present. Enlargement of the fingertips may result in an appearance on physical examination described as "pseudoclubbing," and reflects phalangeal involvement [25].

Clinical History: 29-year-old woman who was in an accident 2 years ago.

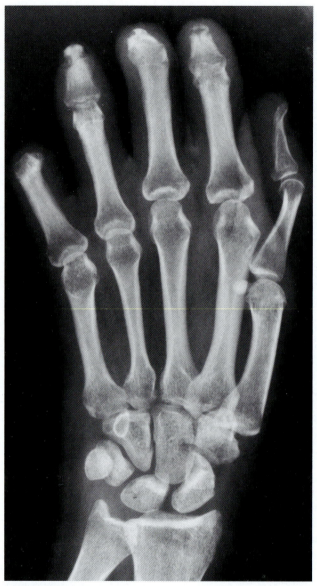

Figure 1-11

Findings: PA radiograph of the hand shows loss of the distal portions of the fingers. The margins of the bone loss are corticated and well healed, with some dystrophic calcification at the tips of the index, middle, and ring fingers. The thumb is spared. There is no osteoporosis and there are no joint changes.

Differential Diagnosis: Thermal injury (burns, frostbite), diabetic neuroarthropathy, leprosy, scleroderma, Lesch-Nyhan disease.

Diagnosis: Burns.

Discussion: Loss of the distal portions of multiple contiguous fingers, including distal phalanges and DIP joints, is usually from a trauma. Sparing of the thumb and normal morphology of the more proximal portions of the hand and wrist makes a systemic or vascular disease unlikely. The presence of dense bone distally would not be expected after traumatic mechanical amputation, but is common following severe burns. Burns cause coagulative tissue necrosis. The depth of the injury is related to the severity and duration of the applied heat. Initially, one can see soft tissue loss and soft tissue edema. Osteoporosis and periostitis may occur in the weeks that follow. Periarticular osseous excrescences are common after extensive burns and may be seen 2 to 3 months after injury. The exact pathogenesis of these ossifications is unknown and seems not to correlate with the severity of the burn.

Clinical History: 45-year-old woman with progressive gastrointestinal symptoms.

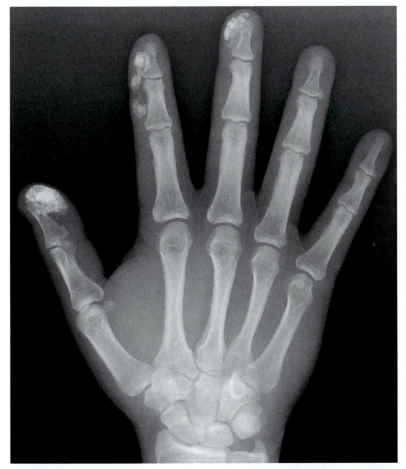

Figure 1-12   A

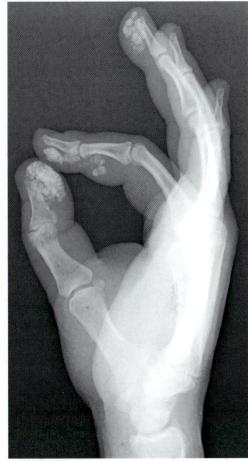

Figure 1-12   B

Findings: PA (**A**) and lateral (**B**) radiographs of the right hand show dense, amorphous calcium hydroxyapatite deposits in the distal portions of several digits.

Differential Diagnosis: Scleroderma, mixed connective tissue disorder.

Diagnosis: Scleroderma.

Discussion: Scleroderma (progressive systemic sclerosis) is a multisystem fibrosing, auto immune, connective tissue disease of variable clinical course. Characteristically, the skin becomes fibrotic, thickened, and taut. Gastrointestinal and renal involvement is prominent, but radiologic manifestations in the musculoskeletal system are present in most patients. These abnormalities are usually seen in the hands and consist of soft tissue atrophy, soft tissue calcification, resorption of the phalangeal tufts, and DIP joint erosions. Osseous destruction and bony erosions are common in the phalangeal tufts. The soft tissue atrophy results in cone-shaped fingertips. Subcutaneous calcifications are typically present in multiple digits and elsewhere in the extremities. The calcium deposits are dystrophic, and consist of calcium hydroxyapatite deposits at sites of local tissue damage. Calcification may also occur in tendons and tendon sheaths, in joint capsules, and even within the joint cavity. Synovial fibrosis without inflammation may cause flexion contractures.

CASE 1-13

Clinical History: 2-year-old girl with bone problems.

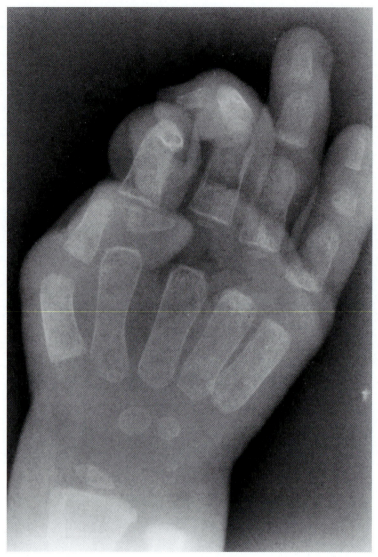

Figure 1-13

Findings: PA radiograph of the hand shows that the metacarpals and phalanges are mildly expanded, with thin, osteopenic cortex and no clearly defined trabecular bone pattern within. The metacarpals are not modeled, resulting in a cylindrical shape. A ground-glass radiolucency can be appreciated.

Differential Diagnosis: Fibrous dysplasia, sickle cell disease, hemoglobinopathies, Gaucher's disease.

Diagnosis: Polyostotic fibrous dysplasia.

Discussion: The age of the patient and the diffuse, polyostotic, dysplastic nature of the abnormalities suggests a congenital condition. The mild expansion of the long bones and thinning of the cortices suggests a space-occupying process in the marrow. Fibrous dysplasia is a nonhereditary condition in which osteoblasts fail to undergo normal morphologic differentiation and maturation, resulting in lesions containing fibro-osseous tissue rather than bone. Lesions may be solitary or multiple, and one or more bones may be involved. Approximately 70% to 80% of cases are monostotic, 20% to 30% are polyostotic, and 2% to 3% are associated with endocrine dysfunction. The typical endocrine abnormality is precocious female sexual development and cutaneous pigmentation (McCune-Albright syndrome). Fibrous dysplasia weakens the structural integrity of the involved bone, predisposing it to fracture or progressive deformity. Such orthopedic complications represent the major morbidity of fibrous dysplasia. Malignant degeneration in fibrous dysplasia is extremely rare, but has been reported in the literature [26].

CASE 1-14

Clinical History: 50-year-old man with acute pain in the index finger following minor trauma.

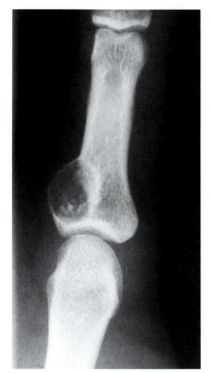

Figure 1-14   A

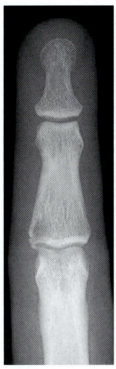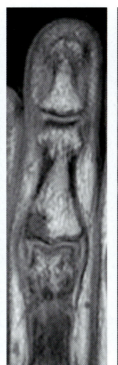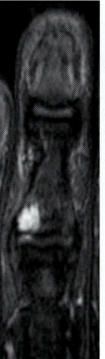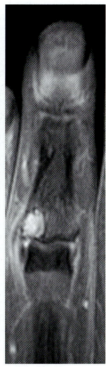

Figure 1-14   B

Findings: PA radiograph of the left index finger (**A**). There is a lucent lesion in the proximal end of the proximal phalanx. Well-defined punctate matrix mineralization is evident, consistent with cartilage, whereas the bulk of the lesion is lucent. The overlying cortex is thinned and mildly expanded. Companion case (**B**), a 47-year-old man with finger pain after a fall. AP radiograph, coronal T1-weighted, coronal T2-weighted fat-suppressed, and coronal T1-weighted gadolinium-enhanced fat-suppressed MR images demonstrates an enhancing, lytic lesion at the base of the middle phalanx.

Differential Diagnosis: None.

Diagnosis: Enchondroma.

Discussion: The lesion has benign characteristics, with a well-defined sclerotic endosteal margin and an intact, although thinned and mildly expanded, cortex. The presence of cartilage calcifications is diagnostic in an adult. Given the clinical history, a nondisplaced pathologic fracture is likely, although not demonstrated on this image. In the companion case, the pathologic fracture is faintly visible. The lack of cartilaginous matrix in the second case does not exclude an enchondroma. The companion case is also enchondroma.

Solitary enchondromas are benign neoplasms, located within the medullary cavity, that are composed of mature hyaline cartilage. They probably arise from cartilaginous rests displaced from the growth plate. The incidence in males and females is equal, and most patients are between 10 and 50 years of age. Typically, the lesions are asymptomatic and discovered incidentally, but many patients present with pathologic fractures. The most common locations for solitary enchondromas are the hands (about 50% of cases), the proximal and distal femur, and the proximal humerus. In the hands, the middle and distal portions of the metacarpals and the proximal portions of the phalanges are typically involved. Radiographically, these lesions are lucent from replacement of bone by nonmineralized cartilage, but the typical mineralization patterns of cartilaginous matrix may be present: dense punctate or flocculent calcifications, or ring-shaped or arc-shaped densities from enchondral ossification of lobular cartilage. Slow, endosteal enlargement causes an expanded, thinned cortex, but cortical penetration is absent. Healing of pathologic fractures tends to be slow, because the thinned cortex overlying an enchondroma will not have a normal endosteal blood supply. The risk of developing chondrosarcoma in a solitary enchondroma of the hand is exceedingly low [27].

Clinical History: 62-year-old man with lumps on his hands.

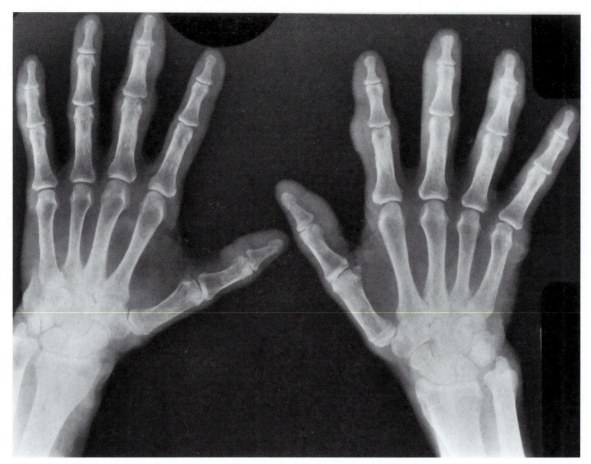

Figure 1-15

Findings: PA radiograph of both hands demonstrates soft tissue prominences, with increased density around most PIP and DIP joints, the fifth MCP and IP joints bilaterally, and the wrists. Erosions with sclerotic margins are noted at the left fifth MCP joint, left third PIP joint, and right second MCP joint.

Differential Diagnosis: Gout, xanthomatosis, psoriasis, multicentric reticulohistiocytosis.

Diagnosis: Tophaceous gout.

Discussion: Gout is defined by the presence of hyperuricemia (serum uric acid concentration greater than 7 mg/dL). Hyperuricemia may be idiopathic or secondary to known conditions, including excess ingestion (in protein), intrinsic overproduction, or reduced renal secretion. There is a familial incidence, but it appears to be controlled by multiple genes. Specific mutations with biochemical defects in purine metabolism leading to hyperuricemia have been found in a few cases. Gout is associated with obesity, diabetes, hyperlipidemia, hypertension, atherosclerosis, alcohol consumption, acute illness, and pregnancy. There is a negative association with rheumatoid arthritis. The prevalence of the symptomatic forms of gout, gouty arthritis, and tophaceous gout has declined dramatically with the increased use of drugs that control hyperuricemia. Gouty arthritis is similar to other crystal-related joint diseases, whereas tophaceous gout has the radiologic appearance of a metabolic deposition disease. Tophaceous gout is the most common metabolic deposition disease. Deposits of monosodium urate crystals are called tophi, and they are generally found in the periarticular soft tissues. The development of tophi requires decades of sustained hyperuricemia and is related to the degree and duration of hyperuricemia. Control of hyperuricemia by drugs has reduced the incidence of tophi in people with gout from over 50% in the 1950s to about 3% today. Deposits near the joints and tendons cause a lumpy-bumpy appearance. These localized areas of swelling may cause the slow development of pressure erosions on adjacent bone. Such erosions will have well-defined sclerotic margins. A shell of new bone may attempt to encompass the deposit, leaving an overhanging edge. The articular spaces may be preserved until late in the disease. Tophaceous gout may occur in combination with episodes of gouty arthritis.

Clinical History: 46-year-old woman with soft mass at the palmar aspect of the wrist.

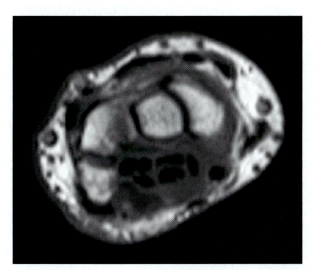

Figure 1-16 A

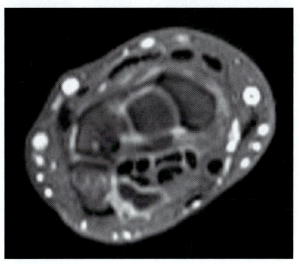

Figure 1-16 B

Figure 1-16 C

Findings: (A) Axial T1-weighted, (B) T2-weighted fat-suppressed, and (C) T1-weighted fat-suppressed post-gadolinium images show a multilobulated, low T1 and high T2 signal mass ventral to the carpal tunnel. The mass demonstrates no significant enhancement on post contrast sequences. The mass has interposed itself into the carpal tunnel adjacent to the median nerve.

Differential Diagnosis: Ganglion cyst, schwannoma, abscess, giant cell tumor of tendon sheath, synovial cyst.

Diagnosis: Ganglion cyst.

Discussion: A ganglion cyst develops along a tendon sheath. It most likely forms due to a herniation of synovial lining in a joint, a tendon sheath, or even a nerve covering. The connection with the original site of formation can be lost as the cyst migrates toward the subcutaneous tissue. A ganglion cyst often contains simple fluid (high T2, low T1 signal). It can also contain hemorrhagic fluid and therefore have heterogenous signal characteristics. Ganglion cysts can be associated with internal derangement (triangular fibrocartilage complex and ligament tears) [28]. It is important to differentiate ganglion cysts from a solid mass. Administering gadolinium helps to make this differentiation. Ganglion cysts will not have central enhancement, whereas solid masses do. Most ganglion cysts demonstrate rim-like enhancement. Because gadolinium diffuses in the extracellular spaces, if there is a long delay between injection and imaging, a cyst may appear to have a thick, enhancing wall, or may even enhance homogeneously.

Clinical History: 70-year-old woman with rapidly progressive pain, swelling and "red bumps" in the skin of both hands.

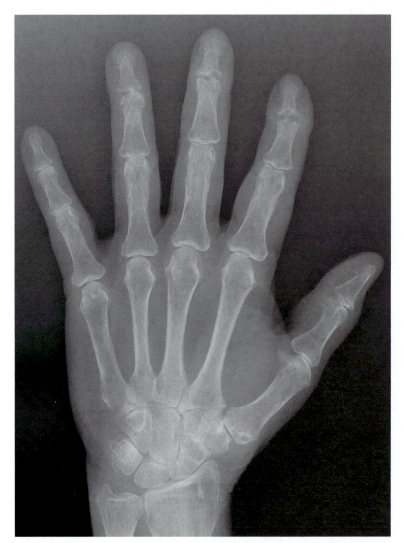

Figure 1-17   A

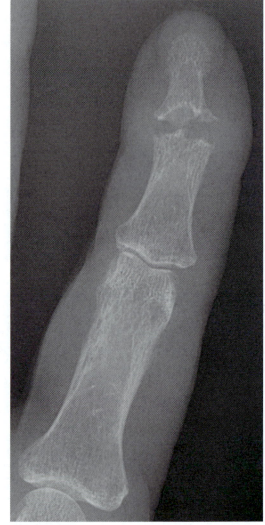

Figure 1-17   B

Findings: (A) PA radiograph of the hand. The soft tissues are diffusely thickened. There are erosions with overhanging edges at multiple joints, seen best at the DIP joints. (B) Detail view of the index finger.

Differential Diagnosis: Multicentric reticulohistiocytosis, erosive osteoarthritis, gout, psoriasis.

Diagnosis: Multicentric reticulohistiocytosis.

Discussion: Metabolic deposition diseases involving the joints, in which the body accumulates a substance it cannot excrete or metabolize, are relatively uncommon. If focal, mass-like deposits are located in the musculoskeletal system, the result is a clinically indolent disease with randomly distributed, slowly enlarging, space-occupying deposits. Chronic erosions with overhanging edges are a classic feature of metabolic deposition disease. In this case, the diffuse soft tissue thickening and the absence of a lumpy-bumpy morphology mitigate against tophaceous gout, the only common form of metabolic deposition disease involving the bones and joints. In the rare condition of multicentric reticulohistiocytosis, lipid-containing macrophages are deposited randomly in the soft tissues around joints and tendons. Skin nodules are common. As with gout and other metabolic deposition diseases, normal bone density and normal joint spaces are associated with intraosseous and juxtaarticular accumulations. Bone erosions with sclerotic margins and overhanging edges are typical, but sometimes a destructive, erosive arthritis ensues [29]. The origin of the abnormal lipid is unknown. Multicentric reticulohistiocytosis may be associated with the development of malignancies and has been described as a paraneoplastic syndrome [30].

Clinical History: 43-year-old woman with difficulty using her hands.

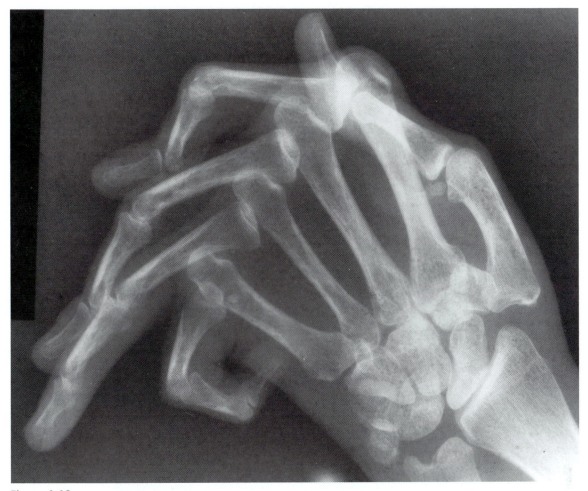

Figure 1-18

Findings: PA radiograph of the left hand shows severe subluxations at the MCP joints, with marked ulnar deviation of the fingers. The carpometacarpal joint of the thumb is dislocated, with proximal retraction of the first metacarpal. The entire carpus is translocated toward the ulna. Boutonniere deformities involve the index and middle fingers, and flexion deformities involve the little finger. Erosions of bone are absent, and there are no hypertrophic changes of bone. Bone density is nearly normal, although perhaps slightly osteopenic.

Differential Diagnosis: Systemic lupus erythematosus (SLE), scleroderma, spondyloarthropathy, rheumatoid arthritis.

Diagnosis: Systemic lupus erythematosus.

Discussion: SLE is a chronic systemic disease whose pathogenesis is related to immune complex deposition. It is more common in women by an 8:1 ratio, and there is a component of genetic susceptibility. The fluorescent antinuclear antibody test is virtually always positive at the onset of clinical disease. Manifestations in the musculoskeletal system are common, and may antedate other systemic manifestations by months or years. Nonerosive symmetric polyarthritis with a distribution similar to that of rheumatoid arthritis is present in 75% to 90% of patients with SLE. The early findings on radiographs are fusiform soft tissue swelling and juxtaarticular osteoporosis, but there should be no joint space narrowing or erosions. A deforming nonerosive arthropathy is also common in patients with SLE. The hands are typically involved at the MCP and IP joints. Thumb, wrist, and foot involvement is more common than shoulder and knee involvement. Ten percent of patients may develop atlantoaxial subluxation. These deformities are initially reducible, and radiographs may appear normal. Fixed deformities and secondary degenerative changes may develop with time. Osteonecrosis may involve the femoral head, femoral condyle, humeral head, and other sites, and it commonly has a symmetric distribution. Myositis, tendon weakening and spontaneous rupture, and soft tissue calcification are other musculoskeletal manifestations.

CASE 1-19

Clinical History: 51-year-old woman with polyarticular arthralgias.

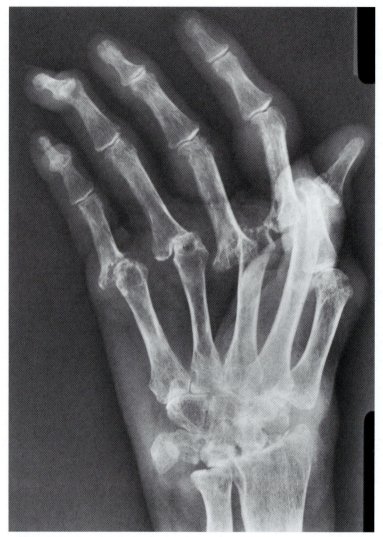

Figure 1-19

Findings: Oblique radiograph of the hand shows diffuse osteoporosis, soft tissue swelling, and late erosive changes at the MCP, intercarpal, and radiocarpal joints. The IP joints of the fingers are virtually spared. Ulnar subluxation and deviation are noted at the second through fifth MCP joints, and the carpus is translocated in the direction of the ulna. Subchondral sclerosis is evident at the radiocarpal joint and at several of the MCP joints.

Differential Diagnosis: Rheumatoid arthritis, ankylosing spondylitis, psoriatic arthritis, osteoarthritis.

Diagnosis: Rheumatoid arthritis (late features).

Discussion: The distribution of disease is that of rheumatoid arthritis in the MCP, intercarpal, and radiocarpal joints. Severe erosive changes are present and, although there is diffuse osteoporosis and a lack of osteophytes, subchondral sclerosis is present at several of the involved joints.

Secondary degenerative changes, such as subchondral sclerosis, may occur if the inflammatory process remits for several years. Both rheumatoid arthritis and primary osteoarthritis are common conditions; patients with both diseases may have confusing radiographic findings. In this case, the distribution of disease is not that of osteoarthritis. The common late radiologic findings of rheumatoid arthritis include chronic generalized osteoporosis, progression of marginal erosions to severe erosions involving subchondral bone, synovial cyst formation, subluxations and abnormalities of alignment, and secondary osteoarthritis. Compressive erosions and remodeling of bone may result from the collapse of osteoporotic bone by muscle tension; this is particularly common at the MCP joints. Malalignment in advanced disease results from the loss of balanced muscular tension and ligamentous involvement by the inflammatory process.

Clinical History: 35-year-old woman with morning stiffness of her hands.

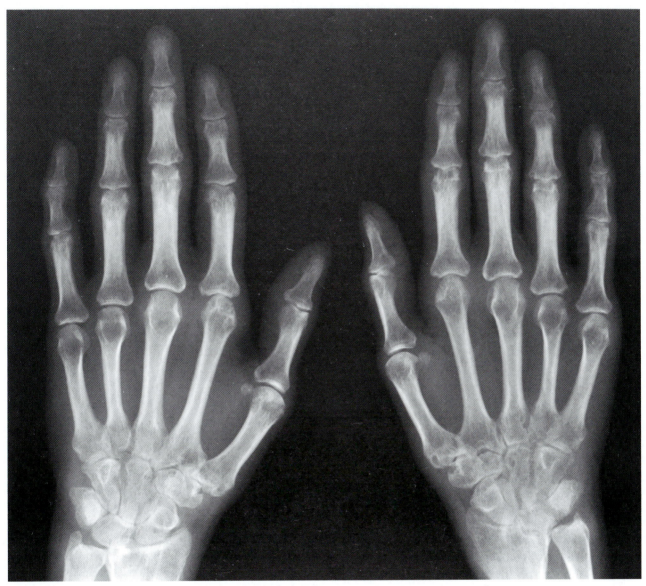

Figure 1-20

Findings: PA radiographs of both hands show juxtaarticular osteoporosis. The cartilage spaces of the carpal, MCP, and PIP joints are diffusely narrowed, and erosions are present, particularly at the MCP joints. There are no hypertrophic bony changes such as osteophytes or subchondral sclerosis.

Differential Diagnosis: Rheumatoid arthritis, ankylosing spondylitis, psoriatic arthritis, osteoarthritis.

Diagnosis: Rheumatoid arthritis (classic features).

Discussion: The underlying pathologic change in rheumatoid arthritis is chronic synovial inflammation with hyperemia, edema, and effusion. Although symmetric clinical involvement is the rule, the clinical involvement may not correlate with the sites of radiologic involvement. The earliest radiographic changes are demonstrated in this case. The earliest sites of erosions are typically at the MCP joints and are seen best on the supinated oblique "ball catcher's" views. As the condition progresses, the radiographic features tend to become much more pronounced and differentiated from other forms of polyarticular arthritis. Rheumatoid arthritis has a prevalence of 1% in the general population; women are affected more than men by a 3:1 ratio. The clinical course is progressive in 70% of cases, with rapid or slow clinical deterioration. In 20% of cases the disease is intermittent, with remissions and exacerbations. In 10% of cases the remissions may last for several years.

Clinical History: 32-year-old woman with arthralgias.

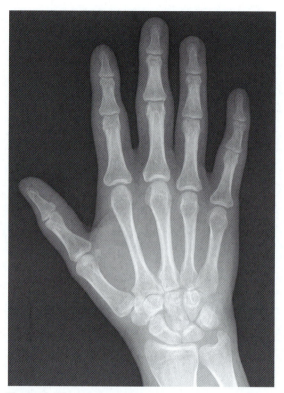

Figure 1-21

Findings: PA view of the right hand shows juxtaarticular osteoporosis involving the ends of the long bones but not the carpal bones. Fusiform soft tissue swelling is evident at several of the PIP joints, particularly at the index and middle fingers, and there may be narrowing of the cartilage space at some of the PIP joints. There is a lack of osteophytes, subchondral sclerosis, and other features of degenerative joint disease, although erosions are not seen on these views.

Differential Diagnosis: Rheumatoid arthritis, ankylosing spondylitis, psoriatic arthritis, osteoarthritis.

Diagnosis: Rheumatoid arthritis (early features).

Discussion: The diagnosis of an acute, symmetric, inflammatory polyarthritis can be made from these radiographs. The presence and bilaterally symmetric distribution of juxtaarticular osteoporosis in the hands and wrists are indicative of hyperemia, suggesting an acute, systemic, inflammatory process. Fusiform periarticular soft tissue swelling, present around the wrists and some of the PIP joints, corresponds to synovial hypertrophy and/or joint effusion, and the diffuse joint space narrowing is typical of joints in which articular cartilage has been dissolved by enzymes released into the joint space. The lack of reactive bone is characteristic of an inflammatory rather than a degenerative process. The presence of marginal bone erosions would absolutely clinch the diagnosis of rheumatoid arthritis, but early in the clinical course, erosions may not be evident. In this case, the diagnosis is clear without these additional features. Bilaterally symmetric clinical involvement is usual, but the severity of radiologic involvement may not necessarily be symmetric, especially when radiographs are obtained early in the clinical course. In the hand, rheumatoid arthritis classically involves the MCP and PIP joints. In the wrist, it usually involves all the carpal compartments.

Rheumatoid arthritis is a systemic autoimmune disease manifested in the musculoskeletal system by inflammatory polyarthritis of the small synovial joints. The typical age at presentation is 25 to 55 years. In 70% of cases, the onset is insidious and occurs over weeks to months; in 20% of cases, the onset occurs over days to weeks; and in 10% of cases, the onset is acute and occurs over hours to days. The acute onset mimics the onset of septic arthritis. The clinical diagnosis is based on criteria that include morning stiffness, symmetric swelling of the PIP, MCP, or wrist joints, rheumatoid nodules, serum rheumatoid factor, and the specific radiographic findings.

Clinical History: 15-year-old boy with chronic disease and short stature.

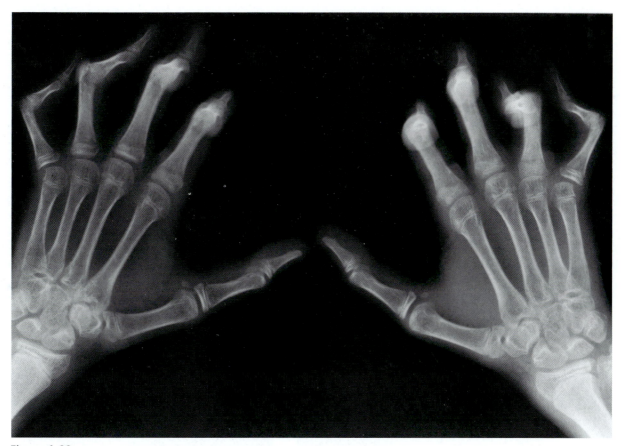

Figure 1-22

Findings: Oblique radiograph of both hands. The growth plates are still open. The bones are osteopenic, and boutonniere deformities are present in all the fingers. The epiphyses are overgrown and mildly dysplastic.

Differential Diagnosis: Still's disease (seronegative juvenile-onset rheumatoid arthritis) and juvenile onset of seropositive adult-type rheumatoid arthritis, seronegative spondyloarthropathies.

Diagnosis: Juvenile idiopathic arthritis (Still's disease, polyarticular appearance).

Discussion: The findings in this case are of systemic polyarticular disease in a child. Juvenile idiopathic arthritis is a designation that includes Still's disease and juvenile onset of seropositive adult-type rheumatoid arthritis, and the seronegative spondyloarthropathies. The radiologic findings in juvenile idiopathic arthritis reflect the effect of a chronic inflammatory arthritis on a growing skeleton, and generally are not specific for a particular clinical entity. The radiographic findings include soft tissue swelling, osteoporosis, periostitis, erosions, ankylosis, and growth disturbances. The earlier the age at onset, the more severe the findings are. Not all findings are likely to be present together, but

combinations of these findings should point to the diagnosis. The disease may remit in adulthood, but permanent muscle-wasting, growth deformities, loss of function from ankylosis, and secondary osteoarthritis are common sequelae.

Approximately 70% of juvenile idiopathic arthritis cases are Still's disease. There are three clinical presentations. Classic systemic disease is usually seen before 5 years of age and is associated with severe systemic manifestations, but mild or absent articular disease. Polyarticular disease may occur with systemic disease or may follow it. Sites of involvement are symmetric and may include the MCP and IP joints of the hand, wrist, elbow, hip, knee, ankle, foot, and cervical spine. The prognosis is generally poor. Pauciarticular or monarticular disease is the most common form of Still's disease. It has a female predominance and is associated with iridocyclitis. Monarticular onset in a knee is the most common presentation, but the ankle, elbow, and wrist are frequent sites. Joint contractures, muscle-wasting, bony ankylosis, growth deformities, epiphyseal overgrowth, and early growth plate closure may follow the articular disease. In the hand, common findings include soft tissue swelling, osteoporosis, bony ankylosis, periostitis, growth disturbances, epiphyseal compression fractures, and joint subluxation.

Clinical History: 62-year-old man with abnormal thyroid function tests.

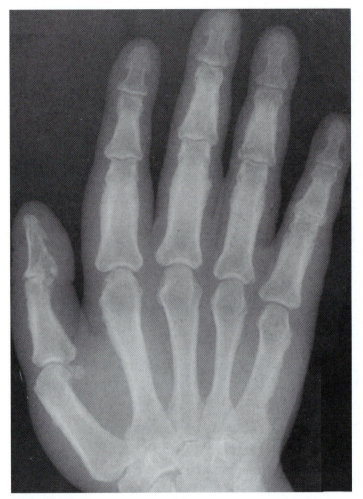

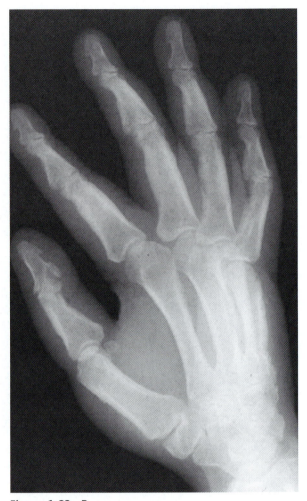

Figure 1-23 A

Figure 1-23 B

Findings: PA and oblique radiographs of the hand demonstrate prominent periosteal reaction along the proximal phalangeal shafts, the radial side of the first and second metacarpal shafts, and the ulnar side of the fifth metacarpal shaft. Diffuse soft tissue swelling is present.

Differential Diagnosis: Hypertrophic pulmonary osteoarthropathy, familial pachydermoperiostosis, thyroid acropachy, sarcoid, venous stasis.

Diagnosis: Thyroid acropachy.

Discussion: Thyroid acropachy is a rare musculoskeletal manifestation of autoimmune thyroid disease. The characteristic appearance is periosteal reaction along the diaphyseal regions of the hand and feet metacarpals, metatarsals, and phalanges. The periosteal reaction is classically seen on the radial side of the first through third digits, and the ulnar side of the fourth and fifth digits. Diffuse soft tissue swelling and clubbing of the digits may also be present. The joints are uninvolved in this disorder and it is typically painless. If only a single digit is involved, the appearance can mimic malignancy [31]. Thyroid acropachy is seen in approximately 1% of patients with Graves' disease. In Graves' disease, acropachy often, but not always, occurs along with dermatopathy and ophthalmopathy. The presence of acropachy and dermatopathy is a marker for severe ophthalmopathy [32].

CASE 1-24

Clinical History: 50-year-old man with increasing hat size.

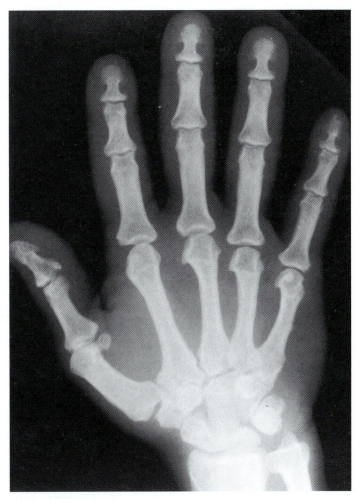

Figure 1-24

Findings: PA radiograph of the right hand shows diffuse thickening of the soft tissues. The phalangeal tufts and the shafts of the long bones, particularly the proximal phalanges, are widened. Alignment, mineralization, and cartilage spaces are normal, but prominent hooks are present at the MCP joints.

Differential Diagnosis: Osteoarthritis, acromegaly, diffuse idiopathic skeletal hyperostosis, hypervitaminosis A, fluorosis.

Diagnosis: Acromegaly.

Discussion: Clinical acromegaly is caused by excess growth hormone in adults. The underlying cause in the vast majority of cases is a pituitary adenoma that produces growth hormone autonomously; however, extrapituitary growth-hormone-secreting tumors, as well as central and peripheral tumors that secrete growth-hormone-releasing hormone also may cause acromegaly. The clinical features of acromegaly are distinctive and include acromegalic facies, enlargement of the hands and feet, prognathism, and oily skin. Commonly associated conditions include carpal tunnel syndrome, osteoarthrosis, hypertension, Raynaud's phenomenon, and diabetes mellitus. Many patients present with the signs and symptoms of a pituitary or hypothalamic mass rather than those of growth hormone excess. Definitive diagnosis is made by direct serum measurements of hormone levels. Growth hormone activates sites of bone remodeling, and may increase bone formation more than bone resorption. As a consequence, the bone mass may actually be elevated, with thickened cortex and increased trabecular bone volume. Periosteal bone formation at the insertions of tendons and ligaments, and periarticular hypertrophy at the insertions of joint capsules, contributes to the increase in skeletal mass. Growth hormone increases chondrocytic activity and leads to hypertrophy of the hyaline articular cartilage. This thickened cartilage lacks the normal biomechanical characteristics of articular cartilage, and is vulnerable to fissuring, ulceration, denudation, and, ultimately, degenerative changes.

Clinical History: 38-year-old man.

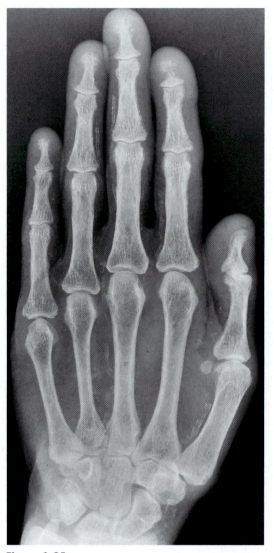

Figure 1-25

Findings: PA radiograph of the left hand. The bones are diffusely osteopenic, with loss of the normal, sharp, cortical outlines around the phalanges, particularly along the radial aspects. Bone loss is also prominent at the phalangeal tufts, and extensive vascular calcification is present. The cartilage spaces are well preserved, and the alignment of the wrist and digits is normal. There are no erosive changes around the joints, and no hypertrophic bone changes.

Differential Diagnosis: Hyperparathyroidism, osteoporosis, rheumatoid arthritis.

Diagnosis: Hyperparathyroidism, secondary to renal failure.

Discussion: Hyperparathyroidism stimulates osteoclastic resorption of bone. The excess parathyroid hormone can be a result of primary or secondary hyperparathyroidism.

Secondary hyperparathyroidism is a response to sustained hypocalcemia that is typically caused by chronic renal failure, as in this case, or gastrointestinal malabsorption. Radiographic changes, including bone resorption, brown tumors, bone sclerosis, and chondrocalcinosis, are seen best in the hands. Bone resorption occurs at all surfaces, including subperiosteal, intracortical (along haversian systems), endosteal, trabecular, subchondral, and subligamentous locations. Subperiosteal bone resorption is virtually diagnostic of hyperparathyroidism. It is seen best and most frequently along the radial aspect of the phalanges of the hands, especially the middle phalanges of the index and middle fingers. Subperiosteal bone resorption may also be evident at the phalangeal tufts. Vascular and soft tissue calcification is common in secondary hyperparathyroidism.

CASE 1-26

Clinical History: Weak 38-year-old woman.

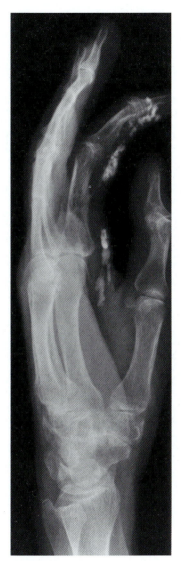 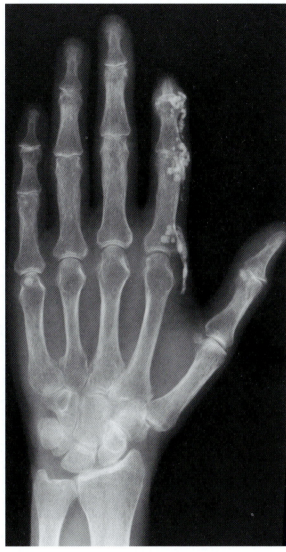

Figure 1-26 A   **Figure 1-26 B**

Findings: (A, B) Lateral and PA radiographs of the right hand demonstrate severe flexion deformity of the index finger, with conglomerate soft tissue calcifications and erosions at the MCP joint. The bones are osteoporotic.

Differential Diagnosis: Polymyositis, dermatomyositis, scleroderma, calcific tendinitis.

Diagnosis: Polymyositis.

Discussion: Polymyositis is a disorder of unknown cause characterized by inflammation and degeneration of muscle [33]. In the most common clinical form of polymyositis, gradually increasing proximal limb weakness, and a later effect on the laryngeal and pharyngeal muscles, may be accompanied by joint manifestations in 20% to 50% of patients. These joint manifestations include arthralgias and

arthritis [34,35], and the clinical and radiographic appearance may be confused with SLE and rheumatoid arthritis. In this particular case, the presence of soft tissue calcification rules out SLE and rheumatoid arthritis as diagnostic possibilities, and suggests scleroderma or related connective tissue diseases, including dermatomyositis or polymyositis. Hydroxyapatite crystal deposition disease (calcific tendinitis) is eliminated by the specific location and distribution of the calcifications—they are not in the expected location of tendons. Calcification in scleroderma and polymyositis may not be distinguishable from each other, but the flexion deformity, MCP erosion, and osteoporosis would be unusual in scleroderma. Moreover, the soft tissue resorptive changes and skin-tightening characteristic of scleroderma are absent.

Clinical History: 5-year-old boy who was very sick as a baby.

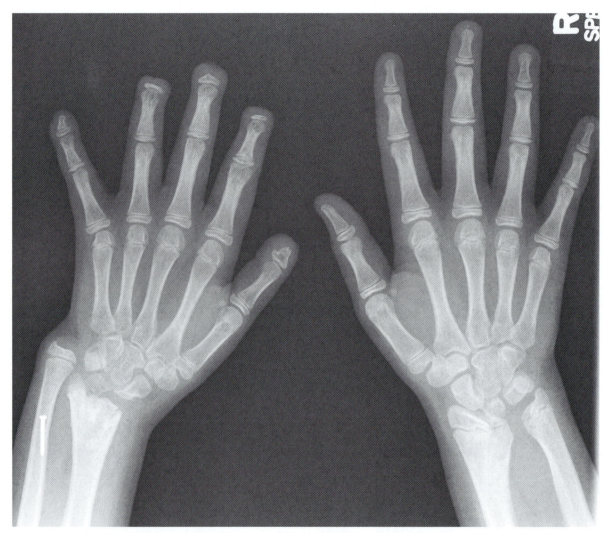

Figure 1-27

Findings: PA radiograph of both hands shows asymmetric absence of the distal portions of the fingers and thumb. The distal bones are smooth. Both wrists have cone-shaped epiphyses and consequent deformities of the distal radioulnar joints. The radius is short relative to the ulna on the left, and the distal right ulna has a tethered physis on the radial side, leading to a slant-like deformity.

Differential Diagnosis: Trauma, burns, frostbite, embolic disease, infection, Lesch-Nyhan syndrome, congenital indifference to pain, child abuse, Munchausen disease by proxy.

Diagnosis: Embolic disease (caused by neonatal meningococcemia).

Discussion: Loss of fingers is most often the result of mechanical or thermal trauma, and the trauma may be accidental or intentional. In this case, however, the presence of coned epiphyses cannot be accounted for by trauma.

A coned epiphysis can be the result of premature closure of the central portion of the physis, following which the peripheral portions of the physis continue to grow. As a result, the metaphysis lengthens around the tethered portion of the epiphysis, and the epiphysis develops into a cone shape. The situation may also be called a cupped metaphysis. This impairment to longitudinal growth also leads to a relative shortening of the affected bone. Because the growth impairment is central, there is no angular deformity. Both loss of fingertips and coned epiphyses may result from vascular infarcts caused by embolic disease [36,37]. Premature closure of the peripheral portion of a growth plate will lead to tethering and asymmetric longitudinal growth. Disseminated intravascular coagulopathy is one complication of neonatal meningococcemia. These long-term sequelae of meningococcemia do not reflect sites of actual infection.

CASE 1-28

Clinical History: 56-year-old man with chronic wrist pain and instability.

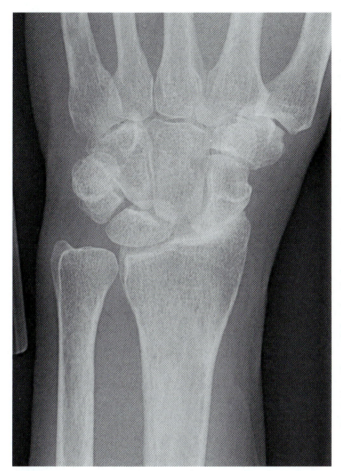

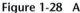

Figure 1-28 A

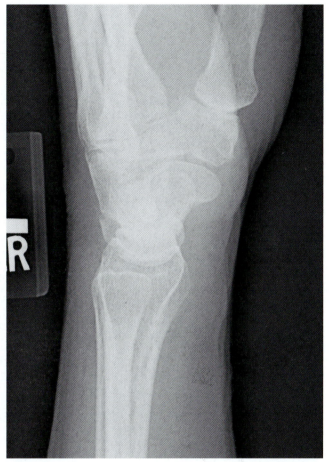

Figure 1-28 B

Findings: (A) PA radiograph of the left wrist shows that the scapholunate joint is grossly widened, and the capitate has migrated proximally into the gap. Joint space narrowing and subchondral sclerosis has developed at the articulation between the scaphoid and radius, and the lunate is slightly rotated. (B) The lateral radiograph shows mild dorsal tilt of the lunate articular surface. Chondrocalcinosis is not visible. There are no erosions. Bone mineralization is normal.

Differential Diagnosis: Pyrophosphate arthropathy, rheumatoid arthritis, osteoarthritis, trauma.

Diagnosis: Pyrophosphate arthropathy with scapholunate advanced collapse (SLAC wrist).

Discussion: Calcium pyrophosphate dihydrate (CPPD) crystal deposition disease is a polyarticular arthritis with deposition of CPPD crystals in articular tissues. CPPD crystals are generated locally in the articular tissues, where asymptomatic deposits may accumulate in cartilage, joint capsules, intervertebral discs, tendons, and ligaments. In cartilage, these deposits may be evident radiographically as chondrocalcinosis. Pyrophosphate arthropathy is the degenerative

result of structural joint damage, caused by chronic CPPD crystal deposition and irreversible destruction of the articular cartilage. The degenerative changes can be identical to those of osteoarthritis, but the distribution of involvement is different. In the wrist, the radiocarpal joint is characteristically involved, whereas in osteoarthritis, the scaphoid-trapezoid-trapezium-first metacarpal articulations are characteristically involved. In severe cases, the process causes gross scapholunate dissociation, in association with degenerative radiocarpal changes. The scaphoid and lunate separate, and the capitate migrates proximally into the resulting gap. This syndrome is called the SLAC wrist. It usually includes pancompartmental degenerative involvement. The shoulder (glenohumeral), knee (especially patellofemoral), elbow, ankle, and foot (talonavicular) are the other common sites of involvement. Chondrocalcinosis need not be present and will be absent if there is no remaining cartilage. Pyrophosphate arthropathy is often, but not necessarily, combined with acute episodes of crystal-induced synovitis. Very severe degenerative changes may lead to an appearance that resembles neuropathic osteoarthropathy.

Clinical History: 52-year-old man with bronze skin and liver disease.

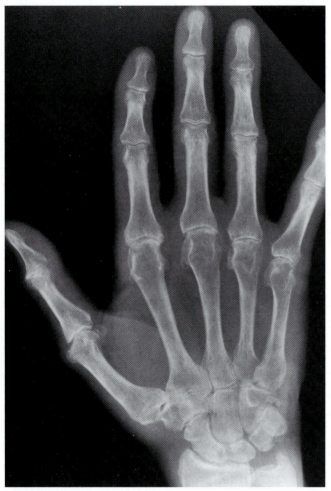

Figure 1-29 A

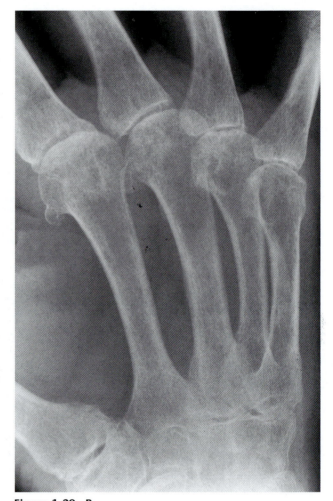

Figure 1-29 B

Findings: (A, B) PA and oblique radiographs of the metacarpals demonstrate flattening of all metacarpal heads, with subchondral sclerosis and joint space loss. Beak-type osteophytes are present on the medial aspects of the second through fifth metacarpals. The IP joints are spared, but there are changes at the basal joints of the thumb and radiocarpal joints. Bone mineralization is mildly decreased. The opposite hand has a similar appearance.

Differential Diagnosis: Hemochromatosis, pyrophosphate arthropathy, osteoarthritis, gout.

Diagnosis: Hemochromatosis.

Discussion: The predominant articular changes are those of a degenerative process, but the distribution is not that of primary osteoarthritis. Pyrophosphate arthropathy, the chronic degenerative form of CPPD deposition disease, may have an identical appearance, but the clinical features suggest hemochromatosis as the underlying cause. As a differential diagnostic point, osteoporosis is usually a feature of hemochromatosis, but typically is not present in pyrophosphate arthropathy. Hemochromatosis results from deposition of iron in various tissues, caused by increased absorption of dietary iron from the gastrointestinal tract (primary), or by increased intake from blood transfusions, alcoholism, or ingestion (secondary). As many as 50% of patients with hemochromatosis may develop arthropathy; the arthropathy is caused by accumulation of iron and/or CPPD crystals in the joints. Arthritis may be the sole manifestation of hereditary hemochromatosis [38]. The classic clinical triad is bronze skin, cirrhosis, and diabetes. Laboratory tests will show an increased serum iron and iron-binding capacity. Phlebotomy does not help the symptoms of advanced arthropathy.

CASE 1-30

Clinical History: 70-year-old man with acute pain and swelling over the dorsal and ulnar aspects of the wrist.

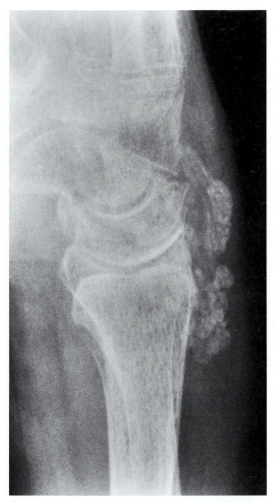

Figure 1-30   A

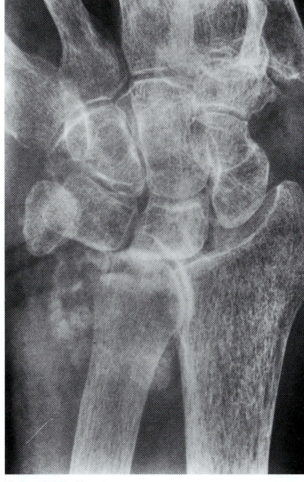

Figure 1-30   B

Findings: (A) Lateral radiograph of the wrist shows amorphous calcification located along the extensor tendons with soft tissue swelling. (B) PA radiograph shows a distended distal radioulnar joint capsule that is made partially visible by calcification. Incidental osteoporosis and osteoarthritis are present.

Differential Diagnosis: Hydroxyapatite deposition disease, synovial chondromatosis, CPPD deposition disease, scleroderma, tumoral calcinosis.

Diagnosis: Hydroxyapatite deposition disease (calcific tendinitis and calcific periarthritis).

Discussion: Amorphous calcification in the soft tissues is characteristic of calcium in the form of hydroxyapatite crystals. Each collection of calcium is more or less uniform in density from the edge to the center, with no evident structural features, and a somewhat irregular shape. The calcifications are distributed along the expected location of the extensor tendons of the wrist and hand. The distal radial-

ulnar joint capsule is similarly involved, where crystals may be grossly visible in the form of milk-of-calcium. Hydroxyapatite crystal deposition may be related to chronic minor trauma and deposition in localized necrotic tissue, and may be associated with a painful inflammatory reaction of acute onset. Generally seen in patients over the age of 40, men and women are affected equally. It is most commonly seen around the shoulder. The main differential diagnostic consideration is synovial chondromatosis. If the calcification represented bone fragments or heterotopic ossification, one would expect a cortical and trabecular structure. Calcification in cartilage may have a punctate, flocculent, or rings-and-arcs morphology if enchondral ossification is occurring, but in this location, the cartilage would be heterotropic. Dystrophic calcification in cartilage may have a lamellated appearance. CPPD crystal deposition occurs in articular cartilage, which would not be expected within tendons. When CPPD crystals are free within the joint capsule, they are generally not visible on radiographs.

Clinical History: 28-year-old man with wrist trauma.

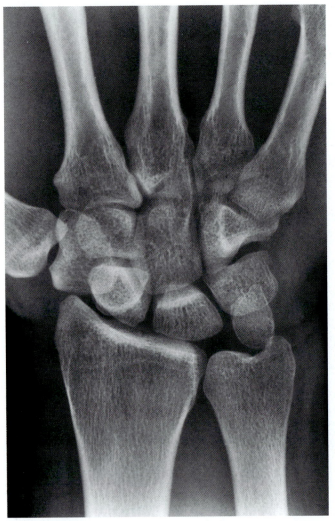

Figure 1-31 A

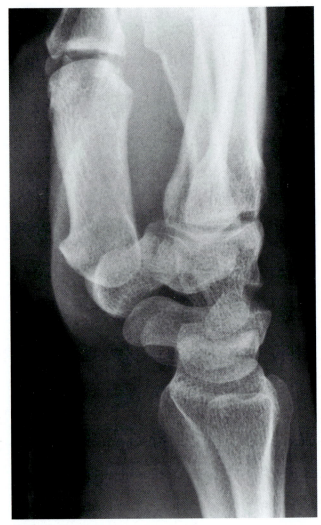

Figure 1-31 B

Findings: (A) PA wrist radiograph shows foreshortening of the scaphoid with a cortical ring sign over its distal pole. The interval between the scaphoid and the lunate is minimally abnormally wide (compare with other carpal bone articulations). (B) Lateral wrist radiograph shows an abnormal scapholunate angle of about 90 degrees.

Differential Diagnosis: None.

Diagnosis: Rotary subluxation of the scaphoid (scapholunate dislocation).

Discussion: The scaphoid bridges the proximal and distal carpal rows, and its long axis is normally oriented approximately 45 degrees on the lateral view from the plane of the carpus, allowing the thumb to be opposed to the fingers. When the ligamentous sling that suspends the scaphoid from the carpus is disrupted, muscle tension from the flexors and extensors of the thumb that cross the carpus brings it proximally, rotating the scaphoid on its short axis. On PA radiographs, the scaphoid will appear as a small round bone. On lateral radiographs, the angle between the long axis of the scaphoid and the long axis of the wrist will be increased to approximately 90 degrees. The injury may be sustained when the hand is extended to break a backward fall. On impact, the hand and wrist undergo hyperextension, ulnar deviation, and intercarpal supination (rotary motion between the proximal and distal carpal rows), loading the ligamentous sling of the carpus in tension from the radial side and causing it to tear.

Clinical History: 27-year-old man who fell backward off scaffolding.

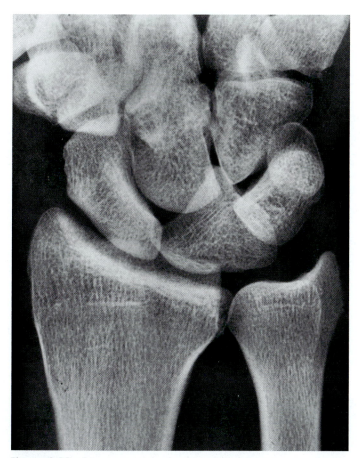

Figure 1-32 A

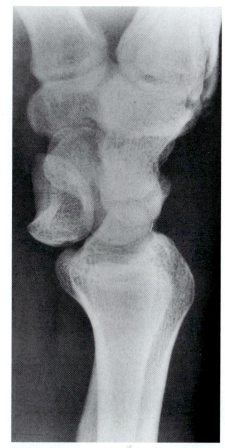

Figure 1-32 B

Findings: (A) PA radiograph shows the lunate as an over-lapping triangular structure. (B) Lateral radiograph of the wrist shows volar dislocation of the lunate with 90-degree rotary displacement. The capitate occupies the normal position of the lunate.

Differential Diagnosis: None.

Diagnosis: Lunate dislocation.

Discussion: On the PA radiograph, one should recognize that the radiographic overlapping of the lunate over the other carpal bones indicates that it is not in the same spatial plane, and the triangular rather than trapezoidal shape indicates that the lunate has rotated out of its normal orientation. The lateral view confirms these findings. Volar dislocation of the lunate is the most severe of the group of perilunate injuries, a consistent pattern of injuries sustained around the lunate when the hand is extended to break a backward fall. On impact, the hand and wrist undergo hyperextension, ulnar deviation, and intercarpal supination. The ligamentous sling of the carpus is loaded in tension from the radial side, and a sequence of injuries may ensue.

- In stage 1 (scapholunate dissociation or rotary subluxation), there is rupture of the proximal ligamentous attachments of the scaphoid; alternatively, the scaphoid may fracture.
- In stage 2 (perilunate dislocation), the capitate dislocates from the lunate dorsally, taking with it the hand and the scaphoid.
- In stage 3 (midcarpal dissociation or triquetral dislocation), the triquetral ligaments fail by tear or avulsion of insertions, separating the triquetrum from the lunate. Although the lunate remains in place, the rest of the carpus is dislocated dorsally, coming to rest on the dorsal surface of the lunate. The lunate is subluxated and tilted volarly, but is not completely dislocated.
- In stage 4 (lunate dislocation), the dorsal radiocarpal ligament tears, allowing the dorsally dislocated carpus to eject the lunate from the radius volarly. The capitate comes to rest in the radial articular surface. The dislocated lunate is also rotated 90 degrees volarly, still held to the radius by its volar ligaments.

The radiologic signs of reduced perilunate injuries may be subtle, particularly in the absence of fractures.

Clinical History: 57-year-old-woman fell on an outstretched hand.

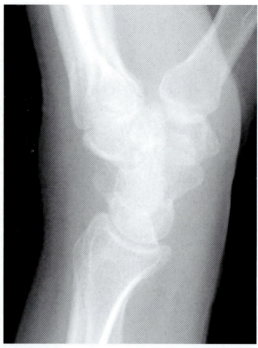

Figure 1-33 A

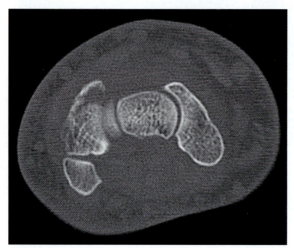

Figure 1-33 B

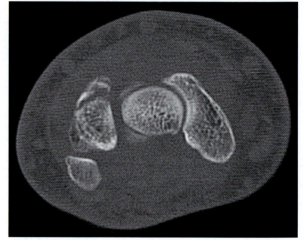

Figure 1-33 C

Findings: (A) Lateral wrist radiograph shows soft tissue swelling and a subtle bony fragment at the dorsal aspect of the proximal carpal row. (B, C) Contiguous axial computed tomography (CT) images demonstrate a minimally displaced fracture of the dorsal triquetral bone.

Differential Diagnosis: None.

Diagnosis: Triquetral fracture.

Discussion: Fractures of the triquetral bone are typically due to a direct blow or to forced dorsiflexion, usually from a fall on the outstretched hand. The mechanism is compressive force from either the hamate or ulnar styloid process. The most common appearance is a "chip" fracture off the dorsal aspect of the bone, which can be treated with immobilization. Displaced fractures of the triquetral body are surgically repaired. The lateral view of the wrist is best to visualize chip fractures. Patients with point tenderness of the triquetral bone, but with no abnormality on standard radiographs, may require CT or MR imaging to delineate the fracture. Fractures off the volar aspect of the triquetral bone have a high association with perilunate ligament injuries [39].

Clinical History: 30-year-old HIV-positive man with acute wrist swelling.

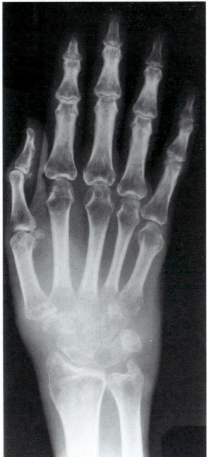

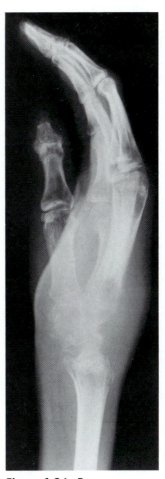

Figure 1-34 A   **Figure 1-34 B**

Findings: (A, B) PA and lateral radiographs of the right hand demonstrate severe juxtaarticular osteoporosis with marked soft tissue swelling about the wrist. Faint periosteal reaction may be noted along the radial aspect of the base of the third metacarpal. A lucency is present in the lunate, but no definite erosions are identified.

Differential Diagnosis: Septic arthritis, trauma, crystal arthropathy.

Diagnosis: HIV-related septic arthritis.

Discussion: Infection with HIV devastates cell-mediated immunity inexorably over a period of years, leading to the acquired immunodeficiency syndrome and death. Musculoskeletal manifestations are less common than manifestations in the central nervous system, the gastrointestinal tract, and the lungs. They include infections, neoplasms, and rheumatologic conditions. Musculoskeletal infections are relatively unusual in patients with HIV infection, with an incidence of approximately 0.3% to 3.5% for various infections of the musculoskeletal system [40]. In the study of

HIV patients conducted by Vassilopoulos et al., septic arthritis was the most commonly reported infection of the musculoskeletal system, usually affecting young men with a median CD4 count of 241. The exact contribution of previous intravenous drug abuse to the pathogenesis of septic arthritis is unclear. *Staphylococcus aureus* was the most commonly isolated agent (31.3%). Numerous common as well as atypical opportunistic pathogens were also identified as causes of septic arthritis. Approximately 90% of patients recovered with appropriate antibiotic treatment. Osteomyelitis may be caused by common and opportunistic organisms, including *S. aureus*, *Salmonella*, tuberculosis, fungus, and bacillary angiomatosis. Half the cases of osteomyelitis were due to atypical mycobacteria, with a mortality rate of approximately 20%. Pyomyositis is an increasingly recognized infection of the striated muscles in HIV-infected patients, described almost exclusively in men with advanced HIV infection (median CD4 count 24). Most cases are due to *S. aureus*, but other common and opportunistic organisms may be found.

Clinical History: 65-year-old-woman who presented with stiffness, weakness, and pain of the right wrist 3 months after sustaining a Colles' fracture in the same extremity.

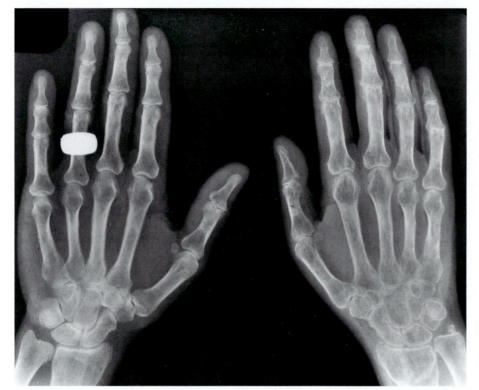

Figure 1-35   A

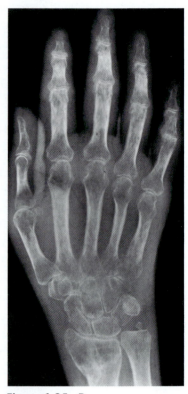

Figure 1-35   B

Findings: (**A**) PA radiograph of both hands demonstrates the well-healed deformity of the right distal radius. There is severe diffuse osteoporosis and decreased muscle mass of the right hand as compared to the left. (**B**) PA radiograph of the right hand taken 2 years after the initial radiographs shows persistent osteopenia and progressive muscle atrophy.

Differential Diagnosis: None.

Diagnosis: Reflex sympathetic dystrophy.

Discussion: The unilateral involvement, lack of erosions and alignment abnormalities, and absence of joint space narrowing suggests that the process is not articular disease.

Reflex sympathetic dystrophy (also called complex regional pain syndrome and Sudeck's atrophy) is a painful swelling of an extremity with rapid onset, typically after an injury. The injury may be a fracture, but often it is minor. The site of swelling and pain is usually in the limb, ipsilateral to the trauma but remote from the site. The incidence of reflex sympathetic dystrophy following trauma has been estimated as 5%. The cause is thought to be neurovascular, but the pathogenesis is unclear. Regional soft tissue swelling and acute osteoporosis is evident at onset. Soft tissue atrophy may follow subsidence of the acute symptoms. The bone usually remains osteoporotic.

Clinical History: 55-year-old woman with rheumatoid arthritis and surgery.

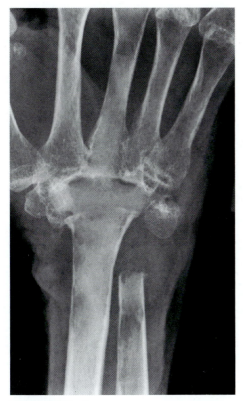

Figure 1-36   A

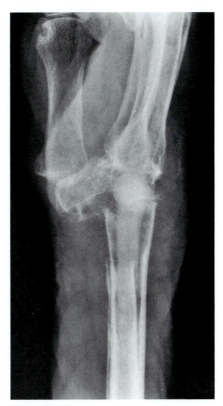

Figure 1-36   B

Findings: (A, B) PA and lateral radiographs of the wrist. The radiocarpal joint and both carpal rows have been resected and replaced by a slightly radiodense implant. The distal radioulnar joint has also been resected. The bones are severely osteoporotic.

Differential Diagnosis: None.

Diagnosis: Silicone arthroplasty of the wrist.

Discussion: The Swanson silicone rubber implant has been a therapeutic option in end-stage arthritis of the carpal joints in rheumatoid arthritis, with pain being the primary surgical indication. The Swanson prosthesis itself has a firm, rubbery consistency and is interposed between the ends of the radius and the third metacarpal, following resection of the radiocarpal, intercarpal, and common carpometacarpal joints. The prosthesis has stems protruding from either side that are inserted by the surgeon into the open ends of the host bones and secured by a mechanical fit. Unlike an arthrodesis, some mobility at the wrist is preserved. Although initially good results are commonly reported, with pain relief in the vast majority and few surgical complications [44], long-term results have been less favorable [45,46]. Problems noted in follow-up after several years included decreasing pain relief, implant fracture, silicone synovitis, and progressive bone resorption. Silicone synovitis is caused by a foreign-body inflammatory reaction to microscopic particles of silicone, and may be evident radiographically as osteolysis. The prevalence of silicone synovitis increases with the duration of the implant, although the clinical significance remains somewhat controversial [47].

Clinical History: 56-year-old man with painful, swollen left hand, 3 months after left shoulder injury.

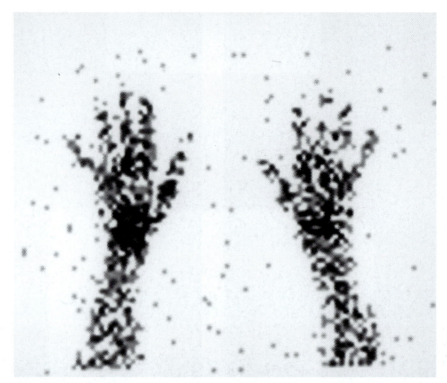

Figure 1-37   A

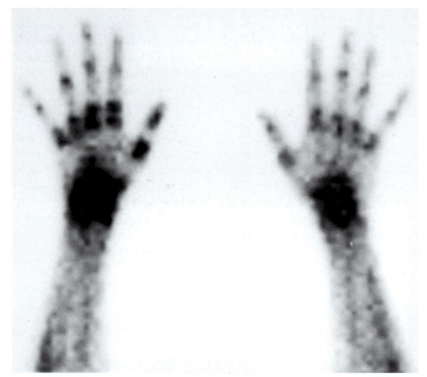

Figure 1-37   B

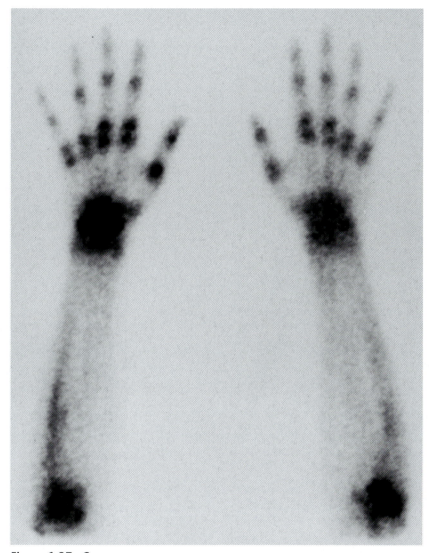

Figure 1-37 C

Findings: (A) Radionuclide angiogram of the hands during three-phase bone scan shows increased flow on the left side. (B) Blood pool image of both hands shows increased activity on the left. (C) Delayed images show increased accumulation of radionuclide in the bone on the left, corresponding to the areas of increased flow and blood pool activity.

Differential Diagnosis: None.

Diagnosis: Reflex sympathetic dystrophy.

Discussion: The three-phase radionuclide bone scan shows the features of reflex sympathetic dystrophy of recent onset. The characteristic scintigraphic abnormalities in reflex sympathetic dystrophy depend on the stage of the disease [41,42,43]. During the acute phase, in which edema and vasomotor instability are manifest clinically with intense burning pain and hypesthesia, there is increased blood flow to the affected limb, seen on the radionuclide angiogram and blood pool images, with increased bone uptake on the delayed scintigraphs. The increased bone uptake is typically greater in the periarticular regions. In very early disease, the bone uptake may be normal if increased bone resorption and/or turnover has not begun. In the second phase, which is characterized by pain and dystrophic changes in the skin and nails with muscle atrophy and osteoporosis, the blood flow and blood pool images typically return to normal, whereas the delayed images remain abnormal. In late, burned-out atrophic disease, when the skin changes, muscle-wasting, and osteoporosis have ceased progression, the scans may be virtually normal. The sensitivity of the bone scan for the diagnosis of reflex sympathetic dystrophy ranges between 60% and 96% with a very high negative predictive value, depending on the criteria used for clinical diagnosis.

Clinical History: 34-year-old man who developed multifocal bone pain over a 1-year period.

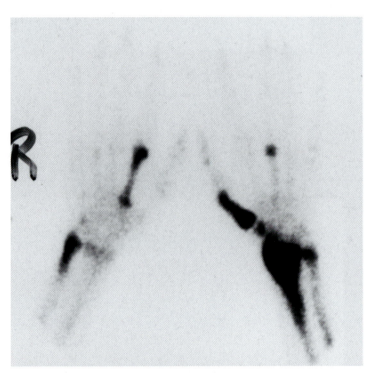

Figure 1-38 A

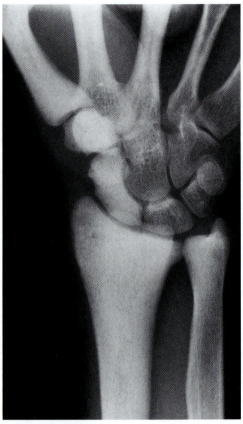

Figure 1-38 B

Findings: (A) Gamma camera views of the hands from delayed images of radionuclide bone scan. Radionuclide accumulation is noted in the right distal ulna and second metacarpal, left radius, ulna, trapezium, and first and third metacarpal heads. (B) PA radiograph of the left wrist show dense sclerosis of the distal radius and ulna, scaphoid, trapezoid, trapezium, and first metacarpal. The differentiation between cortex and medullary space is absent, and very little remaining trabecular bone pattern is seen. However, the bones are not enlarged, and their shape is normal. The remaining bones that are visible have a normal appearance.

Differential Diagnosis: Chronic sclerosing osteomyelitis, osteoblastic lymphoma, osteomyelitis, Paget's disease, sclerosing bone dysplasias.

Diagnosis: Chronic sclerosing osteomyelitis.

Discussion: The abnormal bone scan and corresponding sclerosis raise the differential diagnosis of osteoblastic neoplasm, osteomyelitis, Paget's disease, and sclerosing bone dysplasias. Paget's disease can be eliminated by the lack of bone enlargement and cortical thickening, and sclerosing bone dysplasias can be eliminated by the otherwise normal bone morphology and clinical history. Given the patient's age, lymphoma and osteomyelitis were the primary considerations, and *S. aureus* was cultured from a biopsy specimen of the radius. Hematogenous osteomyelitis is caused most frequently in adults by *S. aureus*. Cortical destruction and periostitis with involucrum formation dominates the early radiographic appearance. In the subacute and chronic stages of osteomyelitis, reactive bone formation may result in dense sclerosis [48], with low-grade clinical symptoms. Foci of bacteria persist within bone cavities that are filled with granulation tissue, and dense reactive bone surrounds the site. The cortex may be thickened as a result of long-term deposition of reactive medullary and periosteal bone. Serpiginous sinus tracts may extend to the skin surface. Chronic osteomyelitis may exist many years after acute osteomyelitis, even if the acute infection was treated appropriately. Systemic antibiotics will be ineffective against organisms sequestered in necrotic bone. Blood cultures are almost always negative, and cultures of the lesions are frequently negative as well.

Clinical History: 31-year-old woman who fell on her outstretched hand.

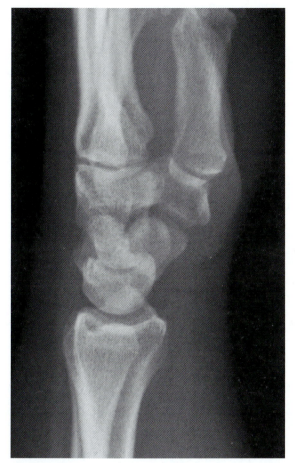

Figure 1-39 A

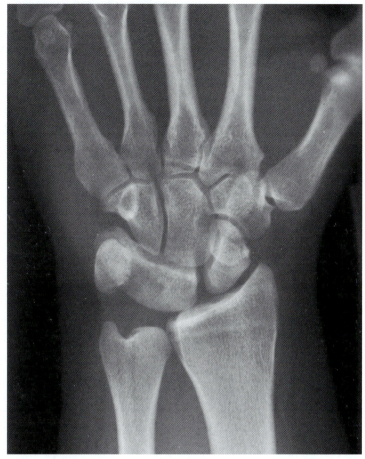

Figure 1-39 B

Findings: (A) Lateral radiograph of the wrist shows an abnormal appearance to the lunate, with slight volar angulation. The scapholunate angle is actually decreased. No fracture is evident. (B) PA radiograph of the wrist shows an incompletely segmented lunate and triquetrum. There is no fracture.

Differential Diagnosis: None.

Diagnosis: Carpal coalition.

Discussion: Carpal coalitions are relatively common anomalies in which two or more carpal bones fail to segment during development, resulting in a congenital fusion. The anomaly results from incomplete cavitation of a common embryologic carpal precursor during the 4th to 8th weeks of intrauterine life [49]. The fusion can be bony, cartilaginous, or fibrous. Carpal coalitions are usually isolated anomalies that involve bones of the same row. The most common coalition is between the lunate and triquetrum. The prevalence of this abnormality is approximately 1%, and it is bilateral in 60%. Carpal coalitions are usually incidental findings, but carpal coalition and associated degenerative arthritis of the incompletely involved joints has been proven as a cause of occult wrist pain [50]. Multiple carpal coalitions or coalitions between bones of the proximal and distal rows are frequently associated with other anomalies, including tarsal coalitions, arthrogryposis, Ellis-van Creveld syndrome, Holt-Oram syndrome, Turner's syndrome, and symphalangism. These coalitions may be familial.

Clinical History: 52-year-old male with chronic wrist pain.

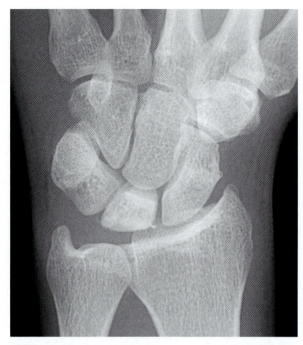

Figure 1-40   A

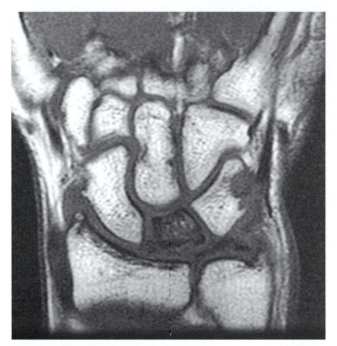

Figure 1-40   B

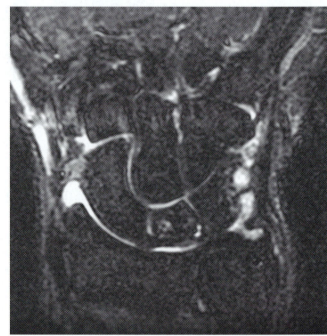

Figure 1-40   C

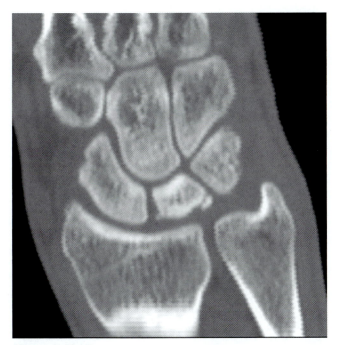

Figure 1-40 D

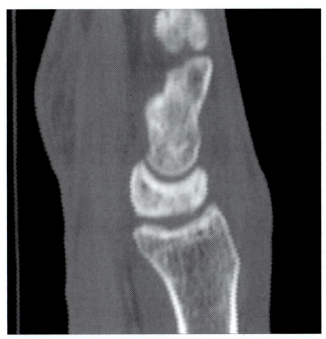

Figure 1-40 E

Findings: (A) PA radiograph of the wrist shows that the lunate is dense, with tiny fragments visible at the proximal articulation with the scaphoid, and perhaps with the triquetrum. (B) Coronal T1-weighted MRI shows mostly low signal in the lunate. (C) Coronal T2-weighted MRI shows effusion in the radiocarpal compartment and focal area of high signal within the lunate. (D) Coronal CT reformation shows sclerosis of the lunate with fragmentation adjacent to the triquetral articulation. (E) Sagittal CT reformation shows sclerosis and flattening of the proximal surface of the lunate.

Differential Diagnosis: Osteonecrosis, trauma.

Diagnosis: Osteonecrosis of the lunate (Kienböck's disease, lunate malacia).

Discussion: In the normal wrist, loading of the hand is transmitted to the forearm through the radiocarpal joint, with approximately one-third of the force passing through each articulating proximal row carpal bone (scaphoid, lunate, and triquetrum). When the ulna is abnormally short with respect to the radius—the so-called ulnar minus variance—loading that would have passed through the triquetrum is passed instead through the lunate. This may result in stress-related osteonecrosis of the lunate [51,52]. A similar process may occur as a result of trauma, as perhaps in this case. It is rare for Kienböck's disease to occur bilaterally [53]. On CT, sclerosis, deformation, and fragmentation are typically seen. On MRI, the lunate tends to be dark on all sequences, presumably as a result of sclerosis. Because the natural history of Kienböck's disease is progressive deformation and fragmentation, high T2-signal is more likely to reflect cystic degenerative change rather than revascularization and remodeling.

Clinical History: 28-year-old woman with persistent wrist pain who fell backward several weeks ago.

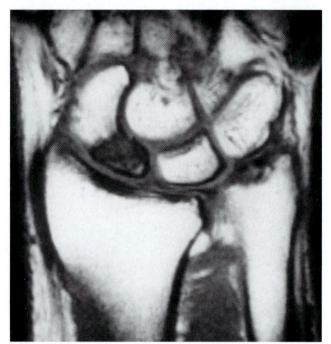

Figure 1-41   A

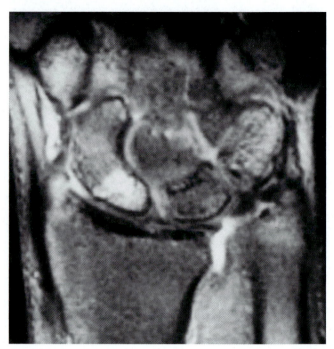

Figure 1-41   B

Findings: (A) Coronal MRI of the wrist (T1-weighted) shows dark signal replacing the normal bright marrow signal of the proximal pole of the scaphoid. The triangular fibrocartilage complex (TFCC) is normally a triangular structure of low signal; in this case, there is irregular intermediate signal within. (B) Coronal MRI (T1-weighted with fat saturation after intravenous gadolinium contrast). Delayed images show enhancement in the proximal pole of the scaphoid. Contrast diffusing into an effusion in the radiocarpal and distal radioulnar joints outlines discontinuities in the TFCC.

Differential Diagnosis: None.

Diagnosis: Osteonecrosis of the proximal pole of the scaphoid following fracture. Tear of the TFCC.

Discussion: Scaphoid fractures comprise about 85% of all isolated carpal bone fractures. The scaphoid bridges the lunate-capitate articulation. With extreme, forceful dorsiflexion between the lunate and capitate, and perhaps impingement of the scaphoid on the dorsal radial rim, the scaphoid starts to bend and the fracture line begins on its volar aspect under tensile loading, propagating transversely through the narrowest region (the scaphoid waist). Most scaphoid fractures have no comminution (70% of cases). Less common are fractures through the proximal (10%) or distal (20%) poles. Because the blood supply to the proximal pole of the scaphoid enters the distal pole and courses proximally across the waist, posttraumatic osteonecrosis of the proximal pole with nonunion is a common complication seen in up to 30% of cases.

CASE 1-42

Clinical History: 1-year-old with generalized disease.

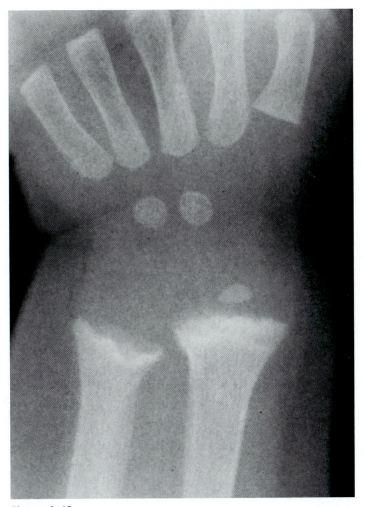

Figure 1-42

Findings: PA radiograph of the distal forearm. The growth plates of the distal radius and ulna are thick and wide. Dense sclerosis is present at the distal metaphyses. The metaphyses have a frayed appearance.

Differential Diagnosis: Healing rickets, hypophosphatasia, renal disease, metaphyseal chondrodysplasia.

Diagnosis: Healing rickets.

Discussion: Rickets is the childhood manifestation of a systemic disease in which the calcification of osteoid is deficient. The final common pathway is the lack of available calcium or phosphorus (or both) for mineralization of osteoid, but a number of different abnormalities in the availability, synthesis, or biologic action of vitamin D and its hormonally active metabolites may be responsible. Because there is continued cartilage growth in the absence of normal mineralization and ossification, the growth plates become widened. This defining radiographic finding will be most apparent in the most active regions of growth. Uncalcified cartilage may become quite bulky and evident on clinical examination. Frequent sites of radiographic abnormalities include the costochondral junctions of the ribs, the distal femur, both ends of the tibia, the proximal humerus, the distal radius, and the distal ulna. Irregular, disorganized mineralization of the zone of provisional calcification creates a frayed appearance. Mechanical stress on the thickened growth plate may lead to widening, cupping, and bowing deformity. The bone texture (trabecular pattern) may appear smudged or coarsened, and there is a delayed appearance of ossification centers. Rachitic bone is less resistant to bending and shearing loads, and insufficiency fractures and bowing deformities are common. Following the initiation of successful treatment of rickets, the uncalcified osteoid calcifies, so that the zone of provisional calcification appears as a wide band that narrows the growth plate to its normal thickness. Ossification of nonmineralized subperiosteal osteoid is apparent as new periosteal bone.

Clinical History: 9-year-old boy with history of trauma.

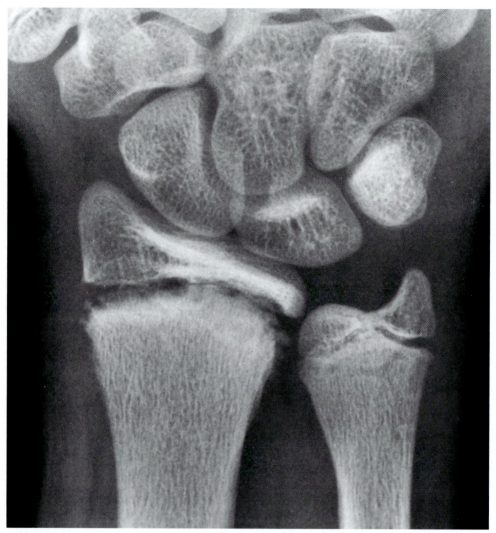

Figure 1-43

Findings: PA radiograph of the wrist. There is widening and irregularity of the zone of provisional calcification of the growth plate of the radius, but the growth plates of the distal ulna and first metacarpal are normal.

Differential Diagnosis: Trauma, rickets.

Diagnosis: Growth plate fracture (Salter type I), healing.

Discussion: The abnormality of the growth plate of the distal radius has a superficial resemblance to rickets—it is widened and there is irregular sclerosis on the metaphyseal side—but the presence of normal growth plates elsewhere (distal ulna, proximal first metacarpal) eliminates systemic or metabolic bone disease as a diagnostic consideration. The growth plate is attached to the metaphysis internally by the interdigitation of bone with the zone of calcified cartilage, and externally by the periosteum. The growth plate is relatively weak when loaded in torsion or shear, but is resistant to tension and compression. When the epiphysis is separated from the metaphysis, the plane of separation through the growth plate is in the zone of cartilage transformation between the calcified and uncalcified layers of cartilage, leaving the germinal cell layers with the epiphysis and the calcified cartilage with the metaphysis. Displacement does not occur unless the periosteum is also torn. The production of growing cartilage by the germinal layers may be uninterrupted by a fracture if the blood supply to the separated epiphysis remains intact. However, the newly formed cartilage will not ossify until vascular ingrowth from the metaphyseal side is reestablished. Thus, after a fracture, the growth plate becomes wider until the normal zone of cartilage transformation is reestablished; once ossification of the widened growth plate begins, its thickness returns to normal.

Clinical History: 2-year-old girl with lethargy.

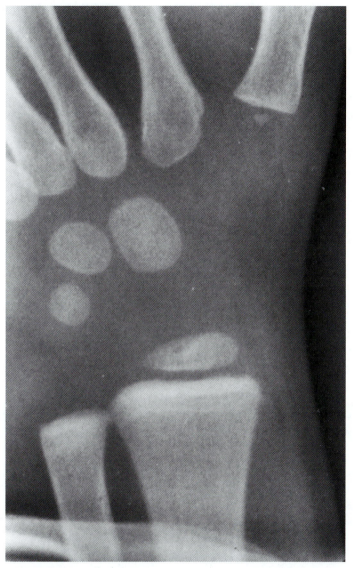

Figure 1-44

Findings: PA radiograph of the wrist. There are dense transverse metaphyseal lines at the distal radius and ulna. The growth plate is of normal thickness, and there is no periosteal bone reaction.

Differential Diagnosis: Heavy metal poisoning, physiologic lines.

Diagnosis: Lead poisoning.

Discussion: Chronic lead poisoning (plumbism) in children results in dense transverse lines across the growing metaphysis, so-called *lead lines* or *lead bands*. Lead interferes with the resorption of the primary spongiosa during growth. New bone is laid down on top of the primary spongiosa, but because normal resorption of the primary spongiosa does not occur during the period of exposure, a dense line becomes evident on radiographs, even if lead is present in only minute amounts. Lead lines are a late manifestation of chronic lead poisoning and are best seen at the knee or distal radius, where growth is the most rapid. Lead lines do not appear until blood lead attains a concentration of 70 to 80 g/dL. Lead lines are not affected by treatment of the underlying lead poisoning; they disappear spontaneously within 4 years [54,55]. Lead toxicity has been reported following retention of lead fragments after gunshot wound. Chronic exposure during growth to other heavy metals, including phosphorus and bismuth, may result in transverse lines similar to those seen with chronic lead poisoning.

Clinical History: 15-year-old girl with wrist pain. No history of trauma.

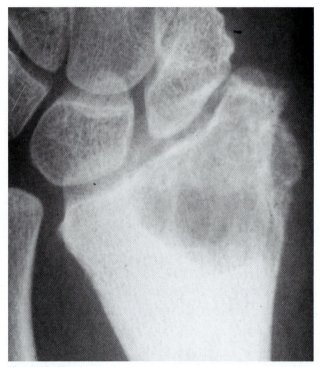

Figure 1-45   A

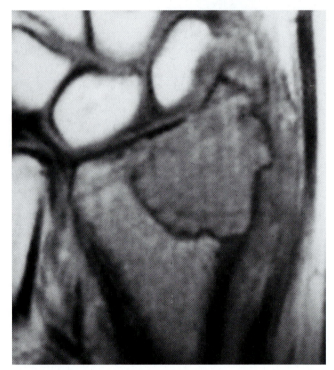

Figure 1-45   B

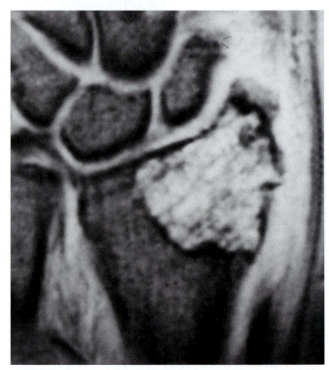

Figure 1-45   C

Findings: (A) Plain film demonstrates a geographic lesion that replaces the radial styloid, abutting the articular surface. There are multiple septations within it, and the margins are lobulated. The lateral margins of the radial styloid are irregular and indistinct, suggesting an associated small soft tissue mass. (B, C) On coronal MR images, T1-weighted isointensity and T2-weighted hyperintensity are noted within the lesion. The radial cortex is buckled, with surrounding soft tissue edema.

Differential Diagnosis: Chondroblastoma, eosinophilic granuloma, Brodie's abscess, giant-cell tumor.

Diagnosis: Chondroblastoma (with pathologic fracture).

Discussion: Chondroblastomas are considered benign neoplasms, although extremely rare occurrences of malignancy [56] and even metastases from histologically benign lesions [57] have been reported. Chondroblastomas occur most commonly before closure of the physis, predominantly in the second decade of life. However, they may be discovered after physeal closure, and should be considered in the differential diagnosis for metaphyseal or end-of-bone lesions when they present the appropriate radiographic features. Chondroblastomas typically present as eccentric, lytic, and well-defined lesions, with sclerotic borders confined almost exclusively to the epiphysis, although extension to the adjacent metaphyseal bone can be observed. Cartilaginous components in this lesion may impart the appearance of a component of calcified matrix in up to 50% of instances. CT may assist further in ascertaining the presence of matrix calcification. Periosteal reaction may be seen in 50% of cases. MRI features consist of foci of low signal intensity within a lesion of higher signal intensity on T2-weighted images, with a lobulated rim of low signal intensity [58]. Often they may resemble enchondroma, as in this case, with small lobulated regions of increased signal intensity separated by fine low signal intensity septations on T2-weighted images. The primary discriminating feature from enchondroma is the characteristic predilection of this lesion to occupy the end of the bone. Other diagnostic considerations include giant-cell tumor and clear-cell chondrosarcoma. The MRI findings should enable differentiation of this lesion from giant-cell tumor. Clear-cell chondrosarcomas typically occur in an older population.

Clinical History: 32-year-old woman with chronic wrist pain.

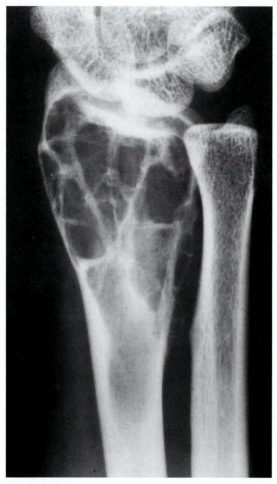

Figure 1-46

Findings: PA radiograph of the wrist. There is a lesion with geographic bone destruction in the distal radius. The lesion extends from the distal shaft to the articular surfaces, both radiocarpal as well as the distal radioulnar. The cortex is thinned and mildly expanded. Prominent bony ridges or struts are seen traversing the lesion. There is no apparent matrix mineralization. The transition between lesion and normal bone is sharp, but with a definite sclerotic rim distally. The cortex appears thin, but intact and mildly expanded on the ulnar side.

Differential Diagnosis: Desmoplastic fibroma, hemophiliac pseudotumor, osteonecrosis, geode, giant-cell tumor.

Diagnosis: Desmoplastic fibroma.

Discussion: The presence of the reinforced ridges or struts of bone suggests that the lesion is indolent, and that the bone has remodeled to accommodate the geographic destruction. Large lesions of low aggressiveness located in the metaphysis but extending to the articular surface in adults are few and include subchondral cyst, hemophiliac pseudotumor,

osteonecrosis, and this lesion, desmoplastic fibroma. Giant-cell tumor, although occurring at this site, would tend to have more aggressive characteristics, and generally not a sclerotic margin or reinforced trabeculae. Desmoplastic fibroma is a rare intraosseous fibrous lesion that is histologically identical to soft tissue fibromatosis (extraabdominal desmoid tumor of soft tissues). They are seen mostly in adolescents and young adults. Their location is typically central in the metaphysis of a long bone, and radiographic characteristics are typically benign [59]. They are geographic, lytic lesions, with a narrow zone of transition but often not a sclerotic rim. There is no matrix mineralization. Endosteal erosion and modest cortical expansion are present, but usually cortical breakthrough is not. The endosteal margins characteristically have thick ridges of bone that may suggest the diagnosis. They may be infiltrative and occasionally locally aggressive, but they have no metastatic potential. Local recurrence is common after intralesional curettage, so en bloc excision is the treatment of choice [60].

Clinical History: 12-year-old boy with arm pain.

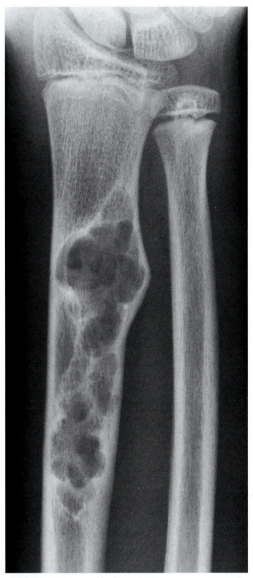

Figure 1-47

Findings: PA radiograph of the forearm. There is a long lesion in the distal radial shaft. The lesion has a bubbly appearance, with a sclerotic margin, mildly expanded cortical shell, and no matrix mineralization.

Differential Diagnosis: None.

Diagnosis: Nonossifying fibroma.

Discussion: The lesion has nonaggressive characteristics: the well-defined sclerotic margin, the mild cortical expansion without cortical thinning, and the lack of cortical penetration or periosteal reaction. The long shape and bubbly appearance are characteristic of nonossifying fibroma (fibroxanthomas). Nonossifying fibromas are nonneoplastic lesions thought to be the result of faulty ossification at the growth plate. A causal relationship with stress or trauma has been suggested but not proven. These lesions are self-limited, with no potential for growth or spread, and regress spontaneously by filling in with bone from the periphery. They are histologically identical to fibrous cortical defects (metaphyseal fibrous defects). Nonossifying fibromas are less common than fibrous cortical defects and occur in older children or adolescents. Located eccentrically within the medullary cavity but still within an expanded cortex, nonossifying fibromas are lucent with a sclerotic margin. Some lesions have a trabeculated, scalloped, multilocular, or bubbly appearance. They range in size from 1 to 7 cm, and the larger ones may fracture or cause pain.

Clinical History: 56-year-old man with swollen, painful joints and chronic cough.

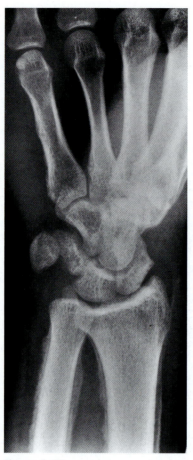

Figure 1-48

Findings: Oblique radiograph of the wrist demonstrates undulating periosteal reaction along the metadiaphysis of the distal radius and distal ulna. The contralateral side has similar findings.

Differential Diagnosis: Hypertrophic osteoarthropathy, melorheostosis, hypervitaminosis A.

Diagnosis: Hypertrophic osteoarthropathy, secondary.

Discussion: Hypertrophic osteoarthropathy is a syndrome characterized by digital clubbing and periostitis of the tubular bones [61]. There are primary and secondary forms of the condition, and there may be incomplete manifestations. Secondary forms may be localized and associated with hemiplegia, aneurysm, infective arteritis, and patent ductus arteriosus, or they may be generalized and associated with a wide variety of conditions, including various chronic and neoplastic pulmonary, cardiac, hepatic, intestinal, and mediastinal diseases, as well as a diverse variety of other malignancies. Hypertrophic osteoarthropathy may occur as one of a number of paraneoplastic syndromes in which the clinical manifestations may precede, coincide with, or follow the diagnosis of the malignancy [62,63]. The clinical presentation as joint disease and the isolated radiographic finding of periosteal reactive bone are typical for hypertrophic osteoarthropathy. Involvement of the diaphysis and metaphysis (but not the epiphysis) is characteristic, and location in the leg and forearm is more common than in the femur, humerus, hands, or feet [64]. In an older patient, the condition is most commonly secondary to bronchogenic carcinoma, although it may also occur in other malignant, benign, or chronic suppurative diseases of the lung; cyanotic heart disease; liver or biliary cirrhosis; or inflammatory bowel disease. The mechanism of the reaction is unknown. In an adolescent or young adult, the condition may be pachydermoperiostosis (primary hypertrophic osteoarthropathy), a condition of unknown etiology that may also include thickening of the skin of the face and hands, and clubbed digits. The primary form of hypertrophic osteoarthropathy represents approximately 3% to 5% of cases. The distinction between primary and secondary hypertrophic osteoarthropathy may be difficult to make radiographically, but findings in the primary form may be more florid, may involve the epiphyses, and may be located in the ribs, pelvis, and skull.

CASE 1-49

Clinical History: 2-week-old infant born to a mother with poor prenatal care, and seen again 3 months later.

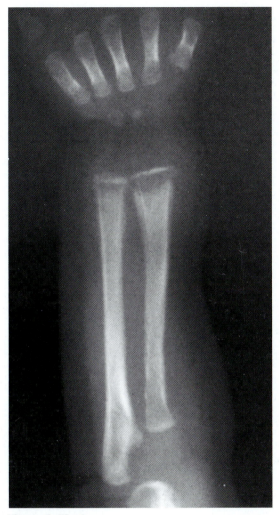

Figure 1-49 A

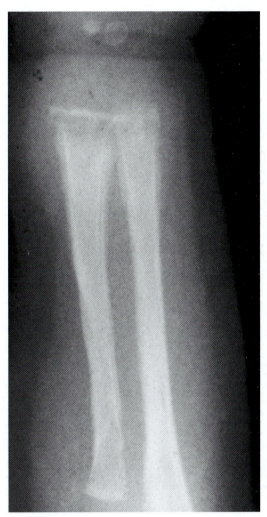

Figure 1-49 B

Findings: (A) PA radiograph of the forearm demonstrates mild periostitis of the metadiaphyseal regions. (B) PA radiograph of the forearm performed 3 months later demonstrates a marked increase in the amount of periostitis, as well as irregularity and widening of the metaphysis, an increase in soft tissue swelling, and a possible focal lucency in the proximal ulna.

Differential Diagnosis: Congenital infections by toxoplasmosis, syphilis, rubella, cytomegalovirus, or herpes simplex; hypervitaminosis A; Caffey's disease.

Diagnosis: Congenital syphilis.

Discussion: Syphilis is a chronic infection caused by the spirochete bacterium *Treponema pallidum*. Congenital syphilis is acquired by transplacental migration of the organism, usually in women who are infected during pregnancy. Heavy infection of the fetus may cause abortion or death shortly after birth. In survivors, invasion of the

developing skeleton, particularly sites of active enchondral ossification, result in the stigmata of congenital syphilis. In the neonate and very young infant, bony abnormalities include osteochondritis, diaphyseal osteomyelitis, and periostitis. Syphilitic osteochondritis is typically seen as symmetric involvement of the sites of enchondral ossification, including the growth plates of long bones, costochondral regions, and sometimes the flat bones and spine. Lucency and osseous irregularity may be seen. In diaphyseal osteomyelitis, focal regions of osteolysis and exuberant periostitis involve the shafts of the long bones. Periostitis may be a manifestation of subperiosteal infection, or may be a reactive process associated with osteomyelitis or healing osteochondritis. These lesions heal promptly with appropriate antibiotic therapy. Although reliable serologic methods for detecting syphilis exist, several epidemiologic factors have contributed to its reemergence as a significant potential cause of congenital infection [65].

Clinical History: 25-year-old woman in motor vehicle crash.

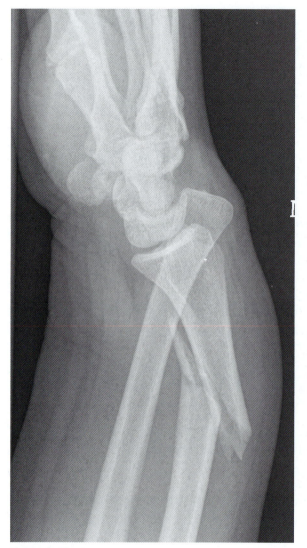

Figure 1-50   A

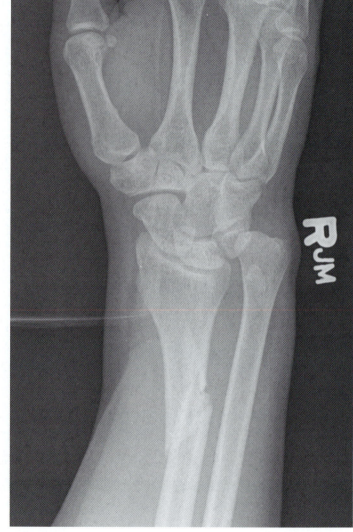

Figure 1-50   B

Findings: (A, B) Lateral and PA radiographs of the wrist. There is a comminuted fracture of the distal radial shaft at the junction of the middle and distal thirds, with volar angulation of the distal fragment and dorsal dislocation of the distal radioulnar joint.

Differential Diagnosis: None.

Diagnosis: Galeazzi fracture-dislocation.

Discussion: A fracture of the radial shaft with dislocation of the distal radioulnar joint is called a Galeazzi's fracture-dislocation. It accounts for approximately 7% of adult forearm fractures [66]. Isolated fractures of the radial shaft in adults are almost always associated with disruption of the distal radioulnar joint. The injury is believed to occur during a fall on an outstretched hand combined with extreme pronation of the forearm. In this case, the distal radioulnar joint dislocation is grossly displaced. In less severe cases, the distal radioulnar joint may only be subluxated or dynamically unstable. CT with the wrist pronated may be required to document the abnormality; in supination, the unstable distal radioulnar joint tends to reduce itself. Treatment typically requires open reduction and internal fixation of the radial shaft fracture, and often direct repair of the distal radioulnar joint [67]. In children, a so-called Galeazzi-equivalent injury may occur as a fracture of the distal radial shaft with displaced epiphyseal separation of the distal ulna (Salter type I); however, unlike the adult injury, the distal ligamentous stabilizers at the distal radioulnar joint will remain intact [68].

Clinical History: 51-year-old woman with pain along the thumb side of the wrist.

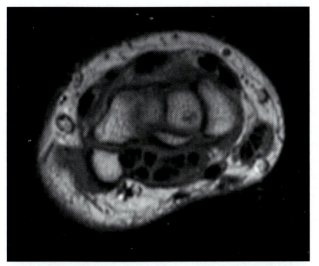

Figure 1-51   A

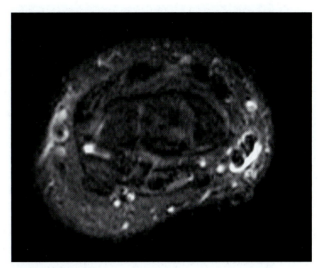

Figure 1-51   B

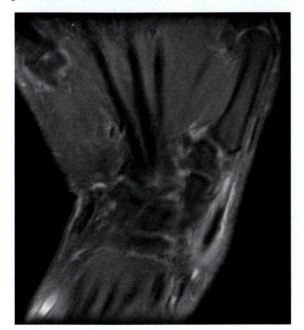

Figure 1-51   C

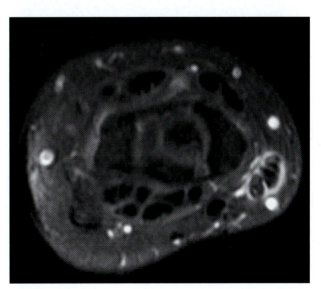

Figure 1-51   D

Findings: Axial T1-weighted (**A**), axial T2-weighted fat-suppressed (**B**) and post-gadolinium coronal (**C**), and axial T1-weighted fat-suppressed (**D**) images of the wrist show thickening and irregularity of the abductor pollicis longus (APL) and the extensor pollicis brevis (EPB). High T2-weighted signal is present around and within these tendons.

Differential Diagnosis: None.

Diagnosis: De Quervain's tendinitis/tenosynovitis.

Discussion: De Quervain's tendonitis and tenosynovitis describes a clinical entity involving inflammation of the abductor pollicis longus and extensor pollicis brevis tendons. These tendons travel through the first dorsal compartment of the wrist. This syndrome is most common in women between the ages of 35 and 55, though it has been reported in new mothers due to overuse [69]. Patients complain of gradual onset of pain over the radial styloid when they abduct or extend the thumb. Clinically, this condition may be difficult to differentiate from osteoarthritis at the base of the thumb. If left untreated, patients may develop fibrosis within the tendon sheath with subsequent limited motion.

Clinical History: 30-year-old man with thumb pain.

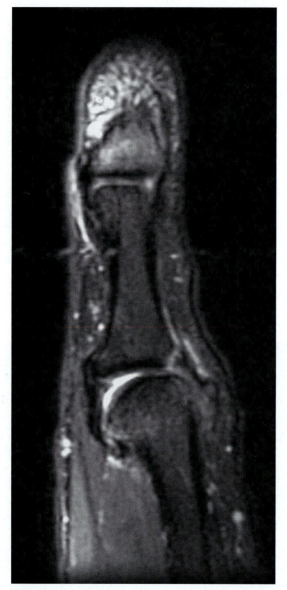

Figure 1-52   A

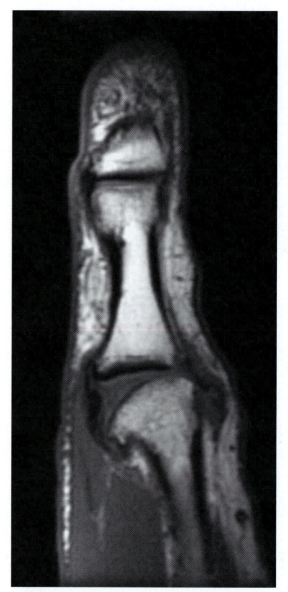

Figure 1-52   B

Findings: (**A**) Coronal T2-weighted fat-saturated and (**B**) T1-weighted images of the thumb show avulsion of the ulnar dorsal base of the thumb proximal phalanx. There is high T2-weighted signal in and around the metacarpophalangeal joint of the first digit. The ulnar collateral ligament of the thumb is disrupted and retracted proximally. There has been interposition of the abductor pollicis aponeurosis between the ruptured ulnar collateral ligament and its distal attachment.

Differential Diagnosis: None.

Diagnosis: Gamekeeper's thumb with a Stener lesion.

Discussion: Gamekeeper's thumb is ligamentous disruption of the ulnar collateral ligament of the thumb's metacar-

pophalangeal joint. The injury mechanism is sudden valgus stress on the thumb, such as during downhill skiing when a pole is improperly planted. Similar mechanisms of injury may also occur in sports such as football, hockey, wrestling, and basketball. Injury of the ulnar collateral ligament can range from partial thickness tear to complete displaced tears [70]. The adductor pollicis aponeurosis is normally superficial to the ulnar collateral ligament. Interposition of the adductor pollicis aponeurosis between the ruptured ulnar collateral ligament and its distal attachment is called a Stener lesion. A Stener lesion will prevent healing of the ligament and result in chronic instability.

SOURCES AND READINGS

1. Tehranzadeh J, Ter-Oganesyan RR, Steinbach LS. Musculoskeletal disorders associated with HIV infection and AIDS. Part II: non-infectious musculoskeletal conditions. *Skeletal Radiol.* 2004; [Epub ahead of print].

2. Pipitone N, Kingsley GH, Manzo A, Scott DL, Pitzalis C. Current concepts and new developments in the treatment of psoriatic arthritis. *Rheumatology* (Oxford). 2003;42(10):1138–1148.

3. Gladman DD. Current concepts in psoriatic arthritis. *Curr Opin Rheumatol.* 2002;14(4):361–366.

4. Bennett DL, Ohashi K, El-Khoury GY. Spondyloarthropathies: ankylosing spondylitis and psoriatic arthritis. *Radiol Clin North Am.* 2004; 42(1):121–134.

5. Gupta KB, Duryea J, Weissman BN. Radiographic evaluation of osteoarthritis. *Radiol Clin North Am.* 2004;42(1):11–41.

6. Belhorn LR, Hess EV. Erosive osteoarthritis. *Semin Arthritis Rheum.* 1993;22:298–306.

7. Greenspan A. Erosive osteoarthritis. *Semin Musculoskelet Radiol.* 2003; 7(2):155–159.

8. Kaandorp CJ, Van Schaardenburg D, Krijnen P, Habbema JD, van de Laar MA. Risk factors for septic arthritis in patients with joint disease. A prospective study. *Arthritis Rheum.* 1995;38:1819–1825.

9. Murray PM. Septic arthritis of the hand and wrist. *Hand Clin.* 1998; 14(4):579–587.

10. Biviji AA, Paiement GD, Steinbach LS. Musculoskeletal manifestations of human immunodeficiency virus infection. *J Am Acad Orthop Surg.* 2002;10(5):312–320.

11. Alpert PL, Munsiff SS, Gourevitch MN, Greenberg B, Klein RS. A prospective study of tuberculosis and human immunodeficiency virus infection: clinical manifestations and factors associated with survival. *Clin Infect Dis.* 1997;24:661–668.

12. Vine JE, Cohen PR. Renal cell carcinoma metastatic to the thumb: a case report and review of subungual metastases from all primary sites. *Clin Exp Dermatol.* 1996;21:377–380.

13. Baran R, Tosti A. Metastatic carcinoma to the terminal phalanx of the big toe: report of two cases and review of the literature. *J Am Acad Dermatol.* 1994;31:259–263.

14. Lambert D, Escallier F, Collet E, et al. Distal phalangeal metastasis of a chondrosarcoma presenting initially as bilateral onycholysis. *Clin Exp Dermatol.* 1992;17:463–465.

15. Cohen PR. Metastatic tumors to the nail unit: subungual metastases. *Dermatol Surg.* 2001;27(3):280–293.

16. Pantoja E, Cross VF, Vitale P, Wendth AJ. Neoplastic involvement of terminal digits masquerading clinically as benign disease. *Rev Interam Radiol.* 1976;1:9–13.

17. Heys SD, Brittenden J, Atkinson P, Eremin O. Glomus tumour: an analysis of 43 patients and review of the literature. *Br J Surg.* 1992;79: 345–347.

18. Dumont J. Glomus tumour of the fingers. *Can J Surg.* 1975;18:542–544.

19. Bhaskaranand K, Naradgi BC. Glomus tumour of the hand. *J Hand Surg [Br].* 2062;27:229–231.

20. Byers P, Mantle J, Salm R. Epidermal cysts of phalanges. *J Bone Joint Surg Br.* 1966;48:577–581.

21. Davids JR, Graner KA, Mubarak SJ. Post-fracture lipid inclusion cyst. A case report. *J Bone Joint Surg Am.* 1993;75:1528–1532.

22. Samlaska CP, Hansen MF. Intraosseous epidermoid cysts. *J Am Acad Dermatol.* 1992;27:454–455.

23. Rivera-Sanfeliz G, Resnick D, Haghighi P. Sarcoidosis of hands. *Skeletal Radiol.* 1996;25:786–788.

24. Gonzalez del Pino J, Diez Ulloa A, Lovic A, Relea MF. Sarcoidosis of the hand and wrist: a report of two cases. *J Hand Surg [Am].* 1997;22:942–945.

25. Lieberman J, Krauthammer M. Pseudoclubbing in a patient with sarcoidosis of the phalangeal bones. *Arch Intern Med.* 1983;143:1017–1019.

26. Yabut SM Jr, Kenan S, Sissons HA, Lewis MM. Malignant transformation of fibrous dysplasia. A case report and review of the literature. *Clin Orthop.* 1988;(228):281–289.

27. Peiper M, Zornig C. Chondrosarcoma of the thumb arising from a solitary enchondroma. *Arch Orthop Trauma Surg.* 1997;166:246–248.

28. el-Noueam KI, Schweitzer ME, Blasbalg R, et al. Is a subset of wrist ganglia the sequela of internal derangements of the wrist joint? MR imaging findings. *Radiology.* 1999;212(2):537–540.

29. Nakajima Y, Sato K, Morita H, et al. Severe progressive erosive arthritis in multicentric reticulohistiocytosis: possible involvement of cytokines in synovial proliferation. *J Rheumatol.* 1992;19:1643–1646.

30. Snow JL, Muller SA. Malignancy-associated multicentric reticulohistiocytosis: a clinical, histological and immunophenotypic study. *Br J Dermatol.* 1995;133:71–76.

31. Chapman ME, Beggs I, Wu PS. Case report: thyroid acropachy in a single digit. *Clin Radiol.* 1993;47(1):58–59.

32. Fatourechi V, Bartley GB, Eghbali-Fatourechi GZ, Powell CC, Ahmed DD, Garrity JA. Graves' dermopathy and acropachy are markers of severe Graves' ophthalmopathy. *Thyroid.* 2003;13(12):1141–1144.

33. Resnick D. Dermatomyositis and polymyositis. In: Resnick D, Niwayama G, eds. *Diagnosis of Bone and Joint Disorders.* 3rd ed. Philadelphia: WB Saunders; 1995:1218–1231.

34. Bunch TW, O'Duffy JD, McLeod RA. Deforming arthritis of the hands in polymyositis. *Arthritis Rheum.* 1976;19:243–248.

35. Schumacher HR, Schimmer B, Gordon GV, Bookspan MA, Brogadir S, Dowart BB. Articular manifestations of polymyositis and dermatomyositis. *Am J Med.* 1979;67:287–292.

36. Hyszczak R, Bartold KP, Eggleston D. Gangrene associated with meningococcemia. *AJR Am J Roentgenol.* 1988;151:203–204.

37. Lowenthal MN. Peripheral gangrene in infancy and childhood. *Br Med J.* 1967;2:700–701.

38. Askari AD, Muir WA, Rosner IA, Moskowitz RW, McLaren GD, Braun WE. Arthritis of hemochromatosis. Clinical spectrum, relation to histocompatibility antigens, and effectiveness of early phlebotomy. *Am J Med.* 1983;75:957–965.

39. Smith DK, Murray PM. Avulsion fractures of the volar aspect of triquetral bone of the wrist: a subtle sign of carpal ligament injury. *AJR Am J Roentgenol.* 1996;166(3):609–614.

40. Vassilopoulos D, Chalasani P, Jurado RL, Workowski K, Agudelo CA. Musculoskeletal infections in patients with human immunodeficiency virus infection. *Medicine* (Baltimore). 1997;76:284–294.

41. Vande Streek P, Carretta RF, Weiland FL, Shelton DK. Upper extremity radionuclide bone imaging: the wrist and hand. *Semin Nucl Med.* 1998;28:14–24.

42. Fournier RS, Holder LE. Reflex sympathetic dystrophy: diagnostic controversies. *Semin Nucl Med.* 1998;28:116–123.

43. Silberstein EB, Elgazzar AH, Fernandez-Ulloa M, Nishiyama H. Skeletal scintigraphy in non-neoplastic osseous disorders. In: Henkin RE, Boles MA, Karesh SM, et al., eds. *Nuclear Medicine.* St. Louis: Mosby; 1996:1182–1185.

44. Schernberg F, Gerard Y, Collin JP, Teinturier P. Arthroplasty of the rheumatoid wrist by silicone implants. Experience with forty cases. *Ann Chir Main.* 1983;2:18–26.

45. Fatti JF, Palmer AK, Greenky S, Mosher JF. Long-term results of Swanson interpositional wrist arthroplasty: part II. *J Hand Surg [Am].* 1991;16:432–437.

46. Jolly SL, Ferlic DC, Clayton ML, Dennis DA, Stringer EA. Swanson silicone arthroplasty of the wrist in rheumatoid arthritis: a long-term follow-up. *J Hand Surg [Am].* 1992;17:142–149.

47. Lanzetta M, Herbert TJ, Conolly WB. Silicone synovitis. A perspective. *J Hand Surg [Br].* 1994;19:479–484.

48. Collert S, Isacson J. Chronic sclerosing osteomyelitis (Garre). *Clin Orthop.* 1982;164:136–140.

49. Delaney TJ, Eswar S. Carpal coalitions. *J Hand Surg [Am]*. 1992;17: 28–31.

50. Marburger R, Burgess RC. Symptomatic lunate-triquetral coalition. *J South Orthop Assoc*. 1995;4:307–310.

51. Gelberman RH, Salamon PB, Jurist JM, Posch JL. Ulnar variance in Kienbock's disease. *J Bone Joint Surg Am*. 1975;57:674–676.

52. Gerwin M. The history of Kienbock's disease. *Hand Clin*. 1993;9:385–390.

53. Morgan RF, McCue FC III. Bilateral Kienbock's disease. *J Hand Surg [Am]*. 1983;8:928–932.

54. Sachs HK. The evolution of the radiologic lead line. *Radiology*. 1981; 139:81–85.

55. Blickman JG, Wilkinson RH, Graef JW. The radiologic "lead band" revisited. *AJR Am J Roentgenol*. 1986;146:245–247.

56. Rogers WB, Mankin HJ. Metastatic malignant chondroblastoma. *Am J Orthop*. 1996;25:846–849.

57. Jambhekar NA, Desai PB, Chitale DA, Patil P, Arya S. Benign metastasizing chondroblastoma: a case report. *Cancer*. 1998;82:675–678.

58. Oxtoby JW, Davies AM. MRI characteristics of chondroblastoma. *Clin Radiol*. 1996;51:22–26.

59. Taconis WK, Schutte HE, van der Heul RO. Desmoplastic fibroma of bone: a report of 18 cases. *Skeletal Radiol*. 1994;23:283–288.

60. Inwards CY, Unni KK, Beabout JW, Sim FH. Desmoplastic fibroma of bone. *Cancer*. 1991;68:1978–1983.

61. Martinez-Lavin M, Matucci-Cerinic M, Jajic I, Pineda C. Hypertrophic osteoarthropathy: consensus on its definition, classification, assessment and diagnostic criteria. *J Rheumatol*. 1993;20:1386–1387.

62. Kurzrock R, Cohen PR. Cutaneous paraneoplastic syndromes in solid tumors. *Am J Med*. 1995;99:662–671.

63. Nashitz JE, Rosner I, Rozenbaum M, Elias N, Yeshurun D. Cancer-associated rheumatic disorders: clues to occult neoplasia. *Semin Arthritis Rheum*. 1995;24:231–241.

64. Pineda C. Diagnostic imaging in hypertrophic osteoarthropathy. *Clin Exp Rheumatol*. 1992;10(suppl 7):27–33.

65. Murph JR. Rubella and syphilis: continuing causes of congenital infection in the 1990s. *Semin Pediatr Neurol*. 1994;1:26–35.

66. Bruckner JD, Alexander AH, Lichtman DM. Acute dislocations of the distal radio-ulnar joint. *J Bone Joint Surg Am*. 1995;77:958–968.

67. Strehle J, Gerber C. Distal radioulnar joint function after Galeazzi fracture-dislocations treated by open reduction and internal plate fixation. *Clin Orthop*. 1993;293:240–245.

68. Imatani J, Hashizume H, Nishida K, Morito Y, Inoue H. The Galeazzi-equivalent lesion in children revisited. *J Hand Surg [Br]*. 1996;21:455–457.

69. Anderson SE, Steinbach LS, De Monaco D, Bonel HM, Hurtienne Y, Voegelin E. "Baby wrist": MRI of an overuse syndrome in mothers. *AJR Am J Roentgenol*. 2004;182(3):719–24.

70. Romano WM, Garvin G, Bhayana D, Chaudhary O. The spectrum of ulnar collateral ligament injuries as viewed on magnetic resonance imaging of the metacarpophalangeal joint of the thumb. *Can Assoc Radiol J*. 2003;54(4):243–248.

CHAPTER TWO
ELBOW, ARM, AND SHOULDER

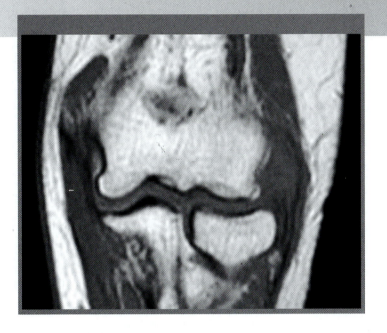

Clinical History: 55-year-old woman who fell off a curb while trying to hail a taxi.

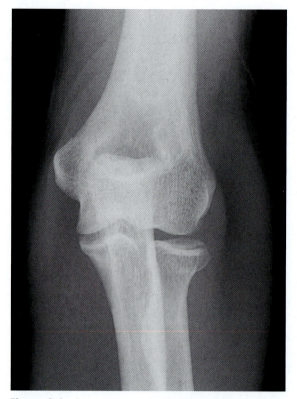

Figure 2-1   A

Figure 2-1   B

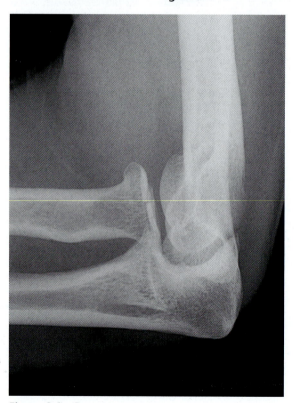

Figure 2-1   C

Findings: (A) Anteroposterior (AP) elbow radiograph shows a minimally impacted fracture of the articular surface of the radial head. (B) Lateral radiograph shows a triangular lucency in the soft tissues anterior to the distal humerus (anterior fat pad sign). The fracture is obliquely oriented and difficult to see. (C) Oblique radiograph shows the fracture.

Differential Diagnosis: None.

Diagnosis: Fracture, radial head.

Discussion: The fat pad sign at the elbow indicates an elbow effusion. Distention of the elbow capsule by fluid lifts up the anterior and posterior fat pads at the superior aspect of the elbow joint, displacing them from their normal positions and rendering them visible radiographically on the lateral view. The displaced anterior fat pad has been likened to a spinnaker sail, so the anterior fat pad is also called the "*spinnaker sail sign*." A small portion of the anterior fat pad is normally visible as a thin, triangular radiolucency with a short base facing the elbow joint. The posterior fat pad is normally fully contained within the olecranon fossa and is not visible. In the setting of acute trauma, the fat pad sign is indicative of fracture, but an effusion from any cause may result in a fat pad sign. Radial head and neck fractures are sustained by younger adults during falls onto an outstretched hand, impacting the radial head against the capitellum. Two types of fractures result: the intra-articular radial head fracture, as in this case, and the radial neck fracture. Radial head fractures may be treated by closed means, open reduction and internal fixation, simple resection of the fragments, or resection with prosthetic implant.

Clinical History: 6-year-old girl who fell.

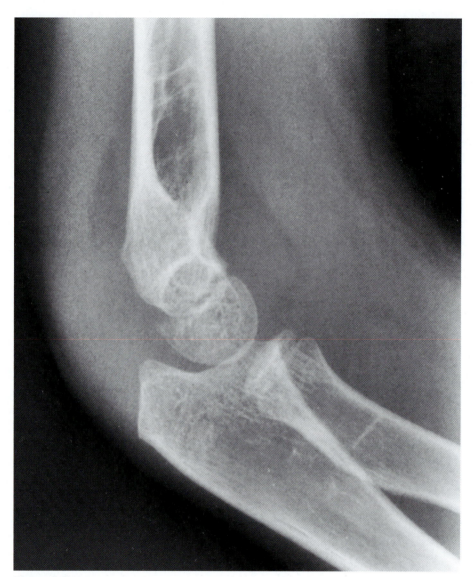

Figure 2-2

Findings: Lateral elbow radiograph. Anterior and posterior fat pad signs are prominent. There is slight posterior angulation of the distal humerus. A line drawn along the anterior cortex of the humerus (anterior humeral line) should intersect the capitellum in its posterior third, but in this case, the line intersects the capitellum in its anterior third. An actual fracture line is not visible on this radiograph.

Differential Diagnosis: None.

Diagnosis: Supracondylar fracture of the distal humerus.

Discussion: The fat pad sign is the clue to the presence of a fracture about the elbow. More than 90% of children or adolescents with a posterior fat pad sign will have a demonstrable fracture, and absence of the fat pad sign in these age groups virtually excludes an intraarticular fracture,

unless the injury is so severe that there is disruption of the elbow joint capsule. The supracondylar fracture comprises 60% of fractures around the elbow in children. Radial head and neck fractures, common in adults, are generally not seen in children. Supracondylar fractures occur with hyperextension of the elbow, usually from a fall. The fracture extends transversely across the distal humerus through the coronoid and olecranon fossae, above the level of the condyles. The distal fragment is angulated posteriorly, so that the anterior humeral line passes anterior to the capitellum. A posterior fat pad sign is almost always present. The fracture is usually complete, but greenstick fractures, torus fractures, or plastic bowing are possible. The typical treatment is closed reduction with casting.

CASE 2-3

Clinical History: 11-year-old boy in a mountain bike accident.

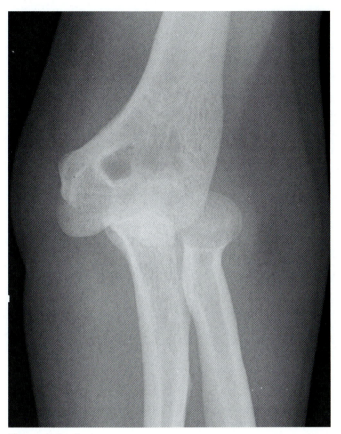

Figure 2-3 A

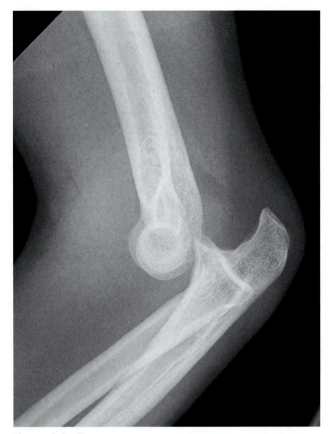

Figure 2-3 B

Findings: (A, B) AP and lateral radiographs of the elbow. Posterior dislocation of the elbow is present, without fractures.

Differential Diagnosis: None.

Diagnosis: Posterior elbow dislocation.

Discussion: The elbow is the most common site of dislocation in a skeletally immature patient, and the third most common site of dislocation in an adult (after shoulder and interphalangeal dislocations). Acute dislocations of the elbow result from falls or sports-related mishaps, with the forces transmitted to a hyperextended elbow. Typically, the ulna dislocates posteriorly relative to the humerus, taking the radius with it. There are frequently no associated fractures, although the coronoid process and radial head in an adult and medial epicondyle in a child should be scrutinized. In children, both the medial epicondyle and the median nerve can become entrapped, preventing a closed reduction. Although posterior elbow dislocations are the most common, dislocation in other directions may occur. There is a rare variant known as a divergent dislocation, in which the radius and ulna separate in different directions. Recurrent dislocations imply instability, usually attributed to rupture of the medial collateral ligaments, avulsion of the brachialis attachment, damage to the anterior capsule, or some combination. Complications associated with elbow dislocations include compromise of the brachial artery, damage to the median or ulnar nerves, and heterotopic ossification (most commonly in the brachialis muscle, anterior to the elbow).

Clinical History: 7-year-old boy with trauma.

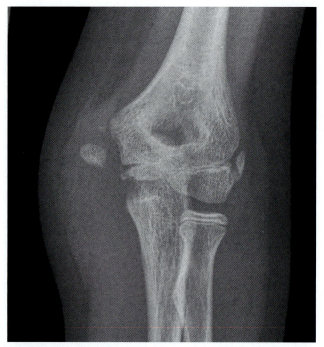

Figure 2-4 A

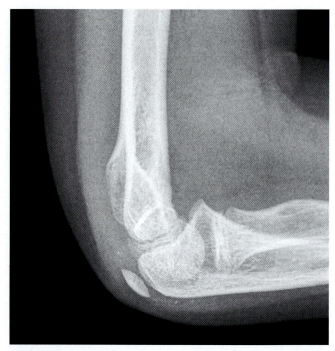

Figure 2-4 B

Findings: (A) AP elbow radiograph shows that the medial epicondyle has been avulsed from the distal humerus, with the fracture plane passing through the apophyseal plate. Soft tissue swelling is present at the site. (B) Lateral elbow radiograph does not show a fat pad sign.

Differential Diagnosis: None.

Diagnosis: Avulsion fracture, medial epicondyle (Salter type I).

Discussion: The medial epicondylar ossification center appears around the age of 5 years. It is the site of origin of the common tendon of the flexor pronator muscle group, and can be avulsed by muscular contraction. This often results in a fracture fragment that is displaced distally or anteriorly. Medial epicondylar injuries are usually seen in the 5-to-15-year age group; after the medial epicondyle fuses in late adolescence, this injury no longer occurs. Medial epicondylar injuries are far more common than lateral epicondyle injuries. An important association to recognize with medial epicondylar injury is damage to the ulnar nerve as it passes the elbow. Injury of the ulnar nerve may result in motor weakness of the flexor carpi ulnaris, flexor digitorum profundus muscle of the fourth and fifth fingers, and intrinsic hand muscles of the fourth and fifth digits, as well as sensory deficits of the fourth and fifth fingers.

Clinical History: 9-year-old boy with trauma.

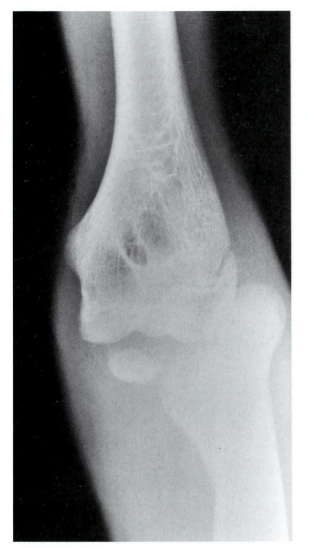

Figure 2-5   A

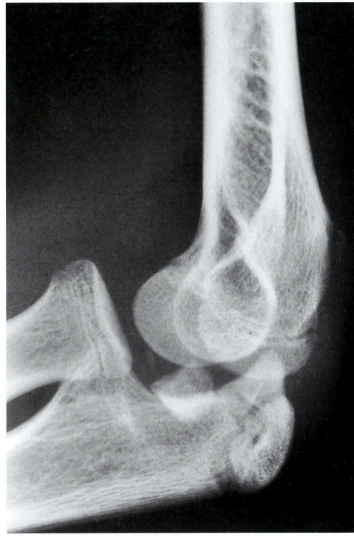

Figure 2-5   B

Findings: (**A, B**) AP and lateral elbow radiographs. The medial epicondyle has been avulsed from the distal humerus during posterior dislocation of the elbow. The fracture plane passes through the apophyseal plate, and the fragment has interposed itself between the trochlea and ulna, preventing reduction of the dislocation.

Differential Diagnosis: None.

Diagnosis: Avulsion fracture, medial epicondyle (Salter type I), with posterior elbow dislocation.

Discussion: Dislocation of the elbow may separate the medial epicondyle from the distal humerus by stress applied through the medial ulnar collateral ligament. The medial epicondylar fragment may then become entrapped in the elbow joint as it opens with valgus stress, requiring surgical reduction. For review, the order of ossification of the epiphyses and apophyses of the elbow can be remembered by the mnemonic CRITOE: Capitellum (less than 1 year), Radial head (5 years), Internal humeral epicondyle (7 years), Trochlea (10 years), Olecranon (10 years), and External humeral epicondyle (12 years). The age at which these centers begin to ossify is variable, but the order in which they close is generally not.

Clinical History: 57-year-old woman with pain at the lateral aspect of the elbow.

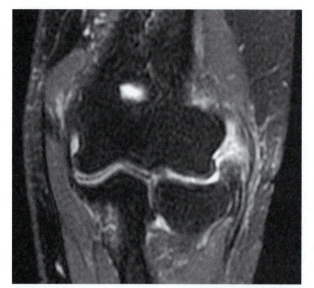

Figure 2-6   A

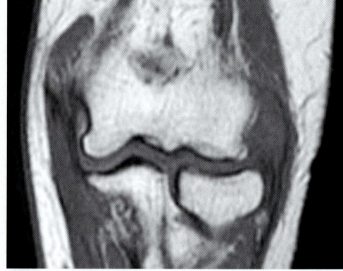

Figure 2-6   B

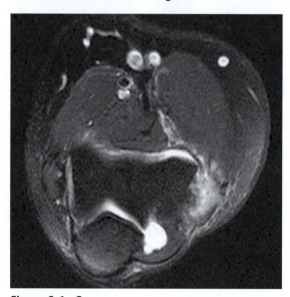

Figure 2-6   C

Findings: Coronal (A) and axial (C) T2-weighted fat-suppressed and coronal T1-weighted (B) images of the elbow show increased signal and thickening within the normally very low signal intensity common extensor tendon.

Differential Diagnosis: Common extensor tendon full-thickness tear, lateral epicondylitis.

Diagnosis: Lateral epicondylitis.

Discussion: Lateral epicondylitis presents as lateral elbow pain that has an insidious onset, beginning gradually after vigorous activity and progressing to pain with activity. Radiographs are frequently normal, although some patients may have evidence of a spur at the lateral epicondyle or calcification of the common extensor tendon. Magnetic Resonance Imaging (MRI) is useful in assessing the degree of tendon damage and associated ligament abnormality. Increased T1-weighted and T2-weighted signal is seen within the tendon with epicondylitis. The tendon is usually thickened, and edema can be present in the adjacent soft tissues. Using both the axial and coronal planes is helpful in assessing these lateral tendons. Additionally, MRI is useful in evaluating additional structures that may explain the lack of response to therapy (e.g., ligamentous injury) [1]. Ultrasonography may also be used to assess for epicondylitis, although it has been found to be less specific than MRI [2].

Clinical History: 21-year-old college baseball player with medial elbow pain.

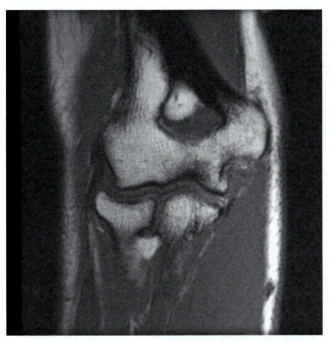

Figure 2-7 A

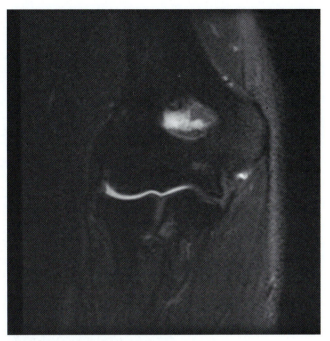

Figure 2-7 B

Findings: (A) Coronal T1-weighted MRI shows globular signal isointense to muscle at the expected humeral origin of the ulnar collateral ligament. The distal portion of the ligament may be seen as a dark, linear structure attaching to the ulna. The overlying common flexor tendon origin is intact at the medial epicondyle. (B) Coronal T2-weighted fat-suppressed MRI shows high signal where the ulnar collateral ligament is torn at its proximal origin.

Differential Diagnosis: Ulnar collateral ligament tear, medial epicondylitis.

Diagnosis: Ulnar collateral ligament tear.

Discussion: The ulnar collateral ligament (UCL, also called medial collateral ligament) originates from the inferior aspect of the medial epicondyle, deep to the common flexor tendon origin, and does not have an attachment to the adjacent medial condyle. The UCL has an important anterior band that inserts at the sublime tubercle at the medial aspect of the coronoid process, and a clinically less important posterior band that inserts along the supinator crest at the lateral aspect of the ulna. Tears of the UCL typically result from repetitive valgus stress, as may occur with pitching a baseball overhand, and may involve the proximal origin, the midsubstance, or the distal insertion. Avulsion fractures of the sublime tubercle may occur through the same mechanism. A tear of the UCL is a much more common injury than medial epicondylitis.

Clinical History: 45-year-old woman with elbow pain following a fall.

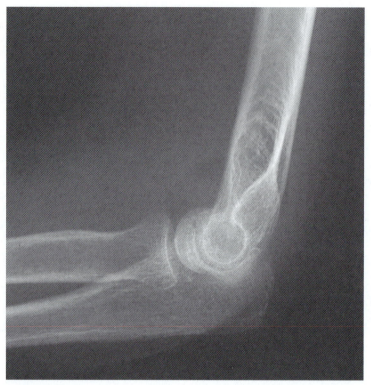

Figure 2-8   A

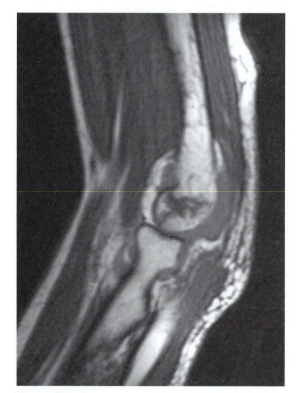

Figure 2-8   B

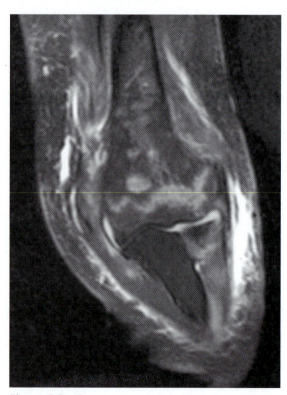

Figure 2-8   C

Findings: (A) Lateral radiograph of the elbow shows anterior and posterior fat pad signs. No fracture was visualized on the AP and oblique views. (B) Sagittal T1-weighted MRI shows a complex intraarticular fracture involving the capitellum. An effusion lifting up the posterior fat pad can be seen. (C) Coronal T2-weighted fat-saturated MRI shows a jagged fracture line traversing the distal humerus, from epicondyle to epicondyle.

Differential Diagnosis: None.

Diagnosis: Distal humerus fracture, radiographically occult.

Discussion: The value of the fat pad sign in identifying patients with elbow fractures has been proven time and again, but it is not perfect. In a recent study, 20 adult elbow trauma cases, with positive fat pad signs but no identified fractures, underwent MRI scans within 0 to 12 days [3]. The authors found that 75% of their patients had identifiable fractures, mostly involving the radial head, but they also noted that actual management was not changed by the additional information in any of the cases. The issues raised by studies like this have been discussed in an editorial by Rogers [4]. If the cost and convenience of MRI in the acute setting were the same as that of radiography, it would clearly be the diagnostic modality of choice, and although management might not change, the diagnostic certainty would have some value to patients and their families, physicians and other providers, insurance companies and other payors, and so forth. Thus, Rogers argues that cost and convenience are the true barriers to the better diagnosis of musculoskeletal trauma.

Clinical History: 33-year-old man with posterior elbow injury.

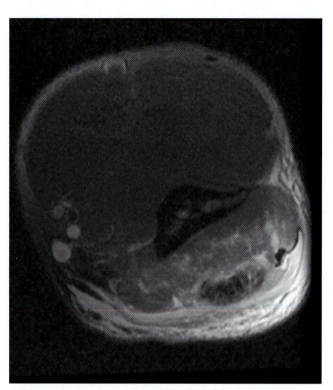

Figure 2-9 A

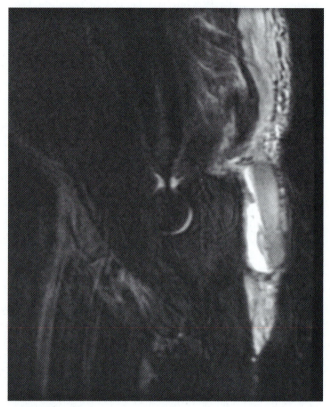

Figure 2-9 B

Findings: (A) Axial proton-density fat-suppressed MRI shows high signal in the triceps compartment, corresponding to edema and hemorrhage in and around the posterior aspect of the muscle. The triceps tendon is thickened and has high signal within it. (B) Sagittal T2-weighted fat-suppressed MRI shows retraction of the triceps tendon, and surrounding edema and hemorrhage. The muscular portion of the triceps insertion has some high signal, but is not detached. Hemorrhage also involves olecranon bursa, with a hematocrit effect.

Differential Diagnosis: None.

Diagnosis: Triceps tendon tear with olecranon bursa hemorrhage.

Discussion: Triceps tendon ruptures are uncommon injuries caused by decelerating counterforce during active extension of the elbow. These injuries are seen mostly in participants of sports that require upper body strength training. Although tears at the musculotendinous junction may occur, in most cases there is a catastrophic failure at the distal insertion. Distal triceps tears are frequently associated with avulsion fractures at the olecranon. On MRI, the detachment of the tendon can be seen directly, with proximal retraction that is best demonstrated on sagittal images. Surrounding hemorrhage and edema will be seen in acute injuries, but clinical diagnosis in the acute phase may be challenging, and many patients will not be imaged until the injuries are subacute or chronic. Treatment in most cases will be surgical repair.

Clinical History: Adult woman with deformity after a fall.

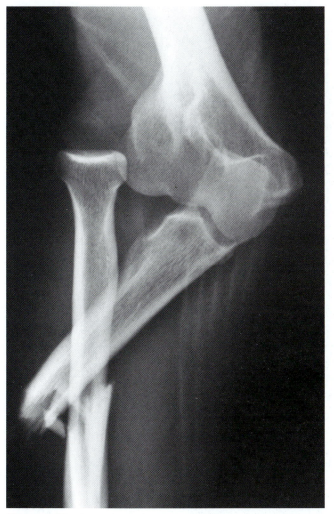

Figure 2-10   A

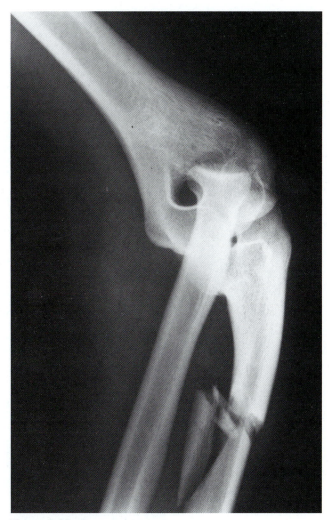

Figure 2-10   B

Findings: (A, B) AP and lateral radiographs of the elbow demonstrate dislocation of the radius and displaced fractures of the middiaphysis of the ulna.

Differential Diagnosis: None.

Diagnosis: Monteggia fracture-dislocation (Bado type III).

Discussion: A Monteggia fracture-dislocation [5] is composed of a fracture of the ulna and a dislocation of the radial head. Various types are based on the site of the fracture and the associated direction of angulation and dislocation (Bado classification). The types are as follows:

- (I) Proximal ulna fracture with anterior angulation and anterior dislocation of the radial head (65%).

- (II) Proximal ulna fracture with posterior angulation and posterior dislocation of the radial head (18%).
- (III) Ulna fracture just distal to coronoid process with lateral dislocation of the radial head (16%).
- (IV) Proximal ulna fracture and fracture of the proximal radius distal to the bicipital tuberosity with anterior dislocation of the radial head (1%).

This adult injury should be sought vigorously in anyone with a demonstrated ulna fracture. The radial head should intersect the capitellum on any view obtained. The radial nerve is damaged in 20% of cases, but most of these injuries are transient.

Clinical History: 2-year-old child refuses to move arm after a trip to the shopping mall.

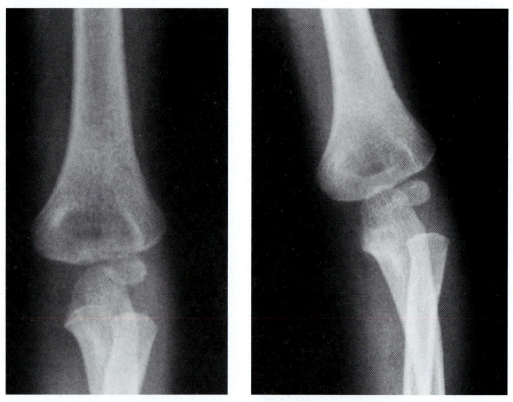

Figure 2-11   A   Figure 2-11   B

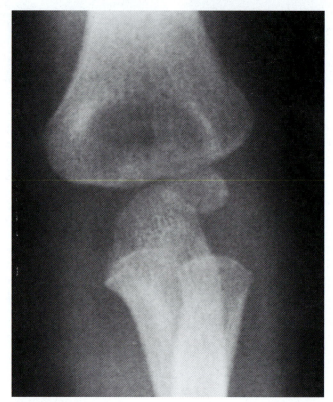

Figure 2-11   C

Findings: (A, B) AP and oblique radiographs of the left elbow demonstrate subtle subluxation of the radius with respect to the capitellum. A line drawn through the short segment of the radial shaft that is proximal to the radial tuberosity should intersect the center of the capitellum on all radiographic projections, but in this case it does not. (C) Photographic detail.

Differential Diagnosis: Subluxation of the radial head, dislocation of the radial head, normal.

Diagnosis: Subluxation of the radial head.

Discussion: Subluxation of the radial head (nursemaid's elbow, pulled elbow) is usually a temporary condition with spontaneous reduction. The usual history is a sudden pull on a forearm held in the pronated position, as might occur when a small child, who is being led by the hand by an adult, stumbles and falls. The adult will pull suddenly on the hand and forearm to prevent the child from striking the ground. The radial head slips under the lax annular ligament. Some authors state that the radiographs are normal, whereas other authors note that there may be subtle signs that indicate subluxation. If the radial head does not intersect the capitellum on all views, it is subluxated or dislocated [6]. The method of reduction involves a combination of flexion and supination (usually against an unhappy, resisting child). A palpable click is felt when the radial head relocates into its normal position. Offering a lollipop to the child and noting the ease of motion at the elbow joint can test the success of the maneuver. Occasionally, the annular ligament can become entrapped and prevent reduction [7]. The orthopedist will cast the child who fails to reduce or has a recurrent subluxation. Isolated radial head dislocation is a rare occurrence, limited to children. One is obligated to search for an associated fracture. Hereditary causes of radial head dislocation exist in, for example, the nail-patella syndrome, but are even more unusual than isolated dislocations. Injuries similar to pulled elbow have been described in adults [8,9].

Clinical History: 2-year-old boy with upper limb deformity since birth.

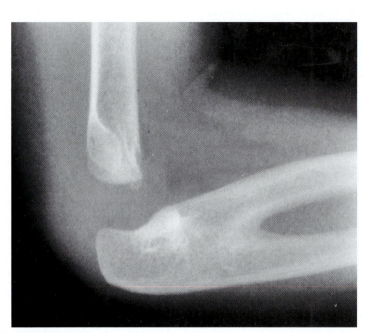

Figure 2-12 A

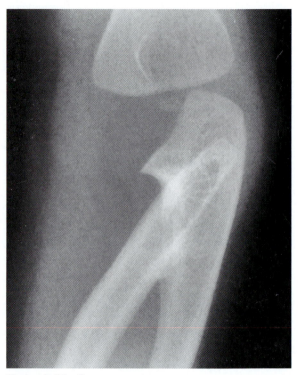

Figure 2-12 B

Findings: (A, B) Lateral and oblique radiographs of the elbow. There is abnormal fusion of the proximal radius and ulna, with continuity of medullary space and cortical margins.

Differential Diagnosis: None.

Diagnosis: Radioulnar synostosis.

Discussion: Two types of radioulnar synostosis have been described [10]. This is a case of "true" or proximal synostosis, where there is smooth fusion along a 2-cm to 6-cm length of the proximal radius and ulna. The other type is typified by congenital dislocation of the radial head. Both types result from a failure of longitudinal segmentation of the proximal forearm, leading to bony or fibrous synostosis. Both types of synostosis may be bilateral in 60% of cases. Sporadic and familial forms are described, but sporadic forms are more common [11]. Associated findings include clubfoot deformities, developmental dysplasia of the hip, thumb hypoplasia, Madelung's deformity, and other segmentation anomalies (including carpal coalition and symphalangism). Associated syndromes include arthrogryposis, multiple hereditary exostoses, and Holt-Oram syndrome, to mention a few. Acquired synostosis can result from trauma, osteomyelitis, or Caffey's disease. Before the osseous bridge is obvious, careful observation for the lateral radial bowing or ulnar tethering may help make an early diagnosis. Although some cases may be treated surgically, a longitudinal study of the natural history of congenital proximal radioulnar synostosis showed that most patients had few or no functional limitations, and were often employed in jobs that demanded extensive use of the forearm [12].

Clinical History: 48-year-old woman with abrupt onset of shoulder pain and weakness. No history of trauma. Symptoms and imaging findings resolved 6 months later.

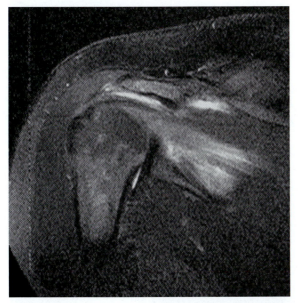

Figure 2-13   A

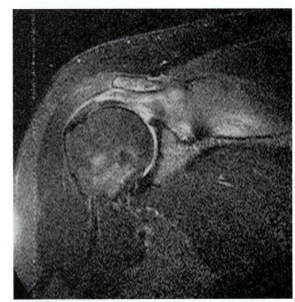

Figure 2-13   B

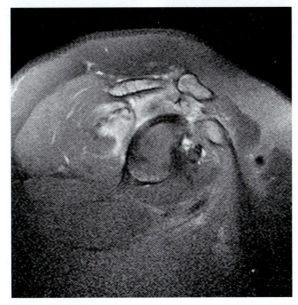

Figure 2-13   C

Findings: (A, B) Coronal oblique and (C) sagittal oblique T2-weighted fat-suppressed images demonstrate edema in the supraspinatus and infraspinatus muscles.

Differential Diagnosis: Parsonage-Turner syndrome, myositis, neuropathy, rotator cuff tear.

Diagnosis: Parsonage-Turner Syndrome.

Discussion: Parsonage-Turner syndrome, also known as acute brachial neuritis, refers to an idiopathic denervation of the shoulder [13]. This can be seen in patients ranging from infants to the elderly, and is more common in men. Up to half of patients had a viral illness or vaccination in the 2 weeks prior to symptom onset. On MRI, increased signal is seen within the shoulder musculature on T2-weighted and inversion recovery images [14]. Muscle enlargement can be present acutely. Muscle atrophy can occur in chronic cases. The muscle edema may or may not follow the nerve distribution, as individual nerves or nerve branches may be involved. The majority of cases resolve spontaneously within a year.

Clinical History: 5-year-old boy with elbow swelling.

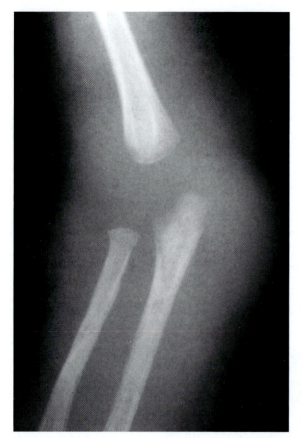

Figure 2-14 A

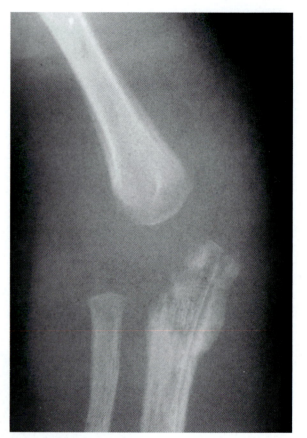

Figure 2-14 B

Findings: (A) Oblique elbow radiograph at presentation reveals soft tissue swelling about the olecranon. Faint periosteal reaction is noted about the proximal olecranon meta-diaphysis, and there is juxtaarticular osteoporosis at the elbow joint. (B) Oblique radiograph taken 4 months later demonstrates a marked increase in the periosteal reaction about the distal humerus and proximal ulna. Juxtaarticular osteoporosis is still present and is most marked in the proximal olecranon.

Differential Diagnosis: Septic Joint, juvenile chronic arthritis, trauma, Lyme arthritis.

Diagnosis: Septic elbow joint.

Discussion: The recovery of an organism from the joint is the only reliable method for distinguishing a septic elbow joint from an aseptic joint. Examples of conditions associated with aseptic or "reactive" arthritis include rheumatic fever, hepatitis, Reiter's syndrome, and some cases involving gonococcus. These immunologic entities commonly occur 2 to 3 weeks after the initial symptoms. Similarly, sterile synovitis can occur secondary to an inflammatory process in the adjacent bone or bursa. Potential sources of infection include the blood, adjacent bones or soft tissues, and direct penetration (accidental or iatrogenic). The classic radiologic sequence of events is as follows: joint effusion and soft tissue swelling (edema and hypertrophy of synovium, with leaky membranes), osteoporosis (hyperemia), joint space loss (chondral loss from inflamed pannus), marginal and central erosions (osseous destruction from inflamed pannus), sclerotic host bone formation (periostitis in this case), and late bony ankylosis (either fibrous or true osseous ankylosis). Bacterial septic arthritis is usually due to *S. aureus* or a streptococcus species. In children, *Haemophilus influenzae* is an important causative organism. Polyarticular involvement is usually secondary to encapsulated organisms such as pneumococcus or *H. influenzae*.

When septic arthritis is secondary to tuberculosis or fungi, then the radiographic findings differ in that there is little or no reparative bone, and the process is more indolent in nature. The hips and knees are more commonly involved than the wrist and elbow. Complications include synovial cyst formation, soft tissue and tendon injury (especially rotator cuff rupture in the shoulder) or abscesses, osteomyelitis, ankylosis, overgrowth of epiphyses from regional hyperemia (if physes are still open), and osteoarthritis.

Clinical History: 29-year-old burn victim with stiff elbow joint.

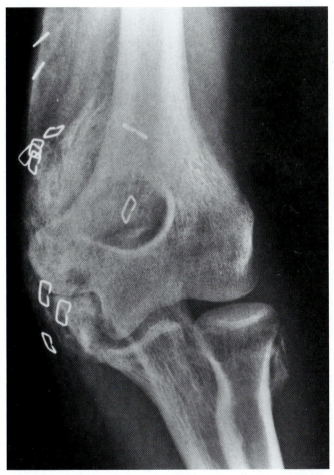

Figure 2-15 A

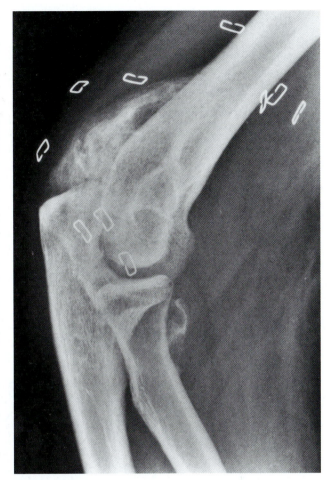

Figure 2-15 B

Findings: (A, B) AP and lateral elbow radiographs show extensive soft tissue ossification at the elbow, enveloping the elbow joint. Flexion and extension at the elbow joint are severely limited. The overlying surgical staples indicate sites of skin grafting.

Differential Diagnosis: Posttraumatic changes, thermal injury, collagen vascular disease.

Diagnosis: Heterotopic ossification after burns.

Discussion: Thermal burns cause coagulative tissue necrosis. The depth of the injury is related to the severity and duration of the applied heat. Initially, one can see soft tissue loss and soft tissue edema. Osteoporosis (30% of cases) may be localized or diffuse, and is explained on the basis of hyperemia, reflex sympathetic response, or alteration in local metabolism. Periostitis may also occur in the weeks that follow, and is thought to be secondary to a local periosteal irritation. Periarticular osseous excrescences, osteophytes, or soft tissue calcification or ossification (23% of cases) are common after extensive burns, and may be seen 2 to 3 months after injury [15,16]. They typically occur in adults along the preexisting connective tissue framework, most commonly around the elbow. The range of motion of involved joints will be limited mechanically. The exact pathogenesis of these ossifications is unknown and does not seem to correlate with the severity of the burn. The hyperemic response seen with burns can elicit bone growth. Contractures are most common about the elbow and within the hand. Articular abnormalities can be local or remote, and result from hyperemia, compression, infection, or thermal injury. Differential considerations of ankylosis from heterotopic ossification include posttraumatic [17], neurogenic, and other etiologies [18].

CASE 2-16

Clinical History: 70-year-old man with shoulder pain and weakness.

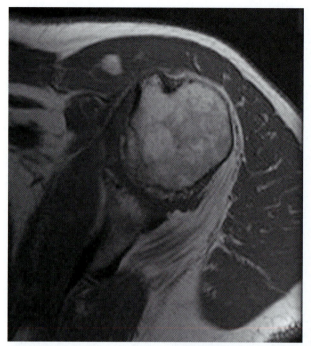

Figure 2-16 A

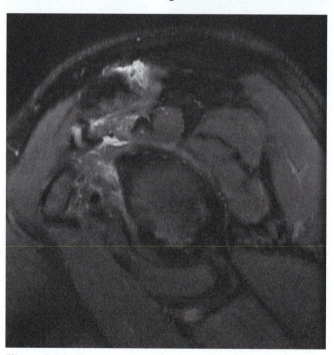

Figure 2-16 B

Figure 2-16 C

Findings: (A) Axial and (B) coronal oblique T1-weighted, and (C) sagittal oblique T2-weighted fat-suppressed MRI images demonstrate disproportionate fatty atrophy of the teres minor, without tendon tear.

Differential Diagnosis: Full-thickness teres minor tendon tear, quadrilateral space syndrome, Parsonage-Turner syndrome.

Diagnosis: Quadrilateral space syndrome.

Discussion: The teres minor muscle is innervated by a distal branch of the axillary nerve that passes posteriorly underneath the teres minor through a space that is also bounded by the teres major muscle (inferiorly), the humerus (laterally), and the long head of the triceps muscle (medially). The posterior humeral circumflex artery also passes through this so-called quadrilateral space [19]. Compression of the nerve within the quadrilateral space causes painful denervation and may lead to focal atrophy of the teres minor muscle. The deltoid muscle may be involved sometimes. Nerve compression is thought to result most often from post-traumatic fibrous bands [20]. On MRI, early changes include muscle edema and swelling. Chronic changes include muscle atrophy and fatty infiltration. Most patients are treated conservatively, but some require surgical decompression of the quadrilateral space [21].

Clinical History: 8-year-old little league pitcher with right elbow pain.

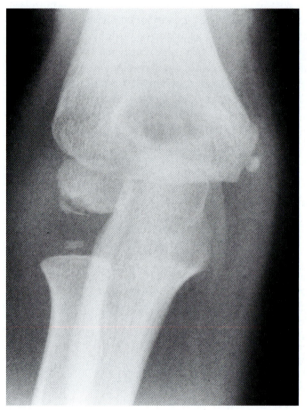

Figure 2-17   A

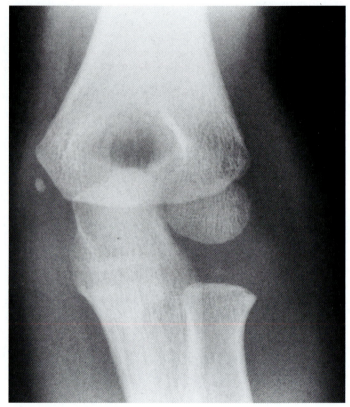

Figure 2-17   B

Findings: (A) AP radiograph of the right elbow (symptomatic). There is an irregular horizontal lucent defect through the ossification center of the capitellum. (B) Radiograph of the left elbow (asymptomatic) is normal.

Differential Diagnosis: Osteochondrosis of the capitellum, osteochondritis dissecans, acute trauma.

Diagnosis: Osteochondrosis of the capitellum.

Discussion: Osteochondrosis of the capitellum, or Panner's disease, is better known as "little leaguer's elbow." The condition is an osteochondrosis of the humeral capitellum that is seen principally in boys between the ages of 5 and 10 years. An osteochondrosis is a general term that has come to refer to the condition resulting from ischemia of a growing epiphysis. The capitellum is the rounded protuberance at the distal humerus that articulates with the proximal radius and is covered with articular cartilage. The blood supply enters from its posterior aspect and is vulnerable to traumatic disruption by indirect repetitive valgus stress or direct compression, sometimes leading to vascular compromise. Although most lesions revascularize and heal without consequence, deformity, bony resorption, or frank fragmentation of the capitellum may occur. Pain and stiffness may limit full extension of the elbow, and a commonly associated clinical finding is joint swelling from effusion and/or synovial hypertrophy. Radiographic findings at the capitellum include the crescentic fissure through the ossification center (as noted in this case), increased density, decreased size, resorption, or frank fragmentation. Hyperemia may lead to premature maturation of the radial head. Unilateral involvement is noted in the throwing arm of little league baseball players, and the condition has also been noted in gymnasts. The main differential consideration is osteochondritis dissecans, a traumatic osteochondral injury seen in an older age group, after the capitellum has essentially stopped growing. Computed tomography (CT) or MRI may be helpful when there is a question of fragmentation.

Clinical History: 74-year-old man with shoulder pain.

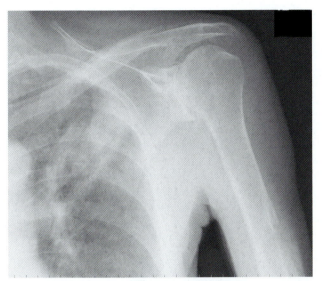

Figure 2-18   A

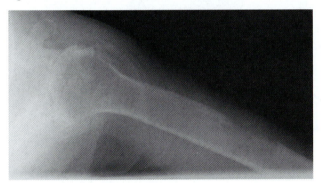

Figure 2-18   B

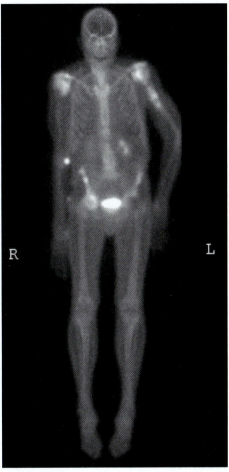

Figure 2-18   C

Findings: (A) AP and (B) axillary radiographs of the left shoulder show a large mass in the left lung apex, and a lytic lesion in the mid humeral shaft. The humeral lesion is centered in the cortex and has provoked little, if any, reactive bone formation. Incidental degenerative changes at the glenohumeral joint are advanced. (C) Radionuclide bone scan demonstrates abnormal radiotracer uptake within the midshaft of the left humerus, right iliac crest, and right acetabulum, which is suspicious for bone metastasis. Increased uptake within the shoulder joints is related to osteoarthritis.

Differential Diagnosis: Metastases, myeloma, lymphoma.

Diagnosis: Metastatic disease from lung carcinoma.

Discussion: Pathologic fractures through bones involved by metastases are common. The most common sites of pathologic fracture are the vertebral bodies, ribs, proximal femur, and proximal humerus. Metastases of lytic, blastic, and mixed radiographic appearance all cause weakening of the bone.

In the long bones, destructive lesions with full-thickness cortical penetration lead to pathologic fractures. Gaps in the cortex weaken the bone by causing uneven and aberrant distribution of the stresses of loading, impeding the normal biomechanical dispersion of force. Weakening is gradual as cortical bone is infiltrated, eroded, and destroyed. Blastic lesions also destroy cortex, and the reactive and the stromal bone that gives blastic lesions their radiodensity is structurally unsound. The bone may fracture under the stresses of normal activity. Cortical weakening makes bone most vulnerable to tensile forces; therefore, in the long bones, pathologic fractures are usually transverse. The onset of pain at a site of metastatic involvement may indicate the presence of microfractures in a weakened cortex. Median survival after discovery of a pathologic fracture through an osseous metastasis is only about 18 months (combined for all primary sites).

Clinical History: 10-year-old girl with left arm pain.

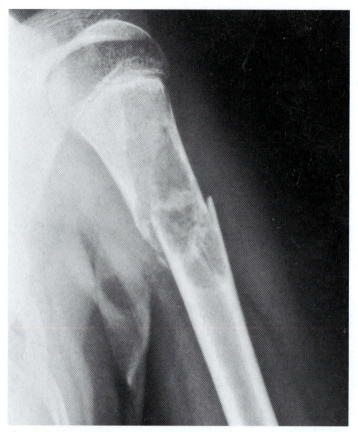

Figure 2-19

Findings: AP radiograph of the humerus. There is a pathologic fracture through a lucent lesion in the metadiaphysis of the humerus. The lesion has a faintly sclerotic border and is centrally located.

Differential Diagnosis: Simple bone cyst, aneurysmal bone cyst, fibrous dysplasia.

Diagnosis: Simple bone cyst, with pathologic fracture.

Discussion: The pathogenesis of a simple bone cyst is not known; the most favored theory is that it results from venous obstruction. Boys are affected more than twice as frequently as girls. Cysts are typically noted in the metaphysis of long bones before the age of 20, and in the pelvis or calcaneus thereafter. Eighty-five percent of humeral or femoral cysts are noted in the proximal metaphysis. Diaphyseal involvement is identified in 4% to 12% of the long bone lesions. Although some authors consider the diaphyseal lesions to be latent, having grown away from the growth plate, an age of less than 10 years is more predictive of a higher recurrence rate (i.e., activity) than is location within bone. Other poor prognostic factors include large size and large numbers of loculations [22]. Simple bone cysts tend to be geographic lucent lesions with a central location, mild cortical thinning, and gentle expansion. In addition, the lesion tends to elongate along the long axis of the bone. CT or MRI may show fluid-fluid levels, septations not seen on radiography, soft tissue changes, and nodular enhancement [23]. A fallen-fragment sign is diagnostic of this entity, but it is reported in only 20% of patients who present with pathologic fractures, and only in those with open physes [24]. The fallen fragment results from a pathologic fracture of the cyst wall, with displacement of a fragment into the cyst itself. Change of position of the fragment within the lesion to the dependent portion indicates that the cyst is fluid-filled rather than solid. A variant of the fallen fragment is the trap-door fragment, in which a periosteal hinge keeps the fragment from falling dependently, but allows it to change position with the patient. Traumatic transformation to aneurysmal bone cyst has been reported [25]. Differential diagnostic considerations in the metaphysis include enchondroma, fibrous lesions, and aneurysmal bone cyst. In the diaphysis, the appearance can be similar to fibrous dysplasia, eosinophilic granuloma, and chondromyxoid fibroma. In the calcaneus, intraosseous lipoma or pseudocyst from rarefied trabeculae should be considered. Complications of simple bone cysts are related to fractures and resultant deformities and/or growth disturbances. Bone cysts have no malignant potential.

CASE 2-20

Clinical History: 12-year-old boy with right arm weakness.

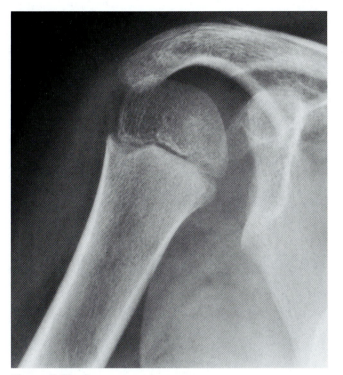

Figure 2-20   A

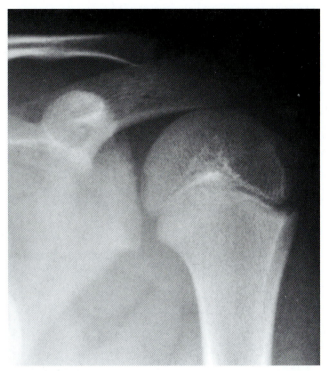

Figure 2-20   B

Findings: (A) AP radiograph of the right shoulder. Hypoplasia and underdevelopment of the humeral head are noted. The concavity of the glenoid is larger than expected. The humeral head is high riding. (B) AP radiograph of the left shoulder. The left shoulder is normal.

Differential Diagnosis: None.

Diagnosis: Brachial plexus palsy (Erb's palsy).

Discussion: Two common forms of obstetrical trauma—clavicle fracture and Erb's palsy—both result in refusal of a newborn to move his arm. Erb's palsy is the result of excessive trauma on the arm, resulting in damage to the C-5 and C-6 roots. A less common injury is Klumpke's paralysis, which results from damage to the C-7, C-8, and T-1 nerve roots. Spontaneous, complete recovery is noted in 90% of cases, representing instances of reversible stretch injury to the nerve roots. Those that completely avulse eventually result in hypoplasia and elevation of the scapula, underdevelopment of the glenoid, and an abnormal coracoid and acromion. Additionally, there is underdevelopment of the remainder of the extremity, including the osseous and soft tissue elements. CT measurements of the amount of humeral torsion (comparable to measurements for tibial torsion) can be undertaken in surgical planning for tendon transfer procedures. Similar to clavicular fractures, brachial plexus palsy in the newborn [26,27,28] may be the result of difficulties during delivery, particularly in infants with shoulder dystocia and macrosomia [29]. Clavicular fractures, however, are a far more common complication, with an incidence of about 2% compared to a mere 0.4% incidence of Erb's palsy. Similar conditions also appear to occur through another mechanism, possibly in utero. The prognosis when no predisposing factor can be identified is worse, with a lengthy recovery time in those cases in which resolution occurred, and a greater proportion with permanent palsy.

Clinical History: 48-year-old man with chronic renal failure, and two companion cases.

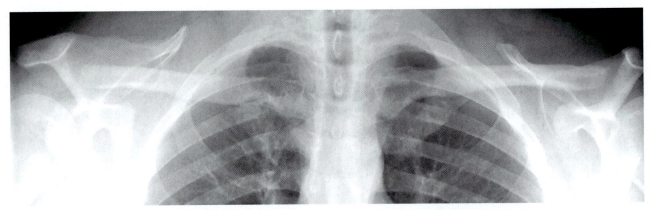

Figure 2-21 A

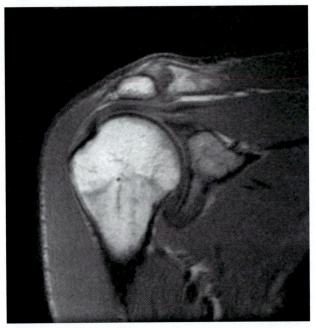

Figure 2-21 B

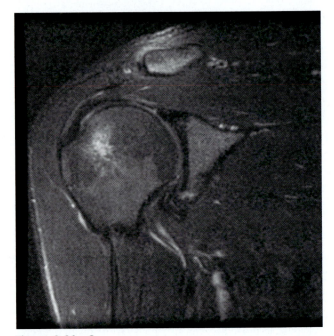

Figure 2-21 C

Findings: (A) AP view of the clavicles demonstrates widening of the acromioclavicular joints, with bony resorption of the distal clavicles. (B) First companion case. Oblique coronal T1-weighted MRI shows bony loss at the distal clavicle and capsular hypertrophy. (C) Second companion case. Oblique coronal T2-weighted MRI with fat saturation shows increased T2 signal in the distal clavicle and surrounding soft tissues.

Differential Diagnosis: Osteolysis of the distal clavicle, acromioclavicular joint separation, acromioclavicular arthritis.

Diagnosis: Osteolysis of the distal clavicle.

Discussion: Osteolysis of the distal clavicle refers to subchondral bony resorption of the distal clavicle. Originally described following direct shoulder trauma, this condition has many etiologies besides posttraumatic, including overuse or repetitive stress (especially weight-lifters), metabolic (hyperparathyroidism), inflammatory (rheumatoid arthritis, infection), collagen vascular disorders, multiple myeloma, and massive essential osteolysis [30]. Radiographs can be normal early in the clinical course. Later changes include irregularity and osteopenia of the distal clavicles, and widening of the acromioclavicular joints. MRI can demonstrate the bone loss and increased T2-weighted signal in the distal clavicle. However, the increased T2 signal is a nonspecific and relatively frequent finding in asymptomatic patients as well [31].

CASE 2-22

Clinical History: 16-year-old boy with shoulder swelling and pain.

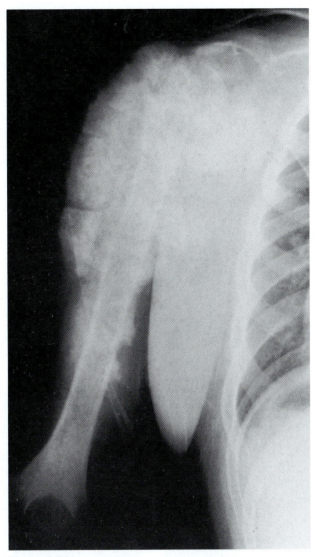

Figure 2-22

Findings: AP radiograph of the humerus. There is a dense, cloud-like lesion centered in the medullary cavity. Involvement of the proximal metaphysis and diaphysis is noted.

Differential Diagnosis: Osteosarcoma, Ewing's sarcoma, lymphoma.

Diagnosis: Osteosarcoma.

Discussion: This is an excellent example of a conventional, high-grade intramedullary osteosarcoma. It is seen most commonly in patients between the ages of 10 and 25. The lesion tends to be permeative, with a wide zone of transition. Ninety percent of the lesions will have some mineralized matrix, which was quite dense in this case, extending into the associated soft tissue mass. This is the third most common location, ranking behind the distal femur and proximal tibia. Osteosarcomas in 50% of cases are osteoblastic on histology,

25% of cases are chondroblastic, and 25% of cases are fibroblastic. It may be difficult radiographically to determine if the increased density seen is truly tumor matrix or elicited periosteal reaction (as in Ewing's sarcoma). Periosteal reaction is a common host bone response, seen in this case inferiorly and medially with a classic Codman's triangle. Osteosarcoma in 90% of cases is monostotic, but up to 10% may have skip metastases, commonly in the same bone. Both radionuclide bone scan and MRI can be used to screen for these metastases. Approximately 10% to 20% of osteosarcoma patients have metastases to lung or bone at presentation. The prognosis of those patients with osseous metastasis is very poor. Relapses typically occur in the first 2 years after initiation of treatment. Treatment of osteosarcoma is usually chemotherapy and en bloc resection of the tumor with prosthetic or allograft reconstruction.

Clinical History: 86-year-old man with right shoulder pain.

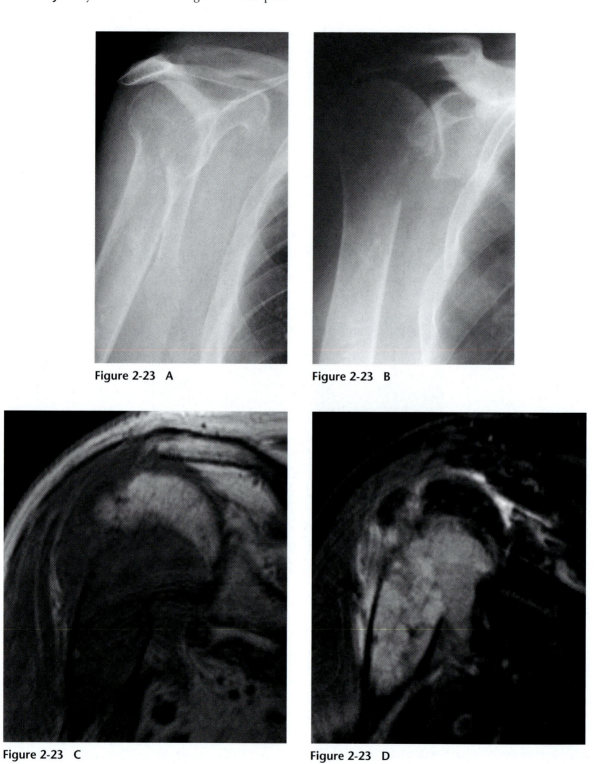

Figure 2-23 A

Figure 2-23 B

Figure 2-23 C

Figure 2-23 D

Findings: (A) Magnified portion of posteroanterior (PA) chest radiograph 6 years prior to presentation shows a chondroid matrix lesion in the proximal humerus. (B) AP shoulder radiograph shows destruction of the medial aspect of the humeral neck, and calcifications with a rings-and-arcs configuration. (C, D) Coronal oblique T1-weighted and T2-weighted fat-suppressed MRI shows a heterogeneous mass involving the entire medullary space, eroding through the medial bone cortex and extending into the shoulder joint.

Differential Diagnosis: Chondrosarcoma, metastasis, lymphoma, malignant fibrous histiocytoma.

Diagnosis: Chondrosarcoma.

Discussion: In this case, the patient had what appeared to be either an enchondroma or low-grade chondrosarcoma for many years prior to presentation. Malignant transformation of an enchondroma into a chondrosarcoma is rare. Pain is the most suggestive symptom for chondrosarcoma in a lesion with cartilaginous calcification. Typical worrisome radiographic features of chondrosarcoma include prominent endosteal scalloping, any degree of cortical thickening or cortical destruction, or an area of lucency in an otherwise mineralized lesion. Associated soft tissue masses are noted more commonly in the flat bones or peripheral lesions. Sixty to seventy percent of the time the tumor contains punctate or flocculent calcification, and ring-shaped ossification characteristic of cartilage tissue. The lucent appearance is due to replacement of normal bone by noncalcified cartilage. On CT, the nonmineralized regions have a myxoid appearance, with attenuation in the range of 10 to 30 Hounsfield units; a high proportion of myxoid material is correlated with a higher histologic grade. On MRI, these regions have very high signal intensity on T2-weighted images, and variable signal on T1-weighted images. A lobular growth pattern is often evident on CT or MRI, and is characteristic of this entity. The bone scan will show increased tracer accumulation. The treatment of chondrosarcoma is surgical. The incidence of metastasis and the prognosis is related to the histologic grade, with 10-year survival ranging from 85% for low-grade lesions to 28% for high-grade lesions. Recurrent lesions will be of a higher grade 10% of the time.

Clinical History: 11-year-old boy with shoulder pain and swelling.

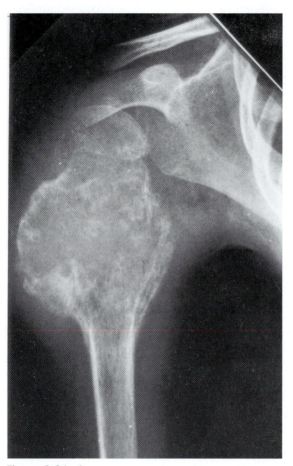

Figure 2-24 A

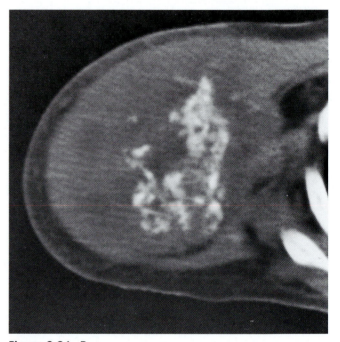

Figure 2-24 B

Findings: (A) AP radiograph of the right shoulder shows an expansile, destructive lesion in the proximal humerus with cortical penetration (blow out). Focal regions of sclerosis are present. The lesion does not appear to cross the growth plate. (B) CT at the level of the central portion of the lesion shows the circumferential cortical penetration and soft tissue extension, with neoplastic and reactive ossification.

Differential Diagnosis: Osteosarcoma, Ewing's sarcoma, lymphoma, aneurysmal bone cyst, giant cell tumor, angiosarcoma.

Diagnosis: Telangiectatic osteosarcoma.

Discussion: Telangiectatic osteosarcomas represent approximately 4% of all osteosarcomas, and display the distinctive pathologic feature of cystic areas filled with hemorrhage in various stages of evolution. They are lined by giant cells and tumor cells, not endothelial cells that would be typical of an aneurysmal bone cyst. The amount of osteoid is quite small. The lesions are destructive and lytic, with large extraosseous masses incompletely surrounded by thin shells of bone [32]. Approximately 25% to 30% of cases have a pathologic fracture at presentation. They grow rapidly and elicit relatively little bone reaction; therefore, their appearance is very similar to that of an aneurysmal bone cyst, giant cell tumor, or angiosarcoma. Fluid levels may be demonstrated on CT or MRI. The distribution of telangiectatic osteosarcoma is similar to that of conventional osteosarcomas. Most arise in the metaphysis; 10% arise in the diaphysis. The femur is involved most frequently, followed by the tibia and humerus. The prognosis is generally considered poorer than that of conventional osteosarcoma, but this has been debated in the recent literature.

Clinical History: 13-year-old girl with shoulder pain and swelling.

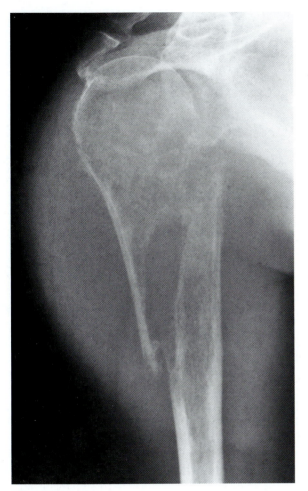 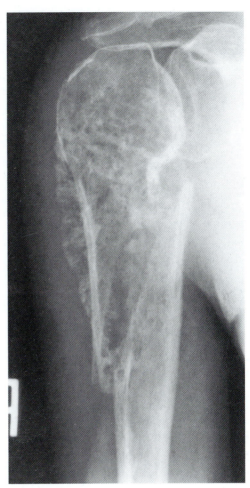

Figure 2-25 A   **Figure 2-25 B**

Findings: (A) AP radiograph of the shoulder at presentation shows an oblique pathologic fracture through the proximal humerus. Marked soft tissue swelling is seen around the shoulder, and the humerus itself is osteopenic. (B) Follow-up examination 2 months after the completion of radiotherapy shows marked diminution in the size of the soft tissue mass, with periosteal bone formation and healing of the fracture.

Differential Diagnosis: Ewing's sarcoma or other round cell malignancy, lymphoma, eosinophilic granuloma, metastasis, infection.

Diagnosis: Ewing's sarcoma.

Discussion: Ewing's sarcoma belongs to the category of small round cell tumors. It is commonly seen before the age of 20, and presents with pain. One-third of patients will present with symptoms simulating infection, including fever, elevated white count, and elevated erythrocyte sedimentation rate. It commonly presents in the femoral metadiaphysis or flat bones as an osteolytic or permeative lesion, with an associated soft tissue mass and periosteal reaction. Sclerotic reactive bone may be present at the periphery, but there is no tumor matrix. Lack of any reactive bone in the soft tissue mass distinguishes this entity from osteosarcoma. The distinguishing pathologic features include a positive stain for glycogen and negative stain for reticulin. In lymphoma, hepatosplenomegaly and mixed osteolytic and osteosclerotic features are identified; additionally, the reticulin stain is positive and the glycogen stain is negative. Metastatic neuroblastoma tends to have larger osteolytic lesions, lacks associated soft tissue masses, and demonstrates an adrenal lesion. Rhabdomyosarcoma usually presents with a complaint of swelling rather than pain. Invasion of the bone is secondary or metastatic. Langerhans cell histiocytosis and infection can be excluded by clinical examination, laboratory test, and possibly MRI. Primitive neuroectodermal tumors differ histologically, but usually not radiologically. Approximately 15% to 30% of Ewing's sarcoma cases have lung and osseous metastases at presentation. Local recurrences occur in 12% to 25% of cases. Treatment consists of radiation therapy, sometimes combined with chemotherapy and surgery.

Clinical History: 19-year-old man with left shoulder pain.

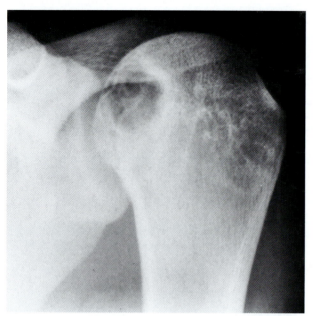

Figure 2-26 A

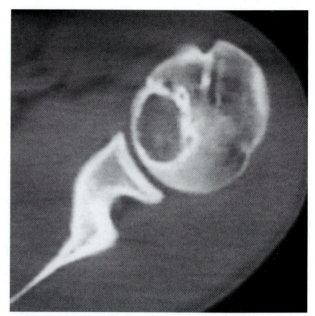

Figure 2-26 B

Findings: (A) AP radiograph of the shoulder shows a lucent lesion with a thin but dense sclerotic margin in the humeral epiphysis, extending into the metaphysis. (B) CT scan of the proximal humerus. The lesion is round in shape and has a well-defined sclerotic margin. Faint matrix mineralization is noted in the lesion.

Differential Diagnosis: Chondroblastoma, Brodie's abscess, eosinophilic granuloma.

Diagnosis: Chondroblastoma.

Discussion: Chondroblastoma (Codman's tumor) is an uncommon benign neoplasm that consists of chondroid tissue mixed with more cellular tissue. Location in the epiphysis or apophysis is characteristic (about 98%), often with extension into the metaphysis. Two-thirds arise in the lower extremities, and half around the knee. Most patients are young: 80% are between 5 and 25 years old. Males are affected twice as often as females. When chondroblastomas occur outside the usual age group, they arise in unusual locations. The presentation is nonspecific, typically consisting of pain. Articular symptoms are commonly encountered, and sterile effusions are noted in up to one-third of cases. The radiographic appearance is an ovoid or rounded lucent epiphyseal lesion that is eccentrically or centrally located. The margins are geographic, usually with a thin, reactive bony rim. Scattered mottled or stippled calcifications, like those of other cartilage tumors, may be present. Extension can occur into the subarticular bone or metaphysis (25% to 50% of cases). Calcification can occur in up to half of the cases, but is commonly subtle enough to require CT for documentation. The associated metaphyseal periostitis seen in up to 50% of cases distinguishes it from the other etiologies of epiphyseal lucent lesions. Cystic or hemorrhagic components are recognized and may be prominent enough to suggest the alternate diagnoses of simple bone cysts or aneurysmal bone cysts (but the location of the lesion should redirect one toward the correct diagnosis). Chondroblastomas treated by curettage usually do not recur, but some are aggressive locally.

The classic differential of an epiphyseal lucent lesion is that of chondroblastoma and a Brodie's abscess. Epiphyseal eosinophilic granuloma is a rare enough entity to be excluded from a general differential. Giant cell tumors can also extend into the epiphysis and contain giant cells, but are distinguished from chondroblastomas by their lack of a sclerotic border. After physeal closure, other differential considerations would include enchondroma, osteoblastoma, and clear cell chondrosarcoma.

Clinical History: 24-year-old man with painless swelling in the right shoulder.

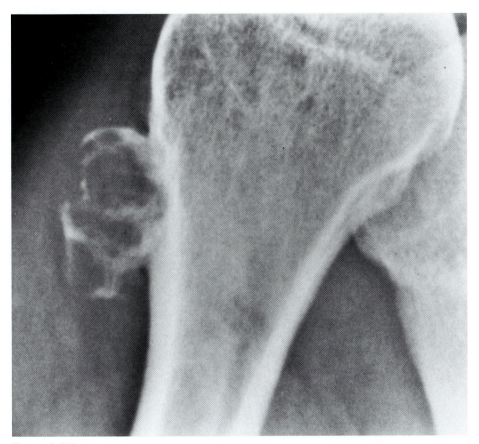

Figure 2-27

Findings: Fluoroscopically positioned radiograph of the proximal humerus. There is a lesion projecting from the cortical surface of the humerus into the soft tissues. The lesion is predominantly lucent, with a lobulated morphology. A well-defined sclerotic rim is present, merging with the underlying cortex. The endosteal surface of the cortex is not affected, and there is no intramedullary component.

Differential Diagnosis: Juxtacortical (periosteal) chondroma, chondrosarcoma, osteochondroma, surface osteosarcoma, posttraumatic deformity, aneurysmal bone cyst.

Diagnosis: Juxtacortical chondroma.

Discussion: Juxtacortical (periosteal) chondroma is a benign, cortically based cartilage lesion that is similar to an enchondroma except for its location on the surface of bone [33]. The lesions consist of mature cartilage, and they are covered with periosteum. On pathologic examination, juxtacortical chondroma can be more cellular than enchondroma and contain double-nucleated chondrocytes, which can lead to a diagnosis of a low-grade chondrosarcoma if the findings are not correlated with the benign radiologic appearance [34]. Most lesions are found in adolescents or young adults, with a male predominance [35]. The most common

sites are the proximal humerus and femur, with two-thirds of lesions involving the metaphysis and the remainder involving the diaphysis. The presenting symptom is usually pain and/or swelling, but many juxtacortical chondromas are discovered incidentally on radiographs obtained for other reasons. The radiographic appearance of a calcified soft tissue mass eroding the associated cortex is classic. Solid periosteal bone formation at the margins of the lesion may produce buttresses and form a cup-like appearance. Calcification of matrix is seen in only one-half of cases and, therefore, need not be present for the diagnosis. Markedly elongated lesions with irregular cortical thickening are not atypical. Reactive medullary sclerosis and periostitis can be identified, and do not necessarily imply malignant degeneration or pathologic fracture; these features are probably a response to the peripheral vascularity. MRI is useful to show the lobulated morphology and T2 hyperintensity that is characteristic of chondroid lesions. Strictly speaking, the juxtacortical chondroma should be a well-defined lesion confined to the cortex, with a maximal diameter that does not exceed 4 cm. Medullary involvement, cortical destruction, and an associated soft tissue mass are features suggestive of chondrosarcoma. Treatment is surgical, and lesions should not recur.

Clinical History: 11-year-old boy with lumpy arm.

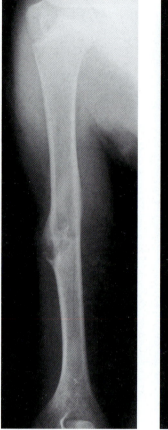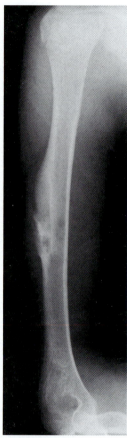

Figure 2-28   A   Figure 2-28   B

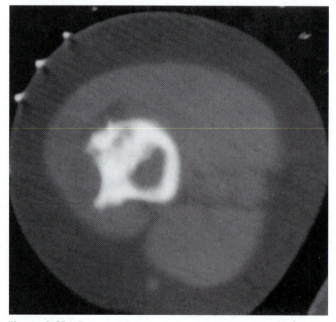

Figure 2-28   C

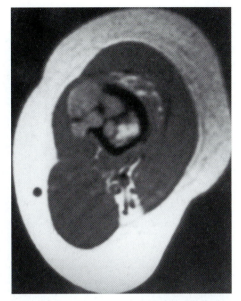

Figure 2-28 D

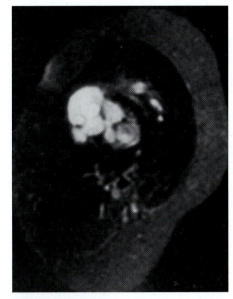

Figure 2-28 E

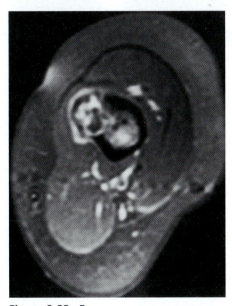

Figure 2-28 F

Findings: (A, B) AP and lateral radiographs demonstrate a cortically based lesion at the humeral diaphysis. The lesion involves the posterolateral cortex and is characterized by lobulated lucency surrounded by thickened cortex. (C) Axial CT image shows the marked cortical thickening associated with the sessile, cortically based lesion. A lower-density soft tissue component surrounds the thickened cortex. (D, E) Axial T1-weighted and axial T2-weighted MRI shows T1 hypointensity and T2 hyperintensity within the lobules of the lesion. The bulk of the lesion is on the cortical surface, but a portion of it projects into the medullary space. (F) Axial T1-weighted MRI obtained after gadolinium injection shows enhancement of portions of the lesion.

Differential Diagnosis: Juxtacortical (periosteal) chondroma, chondrosarcoma, osteochondroma, surface osteosarcoma, posttraumatic deformity, aneurysmal bone cyst.

Diagnosis: Juxtacortical chondroma.

Discussion: The lobulated morphology of the lesion suggests cartilage, a possibility supported by the imaging characteristics (low density on CT, high signal intensity on T2-weighted MRI). The lack of aggressive features and bone destruction suggests an indolent, benign lesion. Location in the cortex, as opposed to the medullary space, should lead one to the correct diagnosis. The solid, heaped-up periosteal reactive bone surrounding the lobules of cartilage is characteristic of this entity.

Clinical History: 87-year-old man with an enlarging shoulder mass.

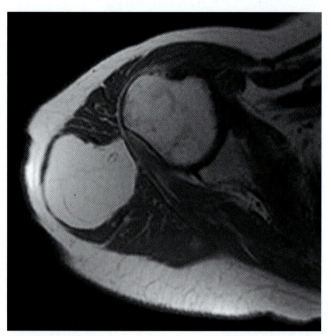

Figure 2-29 A

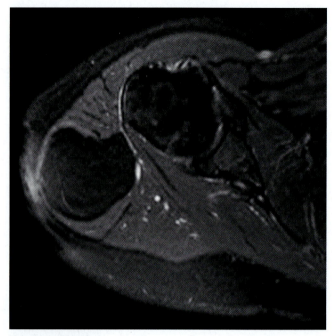

Figure 2-29 B

Findings: Axial T1-weighted (**A**) and T2-weighted fat-suppressed (**B**) MRI of the shoulder demonstrates a well-defined rounded mass within the deltoid muscle. The mass follows the signal intensity of subcutaneous fat on both imaging sequences. Thin septa traverse the lesion, but it is otherwise homogeneous.

Differential Diagnosis: None.

Diagnosis: Intramuscular lipoma.

Discussion: Lipomas are a very common, benign tumor of mesenchymal origin that are most frequent in the subcutaneous soft tissues of the extremities in women. They are usually painless, freely moveable soft tissue masses that can be distorted easily by mild pressure. Painful lipomas are known by the eponym "*lipoma dolorosa*," and are characterized by a migratory pain syndrome associated with multiple lipomas.

The general classification is by site (subcutaneous or deep). Deep lipomas within a limited fascial compartment can sometimes be hard on physical examination due to local infiltration and distention of the compartment. Subcutaneous lipomas may be indistinguishable from the native fat on imaging [36].

Both osseous and cartilaginous elements can be seen radiographically and pathologically in benign lipomas, but increase the likelihood that the lesion is actually a liposarcoma. A Hounsfield unit measurement with negative value is diagnostic of a fatty constituent. On MRI, T1-weighted hyperintensity and fat-suppressed sequence hypointensity are suggestive, but they can also be seen with the presence of intracellular methemoglobin. An uncomplicated lipoma should not enhance on CT or MRI and appears avascular at angiography. Periosteal and synovial lipomas are uncommon. Within the joint, a discrete round or oval fat-containing lesion is noted, and should be distinguished from lipoma arborescens, a form of synovial metaplasia seen in osteoarthritis, rheumatoid arthritis, or after trauma. Treatment is surgical resection.

Clinical History: 75-year-old man with injury sustained while pulling cactus out of his yard.

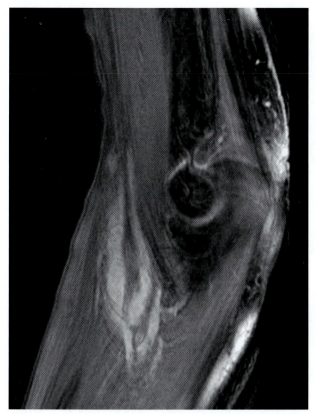

Figure 2-30 A

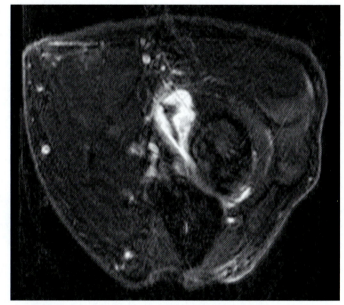

Figure 2-30 B

Findings: (A) Sagittal T2-weighted fat-suppressed MRI shows a proximally retracted biceps tendon, surrounded by fluid. (B) Axial inversion recovery MRI shows the abnormal biceps tendon surrounded by high-signal fluid.

Differential Diagnosis: High-grade partial-thickness or full-thickness tear of the biceps tendon.

Diagnosis: Complete rupture of the biceps tendon.

Discussion: Biceps tendon tears occur during flexion against strong resistance. These are most commonly seen in the dominant arm of middle-aged males who smoke tobacco [37]. The complete tear typically occurs at its insertion at the bicipital tuberosity of the proximal radius. In complete tears, proximal retraction of the tendon by muscle action results in a mass or bulbous swelling of the proximal arm; swelling at the distal arm may be minimal because of the tense antecubital fascia. Degenerative thickening of the biceps tendon may be present. MRI of complete biceps tendon ruptures will always show the absence of the tendon distally, and nearly always shows a fluid-filled tendon sheath. Less common findings include an antecubital fossa mass, muscle edema, and atrophy [38]. Partial tears show high signal intensity within the tendon, fluid in the biceps tendon sheath, and thinning or thickening of the distal tendon, but the tendon will remain in continuity with its insertion. Biceps tendon ruptures are treated surgically, but some loss of function, particularly with activities requiring repetitive supination, is common [39].

Clinical History: 45-year-old woman with progressive difficulty in rotating her shoulder after an injury. She had previously undergone surgical repair of her rotator cuff.

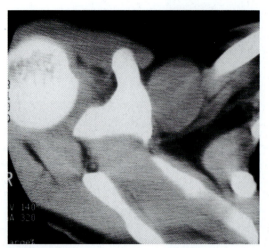

Figure 2-31   A

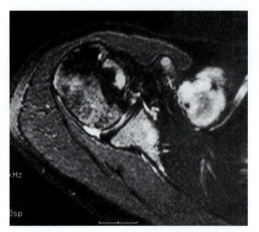

Figure 2-31   B

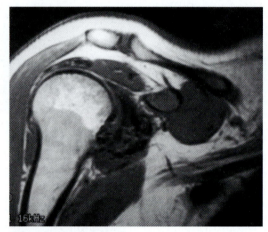

Figure 2-31   C

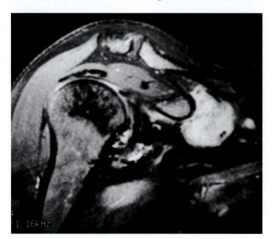

Figure 2-31   D

Findings: (A) Axial CT scan (soft tissue windows) shows a globular 3-cm mass, isodense to muscle, in the infraclavicular region, medial to the coracoid process. The lesion is not calcified. (B) Axial T2-weighted MRI demonstrates the rounded lesion located medial to the coracoid process and inferior to the clavicle. The lesion has high signal intensity. (C, D) Coronal T1-weighted MRI before and after intravenous injection of gadolinium shows avid enhancement in the lesion. The abnormal appearance of the epiphysis is related to prior surgery.

Differential Diagnosis: Ganglion cyst, fibromatosis, postsurgical scarring, soft tissue sarcoma.

Diagnosis: Fibromatosis (extraabdominal desmoid tumor).

Discussion: Fibromatosis is a neoplastic process that arises in fascial and musculoaponeurotic coverings, sometimes at a site of previous trauma or surgery [40]. Described initially in the abdominal wall, it is commonly divided into superficial and deep forms [41]. Deep forms include extraabdominal, abdominal, and intraabdominal, which refer to their location relative to the abdominal wall. The extraabdominal form of deep fibromatosis is of concern in this case. The age of peak incidence is between 25 and 35 years, and there is no clear sex predominance. The tumors are usually solitary, but as many as 15% of patients have synchronous multicentric lesions in the same extremity. Commonly involved sites include the shoulder area, upper arm, thigh, neck, pelvis, forearm, and popliteal fossa, in decreasing order of prevalence. Fibromatosis is nonencapsulated and has an infiltrative growth pattern that may be locally invasive. Lesions may grow to large size and become adherent to adjacent structures such as bone or neurovascular bundles. Fibromatosis is composed of well-differentiated fibroblasts embedded in an abundant collagenous matrix. Because of variable degrees of cellularity, matrix water content, and infiltration, attenuation on CT scans and signal intensity on MRI may be variable [42]. Enhancement may be heterogeneous. Associated osseous findings can include periostitis and pressure erosion. Treatment is surgical resection, but local recurrence is frequent unless wide margins can be obtained.

Clinical History: 16-year-old boy with shoulder pain for 1 month.

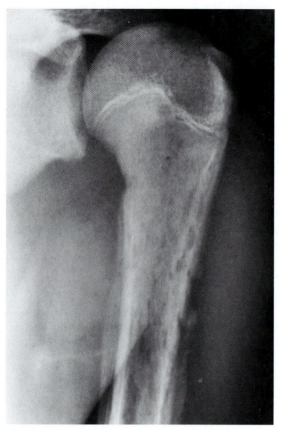

Figure 2-32   A

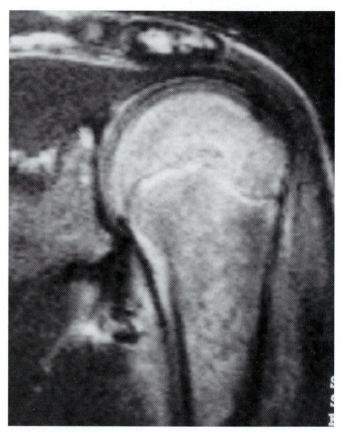

Figure 2-32   B

Findings: (A) AP radiograph of the shoulder. There is permeated destruction of the proximal humeral metaphysis extending into the shaft, with a single layer of periosteal reaction enveloping the region of abnormality. Penetration of the cortex is present along the medial aspect of the metaphysis. (B) Coronal T2-weighted MRI shows marrow edema, permeated cortical destruction, and subperiosteal fluid medially. Note the well-defined dark line of enveloping periosteal new bone surrounding the proximal humerus. There is a small amount of fluid in the glenohumeral joint capsule.

Differential Diagnosis: Infection, Ewing's sarcoma, osteosarcoma, lymphoma.

Diagnosis: Acute osteomyelitis.

Discussion: Acute hematogenous osteomyelitis is generally a disease of children that occurs when the physes are open. Bacteria from a remote source of infection are carried into the bone via the nutrient artery and become deposited in the metaphysis, where blood flow slows as arterial branches loop in a hairpin turn and enter large sinusoidal veins. Once colonies begin to grow, they may spread across the physis into the epiphysis and throughout the medullary cavity. As the acute inflammatory reaction proceeds, edema and accumulated pus increase the intramedullary pressure, leading to decreased blood flow, thrombosis, and necrosis. Pus may extrude through the cortex into the subperiosteal space via haversian and Volkmann's canals, elevating the periosteum and stripping away the cortical blood supply. Reactive periosteal bone forms a shell around the necrotic cortex. The most common pathogen is *S. aureus*. Radiographic changes tend to occur late in the pathophysiologic process, but MRI is sensitive very early in the course and precise in delineating the anatomic extent [43]. Osteomyelitis usually responds to systemic antibiotics, but collections of pus must be drained surgically. Pathogenic bacteria may remain sequestered for decades within avascular pockets of necrotic bone, where they are inaccessible to systemic antibiotics.

Clinical History: 46-year-old man with three-year history of pain and weakness.

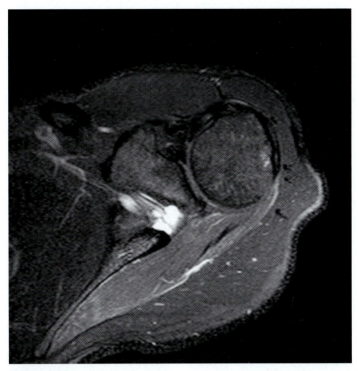

Figure 2-33

Findings: Axial T2-weighted fat-suppressed MRI shows a multiloculated, hyperintense mass in the spinoglenoid notch, with extension into the suprascapular notch. There is increased signal in the teres minor muscle.

Differential Diagnosis: Ganglion cyst, synovial cyst, schwannoma, neurofibroma.

Diagnosis: Ganglion cyst.

Discussion: Suprascapular nerve entrapment occurs most commonly in the suprascapular notch [44]. In this location, the nerve carries fibers to the supraspinatus muscle, infraspinatus muscle, glenohumeral joint, acromioclavicular joint, and anterior two-thirds of the shoulder joint capsule. The second most common location for impingement, as illustrated in this case, would be the spinoglenoid notch, adjacent to the infraspinatus muscle. Clinical features include shoulder pain and weakness, with limited external rotation and abduction of the humerus. Radiographic features in chronic cases include fatty atrophy of the infraspinatus muscle, with or without involvement of the supraspinatus muscle. Etiologies for entrapment include scapular fracture, ligamentous hypertrophy, glenohumeral dislocation, ganglia, tumors, developmental notch abnormalities, and excessive traction on the suprascapular, inferior transverse, or spinoglenoid ligaments, as seen in manual laborers or weight-lifters.

If the ganglion occurs in the suprascapular notch, then both the supraspinatus and infraspinatus muscles are usually involved. If the ganglion occurs more distally in the spinoglenoid notch, then the infraspinatus alone is typically involved.

These lesions are typically hypointense or isointense on T1-weighted MRI, and hyperintense on T2-weighted MRI. They are multiloculated but are typically discrete. The lesion in this case had a neck communicating with a torn glenoid labrum, thought to be the etiology of these cysts.

Ganglion cysts are benign cystic lesions that are attached to a tendon sheath, tendon, muscle, or cartilage. They are typically found in the hands, feet, or wrists. Ganglion cysts are thought to develop as a result of tissue degeneration or synovial herniation. They may or may not communicate with the associated joint or tendon sheath. Ganglion cysts are commonly considered by patients to be unsightly, and this may lead to treatment by surgical excision. Depending on location, their physical mass also may cause significant neurologic impairment. Well-documented conditions include ganglion cysts at the region of the proximal tibiofibular articulation causing footdrop, and ganglion cysts in the suprascapular notch causing atrophy of the infraspinatus muscle. Ganglion cysts that are associated with the cruciate ligaments may cause limitation of motion in the knee, and meniscal cysts may cause swelling, pain, and limitation of motion. If the ganglion cyst is adjacent to a bone, it can erode or elicit a periosteal reaction.

Clinical History: 55-year-old man crashed on motorbike.

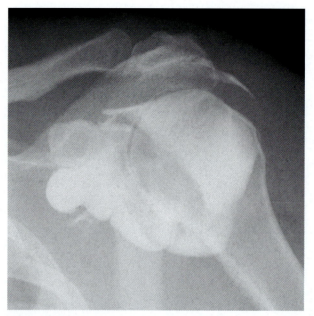

Figure 2-34   A

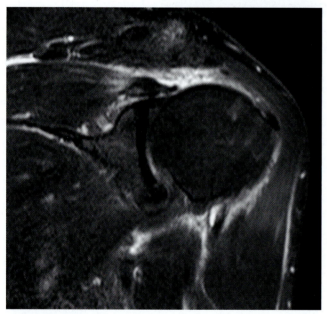

Figure 2-34   B

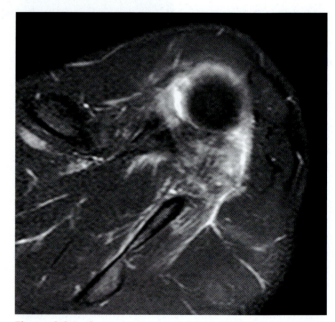

Figure 2-34   C

Findings: (A) AP arthrogram shows intravasation of contrast into the expected location of the supraspinatus tendon. (B) Oblique coronal T2-weighted fat-suppressed MRI shows fluid in the expected location of the supraspinatus tendon and 4 cm of medial retraction of the tendon stump. (C) Axial T2-weighted fat-suppressed MRI through the upper humeral head shows fluid where normal dark-signal tendon should be.

Differential Diagnosis: None.

Diagnosis: Rotator cuff tear involving supraspinatus tendon.

Discussion: The tendons of the rotator cuff may tear as a result of acute or repetitive trauma, mechanical impingement, degeneration, focal ischemia, or some combination of these. More than 90% of rotator cuff tears are spontaneous ruptures through an abnormal tendon, and present as chronic weakness and pain.

Patte [45] has introduced the following grading system:

- (I) Partial-thickness and full-thickness tears that measure less than 1 cm in sagittal dimension.
- (II) Full-thickness supraspinatus tears that measure less than 2 cm in sagittal dimension.
- (III) Full-thickness supraspinatus (and infraspinatus or subscapularis) tears that measure greater than 4 cm in sagittal dimension.
- (IV) Massive full-thickness tears with secondary glenohumeral osteoarthritis.

Partial tears are more common than complete tears, tendon insertion articular side tears are more common than bursal side tears at the myotendinous junction, and intrasubstance tears are the least common. Rotator cuff tears can be demonstrated by arthrography, sonography, or MRI. On arthrography, contrast medium leaks through full-thickness tears into the subdeltoid-subacromial bursa. On MRI or sonography, tears result in a discontinuity that may fill with fluid or granulation tissue. The involved muscle belly, most often the supraspinatus muscle, may retract, and the humeral head may subluxate superiorly. Partial-thickness tears may involve either the inferior or superior surfaces of the cuff, or they may be entirely within the substance of the tendons. Chronic tears can be identified by narrowing of the acromiohumeral distance to less than 0.6 cm, reversal of the normal inferior acromial convexity secondary to repeated impaction, and cystic changes and sclerosis of both the humeral head and acromion undersurface.

Clinical History: 27-year-old man with rugby injury, and a companion case.

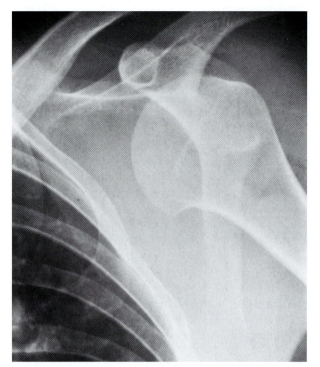

Figure 2-35   A

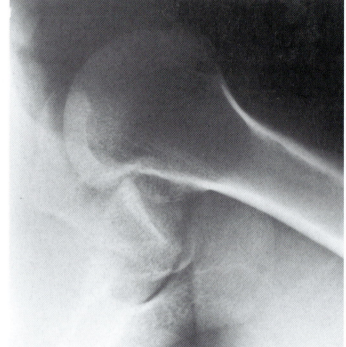

Figure 2-35   B

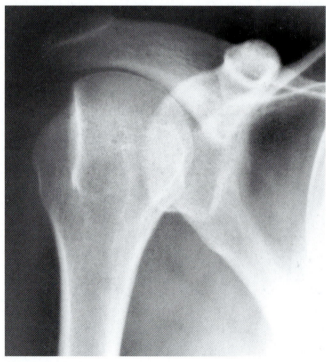

Figure 2-35   C

Findings: (A) AP radiograph of the shoulder. The humeral head is located in a subcoracoid position. (B) Axillary lateral shoulder radiograph. The humeral head is located anterior to the glenoid process. (C) Companion case. AP radiograph of the shoulder in internal rotation shows a defect in the posterolateral aspect of the humeral head.

Differential Diagnosis: None.

Diagnosis: Anterior (subcoracoid) shoulder dislocation. The companion case shows an impaction fracture of the humeral head from previous anterior shoulder dislocation (Hill-Sachs lesion).

Discussion: The stability of the glenohumeral joint depends on the surrounding capsule and ligaments; the glenohumeral contact surface area is only one-third the cross-sectional area of the humeral head, similar to the relationship of a golf ball to a tee. Therefore, shoulder dislocation is a common injury in adults. In about 95% of cases of glenohumeral dislocation, the humeral head dislocates anteriorly and ends up anterior, inferior, and medial to the glenoid process, in a subcoracoid location. Impaction of the anterior inferior surface of the glenoid labrum on the posterolateral aspect of the humeral head after it dislocates may cause a depressed humeral head fracture called the Hill-Sachs lesion. A large Hill-Sachs lesion may cause the glenoid process to catch during rotation of the shoulder, and result in recurrent dislocations. Visualization of the defect is optimized with internal rotation, positioning the lesion in profile. Less dramatic, but perhaps more important than the dislocation itself, is the concomitant soft tissue injury, anterior capsulolabral tears, in which the glenoid labrum and shoulder capsule becomes detached from the glenoid process (Bankart lesion). This injury is present in over 90% of young patients [46,47], and is sometimes associated with an avulsion fracture of the anterior inferior margin of the glenoid process (Bankart fracture). If not repaired, these injuries usually result in posttraumatic anterior shoulder instability or recurrent dislocations. Concomitant rotator cuff disruption occurs in about one-third of patients over the age of 40 who suffer a traumatic anterior shoulder dislocation for the first time [48]. These rotator cuff tears may result in prolonged morbidity, or the need for surgical repair. A brachial plexus injury together with rotator cuff tear has also been recognized as a concurrent injury combination [49]. Acute dislocations are treated with closed reduction. The most common surgical repair for anterior dislocations is the Bankart repair, in which the anterior capsular mechanism is reattached to the glenoid process.

Clinical History: 32-year-old woman in a rollover automobile accident.

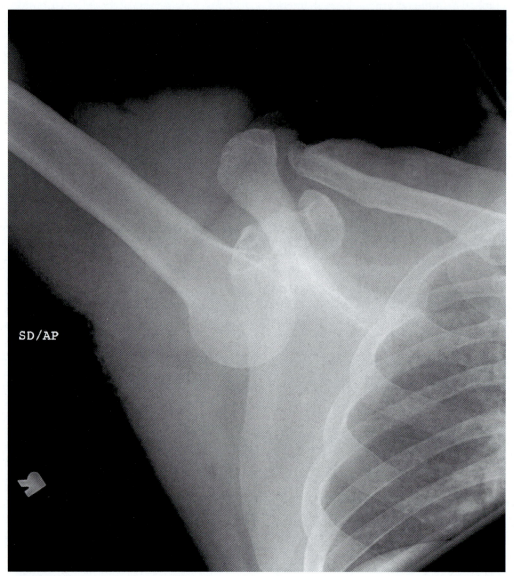

Figure 2-36

Findings: AP radiograph of the right shoulder. The humeral head is located in a subcoracoid position, with the humeral shaft extended superiorly. She was unable to bring the arm down.

Differential Diagnosis: None.

Diagnosis: Luxatio erecta (inferior glenohumeral dislocation).

Discussion: Dislocation of the glenohumeral joint should be immediately obvious; however, the location of the humeral head and the mechanism of injury may require a little more consideration. This patient arrived in the emergency room with her forearm resting on the top of her head, and could not be coaxed by the radiologic technologist to bring it down to her side for proper positioning. Luxatio erecta, or inferior glenohumeral dislocation, is a rare form of shoulder dislocation [50]. It is caused by hyperabduction of the arm while in the overhead position. As with the common anterior dislocation, the humeral head comes to rest in an anterior subcoracoid position, but the humeral shaft will be extended superiorly or parallel to the scapular spine, rather than inferiorly and parallel to the chest wall. Either a fracture of the greater tuberosity or a tear of the rotator cuff is associated with this injury in 80% of patients. Sixty percent may have some degree of neurologic compromise, most commonly to the axillary nerve, and 3% may have significant vascular compromise to the limb [51].

Clinical History: 22-year-old student with ice hockey injury.

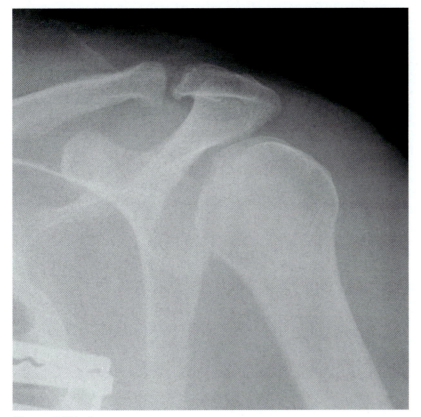

Figure 2-37   A

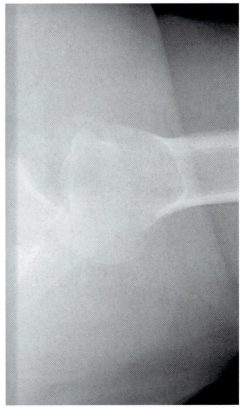

Figure 2-37   B

Findings: (A) AP radiograph of the shoulder. The humeral head is in extreme internal rotation, and the humeral head is positioned too far laterally relative to the glenoid process. There is a fine cortical line along the medial aspect of the humeral head that parallels the medial cortex. (B) Axillary lateral view. The humeral head is impacted on the posterior aspect of the glenoid process.

Differential Diagnosis: None.

Diagnosis: Posterior shoulder dislocation.

Discussion: Size incongruity between the glenoid fossa and the humeral head predisposes this joint to dislocation. The surrounding capsular structures, in large measure, are responsible for maintaining the stability of this articulation. Anterior dislocations are by far the most common variety of dislocation. Posterior dislocations are uncommon and constitute no more than 5% of all cases. The radiographic findings may be subtle. Axillary or Y-views are diagnostic and demonstrate posterior displacement of the humeral head relative to the glenoid fossa. The humeral head tends to be fixed in internal rotation. This may be detected on the frontal views. The glenohumeral joint space is widened (greater than 6 mm) [52]. A reverse Hill-Sachs deformity should be sought and, when present, provides further evidence to support acute or prior posterior dislocation. More than 50% of posterior dislocations of the shoulder are not recognized initially. In 75% of cases, two parallel lines of cortical bone may be recognized on the medial aspect of the humeral head. One line represents the medial cortex of the humeral head, but the other represents the margin of a trough-like impaction fracture of the anterior aspect of the humeral head [53], where the posterior margin of the glenoid impinges on it.

Clinical History: 17-year-old boarding school student with bilateral shoulder pain and nocturnal episodes.

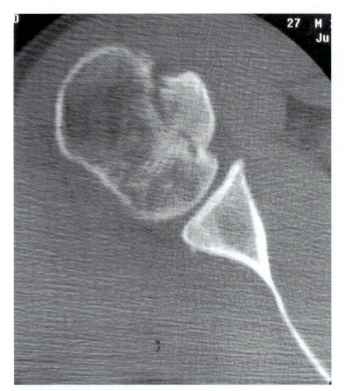

Figure 2-38 A

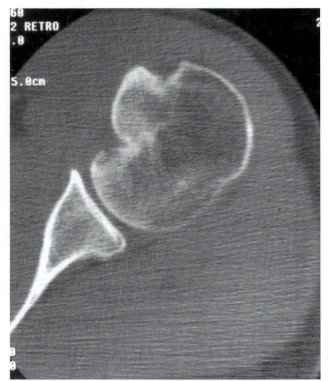

Figure 2-38 B

Findings: (A, B) Axial CT scans of each shoulder at the level of the mid glenohumeral joints. Both glenohumeral joints are normally located. There are bilateral, symmetric, impaction fractures of the anterior aspects of the humeral heads. There is a nondisplaced avulsion fracture of the lesser tuberosity on the right.

Differential Diagnosis: Bilateral shoulder dislocation, secondary to seizures or trauma.

Diagnosis: Seizure disorder, with recurrent bilateral posterior shoulder dislocations.

Discussion: The anterior humeral head impaction fracture is known as a reverse Hill-Sachs lesion, or a trough fracture. Posterior dislocation of the glenohumeral joint allows the posterior rim of the glenoid process to impact into the softer cancellous bone of the humeral head. Trough fracture deformities are seen much better on CT than radiography, as are associated fractures such as avulsions of the lesser tuberosity that otherwise may not be apparent [54]. In this case, the student was having unwitnessed grand mal seizures during the night, resulting in recurrent bilateral posterior shoulder dislocations. Bilateral posterior shoulder dislocation is an uncommon complication of seizure activity [55]. Other orthopedic injuries associated with seizures include dislocations of the hip [56], central fractures of the acetabulum [57], thoracic burst fractures [58], anterior shoulder dislocations, manubriosternal fracture-dislocation, and fractures of the proximal femur and humerus. Other causes of uncontrolled myoclonus may cause injuries similar to those sustained during seizures. Posterior shoulder dislocations may also be caused by trauma, most commonly falls.

Clinical History: 31-year-old man with joint problems.

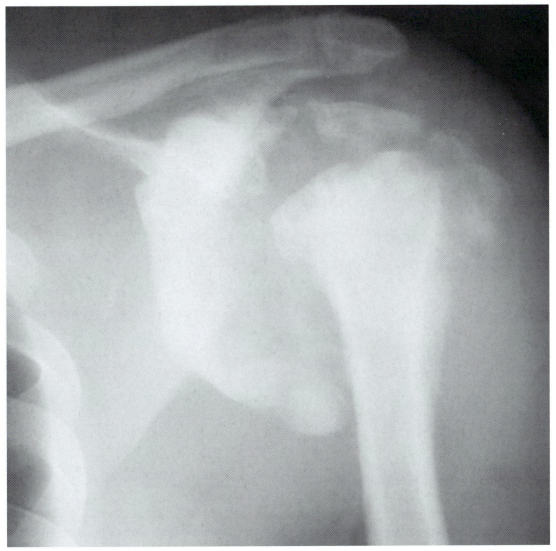

Figure 2-39

Findings: AP radiograph of the left shoulder shows marked deformity of the glenoid with osteolysis, marked productive change, extensive soft tissue calcification, and fragmentation with periosteal reaction about the proximal humerus. The humeral head is missing. There is no destructive change in the adjacent bones.

Differential Diagnosis: Neuropathic arthropathy, septic arthritis, tuberculosis, metastasis, primary bone malignancy.

Diagnosis: Neuropathic arthropathy (Charcot joint).

Discussion: Destruction of the glenohumeral joint may result from infection, tumor, and neuropathic arthropathy. Septic arthritis would typically be accompanied by osteomyelitis of the adjacent bone, and tumors that cause this degree of joint resorption might be expected to show destructive changes in the adjacent bones. Tuberculosis could have a similar appearance, but in this case, the clinical history suggests neurologic disease. Although the most common cause of neuropathic arthropathy in the upper extremities is syringomyelia, other causes include multiple sclerosis, myelomeningocele, spinal cord injury, Charcot-Marie-Tooth disease, alcoholism, amyloidosis, congenital indifference to pain, dysautonomia, and iatrogenic steroid injection. Neuropathic arthropathy may be considered an end-stage degenerative arthropathy, with characteristic findings of debris, increased density, disorganization, joint distension, and dislocation (or more concisely, the five D's). While the hypertrophic form of this condition is more common in the lower extremities, the atrophic form, as in this case, is more common in the upper extremities.

Clinical History: 62-year-old woman with chronic shoulder deformity several weeks after trauma.

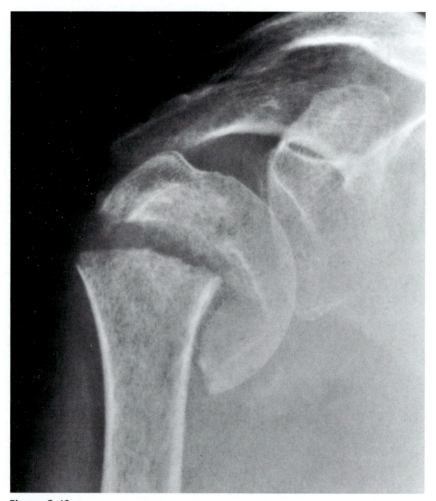

Figure 2-40

Findings: There is a fracture of the humeral neck with medial rotation of the humeral head. Sclerotic, sharp borders are noted. Diffuse osteoporosis is present.

Differential Diagnosis: None.

Diagnosis: Fracture nonunion, surgical neck of the humerus.

Discussion: The three phases of bone healing (inflammatory, reparative, and remodeling) can be modified or arrested by an alteration in the local environment. The inflammatory phase is elicited by the hematoma and necrotic material in the fracture bed. An influx of plasma cells and leukocytes is the result. The reparative phase ensues, with fibrovascular ingrowth into the clot, which establishes an organized framework for mineralization. Callous formation stabilizes the fracture fragments for the next stage, remodeling. The remodeling phase is characterized by resorption of the excess callus according to the principles of the piezoelectric effect.

Cortical bone heals with callus, whereas cancellous bone heals by endosteal apposition. Local factors that slow the progression through the sequence include severe trauma, poor immobilization, infection, osteonecrosis, contact with synovial fluid (which contains fibrinolysins), interposed tissue, underlying pathology, and prior radiation. Systemic factors that slow the progression include old age, malnutrition, steroid use, and metabolic derangements. If the healing process is delayed, the fracture has *delayed union*. If healing fails to progress, the diagnosis of nonunion is raised. Usually a fibrous union or pseudoarthrosis is present. A pseudoarthrosis is defined by a synovial-lined cavity, perpetuated by motion at the fracture site. A pseudoarthrosis need not be present to suggest a nonunion. Radiographically, the ends of the fracture site are osteoporotic, with atrophic or sclerotic margins. Pseudoarthroses are commonly present at the humeral diaphysis or femoral neck, both of which are subjected to considerable motion.

CASE 2-41

Clinical History: 40-year-old man with history of anterior shoulder dislocation.

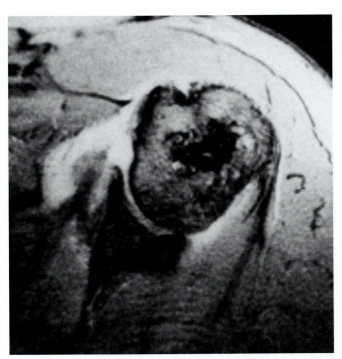

Figure 2-41 A

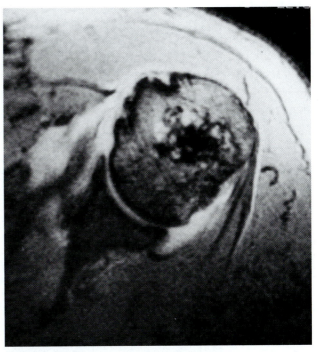

Figure 2-41 B

Findings: (A, B) Axial T2-weighted MRI demonstrates 2 cm of retraction and balling up of the distal subscapularis muscle. A joint effusion is present. The hypointense marrow signal in the humeral head likely represents sclerosis from prior impaction injury during dislocation.

Differential Diagnosis: None.

Diagnosis: Subscapularis rupture.

Discussion: Most subscapularis ruptures occur in the setting of gross rotator cuff tears, and follow rupture of the supraspinatus or infraspinatus tendons; isolated rupture is uncommon but well documented [59]. Clinical signs suggestive of isolated subscapularis tendon tears include increased external rotation and decreased strength of internal rotation. Patients will complain of anterior pain and weakness, particularly when the arm is used above or below the shoulder level. Patients generally do not experience instability. The mechanism of injury is usually a discrete episode of trauma, with traumatic hyperextension or external rotation of the abducted arm.

The axial images on CT arthrography or MRI are most sensitive in detecting subscapularis tendon abnormalities. A partial tear is manifest as thickening or fraying of the tendon. A complete tear is typically associated with tendon retraction and fluid intravasation into the prior tendon site. After partial tear, fatty infiltration is common in the subscapularis muscle. The MRI appearance of subscapularis tendon tears will show the subscapularis tendon to have poorly defined contours and abnormal high signal on T2-weighted images [60]. Most cases will show discontinuity and frank retraction of the tendon, whereas a few may show thickening of the distal portion of the tendon or calcification. An important association with subscapularis rupture includes dislocation of the biceps tendon from its groove, particularly medial dislocation of the tendon. Bony abnormalities are uncommon.

Clinical History: 49-year-old woman with constant shoulder pain.

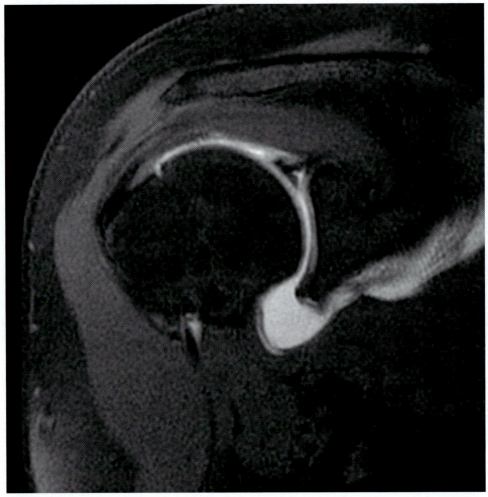

Figure 2-42

Findings: Coronal oblique T1-weighted fat-suppressed MRI after intraarticular administration of dilute gadolinium shows extension of contrast into the superior glenoid labrum.

Differential Diagnosis: None.

Diagnosis: Superior labral anterior to posterior (SLAP) tear.

Discussion: Injuries of the labrum and associated capsular structures are often related to sports activities. The SLAP tear consists of detachment of the labral-capsular-bicipital tendon complex from the superior aspect of the glenoid process. The mechanism of injury consists of traction on the long head of the biceps tendon during sudden arm abduction (e.g., sports that require throwing). This injury does not necessarily result in instability. Pain and clicking are usually the reported symptoms.

One grading system for SLAP lesions is as follows:

- (I) Irregularity of the superior labrum with an intact biceps tendon (10%).
- (II) Avulsion of the labral-biceps-capsular complex (40%).
- (III) Bucket-handle tear of the superior labrum with an intact labral-biceps-capsular complex seen by arthrography as grouped tissue surrounded by contrast ("*cheerio sign*") (30%).
- (IV) Bucket-handle tear of the superior labrum with extension into the proximal biceps tendon (20%).

Labral and capsular injuries are best shown by MRI arthrography or CT arthrography. A major diagnostic differential is between a SLAP lesion and isolated injury to the biceps tendon. Treatment consists of excision of part of the glenoid labrum and associated ganglia or cysts, which can insinuate as far as the suprascapular notch or spinoglenoid notch and cause entrapment neuropathies.

CASE 2-43

Clinical History: 25-year-old college student with seat belt shoulder restraint injury, and a companion case.

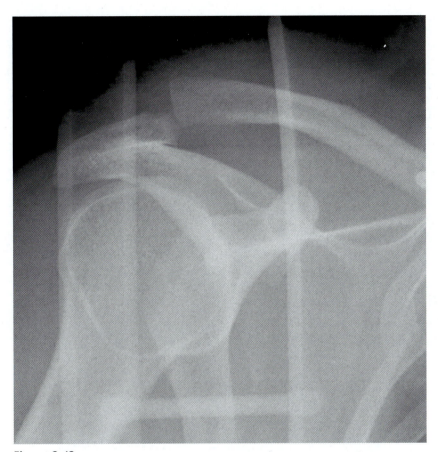

Figure 2-43

Findings: AP radiograph of the right acromioclavicular joint shows superior subluxation of the distal clavicle relative to the acromion process. No fracture is seen.

Differential Diagnosis: None.

Diagnosis: Acromioclavicular subluxation (AC separation, grade 2).

Discussion: Acromioclavicular injuries involve disruption of the acromioclavicular and coracoclavicular ligaments. Acromioclavicular subluxation can result from a direct blow if the arm is adducted at the time of injury, or from an indirect transmission of the forces through the glenohumeral joint to the acromion if the shoulder is in the protected stance of flexion and abduction. The inferior surfaces of the acromion process and the distal clavicle are normally at the same level on AP radiographs. In a grade 1 injury, the acromioclavicular ligaments are stretched but not disrupted; radiographs are normal or show a slight increase in the joint space and associated soft tissue swelling. When the acromioclavicular ligaments (and usually the trapezius and deltoid aponeuroses as well) are completely torn (grade 2), the distal clavicle subluxates superiorly. If the coracoclavicular ligaments are also torn, or the coracoid avulses (grade 3), the clavicle dislocates and the space between clavicle and coracoid process widens. Stress views may be needed to elicit the subluxation and are obtained with angled frontal radiographs while the patient holds hand weights. It is recommended that both acromioclavicular joints be included on the radiographs because there may be normal joint laxity in asymptomatic patients. If the distance between the superior aspect of the coracoid and the inferior aspect of the clavicle differs by more than 2 mm to 4 mm relative to the opposite comparison side, the diagnosis is made. Rarely, the clavicle will dislocate inferiorly, entrap superiorly, or dislocate in association with the sternoclavicular joint (floating clavicle). Posttraumatic coracoclavicular ligament calcification or ossification is common and is usually asymptomatic. The most common complication is osteoarthritis. The most problematic complication is posttraumatic osteolysis of the distal clavicle, which can have an active lytic phase for up to 18 months and mimic infection.

CASE 2-44

Clinical History: 58-year-old woman with shoulder pain for many years.

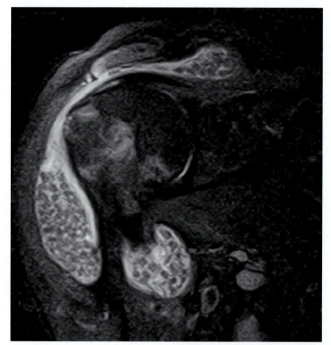

Figure 2-44   A

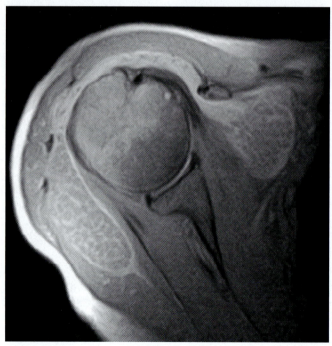

Figure 2-44   B

Figure 2-44   C

Findings: Coronal oblique T2-weighted fat-suppressed (**A**), coronal oblique T1-weighted (**B**) and axial T2-weighted (**C**) MRI demonstrates numerous, tiny, intermediate signal intensity masses within the subacromial-subdeltoid bursa.

Differential Diagnosis: None.

Diagnosis: Synovial osteochondromatosis.

Discussion: Synovial metaplasia occurs most commonly in the joints, but also in the tendon sheaths and bursae. Typically, this is a monoarticular process seen in men between the ages of 20 and 50. Commonly involved joints include the knee, hip, and elbow, but the shoulder is depicted in this case. The patient complains of a chronic history of joint locking. Joint effusion is typically not seen, but, when present, aspiration will yield bloody material. Secondary osteoarthritis is very common. These bodies can extrude outside the joint and persist in a periarticular location. After surgical debridement, recurrences are not uncommon, though malignant degeneration is rare [61,62,63]. The cartilaginous nodules begin their life cycle as synovial villonodular projections that become pedunculated, break off, and ossify. Growth may continue by nourishment through the synovial fluid, but individual bodies do not typically exceed 3 cm in size. Radiography may reveal soft tissue prominence, specks of calcification, peripherally dense lesions, or mature central ossific trabeculations. In the 15% that do not calcify or ossify, arthrography or MRI is most useful for their demonstration.

Clinical History: 43-year-old woman with polyarticular arthritis, and a companion case.

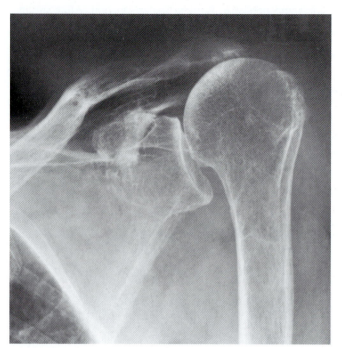

Figure 2-45   A

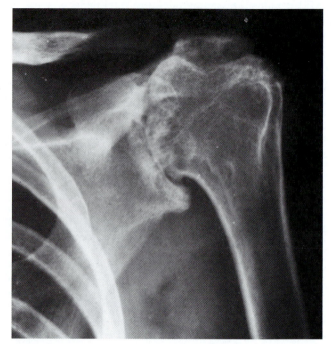

Figure 2-45   B

Findings: (A) AP shoulder radiograph. The bones are diffusely osteoporotic. The humeral head is subluxated superiorly, with adaptive change at the inferior surface of the acromion. Bony hypertrophy is virtually absent, but there are no erosions. There are no soft tissue calcifications. (B) Companion case. AP radiograph of the shoulder of a different patient shows more marked subchondral cyst formation and bony eburnation on both sides of the glenohumeral joint. Elevation of the humerus is secondary evidence of a chronic rotator cuff tear.

Differential Diagnosis: None.

Diagnosis: Rheumatoid arthritis.

Discussion: Involvement of the shoulder in rheumatoid arthritis is common [64]. The shoulder capsule surrounds the articular surfaces of the humeral head and glenoid process, and extends medially beneath the coracoid process and inferiorly well below the glenoid process. Chronic inflammation of the synovium may lead to extensive involvement of the adjacent structures, including the glenohumeral joint itself, the rotator cuff, the acromioclavicular joint, and the adjacent thoracic cage. Inflammatory changes of the subdeltoid-subacromial bursa, the subcoracoid bursa, and the extensive tendon sheaths around the shoulder may contribute to the process. At the glenohumeral joint, the presence of inflamed synovium results in progressive destruction of the cartilage surfaces, and marginal and subchondral erosions. Erosions of the humerus tend to be more prominent than erosions of the glenoid process, and are particularly characteristic of advanced disease. Inflamed synovial tissue may eventually damage adjacent tendons, so that rotator cuff tear or atrophy is common. The result is superior subluxation of the humeral head relative to the glenoid process, and the development of adaptive change at the inferior surface of the acromion process. This surface develops a concavity to fit the top of the humeral head, along with sclerosis, subchondral cyst formation, and osteophyte formation. Unlike most joints that are involved by rheumatoid arthritis, secondary degenerative changes with sclerosis and osteophyte formation are not unusual at the shoulder. When medical therapy fails, total shoulder replacement is an option.

CASE 2-46

Clinical History: 39-year-old man with episodic shoulder pain.

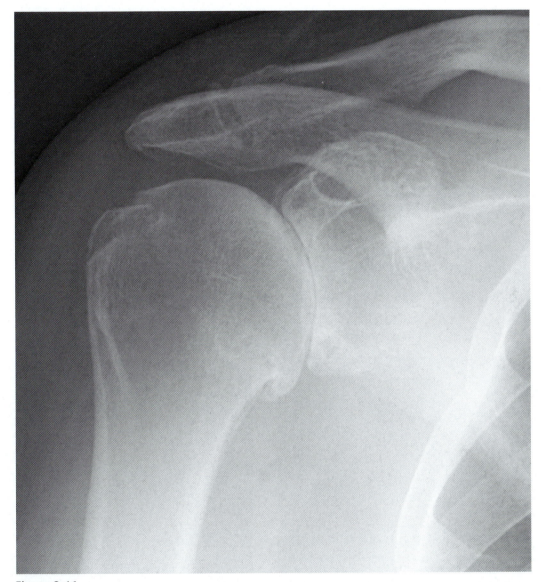

Figure 2-46

Findings: AP radiograph of the shoulder. Arthritic changes are present at the glenohumeral joint with cartilage space narrowing, subchondral sclerosis, and prominent osteophyte formation. The joint surface is enlarged and remodeled, but the humeral head is not subluxated and there are no erosions or soft tissue calcifications. The acromioclavicular joint is not involved.

Differential Diagnosis: Pyrophosphate arthropathy, neuropathic arthropathy, posttraumatic arthropathy.

Diagnosis: Pyrophosphate arthropathy.

Discussion: The radiographic findings are those of degenerative joint disease; however, osteoarthritis at the glenohumeral joint is unusual except in the setting of pre-existing disease. Pyrophosphate arthropathy is the end-stage degenerative joint disease associated with calcium pyrophosphate dihydrate crystal deposition disease. Abnormalities that may be seen in this condition at the glenohumeral joint include chondrocalcinosis, cartilage space narrowing, subchondral sclerosis, subchondral cyst formation, and osteophyte formation. Osteophytes are characteristically florid on the humeral side, as in this case, with a drooping appearance on the AP projection. If the articular cartilage has been destroyed, chondrocalcinosis will be absent. Rotator cuff tears and calcific deposits in the joint capsule, tendons, and bursae may be associated abnormalities. Occasionally, destructive bone changes may be severe and progressive, resembling neuropathic arthropathy.

Clinical History: 39-year-old woman with shoulder pain.

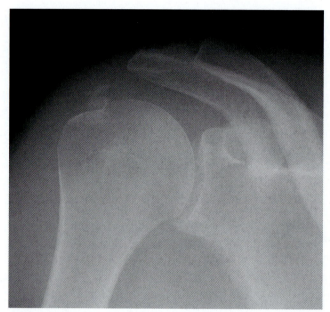

Figure 2-47   A

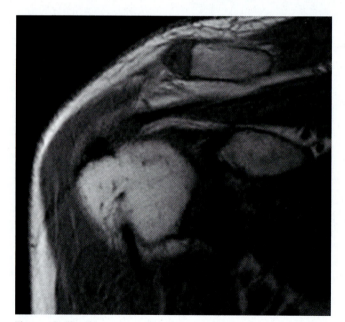

Figure 2-47   B

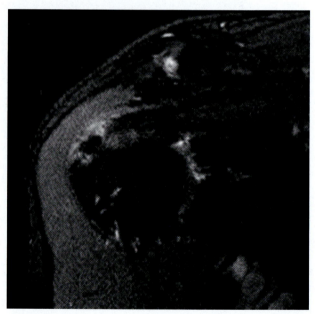

Figure 2-47   C

Findings: External rotation radiograph (**A**), coronal oblique T1-weighted MRI (**B**), and coronal oblique T2-weighted fat-suppressed MRI (**C**) of the right shoulder demonstrates calcium hydroxyapatite deposit in the supraspinatus tendon of the rotator cuff. Calcium deposits have low T1-weighted and T2-weighted signal on MRI. A mild amount of high signal is seen surrounding the calcium deposit on the T2-weighted MRI, indicating inflammation or edema.

Differential Diagnosis: Calcific tendinitis, calcific bursitis, intraarticular loose body.

Diagnosis: Calcific tendinitis.

Discussion: Soft tissue calcium deposits appear on radiographs as amorphous densities, often sharply defined or angular in shape, and never having a cortex or a trabecular bone pattern, or a calcification pattern of cartilage. Recurrent episodes of calcific tendinitis or calcific bursitis are commonly associated with hydroxyapatite deposits. Most patients are adults in their 40s and 50s who present with acute pain, swelling, and tenderness. Symptoms respond rapidly to nonsteroidal anti-inflammatory agents. The shoulder is a common site of involvement, usually at the supraspinatus tendon. Tendons may go on to atrophy and rupture, but it is unclear whether the deposits initially caused the local tissue damage, or whether preexisting tissue damage allowed the deposits to accumulate. The calcific deposits around the shoulder are bilateral in about half the cases, and they may migrate to contiguous structures. After clinical resolution, the deposits may disappear. The process is usually monoarticular, but multiple joints may be involved at the same time or in succession. Other common sites of involvement include the long head of the biceps tendon, the extensors of the wrist, the myotendinous attachments along the linea aspera of the femur (thigh adductors), at the medial border of the proximal tibia (pes anserinus), the olecranon bursa, the trochanteric bursa, and the ischial bursa.

Clinical History: (A) 39-year-old man with chronic renal failure. (B, C, D) 58-year-old female on hemodialysis with enlarging posterior shoulder and back mass.

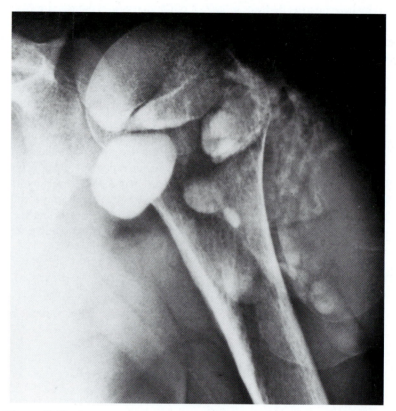

Figure 2-48   A

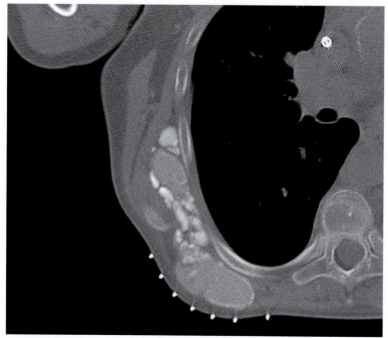

Figure 2-48   B

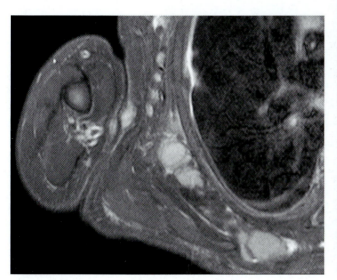

Figure 2-48   C

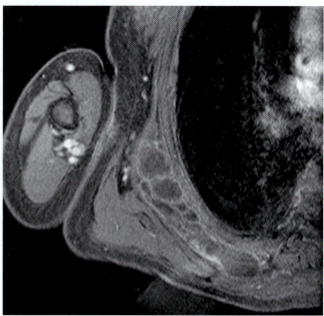

Figure 2-48   D

Findings: (A) AP radiograph of left shoulder shows calcific densities overlying the region of the shoulder. The calcifications are rounded and amorphous. The underlying bone appears intact. A few fluid levels are present. Companion case: (B) Axial unenhanced CT in preparation for a CT-guided biopsy demonstrates multiloculated calcific collections of varying density. (C) Axial inversion recovery MRI shows some of the loculations to have fluid signal intensity. (D) Axial gadolinium enhanced T1-weighted, fat-suppressed MRI shows no enhancement.

Differential Diagnosis: None.

Diagnosis: Periarticular calcinosis in chronic hemodialysis (metastatic calcification, secondary tumoral calcinosis).

Discussion: Metastatic soft tissue deposits of calcium hydroxyapatite crystals around joints may be found in patients with chronic renal failure who are managed on hemodialysis or continuous ambulatory peritoneal dialysis [65]. The particular condition that appears to result in the deposition of calcium is a combination of hyperphosphatemia, hypercalcemia, and increased calcium-phosphorus product. On radionuclide bone scans, the deposits of calcium will show tracer accumulation, often before visualization on radiographs [66]. Because the crystals are often in an aqueous suspension (milk of calcium), CT and upright radiographs may demonstrate fluid-sediment levels [67]. Other dialysis-related bone conditions include aluminum toxicity, which has the appearance of osteomalacia, and amyloid arthropathy.

Clinical History: 52-year-old man on long-standing renal dialysis with shoulder pain.

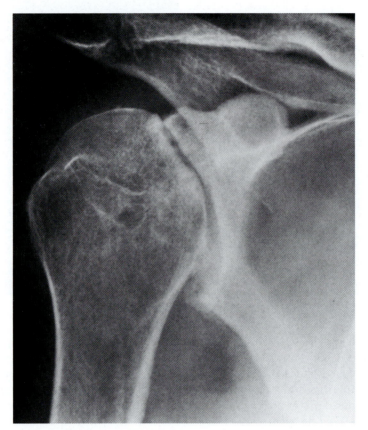

Figure 2-49   A

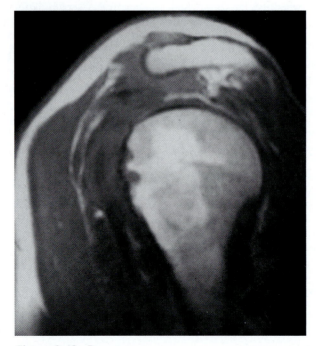

Figure 2-49   B

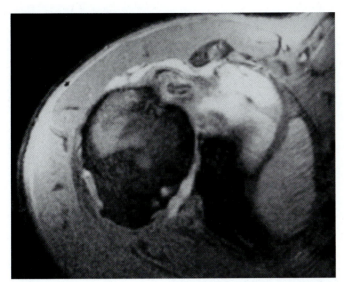

Figure 2-49   C

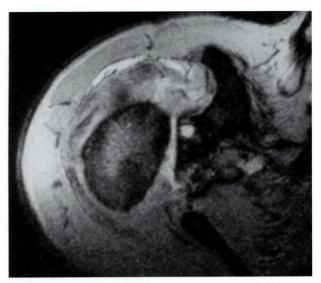

Figure 2-49   D

Findings: (A) AP radiograph demonstrates a loss of the normal glenohumeral joint space, with superior migration of the humeral head. The articular margins are irregular and sclerotic. The acromiohumeral distance is preserved in this case. (B) T1-weighted sagittal MRI demonstrates synovial material that is isointense to muscle. (C, D) T2-weighted axial MRI demonstrates that the material is isointense to hyperintense to muscle. A small joint effusion is noted. Subchondral cyst formation is present on both sides of the joint. The articular cartilage is absent, and there is secondary irregularity of the cortical surface of the humerus and glenoid. Extensive low-to-intermediate signal intensity intracapsular material is present.

Differential Diagnosis: Amyloid arthropathy, pyrophosphate arthropathy, pigmented villonodular synovitis, synovial osteochondromatosis, rheumatoid arthritis, tuberculosis.

Diagnosis: Amyloid arthropathy.

Discussion: Amyloid arthropathy is related to the duration of therapy and the patient's age at the start of hemodialysis. Renal transplantation halts the process. Cystic changes and erosive-type osteoarthropathy may occur in association with amyloid deposition [68]. Several forms of amyloidosis [69] have been described:

- Primary (common involvement of the heart, synovium, muscle, tongue, and perivascular connective tissue, associated with multiple myeloma).

- Secondary (common involvement of the liver, spleen, kidneys, and adrenals, associated with rheumatoid arthritis, neoplasms, sepsis, inflammatory disorders, Crohn's disease, intravenous drug abuse, and cystic fibrosis).
- Hereditary-familial (common manifestations as neuropathies, nephropathies, and cardiomyopathies).
- Senile (patients with chronic disorders, typically rheumatoid arthritis).
- Localized amyloid tumors (common involvement in the larynx, tracheobronchial system, and skin).

Amyloid can occur in children and is most commonly secondary to juvenile chronic arthritis. Radiographic findings typical of this disease process include osteoporosis, soft tissue nodules and swelling, subchondral cysts, erosions, joint subluxations, and contractures similar to rheumatoid arthritis [70]. Additional manifestations include lytic lesions, pathologic fractures, osteonecrosis, and neuropathic osteoarthropathy [71,72]. MRI can be used to distinguish amyloidosis from other arthropathies. Typically, the lesions are homogenously isointense to muscle on all pulse sequences. With short tau inversion recovery imaging, there is only a minimal increase in signal intensity relative to normal muscle, in contrast to all other myopathies, in which there is markedly increased signal intensity in acute stages. In amyloid, the muscles tend to be enlarged, with obscuration of the normal boundaries and a coarse reticulated pattern in the soft tissues.

Clinical History: 52-year-old man in high-speed automobile accident.

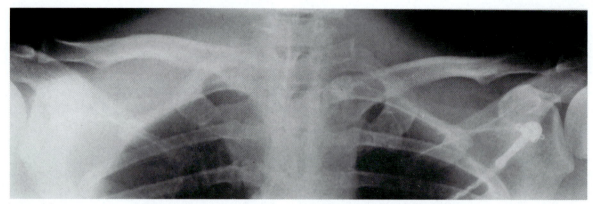

Figure 2-50   A

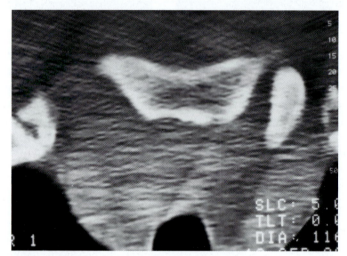

Figure 2-50   B

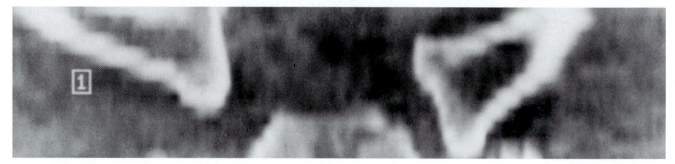

Figure 2-50   C

Findings: (A) AP chest radiograph (detail). The medial clavicles are asymmetric, with the right being superior to the left in position. (B) Axial CT scan. The right sternoclavicular joint is much wider than the left. (C) Coronal CT reformation. The right sternoclavicular joint is dislocated superiorly.

Differential Diagnosis: None.

Diagnosis: Superior dislocation of the right sternoclavicular joint.

Discussion: Sternoclavicular dislocations are exceedingly rare. Indirect trauma propagated along the clavicular long axis can result in anterior or posterior dislocation of the joint. Direct trauma to the sternoclavicular joint results in posterior dislocation. Reduction of a posterior dislocation is an orthopedic emergency, because the dislocated medial head of the clavicle can impinge on the great vessels, phrenic nerve, esophagus, or trachea. Pneumothorax or hemothorax may also be associated with this condition. Anterior dislocations of the sternoclavicular joint result from a forcible backward traction on the scapula, which torques the clavicle and exceeds the tolerance of the joint capsule and ligaments. Complications are unusual. Dislocation needs to be distinguished from avulsion of the medial clavicular epiphysis [73,74], which is the last growth plate to fuse at about 25 years of age. Both result in pain and a prominent soft tissue bump. CT may be required for definitive diagnosis.

Clinical History: 52-year-old man with chest pain and history of smoking.

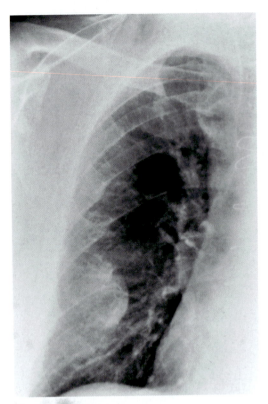

Figure 2-51   A

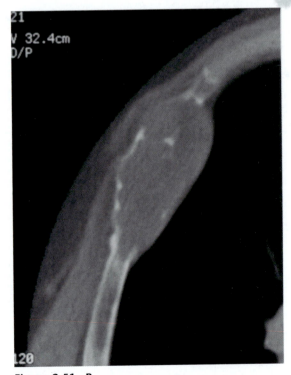

Figure 2-51   B

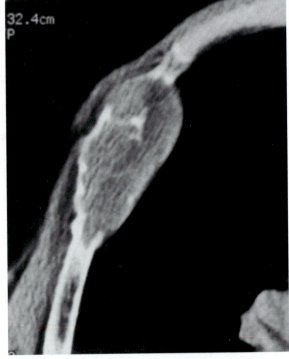

Figure 2-51   C

Findings: (**A**) AP radiograph (detail) of the right ribs demonstrates a pleural-based mass (smooth, well-defined superior margins, indistinct inferior margins) with a loss of the normal anterior right fifth rib. (**B, C**) Axial CT (bone and soft tissue settings) shows an expansile soft tissue mass in the rib that has largely destroyed the normal cortical margin. The lesion does not involve the costal cartilage.

Differential Diagnosis: Metastasis, myeloma, lymphoma, Ewing's sarcoma, plasmacytoma, eosinophilic granuloma, hemophiliac pseudotumor, giant cell tumor, brown tumor.

Diagnosis: Brown tumor.

Discussion: A focal, destructive lesion of bone with cortical breakthrough suggests an aggressive process. In this clinical setting, metastasis or marrow element malignancy would be the leading consideration. If the underlying disorder of hyperparathyroidism is known, then brown tumor would be a leading diagnosis. Brown tumors are typically solitary, expansile, eccentric or cortical lucent lesions that can cause pain due to a pressure phenomenon or pathologic fracture. The lesions provoke little, if any, reactive bone and consist of hemorrhage, multinucleated giant cells, and proliferating fibrous tissue. With successful treatment of the underlying metabolic condition, the lesions can be observed to become sclerotic and heal. Although brown tumors are more common in primary hyperparathyroidism, secondary hyperparathyroidism is more prevalent than primary hyperparathyroidism [75]. Therefore, brown tumors are seen more commonly in conjunction with secondary hyperparathyroidism.

Clinical History: 70-year-old male with an enlarging back mass.

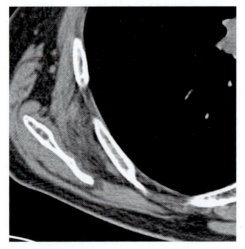

Figure 2-52   A

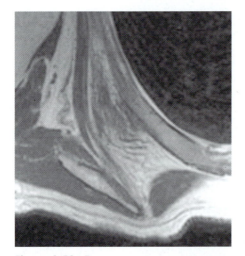

Figure 2-52   B

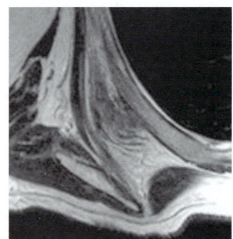

Figure 2-52   C

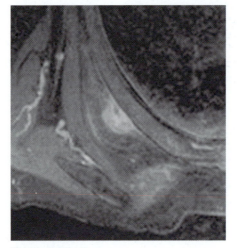

Figure 2-52   D

Findings: (**A**) Axial CT image demonstrates a semicircular mass deep to the scapula. The lesion abuts the chest wall, but does not erode the bone or involve the subpleural space. The lesion is predominantly fatty, but also has strands of soft tissue attenuation. (**B, C, D**) Axial T1-weighted, T2-weighted, and T1-weighted fat-suppressed gadolinium-enhanced MRI demonstrates heterogenous signal and enhancement, arranged in bands.

Differential Diagnosis: Liposarcoma, atypical lipoma, elastofibroma, hemangioma, fibromatosis.

Diagnosis: Elastofibroma.

Discussion: The appearance and location is characteristic of an elastofibroma. An elastofibroma is a benign fibrous proliferation of adulthood [76]. Other lesions in this category include nodular fasciitis, proliferative fasciitis, proliferative myositis, and keloid formation. The etiology is thought to be a degenerative response to chronic, repetitive trauma in the upper limb girdle, and the lesion is seen most commonly in weight-lifters or laborers who require strong upper body strength. Although they tend to be unilateral, when they occur bilaterally the appearance is virtually diagnostic. Elastofibromas have many of the imaging characteristics of fat-containing tumors, including liposarcoma and hemangioma. The radiologic appearance is that of semicircular, heterogeneous, low-attenuation mass that respects the normal contours of the chest wall or scapula. On MRI, the lesion tends to be heterogeneous, but always has portions with the signal intensity of fat. Enhancement is the rule for all fibromatosis or fibrous proliferative lesions, benign or malignant [77]. On sonography, the fibroelastic strands are hypoechoic, and the characteristic location between the serratus anterior muscles and the chest wall may be identified. Occasionally, biopsy must be used in unilateral lesions to exclude liposarcoma. The prevalence of elastofibroma on autopsy series is 11% to 24%. In one large CT series of adults, the prevalence was 2% [78].

Clinical History: 25-year-old man with painless winging of the scapula. He underwent prophylactic therapeutic irradiation (approximately 20 Gy) to the lungs for Wilms' tumor in early childhood. The radiation field included both scapulae.

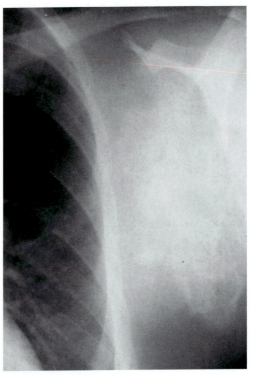

Figure 2-53   A

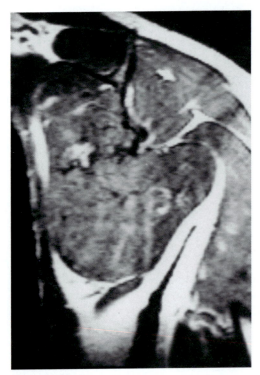

Figure 2-53   B

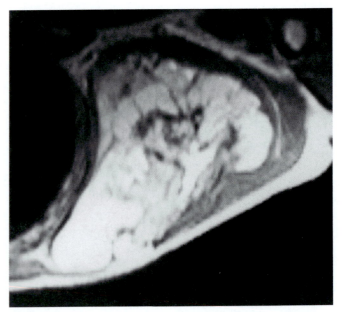

Figure 2-53   C

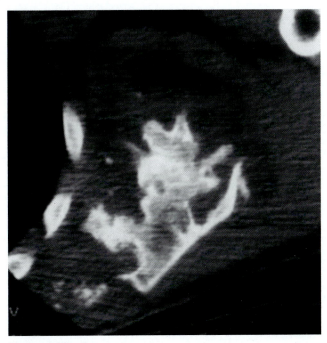

Figure 2-53 D

Findings: (A) Lateral scapular radiograph. There is a mineralized mass arising from the anterior surface of the scapula, displacing it from the chest wall. (B) Coronal T1-weighted MRI shows the lesion adjacent to the chest wall. It has intermediate signal intensity. (C) Axial T2-weighted MRI shows high signal intensity in the nonmineralized portion of the lesion, consistent with hyaline cartilage. (D) Axial CT scan through the mid scapula. The mass is ossified, but it has a large nonmineralized component of low attenuation relative to muscle.

Differential Diagnosis: Osteochondroma, chondrosarcoma.

Diagnosis: Radiation-induced osteochondroma.

Discussion: The morphologic features of this lesion are typical for osteochondroma. The ossified portion of the lesion has a medullary space and cortex that are contiguous with the bone from which it arises. The nonmineralized cartilaginous cap has attenuation noted on CT that is similar to water, and is bright on T2-weighted MRI. Solitary osteochondromas are not true neoplasms, but rather are aberrations of normal growth. Osteochondromas may arise after a variety of traumas to the perichondrial ring of the growing physis, including therapeutic irradiation. Those induced by radiation

are indistinguishable from those that occur in other circumstances, and the prevalence among long-term survivors of childhood cancer treated by radiation is approximately 6% to 12% [79,80]. Malignant degeneration to chondrosarcoma is extremely rare [81]. In patients who receive radiotherapy by 2 years of age, induced tumors are usually benign. The most common neoplasms are exostoses (osteochondromas), which are histologically and biologically indistinguishable from those that occur naturally. Malignant tumors typically occur in older patients who have received radiotherapy. Osteosarcoma, fibrosarcoma, malignant fibrous histiocytoma, chondrosarcoma, and other unusual sarcomas are much less likely to occur as the result of radiation than are benign tumors. The following criteria must be satisfied to make the diagnosis of a radiation-induced sarcoma:

- (i) The sarcoma arises within the irradiated field.
- (ii) The latent period is at least 4 years.
- (iii) The sarcoma is histologically different from a previous tumor, or the radiation was delivered in the absence of a malignant diagnosis.

The latent period averages 11 years. The presence of pain, soft tissue mass, and progression on serial films should raise suspicion and lead to biopsy.

SOURCES AND READINGS

1. Fritz RC. MR imaging of sports injuries of the elbow. *Magn Reson Imaging Clin N Am.* 1999;7(1):51–72.

2. Miller TT, Shapiro MA, Schultz E, Kalish PE. Comparison of sonography and MRI for diagnosing epicondylitis. *J Clin Ultrasound.* 2002;30(4):193–202.

3. O'Dwyer H, O'Sullivan P, Fitzgerald D, Lee MJ, McGrath F, Logan PM. The fat pad sign following elbow trauma in adults: its usefulness and reliability in suspecting occult fracture. *J Comput Assist Tomogr.* 2004;28:562–565.

4. Rogers LF. To see or not to see, that is the question: MR imaging of acute musculoskeletal trauma. *AJR.* 2001;176:1.

5. Ring D, Jupiter JB, Waters PM. Monteggia fractures in children and adults. *J Am Acad Orthop Surg.* 1998;6(4):215–224.

6. Frumkin K. Nursemaid's elbow: a radiographic demonstration. *Ann Emerg Med.* 1985;14:690–693.

7. Triantafyllou SJ, Wilson SC, Rychak JS. Irreducible "pulled elbow" in a child. A case report. *Clin Orthop.* 1992;284:153–155.

8. Adeniran A, Merriam WF. Pulled elbow in an adult patient. *J Bone Joint Surg Br.* 1994;76:848–849.

9. Prendergast M. Hysteria or pulled elbow. *Lancet.* 1994;343:926.

10. Sachar K, Akelman E, Ehrlich MG. Radioulnar synostosis. *Hand Clin.* 1994;10:399–404.

11. Spritz RA. Familial radioulnar synostosis. *J Med Genet.* 1978;15:160–162.

12. Cleary JE, Omer GE Jr. Congenital proximal radio-ulnar synostosis. Natural history and functional assessment. *J Bone Joint Surg Am.* 1985;67:539–545.

13. Miller JD, Pruitt S, McDonald TJ. Acute brachial plexus neuritis: an uncommon cause of shoulder pain. *Am Fam Physician.* 2000;62:2067–2072.

14. Helms CA, Martinez S, Speer KP. Acute brachial neuritis (Parsonage-Turner syndrome): MR imaging appearance—report of three cases. *Radiology.* 1998;207(1):255–259.

15. Holguin PH, Rico AA, Garcia JP, Del Rio JL. Elbow ankylosis due to postburn herterotopic ossification. *J Burn Care Rehabil.* 1996;17:150–154.

16. Richards AM, Klaassen MF. Heterotopic ossification after severe burns: a report of three cases and review of the literature. *Burns.* 1997;23:64–68.

17. Ilahi OA, Strausser DW, Gabel GT. Posttraumatic heterotopic ossification about the elbow. *Orthopedics.* 1998;21:265–268.

18. Goodman TA, Merkel PA, Perlmutter G, Doyle MK, Krane SM, Polisson RP. Heterotopic ossification in the setting of neuromuscular blockade. *Arthritis Rheum.* 1997;40:1619–1627.

19. Chautems RC, Glauser T, Waeber-Fey MC, Rostan O, Barraud GE. Quadrilateral space syndrome: case report and review of the literature. *Ann Vasc Surg.* 2000;14(6):673–676.

20. Helms CA. The impact of MR imaging in sports medicine. *Radiology.* 2002;224(3):631–635.

21. Lester B, Jeong GK, Weiland AJ, Wickiewicz TL. Quadrilateral space syndrome: diagnosis, pathology, and treatment. *Am J Orthop.* 1999;28(12):718–722, 725.

22. Capanna R, Dal Monte A, Gitelis S, Campanacci M. The natural history of unicameral bone cyst after steroid injection. *Clin Orthop.* 1982;166:204–211.

23. Margau R, Babyn P, Cole W, Smith C, Lee F. MR imaging of simple bone cysts in children: not so simple. *Pediatr Radiol.* 2000;30(8):551–557.

24. Struhl S, Edelson C, Pritzker H, Seimon LP, Dorfman HD. Solitary (unicameral) bone cyst. The fallen fragment sign revisited. *Skeletal Radiol.* 1989;18:261–265.

25. Johnston CE 2nd, Fletcher RR. Traumatic transformation of unicameral bone cyst into aneurysmal bone cyst. *Orthopedics.* 1986;9:1441–1447.

26. Gherman RB, Ouzounian JG, Miller DA, Kwock L, Goodwin TM. Spontaneous vaginal delivery: a risk factor for Erb's palsy? *Am J Obstet Gynecol.* 1998;178:423–427.

27. Ouzounian JG, Korst LM, Phelan JP. Permanent Erb palsy: a traction-related injury? *Obstet Gynecol.* 1997;89:139–141.

28. Jennett RJ, Tarby TJ, Kreinick CJ. Brachial plexus palsy: an old problem revisited. *Am J Obstet Gynecol.* 1992;166:1673–1676.

29. Peleg D, Hasnin J, Shalev E. Fractured clavicle and Erb's palsy unrelated to birth trauma. *Am J Obstet Gynecol.* 1997;177:1038–1040.

30. Gordon BH, Chew FS. Isolated acromioclavicular joint pathology in the symptomatic shoulder on magnetic resonance imaging: a pictorial essay. *J Comput Assist Tomogr.* 2004;28:215–222.

31. Fiorella D, Helms CA, Speer KP. Increased T2 signal intensity in the distal clavicle: incidence and clinical implications. *Skeletal Radiol.* 2000;29(12):697–702.

32. Murphey MD, Robbin MR, McRae GA, Flemming DJ, Temple HT, Kransdorf MJ. The many faces of osteosarcoma. *Radiographics.* 1997;17:1205–1231.

33. Fechner RE, Mills SE. *Tumors of the bones and joints.* Washington, DC: Armed Forces Institute of Pathology. 1993:84–85.

34. Brien EW, Mirra JM, Luck JV Jr. Benign and malignant cartilage tumors of bone and joint: their anatomic and theoretical basis with an emphasis on radiology, pathology and clinical biology: II. Juxtacortical cartilage tumors. *Skeletal Radiol.* 1999;28(1):1–20.

35. Unni KK. *Dahlin's bone tumors: general aspects and data on 11,087 cases.* 5th ed. Philadelphia: Lippincott-Raven Publishers; 1996:25–45.

36. Roberts CC, Liu PT, Colby TV. Encapsulated versus nonencapsulated superficial fatty masses: a proposed MR imaging classification. *Am J Roentgenol.* 2003;180(5):1419–1422.

37. Safran MR, Graham SM. Distal biceps tendon ruptures: incidence, demographics, and the effect of smoking. *Clin Orthop.* 2002;(404):275–283.

38. Falchook FS, Zlatkin MB, Erbacher GE, Moulton JS, Bisset GS, Murphy BJ. Rupture of the distal biceps tendon: evaluation with MR imaging. *Radiology.* 1994;190:659–663.

39. Davison BL, Engber WD, Tigert LJ. Long term evaluation of repaired distal biceps brachii tendon ruptures. *Clin Orthop.* 1996;333:186–191.

40. Satsuma S, Yamamoto T, Kobayashi D, et al. Extraabdominal desmoid tumor in a surgical scar of a patient with Sprengel's deformity. *J Pediatr Surg.* 2003;38(10):1540–1542.

41. Edmonds LD, Ly JQ, LaGatta LM, Lusk JD, Beall DP. Quiz case. Extraabdominal desmoid tumor of the upper arm. *Eur J Radiol.* 2003;48(3):312–315.

42. Robbin MR, Murphey MD, Temple HT, Kransdorf MJ, Choi JJ. Imaging of musculoskeletal fibromatosis. *Radiographics.* 2001;21(3):585–600.

43. Schweitzer ME, Morrison WB. MR imaging of the diabetic foot. *Radiol Clin North Am.* 2004;42(1):61–71.

44. Zehetgruber H, Noske H, Lang T, Wurnig C. Suprascapular nerve entrapment. A meta-analysis. *Int Orthop.* 2002;26(6):339–343.

45. Patte D. Classification of rotator cuff lesions. *Clin Orthop.* 1990;254:639–645.

46. Taylor DC, Arciero RA. Pathologic changes associated with shoulder dislocations. Arthroscopic and physical examination findings in first-time, traumatic anterior dislocations. *Am J Sports Med.* 1997;25:306–311.

47. Suder PA, Frich LH, Hougaard K, Lundorf E, Wulff Jakobsen B. Magnetic resonance imaging evaluation of capsulolabral tears after traumatic primary anterior shoulder dislocation. A prospective comparison with arthroscopy of 25 cases. *J Shoulder Elbow Surg.* 1995;4:419–428.

48. Pevny T, Hunter RE, Freeman JR. Primary traumatic anterior shoulder dislocation in patients 40 years of age and older. *Arthroscopy.* 1998;14:289–294.

49. Gonzalez D, Lopez R. Concurrent rotator-cuff tear and brachial plexus palsy associated with anterior dislocation of the shoulder. A report of two cases. *J Bone Joint Surg Am.* 1991;73:620–621.

50. Yamamoto T, Yoshiya S, Kurosaka M, Nagira K, Nabeshima Y. Luxatio erecta (inferior dislocation of the shoulder): a report of 5 cases and a review of the literature. *Am J Orthop.* 2003;32(12):601–603.

51. Karaoglu S, Guney A, Ozturk M, Kekec Z. Bilateral luxatio erecta humeri. *Arch Orthop Trauma Surg.* 2003;123(6):308–310.

52. Arndt JH, Sears AD. Posterior dislocation of the shoulder. *AJR Am J Roentgenol.* 1965;94:81–86.

53. Cisternino SJ, Rogers LF, Stufflebam BC, Kruglik GD. The trough line: a radiographic sign of posterior shoulder dislocation. *AJR Am J Roentgenol.* 1978;130:951–954.

54. Wadlington VR, Hendrix RW, Rogers LF. Computed tomography of posterior fracture-dislocations of the shoulder: case reports. *J Trauma.* 1992;32:113–115.

55. Elberger ST, Brody G. Bilateral posterior shoulder dislocations. *Am J Emerg Med.* 1995;13:331–332.

56. Rath E, Levy O, Liberman N, Atar D. Bilateral dislocation of the hip during convulsions: a case report. *J Bone Joint Surg Br.* 1997;79:304–306.

57. Van Heest A, Vorlicky L, Thompson RC Jr. Bilateral central acetabular fracture dislocations secondary to sustained myoclonus. *Clin Orthop.* 1996;324:210–213.

58. McCullen GM, Brown CC. Seizure-induced thoracic burst fractures. A case report. *Spine.* 1994;19:77–79.

59. Mansat P, Frankle MA, Cofield RH. Tears in the subscapularis tendon: descriptive analysis and results of surgical repair. *Joint Bone Spine.* 2003;70(5):342–347.

60. Tung GA, Yoo DC, Levine SM, Brody JM, Green A. Subscapularis tendon tear: primary and associated signs on MRI. *J Comput Assist Tomogr.* 2001;25(3):417–424.

61. Hermann G, Klein MJ, Abdelwahab IF, Kenan S. Synovial chondrosarcoma arising in synovial chondromatosis of the right hip. *Skeletal Radiol.* 1997;26:366–369.

62. De Ferm A, Lagae K, Bunker T. Synovial osteochondromatosis: an unusual cause for subacromial impingement. *Acta Orthop Belg.* 1997;63:218–220.

63. Buess E, Friedrich B. Synovial chondromatosis of the glenohumeral joint: a rare condition. *Arch Orthop Trauma Surg.* 2001;121(1–2):109–111.

64. Resnick D. *Diagnosis of bone and joint disorders.* 4th ed. Philadelphia: WB Saunders; 2002:917–921.

65. Kuriyama S, Tomonari H, Nakayama M, Kawaguchi Y, Sakai O. Successful treatment of tumoral calcinosis using CAPD combined with hemodialysis with low-calcium dialysate. *Blood Purif.* 1998;16:43–48.

66. Ejaz AA, Nisar N, Ghandhi VC, Eilers DB, Shirazi PH, Ing TS. Metastatic soft tissue calcification in chronic renal failure detected by radionuclide imaging. *Clin Nucl Med.* 1995;20:505–507.

67. Gordon LF, Arger PH, Dalinka MK, Coleman BG. Computed tomography in soft tissue calcification layering. *J Comput Assist Tomogr.* 1984;8:71–73.

68. Sheldon PJ, Forrester DM. Imaging of amyloid arthropathy. *Semin Musculoskelet Radiol.* 2003;7(3):195–203.

69. Kurer MHJ, Baillod RA, Madgwick JCA. Musculoskeletal manifestations of amyloidosis: a review of 83 patients on haemodialysis for at least 10 years. *J Bone Joint Surg Br.* 1991;73B:271–276.

70. Penrod BJ, Resnik CS. Amyloid arthropathy. *Arthritis Rheum.* 1997;40:1903–1905.

71. Kaplan P, Resnick D, Murphey M, et al. Destructive noninfectious spondyloarthropathy in hemodialysis patients: a report of four cases. *Radiology.* 1987;162:241–244.

72. Murphey MD, Sartoris DJ, Quale JL, Pathria MN, Martin NL. Musculoskeletal manifestations of chronic renal insufficiency. *Radiographics.* 1993;13:357–379.

73. Cope R. Dislocations of the sternoclavicular joint. *Skeletal Radiol.* 1993;22:233–238.

74. Lewonowski K, Bassett GS. Complete posterior sternoclavicular epiphyseal separation. A case report and review of the literature. *Clin Orthop.* 1992;281:84–88.

75. Pai M, Park CH, Kim BS, Chung YS, Park HB. Multiple brown tumors in parathyroid carcinoma mimicking metastatic bone disease. *Clin Nucl Med.* 1997;22:691–694.

76. Kudo S. Elastofibroma dorsi: CT and MR imaging findings. *Semin Musculoskelet Radiol.* 2001;5(2):103–105.

77. Schick S, Zembsch A, Gahleitner A, et al. Atypical appearance of elastofibroma dorsi on MRI: case reports and review of the literature. *J Comput Assist Tomogr.* 2000;24(2):288–292.

78. Brandser EA, Goree JC, El-Khoury GY. Elastofibroma dorsi: prevalence in an elderly patient population as revealed by CT. *AJR Am J Roentgenol.* 1998;171:977–980.

79. Libshitz HI, Cohen MA. Radiation-induced osteochondromas. *Radiology.* 1982;142:643–647.

80. Jaffe N, Ried HL, Cohen M, McNeese MD, Sullivan MP. Radiation induced osteochondroma in long-term survivors of childhood cancer. *Int J Radiat Oncol Biol Phys.* 1983;9:665–670.

81. Mahboubi S, Dormans JP, D'Angio G. Malignant degeneration of radiation-induced osteochondroma. *Skeletal Radiol.* 1997;26(3):195–198.

CHAPTER THREE
SPINE

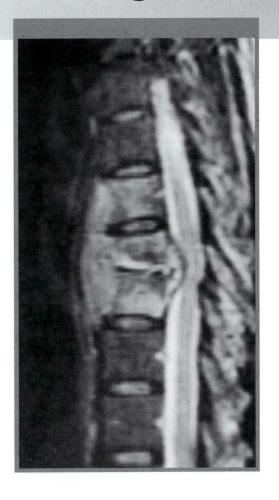

Clinical History: 35-year-old woman in an automobile accident.

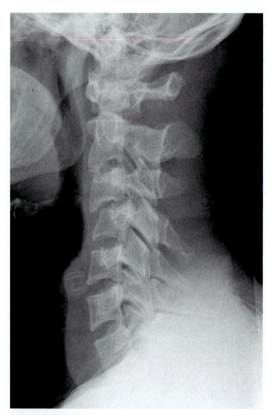

Figure 3-1 A

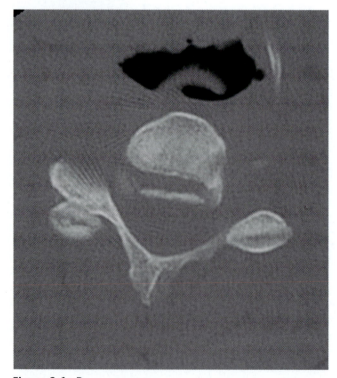

Figure 3-1 B

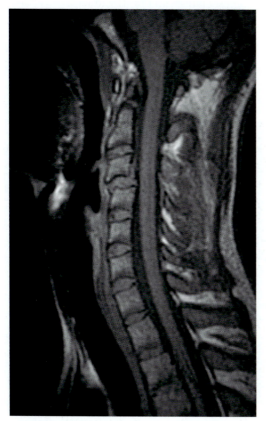

Figure 3-1 C

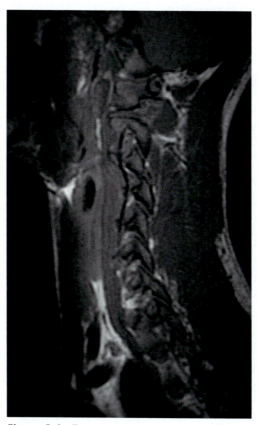

Figure 3-1 D

Findings: (**A**) Lateral radiograph of the cervical spine. There is 25% forward subluxation of C3 over C4. The interior facet of C3 is dislocated over the superior facet of C4, leaving it partially uncovered. Rotatory displacement is evident by the differences in the radiographic overlap of the facets above and below the level of injury. A focal kyphosis is present, and there is soft tissue swelling. (**B**) CT (bone windows) at the C3–C4 level shows the right inferior articular process of C3 is anterior to the right superior articular process of C4, but a normal relationship is present on the left. (**C**) Sagittal Proton Density (PD) MRI in the midline shows forward subluxation of C3 over C4 with a widening of the disc space. (**D**) MRI on the right shows the C3 facet dislocated over C4.

Differential Diagnosis: None.

Diagnosis: Unilateral facet dislocation (unilateral locked facet).

Discussion: The plain film is diagnostic in this case. C3 is anteriorly subluxated approximately 25% of a vertebral body width in conjunction with minimal distraction of the C3–4 disc space and a solitary "jumped" facet (the more superior facet is anterior to its articulating inferior facet). These findings are corroborated on CT and MRI. Unilateral facet dislocation occurs with hyperflexion and rotation [1]. Axial rotation and lateral bending are normally coupled in the middle and lower cervical spine because of the angle of the facet joints. With lateral bending, the facet joint on the concave side of the bend is compressed and essentially fixed, and the contralateral articular mass rides forward and up and dislocates into the intervertebral foramen. The superior portion of the inferior facet is frequently fractured, presumably from impaction. The ligaments are disrupted on the side of the dislocation. Unilateral facet dislocation is recognized by forward subluxation of the vertebral body, as shown here, combined with the dislocation of the facet. Sometimes the dislocated inferior facet can be seen projecting into the vertebral foramen (not shown), and the superior facet of the level below is uncovered or "naked" (shown on the plain radiographs). Soft tissue swelling is often present. The fanning of the spinous processes and widening of the disc space are indicative of the hyperflexion component of the injury. The CT can show the clockwise rotation of one vertebral body relative to the level below. In addition, the "reverse hamburger bun" sign can be demonstrated as replacement of the normal, flat, articulating surfaces with the convex surfaces in apposition [2]. CT can also define an associated articular process fracture, seen in up to 73% of cases. MRI would show the associated hemorrhage tracking along the anterior and posterior longitudinal ligaments. MRI can also identify associated soft tissue injuries [3] and serve as a screen to identify intimal injury of the vertebral artery.

Clinical History: Adult female automobile accident victim, acute presentation, and posttreatment.

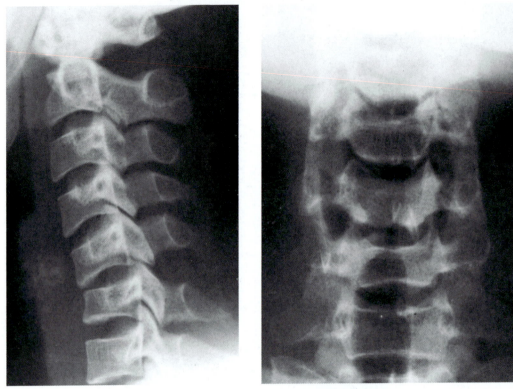

Figure 3-2   A   Figure 3-2   B

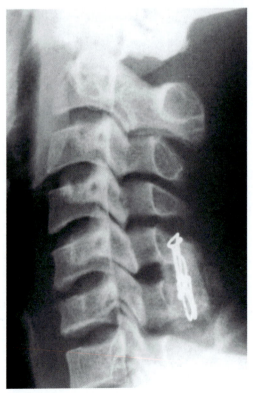

Figure 3-2   C

Findings: **(A)** Lateral radiograph of the cervical spine. There is narrowing of the C5–6 anterior disc space and widening of the posterior disc space. Marked widening is present between the C5 and C6 spinous processes. Mild prevertebral soft tissue swelling is present. No fracture is identified. **(B)** Anteroposterior (AP) radiograph of the cervical spine. The alignment in this projection is normal. **(C)** Lateral radiograph of the cervical spine, taken after treatment, shows normal alignment. The spinous processes of C5 and C6 have been wired together and fused with bone graft.

Differential Diagnosis: None.

Diagnosis: Hyperflexion sprain.

Discussion: When the neck is forcibly flexed, the cervical spine is distracted posteriorly and compressed anteriorly [4]. If the forces are relatively small, the injury may consist of a posterior ligamentous sprain (hyperflexion sprain) and possibly a compression fracture of the vertebral body. The radiographic hallmarks of a hyperflexion injury are a focal kyphosis in conjunction with narrowing of the anterior disc space, widening of the posterior disc space, and splaying of the spinous processes. Hyperflexion sprain results in a tear of the posterior longitudinal ligament complex (including the posterior longitudinal ligament, supraspinous and interspinous ligaments, joint capsule, and ligamentum flavum) [5]. This disruption allows anterior subluxation of the vertebral body by 1 to 3 mm in conjunction with mild subluxation of the facet joints. The radiographic findings may be subtle. Straightening of the cervical spine in the acute setting may be secondary to muscular trauma, and a focal kyphosis may ensue at a later time. Critical examination of the kyphotic level reveals an abnormal anterior subluxation of the superior vertebra, focal narrowing of the anterior disc space, widening of the posterior disc space, mild subluxation of the facet joints, and increased splaying of the spinous processes. Injury can occur at more than one level, and tends to spare levels with preexisting degenerative disease. This type of injury is associated with delayed instability in up to 50% of cases.

Clinical History: 22-year-old woman with chronic neck pain. She was in an automobile accident 2 years earlier.

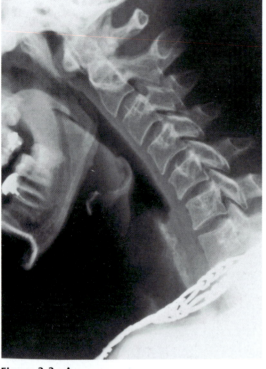

Figure 3-3   A

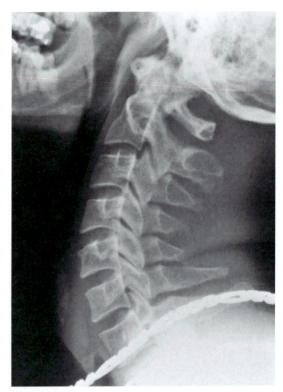

Figure 3-3   B

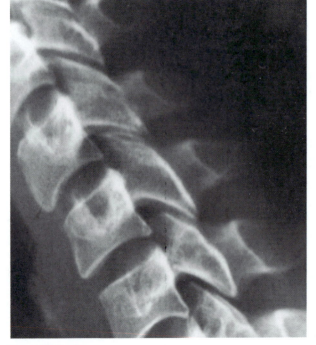

Figure 3-3   C

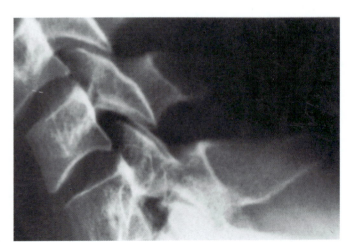

Figure 3-3   D

Findings: (A, B) Flexion-extension lateral cervical spine. A focal kyphosis is present at C5–6. The intervertebral disc space is narrowed anteriorly and widened posteriorly, and the spinous processes are splayed apart. The superior facets of C6 are partially uncovered. There are no fractures. Spot radiographs obtained during fluoroscopy show normal alignment in mild flexion (C) and kyphosis and posterior widening of the C5–6 intervertebral disc space with slightly more flexion (D).

Differential Diagnosis: Hyperflexion sprain, degenerative disc disease.

Diagnosis: Hyperflexion sprain, delayed diagnosis.

Discussion: At C5–6, there is subtle narrowing of the anterior disc space, and widening of the posterior disc space and spinous processes. No fractures are identified; therefore, this is considered a purely ligamentous injury. In severe hyperflexion sprain, damage to the posterior longitudinal ligament and the intervertebral discs, particularly the cartilage endplates [6], may result in an unstable injury. These injuries may be overlooked at the initial presentation [7], or the severity of the injury may not be appreciated, resulting in delayed diagnosis and treatment [8]. The preferred treatment is posterior wiring and fusion. Disruption of the posterior ligament complex may be evident on radiographs as a focal kyphosis localized to the level of the sprain, with fanning of the spinous processes. Anterior wedging is characteristic of hyperflexion sprains, as opposed to hyperextension sprains, which have posterior wedging. The abnormalities are accentuated with flexion and reduced with extension. The anterior compression fracture may be evident as loss of height, buckling of the anterior cortex, and disruption of the endplate. Prevertebral soft tissue swelling tends to be minimal and focal, reflecting the integrity of the anterior longitudinal ligament. If the direction of force is slightly to one side, the injuries may be eccentric. Fluoroscopy may demonstrate dynamic instability that is virtually inapparent on radiographic or other images obtained while the patient is in a single position.

Clinical History: 54-year-old man with chronic neck pain. He was involved in an automobile accident at age 20.

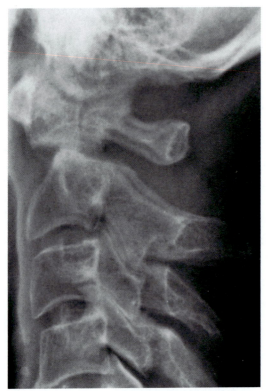

Figure 3-4   A

Figure 3-4   B

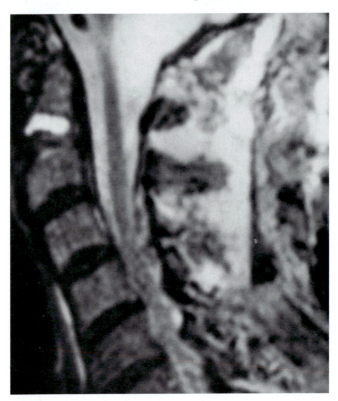

Figure 3-4   C

Findings: (A, B) Lateral cervical spine flexion-extension series. There is gross instability of C1 over C2 in both flexion and extension, resulting from an ununited odontoid fracture. Sclerotic, remodeled fracture margins with pseudoarthrosis are evidence of the chronicity of the lesion. The margins of the spinal canal at C1 and C2 are malaligned. (C) Sagittal T2-weighted MRI demonstrates a neutral position of the dens at the time of imaging, with T2 hyperintense fluid interposed between the C2 body and the dens. Extensive ligamentous edema is noted in the posterior neck musculature.

Differential Diagnosis: None.

Diagnosis: Nonunion of odontoid fracture (os odontoideum).

Discussion: Fractures of the odontoid process of C2 (dens) occur transversely across the base, probably as a result of hyperextension, hyperflexion, or lateral flexion [9]. The Anderson classification for fractures of the dens is as follows:

- (I) Superolateral odontoid, avulsed by the intact alar ligament, an exceedingly rare lesion.
- (II) Base of dens, "high dens fracture."
- (III) Superior axis, caudal to the odontoid base, "low dens fracture."

The odontoid is composed primarily of cortical bone, so this fracture heals less well than fractures through portions of the vertebra that are primarily cancellous. Schatzker et al. [10] report nonunion in 64% of type II fractures, and 100% of those with 5 mm or more of distraction.

An odontoid fracture that has progressed to atrophic nonunion is called an os odontoideum. Like nonunions elsewhere, the margins of the fracture line become corticated; a fibrous union or a pseudoarthrosis may be present. Although some authorities argue that the os odontoideum is a developmental variant in which the odontoid process does not fuse to the body of C2, the site of the synchondrosis between the odontoid process and the body of C2 is not located here. Because of present or potential mechanical instability, surgical fusion of C1 and C2 is the common method of management.

This is a complex case because the sclerotic dens margin suggests chronicity, whereas the prevertebral soft tissue swelling indicates a superimposed acute injury. The instability of the upper cervical spine leaves the spine vulnerable to catastrophic injury with relatively minor trauma.

Clinical History: 43-year-old automobile accident victim.

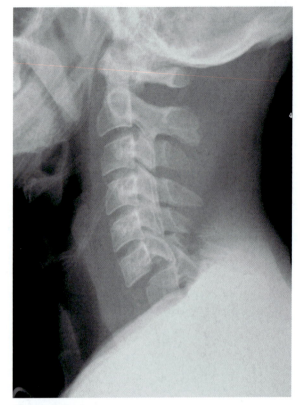

Figure 3-5   A

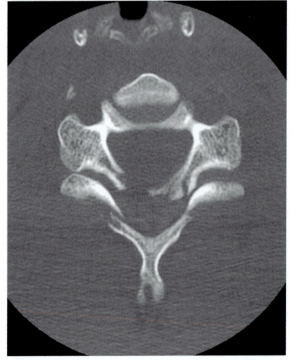

Figure 3-5   B

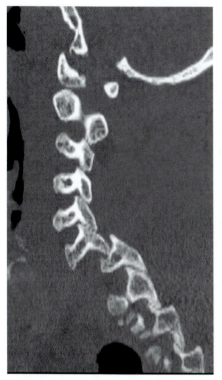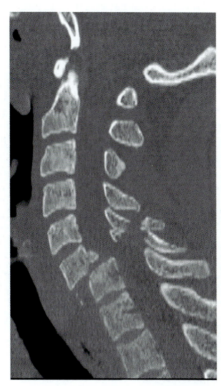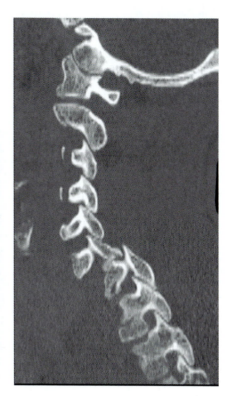

Figure 3-5 C

Findings: (A) Lateral radiograph of the cervical spine. The cervical spine is disrupted at C6–C7, with approximately 50% of the body of C6 displaced anteriorly relative to C7. The superior articular facets of C7 are not covered by the inferior articular facets of C6 (naked facet sign). Rotatory displacement is absent. (B) Axial CT at the level of the C6–C7 disc space shows forward displacement of C6 over C7. Laminar fractures are present. (C) Sagittal CT reformats through the left lateral masses, the midline, and the right lateral masses show the dislocated C6–C7 facets, the forward subluxation of the vertebral bodies, and spinous process fractures.

Differential Diagnosis: None.

Diagnosis: Bilateral facet dislocation (bilateral locked facets).

Discussion: The plain film evidence of greater than 50% anterolisthesis of C6 relative to C7 is diagnostic of this entity. CT is usually recommended to characterize the injury, identify the fractures, and locate any fragments.

The major injury vector in bilateral facet dislocation is hyperflexion of large magnitude without axial compression [11]. Bilateral facet dislocation is a tension injury that propagates from posterior to anterior. Complete disruption of the ligaments and forward displacement of one involved vertebra over another allows the inferior articular facets of the superjacent vertebra to dislocate into the intervertebral foramen. In addition to disruption of the posterior longitudinal complex, seen in unilateral facet dislocation, the disc and anterior longitudinal ligament are disrupted, allowing the superior vertebra to be subluxated anteriorly by about 50% of the width of its body. When the facets are subluxated (perched) but not completely dislocated ("partial dislocation"), the anterior subluxation is greater than the 3 mm seen in a flexion strain, but less than the 50% seen in the complete dislocation. There may be accompanying fractures of the articular processes of the subjacent vertebra, but these are commonly detected only with CT. The spine is unstable, and there is a high association with cord contusion. MRI is better than CT for demonstrating possible cord injury and other soft tissue abnormalities [12].

Clinical History: 33-year-old man who was the front seat passenger in an automobile accident.

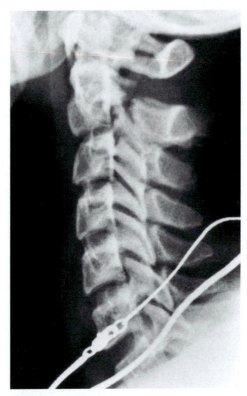

Figure 3-6   A

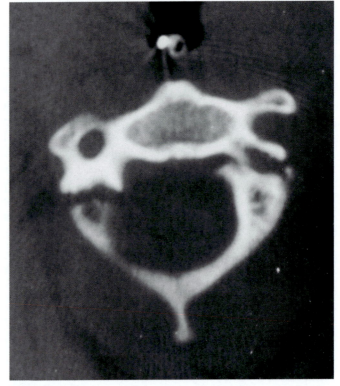

Figure 3-6   B

Findings: (A) Lateral radiograph of the cervical spine. The patient has been intubated. Horizontal fractures through the pars interarticularis allowed the anterior portion of C2 to incline forward. The posterior arch fragment of C2 is displaced posteriorly, resulting in a segmental widening of the spinal canal. (B) Axial CT demonstrates the mild distraction at the fracture sites. The fractures have a transverse morphology in the axial plane from tensile loading. Evaluation of the prevertebral soft tissues is unreliable in the presence of an endotracheal tube.

Differential Diagnosis: None.

Diagnosis: Traumatic C2 spondylolisthesis.

Discussion: In traumatic C2 spondylolisthesis (hangman's fracture), there are bilateral pars interarticularis fractures with forward subluxation of C2 over C3 [13]. The pars interarticularis is the bridge of bone that occupies the position in the articular mass between the superior and inferior articular facets.

An individual subjected to judicial hanging drops feet first through a trap door with a rope secured around the neck and the hangman's knot located under the chin. When he or she reaches the end of the rope, the upper cervical spine is pulled violently into hyperextension and simultaneously subjected to massive distractive forces from the downward inertia of the body. The ligaments of the anterior column tear at the C2–3 level, and the posterior elements are fractured at the pars interarticularis. Similar fractures of the C2 posterior elements may also occur when an axial load (compressive rather than distractive) is applied with the neck hyperextended. This may occur in a motor vehicle accident in which the passenger slides forward and strikes the forehead, forcing the neck into hyperextension.

The Effendi classification is as follows:

- (I) Minimal to no displacement of C2.
- (II) Anteriorly displaced C2 anterior elements, with narrowing of the C2–3 disc space.
- (III) Anteriorly displaced C2 anterior elements, flexed attitude, and bilateral facet dislocation of C2–3.

There are associated injuries in 14% of cases, half of which involved the C1 posterior arch or dens.

The resulting neurologic deficits are often absent or minimal because of the typically capacious spinal canal at this level, and the fact that the fragments spread circumferentially (with the exception of the type III variant).

Clinical History: 27-year-old man with quadriplegia after rescue from an automobile accident, and a companion case.

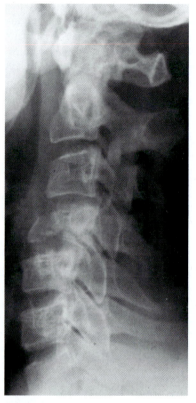

Figure 3-7   A

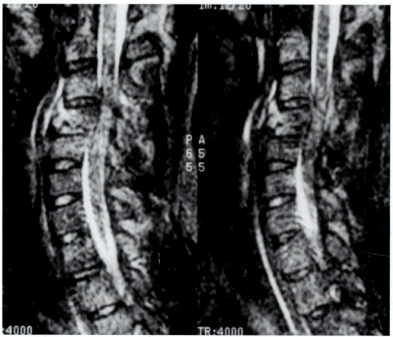

Figure 3-7   B

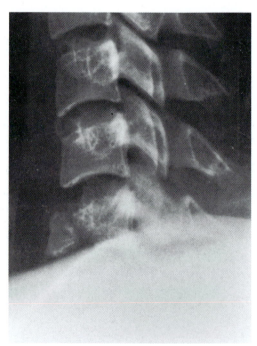

Figure 3-7   C

Findings: (A) Lateral radiograph of the cervical spine. A fracture of the body of C4 is present with anterior soft tissue swelling. The major portion of the C4 vertebra remains in normal alignment, whereas the anteroinferior teardrop fragment is rotated anteriorly. Mild soft tissue swelling is evident by a contour abnormality of the anterior prevertebral soft tissues. (B) Sagittal T2-weighted MRI at the midline shows the fracture at C4. The spinal canal is narrowed, with impingement on the spinal cord. (C) Companion case. Lateral radiograph of the cervical spine shows a displaced teardrop fragment of the body of C6, which is also compressed.

Differential Diagnosis: None.

Diagnosis: Hyperflexion teardrop fracture.

Discussion: The hyperflexion teardrop injury is the result of axial compression with hyperflexion caused by large forces, leading to a fracture-dislocation [14]. An example of this type of loading might be diving into shallow water with the chin tucked, flexing the neck [15]. Massive posterior distractive forces disrupt the posterior ligament complex and dislocate the facet joints. The anterior and middle columns are disrupted, with tears of the longitudinal ligaments and the intervertebral disc. A triangular fragment (teardrop fragment) is sheared off the anteroinferior corner of the dislocating vertebral body. The result is complete disruption of the cervical spine, with the superior portion displaced posteriorly and angulated anteriorly. The injury is recognized radiographically by focal kyphosis, posterior dislocation, distraction of the posterior elements, and wedging deformity of the vertebral body with teardrop fragment off the anteroinferior corner. The teardrop fragment usually remains aligned with the vertebral column inferior to the level of injury, whereas the remainder of the vertebral body and the vertebral column superior to the injury will be displaced posteriorly. This retrolisthesis may result in widening of the facet joints and disruption of the spinolaminar line. Sagittal fractures of the vertebral body and laminae, caused by the axial loading, are commonly associated. Diffuse, marked, anterior prevertebral soft tissue swelling is always present. The most common site of involvement is C5. The hyperflexion teardrop fracture-dislocation is a highly unstable injury and the spinal cord is always injured. Although paraplegia or quadriplegia can result, the characteristic injury associated with this fracture is the anterior cord syndrome, which consists of complete motor paralysis coupled with a loss of pain, temperature, and touch, but preservation of the posterior column functions of vibration and position.

Clinical History: 36-year-old man in an automobile accident, and a companion case.

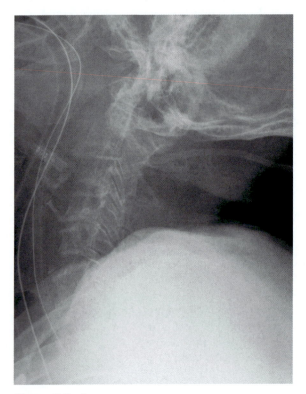

Figure 3-8   A

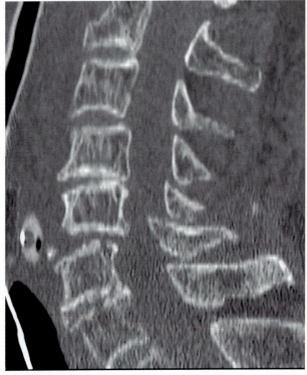

Figure 3-8   B

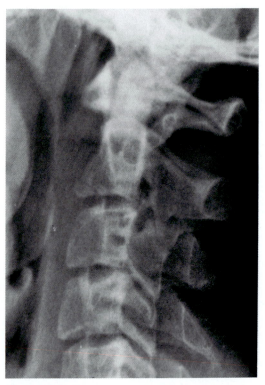

Figure 3-8   C

Findings: (A) Lateral radiograph of the cervical spine. Anterior soft tissue swelling is present. At the C5–C6 level, the intervertebral disc space is widened anteriorly and narrowed posteriorly. There is retrolisthesis of C5 relative to C6. A small fragment of the C5 body remains aligned with the anterior aspect of C6. (B) Sagittal CT reformation shows the misalignment of C5 over C6. (C) Companion case. Lateral radiograph of the cervical spine shows anterior soft tissue swelling and a nondisplaced fracture of the anteroinferior corner of the body of C2. Alignment is normal.

Differential Diagnosis: None.

Diagnosis: Hyperextension sprain at C5–C6 with teardrop fragment (companion case, hyperextension sprain at C2–C3 with tear drop fragment).

Discussion: Widening of the anterior disc space and narrowing of the posterior disc space is the hallmark for a hyperextension injury. Axial loading with hyperextension places the anterior column under tension, and the posterior column under compression [16]. Structures of the spine fail in sequence, depending on the magnitude of the loading: tear of the anterior longitudinal ligament, disruption of the intervertebral disc, and tear of the posterior longitudinal ligament. A tension fracture of the anterior inferior corner of the vertebral body may occur instead of disc disruption, as in this case. If present, the triangular fracture fragment may be called a teardrop fragment, and the injury may be called a hyperextension teardrop fracture, but the significance of this fragment is the accompanying ligamentous injury. The anteroinferior avulsion may remain undisplaced, or may be rotated anteriorly from the vertebral body on an intact hinge of anterior longitudinal ligament. If the spine reduces after the injury, the teardrop fragment may be the best radiographic clue to the presence of the more serious injury. Compression fractures of the posterior elements are common, including fractures of the lamina and lateral masses. One or both facet joints may become dislocated. If only ligaments are disrupted and the spine relocates on the rebound, radiographs may show a normally aligned spine without fracture in an acutely quadriplegic patient. Marked prespinal soft tissue swelling should be present.

This injury is most commonly seen in older patients with osteopenia or cervical spondylosis [17]. The prevertebral soft tissue swelling can be minimal in older patients.

Clinical History: 70-year-old man who fell.

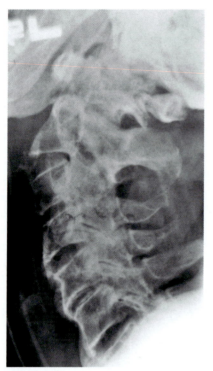

Figure 3-9 A

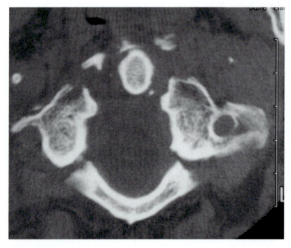

Figure 3-9 B

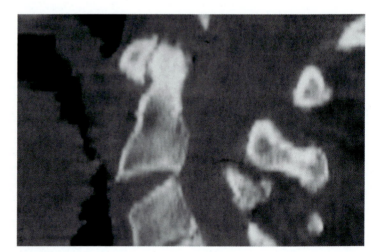

Figure 3-9 C

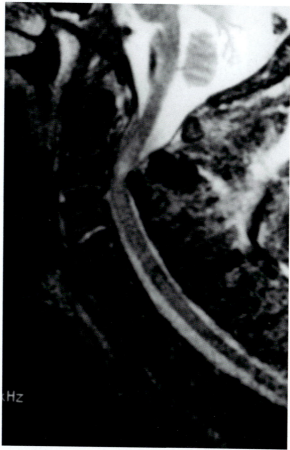

Figure 3-9 D

Findings: (**A**) Lateral radiograph of the cervical spine demonstrates widening of the C1 ring. Increased distraction of the C2–3 disc space is noted, with an accentuated, focal lordosis. There are incidental findings of diffuse idiopathic skeletal hyperostosis (DISH). (**B**) Axial CT demonstrates Jefferson burst fracture at C1. (**C**) Detail of sagittally reformatted CT image shows the increased distraction and lordosis at C2–3 and the displacement of the posterior arch of C1. (**D**) Sagittal T2-weighted MRI at the midline demonstrates mechanical impingement on the posterior aspect of the cervical spinal cord at the C2–3 level. High signal in the cord itself indicates contusion.

Differential Diagnosis: None.

Diagnosis: Complex C1–2 fractures.

Discussion: Mimics of a Jefferson fracture include the isolated posterior C1 arch fracture (which can be distinguished by the lack of prevertebral soft tissue swelling), and the congenital fusion failure of posterior C1 arch. These can be differentiated by CT.

This case illustrates the importance of careful screening after identifying one injury [18]. Distraction of the C2–3 disc space is most suggestive of a concurrent hyperextension injury.

The classic axial load injury is the Jefferson fracture, which consists of a disruption of the anterior and posterior arches of C1. The fractures can be unilateral or bilateral. The transverse ligament can be intact or disrupted, resulting in widening of the anterior or lateral atlantodental interval. If there is a vertical fracture through one of the articular masses, the medial fragment may maintain its normal relationship with the dens while the lateral fragment migrates laterally.

The odontoid view is most helpful by showing the increase in the atlantodental interval. The lateral view obscures the anterior arch and simply shows the prevertebral soft tissue swelling, and sometimes the posterior arch disruption.

Cervical spine fractures in the elderly are relatively common, comprising 23% of cervical spine fractures in one study [19]. Virtually all fractures in the elderly age group involve the atlantoaxial complex [20], with the most common lesion being a fracture of the odontoid process or a combination of fractures of both C1 and C2, as in this case. The injuries are associated with considerable morbidity and mortality, mostly from coexisting respiratory disease [21]. Treatment with a rigid collar, a halo brace, or surgical stabilization may be successful according to circumstance.

Clinical History: Unconscious 13-year-old girl after a motor vehicle accident, and a companion case.

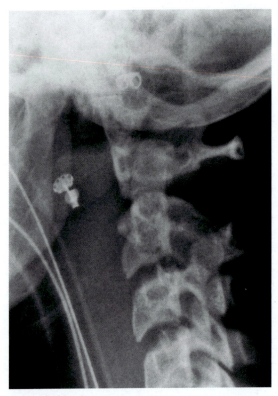

Figure 3-10 A

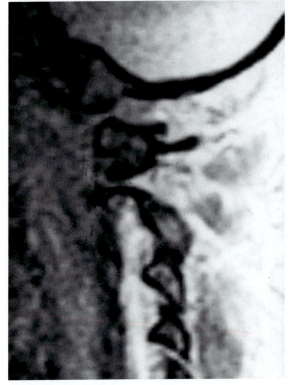

Figure 3-10 B

Findings: (A) Lateral radiograph of the cervical spine. The prevertebral soft tissues are massively enlarged, even with intubation of the patient. The integrity of the craniocervical junction is difficult to assess, but the upper cervical spine appears intact. (B) Companion case: 42-year-old woman ejected from rollover motor vehicle accident. Sagittal T2-weighted MRI through the left atlantooccipital joint demonstrates marked forward subluxation of the occipital condyle. The appearance of the right atlantooccipital joint (not shown) is similar.

Differential Diagnosis: None.

Diagnosis: Atlantooccipital dislocation.

Discussion: The craniocervical junction is evaluated on radiographs with lateral and open mouth views. Soft tissue swelling is an invariable finding in the acute presentation, as seen here. The superior facets of the lateral masses of C1 should articulate with the occipital condyles. Although there are several indirect radiographic methods for assessing the craniocervical junction, they depend on accurately positioned radiographs, which are often difficult to obtain in the acute setting with multiple injuries. When injury is suspected by the mechanism of trauma and the presence of soft tissue swelling, even if the relationship of the occipital condyles to the superior facets of the atlas appears normal on radiographs, direct imaging with cross-sectional methods (CT or MRI) is still indicated.

Traumatic atlantooccipital dislocation has generally been considered to be incompatible with life, but many patients have survived this injury [22–25]. As CT is being used more frequently to screen for cervical spine injuries, less severe forms of atlantooccipital dislocation are being recognized. Early diagnosis is crucial in order to avoid life-threatening diagnostic manipulations, such as attempts at flexion-extension views, and to provide adequate treatment. This is a particular concern in patients with multiple traumas. Unrecognized traumatic atlantooccipital dislocation may contribute to deterioration and rapid demise of patients who arrive from the scene alert and neurologically intact. Patients who survive these injuries often have severe spinal cord injury, but there are reports of recovery with good neurologic outcome [26]. Cerebral trauma is frequently associated. Treatment is halo immobilization and surgical fusion of the occiput to C1 and C2.

Clinical History: 57-year-old man with a stiff, painful neck.

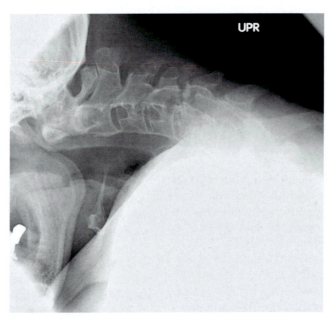

Figure 3-11   A

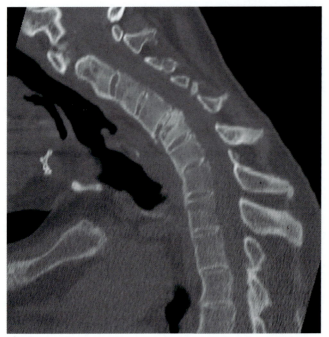

Figure 3-11   B

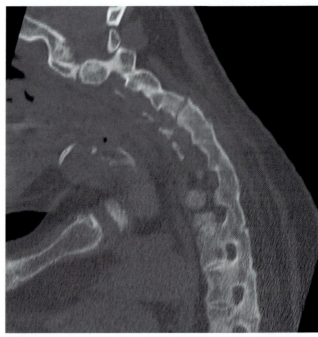

Figure 3-11   C

Findings: (A) Lateral radiograph of the cervical spine shows severe cervical kyphosis, but vertebral heights are normal. There is ankylosis of the facet joints and intervertebral disc joints, and the anterior corners of the vertebral bodies are squared off. The bones are osteoporotic. In addition, there is a minimally displaced fracture that extends through the entire vertebral column at the C4–C5 level. (B, C) Sagittal reformatted images from CT show the fracture plane extending through the upper portion of the body of C5 and then through the fused posterior elements of C4 and C5.

Differential Diagnosis: Ankylosing spondylitis, juvenile idiopathic arthritis, DISH.

Diagnosis: Ankylosing spondylitis, with fracture.

Discussion: The combination of ankyloses of the facet joints and syndesmophytes is diagnostic of this disorder. The delicacy of the syndesmophytes and the presence of osteopenia are key differential features relative to DISH. Preservation of vertebral body height and intervertebral disc spaces are key differential features relative to juvenile idiopathic arthritis. Syndesmophyte formation in ankylosing spondylitis is the result of inflammation that leads to ossification of the outer layers of the annulus fibrosis. The resulting bridges of bone that fuse the adjacent vertebral bodies should not extend beyond the endplates. Ankylosing spondylitis affects the synovial articulations, cartilaginous articulations, and entheses. In synovial joints, the inflammatory process is a synovitis that is pathologically similar to rheumatoid arthritis, but less intense. Inflammatory fibroplasia of synovium can transform into chondroid metaplasia that then ossifies, resulting in ankylosis; this is a major feature of this disease, unlike rheumatoid arthritis.

Similar pathologic abnormalities occur in cartilaginous articulations. Swollen fibrocytes in the outer annulus fibrosis layers at the attachment of Sharpey's fibers undergo chondroid metaplasia and ossify, resulting in the smooth, flowing appearance of syndesmophyte formation. Pain diminishes or disappears as the spine fuses, but the fused spine becomes osteoporotic and fragile and is subject to insufficiency fractures. Fusion usually begins at the lumbosacral junction and extends superiorly.

The enthesopathy is a feature that distinguishes ankylosing spondylitis and the other seronegative spondyloarthropathies from other inflammatory forms of arthritis. In the spondyloarthropathies, inflammation at sites of ligamentous attachments may heal with the formation of osseous excrescences. The typical onset of ankylosing spondylitis is insidious low back pain and stiffness in adolescent White men. In the severe classic form, there is gross ankylosis and deformity of the spine; in mild forms, there may only be occasional arthralgias. In most cases, ankylosing spondylitis is a benign, self-limited, and undiagnosed disease with absent or minimal radiographic changes. The overall sex distribution is probably equal, but men generally have severe, progressive disease and women have mild, self-limited disease. The disease progresses most rapidly during the first 10 years after presentation. Ankylosis and peripheral arthritis may result in permanent functional loss.

CASE 3-12

Clinical History: 43-year-old woman with polyarticular arthritis, and a companion case.

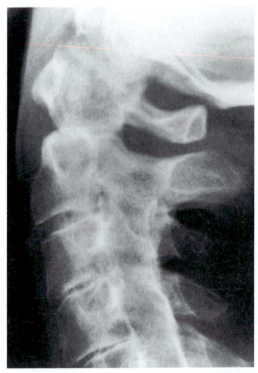

Figure 3-12   A

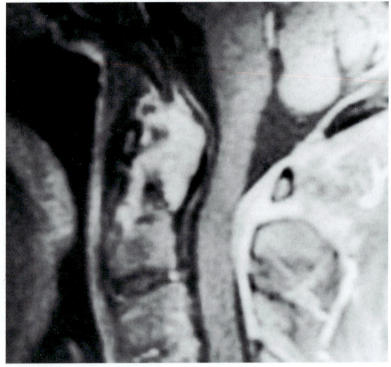

Figure 3-12   B

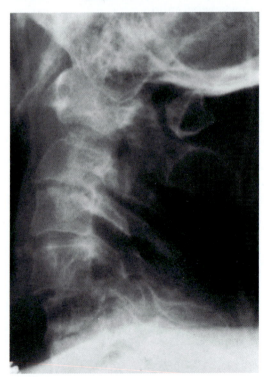

Figure 3-12   C

Findings: (**A**) Lateral cervical spine (neutral position). The atlantoaxial distance is difficult to assess since there is marked irregularity of the odontoid. Generalized osteoporosis is present. The visualized facets are fused. (**B**) Sagittal T1-weighted MRI with gadolinium demonstrates marked erosion of the odontoid, with an effective increase in the atlantoaxial distance. Marked enhancement of pannus is identified. Companion case. (**C**) Lateral cervical spine. There is axial migration of the C2 vertebral body with absence of the dens. Subluxation is most prominent at C5–6. Whittling of the C3, C4, and C5 spinous processes is noted. Disc space narrowing with associated endplate is present at C6–7, but also at the uncommon C3–4 level.

Differential Diagnosis: Rheumatoid arthritis, ankylosing spondylitis, juvenile idiopathic arthritis.

Diagnosis: Rheumatoid arthritis.

Discussion: In the cervical spine, multilevel subluxation, osteopenia, and erosions at sites of ligamentous attachments without evidence for reparative bone is characteristic of rheumatoid arthritis. Erosion of the odontoid and instability of the atlantoaxial articulation is a classic presentation for rheumatoid arthritis. Other etiologies for these two findings might include congenital hypoplasia of the odontoid with ligamentous instability, amyloid, or perhaps an atypical infection. Atlantoaxial subluxation is the dominant and the first cervical spine finding, and may occur without radiographic evidence for erosions [27]. A measurement of greater than 2.5 mm between the inferior aspect of the posterior C1 arch and anterior dens is diagnostic. It typically results from disruption of the transverse ligament by pannus formation, as demonstrated here by MRI. Axial migration of the C2 vertebral body is not uncommon as the odontoid dissolves and a potential space is created.

In the lower cervical spine, subluxations are most prominent at the C3–4 and C4–5 levels. Anterior subluxation is most common, and the levels of involvement are commonly discontinuous. Apophyseal joint space narrowing and erosions are can lead to instability or fibrous union. Discovertebral narrowing, erosion, and late subchondral sclerosis without osteophyte formation can be seen. Whittling of the spinous processes at the insertion of the supraspinous ligaments may be identified. Generalized osteoporosis may be secondary to the disease process or the use of steroids. Compared with other patients with rheumatoid arthritis, those with cervical involvement tend to have a positive rheumatoid factor, higher C-reactive protein level, and progression of peripheral joint disease.

CASE 3-13

Clinical History: 42-year-old woman with polyarticular disease.

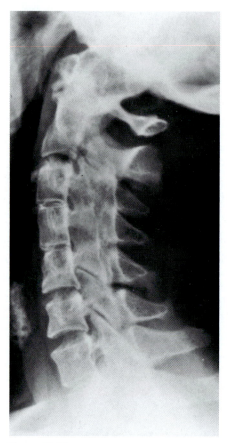

Figure 3-13

Findings: Lateral radiograph of the cervical spine demonstrates fusion of the C3, C4, and C5 facets, with hypoplasia of the respective vertebral bodies and calcification of the intervertebral discs.

Differential Diagnosis: Ankylosing spondylitis, juvenile chronic arthritis, DISH.

Diagnosis: Juvenile idiopathic arthritis.

Discussion: Diffuse ankylosis of the facet joints in the cervical spine is associated with two conditions: ankylosing spondylitis and juvenile idiopathic arthritis. Distinguishing between the two on radiographs is often possible because ankylosing spondylitis is a disease that involves the mature skeleton, whereas juvenile idiopathic arthritis, by definition, involves the immature, growing skeleton. In the latter, stigmata of the disease process itself and of the effects of the disease on skeletal development should be evident. Thus, diffuse ankylosis of the facet joints in combination with hypoplasia of the vertebral bodies and intervertebral discs is virtually diagnostic for juvenile idiopathic arthritis. In ankylosing spondylitis, the vertebral body and intervertebral disc heights remain normal, even in the presence of ankylosis of the facet joints and syndesmophyte formation, because the spine has already developed fully at the time the disease process affects it.

The cervical spine is more commonly involved with juvenile idiopathic arthritis than other spinal levels [28]. The most common finding is that of atlantoaxial instability; however, other considerations for this finding in a child would include Down's syndrome, odontoid hypoplasia, and Grisel's syndrome (infectious laxity as an extension of a peripharyngeal process).

The apophyseal joint fusion is most common at the C2–3 and C3–4 levels, as seen in this case. Because this occurs before full growth potential, the constellation of ankylosis and vertebral body and disc hypoplasia is diagnostic.

Other etiologies of apophyseal joint fusion can be excluded by their secondary findings. In addition, enthesopathy and tarsal disease within the first year of presentation is diagnostic of juvenile ankylosing spondylitis, with or without the presence of axial disease. Klippel-Feil syndrome (congenital fusion anomaly) may be difficult to distinguish unless posterior element fusion is a dominant feature. Fibrodysplasia ossificans progressiva should have an element of soft tissue ossification.

CASE 3-14

Clinical History: 25-year-old man with back pain in the upper cervical region for several months.

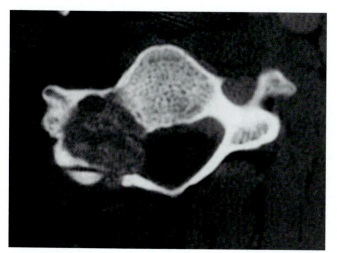

Figure 3-14 A

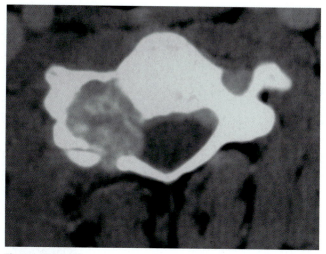

Figure 3-14 B

Findings: (A, B) CT (bone and soft tissue windows). CT shows an expansile lesion in the right lateral mass of a cervical vertebra (C4), extending into the spinal canal, transverse foramen, and vertebral body. Focal destruction of the cortex is present. The lesion is well circumscribed, but does not have reactive margin of bone. The lesion is mineralized.

Differential Diagnosis: Osteoblastoma, aneurysmal bone cyst, osteosarcoma, brown tumor, fibrous dysplasia.

Diagnosis: Osteoblastoma.

Discussion: Differential considerations in this case include osteoid osteoma (if the lesion were less than 2 cm), osteosarcoma (if the lesion had a more aggressive appearance or associated soft tissue mass), aneurysmal bone cyst (which can be seen in conjunction with an osteoblastoma; therefore, the pathologist ultimately distinguishes between the two), giant cell tumor (if the lesion were less well-defined), and a brown tumor (if the patient had other clinical evidence for hyperparathyroidism).

Osteoblastomas are uncommon lesions considered by some to be giant osteoid osteomas because of their histologic resemblance [29]. They affect young people—80% occur in patients younger than 30 years old—and there is a male predominance. About half are located in the spine and most of the remainder in the femur and tibia; 9% are located in the cervical spine [30,31]. Of those in the spine, most are in the posterior elements, but a few also involve the vertebral body, and very few involve the vertebral body alone.

The radiographic appearance is a partially lucent expansile lesion, with well-defined thin sclerotic margins and a variable amount of matrix mineralization. The lucent area of geographic bone destruction corresponds to replacement of bone by nonmineralized tumor tissue. The tumor osteoid may have densely solid or ground-glass mineralization. Large lesions may have an expanded cortical shell from slow endosteal cortical erosion, balanced against an enlarging layer of periosteal new bone. Cortical penetration into the soft tissues is absent, but tomography may be required to demonstrate the cortical shell. The tumor tissue may have high attenuation on CT from the diffuse mineralization. Osteoblastomas are hot on bone scan. They usually grow slowly and respond well to excision; radiation is useful when the lesion is difficult to excise. Very few have been reported to become locally aggressive. In the cervical spine, lesions in close proximity to the vertebral artery require complex therapeutic solutions [32].

CASE 3-15

Clinical History: 53-year-old man with neck pain for several weeks.

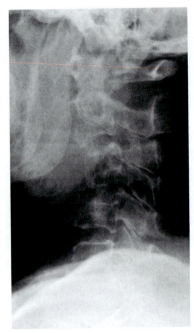

Figure 3-15   A

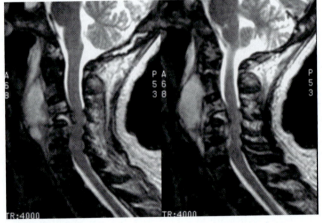

Figure 3-15   B

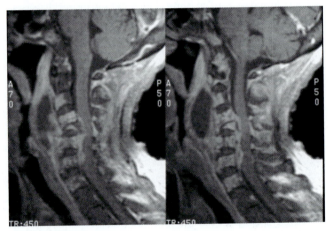

Figure 3-15   C

Findings: (A) Lateral radiograph of the cervical spine through a cervical collar. The C4 vertebral body has dissolved and the C3–4 and C4–5 disc spaces are narrowed. Marked prevertebral soft tissue swelling is identified. (B) Sagittal T2-weighted MRI shows partial collapse of C4 and C5, with prevertebral fluid collection and posterior mass effect on the spinal cord. The abnormality extends along several levels. (C) Sagittal T1-weighted MRI after gadolinium shows enhancement involving most of the cervical spine, with no enhancement of the prevertebral collection.

Differential Diagnosis: Pyogenic diskitis, tuberculous spondylitis, metastasis, lymphoma, massive vertebral osteolysis (Gorham's disease), trauma.

Diagnosis: Tuberculous spondylitis.

Discussion: At first glance, one might suspect osteolytic destruction secondary to tumor or Gorham's disease, but the large prevertebral fluid collection would be expected only with infection. Pyogenic infections typically arise in the disc space and provoke reactive bone formation, whereas tuberculosis tends to provoke little, if any, reactive bone formation. The large retropharyngeal abscess and the multilevel involvement would also be very unusual in pyogenic diskitis. Although tuberculosis is becoming more common in North America, involvement of the cervical spine remains rare, comprising only 3% to 5% of cases of tuberculosis of the spine. Patients present with neck pain and may have a kyphotic deformity. In children, the disease is frequently extensive, with paraspinal abscess formation [33], while in adults it is more commonly localized to one or two segments. Cord compression is common, and patients may develop reversible quadriparesis as a result [34]. The treatment of tuberculous spondylitis in the cervical spine is similar to treatment of tuberculosis elsewhere in the spine, and consists of antituberculous chemotherapy and, when necessary, surgical resection of abscesses and mechanical stabilization.

Clinical History: 13-year-old boy with short stature.

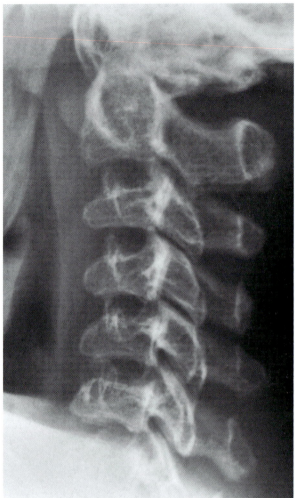

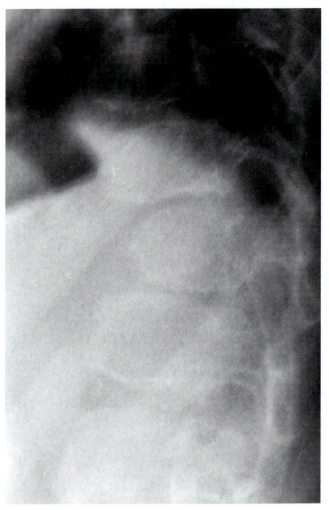

Figure 3-16 A   **Figure 3-16 B**

Findings: (A) Lateral radiograph of the cervical spine. There is flattening of the visualized cervical vertebral bodies and hypoplasia of the odontoid process. (B) Lateral radiograph of the thoracic spine. There is hypoplasia of the T11 vertebral body with a central beak deformity.

Differential Diagnosis: Mucopolysaccharidoses (dysostosis multiplex), spondyloepiphyseal dysplasia.

Diagnosis: Morquio's syndrome.

Discussion: Morquio's syndrome, or mucopolysaccharidosis IV A, is an autosomal recessive deficiency of the enzyme N-acetylgalactosamine-6-sulfatase, and has a frequency of 1 in 100,000 births [35]. The key radiologic feature in this case is flattening of the cervical vertebral bodies at every level (universal platyspondyly). In addition, the findings of hypoplastic odontoid with secondary atlantoaxial instability are common in this condition. Although it would be unrealistic for a radiologist to make a specific biochemical and genetic diagnosis from these radiographs, one should recognize that a systemic, congenital disease is present. Morquio's syndrome is one of the mucopolysaccharidoses, or diseases caused by inborn errors of complex carbohydrate metabolism. The skeletal features of all these conditions have been collectively called dysostosis multiplex, and are the manifestation of storage of abnormal complex carbohydrate substances that cannot be metabolized further because of enzyme deficiencies. The mucopolysaccharidoses share the findings of macrocephaly; "canoe paddle shaped" ribs; focal kyphosis with distinctive centrally beaked, diminutive retrolisthesed L1 or L2 vertebral body; flared pelvis; and shortened, broadened long bones [36].

In Morquio's syndrome, the platyspondyly tends to be more widespread and marked than in the other mucopolysaccharidoses, which is a possible clue to the specific diagnosis.

CASE 3-17

Clinical History: Asymptomatic 11-year-old boy.

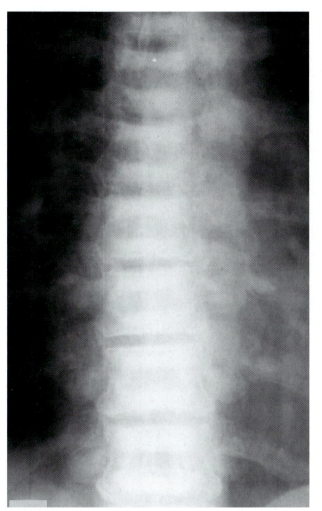

Figure 3-17 A

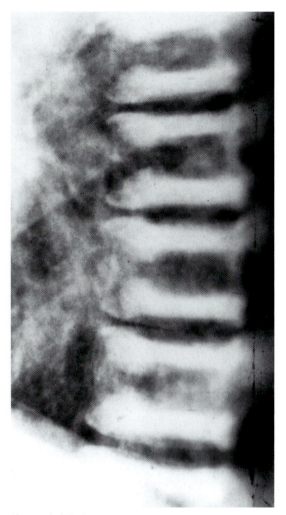

Figure 3-17 B

Findings: (A) AP and (B) lateral radiograph of the thoracic spine shows that the vertebral bodies have a uniform "sandwich" appearance, with sharply demarcated sclerosis abutting the endplates. The vertebral body heights and alignment are normal.

Differential Diagnosis: Osteopetrosis, renal osteodystrophy, degenerative disc disease.

Diagnosis: Osteopetrosis.

Discussion: The sandwich appearance of vertebral bodies results from horizontal layers of increased bony density involving the upper and lower ends of the vertebral body, with a less dense central portion. This appearance is distinguished from the rugger jersey spine of renal osteodystrophy by the sharpness of the margin between sclerotic and less sclerotic bone and, of course, by the absence of other features of renal osteodystrophy. Discogenic sclerosis may also have the appearance of horizontal stripes of sclerosis, but is seen only in

combination with degenerative disc disease in older patients. The exact pathogenesis of the layers of sclerotic bone in osteopetrosis is unknown, but this appearance is classic for the autosomal dominant osteopetrosis with delayed manifestations that was originally described by Albers-Schoenberg [41]. The sandwich appearance may also be thought of as a variation of the bone-in-bone appearance that may be seen in the pelvis or the long bones. A central core of more primitive, coarsely fibrillar, and cellular osseous tissue becomes surrounded by dense new bone during growth that is not able to remodel into normal trabecular and cortical bone. Osteopetrosis is a group of heritable diseases characterized by reduced bone resorption from osteoclast failure [42]. Many genetic defects may cause osteoclast failure, and each has different underlying biochemical and histopathologic abnormalities. The final common effect is that bone remodels incompletely or not at all.

Clinical History: 26-year-old patient with congenital ichthyosis.

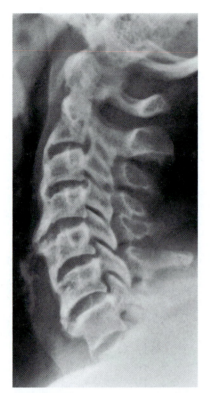

Figure 3-18   A

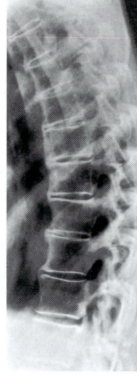

Figure 3-18   B

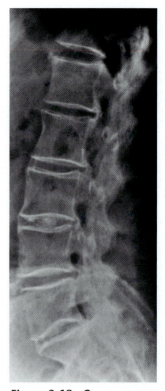

Figure 3-18   C

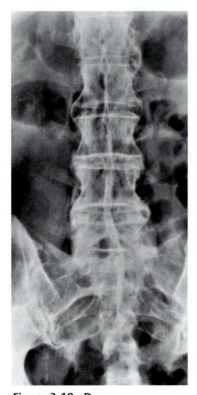

Figure 3-18   D

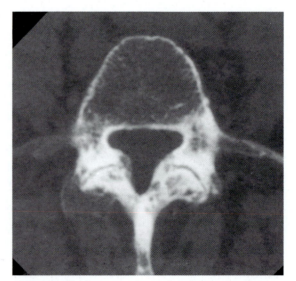

Figure 3-18   E

Findings: (A, B) Lateral radiographs of the cervical and thoracic spine demonstrate flowing ossification of the anterior longitudinal ligament at multiple contiguous levels. (C, D) lateral and AP radiographs of the lumbar spine demonstrate mild anterior longitudinal ligament ossification, but severe facet arthropathy. Ankylosis of the interspinous ligament of the lower lumbar vertebrae is present. (E) Axial CT through the L4–5 facet joint shows severe facet arthropathy with dominant hyperostotic changes.

Differential Diagnosis: DISH, degenerative joint disease, spondyloarthropathy, hypertrophic osteoarthropathy, retinoid toxicity, fluorosis.

Diagnosis: Retinoid toxicity.

Discussion: Congenital ichthyosis is a severe disorder of skin keratinization that responds to treatment by oral retinoids. Retinoids, a class of pharmaceutical agents derived from vitamin A, are highly effective in various dermatologic conditions, including acne, severe psoriasis, and severe disorders of keratinization [37]. Although ichthyosis itself has no skeletal manifestations, the retinoids used to treat it may have adverse effects on the skeleton. Retinoid-induced changes in bone are similar to those described in hypervitaminosis A. Retinoids may also have a severe teratogenic effect, thus limiting their use in females of child-bearing potential. Chronic use of retinoids in children may cause premature closure of growth plates, which inhibits growth [38,39]. Isotretinoin is among the more commonly used retinoids for oral use. Isotretinoin (13-*cis*-retinoic acid [Accutane]) in high doses given over prolonged periods, such as for treatment of congenital ichthyosis, may result in various skeletal changes. Some of these findings are similar to those of DISH. Although ligamentous calcifications are seen in both conditions, they are less dramatic with isotretinoin therapy. Additional findings with long-term isotretinoin therapy include osteoporosis, osteophytosis, and growth arrest. The osteophytosis is more pronounced in the lumbar spine. The mechanism of action may be related to effects on preosteoclasts via cytokines. Bone scintigraphy may play a useful role in identifying patients with early bone changes [40].

Clinical History: 19-year-old man with back pain.

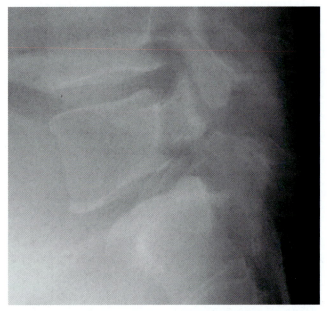

Figure 3-19 A

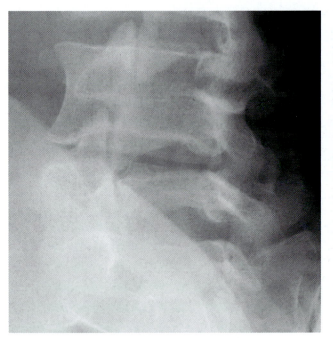

Figure 3-19 B

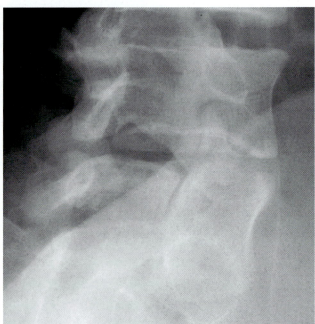

Figure 3-19 C

Findings: (A) Lateral view of the lumbosacral junction. The L5 vertebral body is anteriorly subluxed on the S1 vertebra approximately one-quarter of the vertebral body length (Grade 1 anterolisthesis). There is a focal bony defect in the pars interarticularis of the posterior elements at the L5 level. (B, C) Right and left oblique views of L4 and L5 levels show a normal "Scottie dog" configuration to the L4 level, and an amputation through the neck of the L5 Scottie dog.

Differential Diagnosis: None.

Diagnosis: Bilateral spondylolysis defect with anterolisthesis.

Discussion: The pars interarticularis is the portion of the vertebral body lamina that connects the superior facet to the inferior facet. When defects are present in this region on both sides of a vertebral body, it allows the vertebra to slip anteriorly (anterolisthesis or spondylolisthesis). Mechanisms leading to the defect are proposed to be heredity and repetitive microtrauma, leading to completed stress fractures. Spondylolysis is the most common cause of back pain in athletically active adolescents [43]. Conservative treatment with bracing is the favored initial treatment of adolescents, because some will go on to heal [44]. Approximately 95% of spondylolysis defects are found at the L5 level. On lateral radiographs, a focal lucency in the posterior elements can sometimes be seen. On oblique radiographs, the normal posterior elements form a Scottie dog outline. When a spondylolysis defect is present, the Scottie dog can appear to have a collar or a focal lucency in the neck region.

Clinical History: 24-year-old man in high-speed automobile accident.

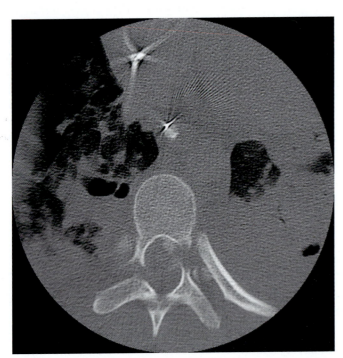

Figure 3-20   A

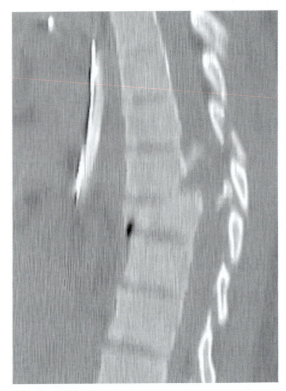

Figure 3-20   B

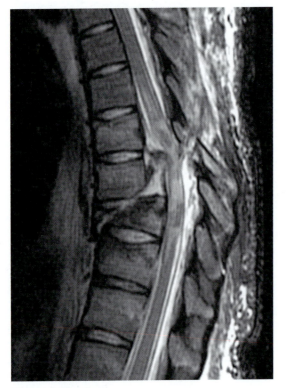

Figure 3-20   C

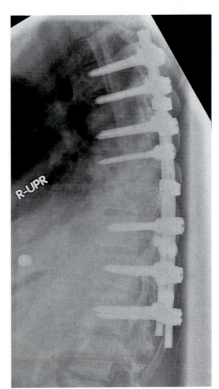

Figure 3-20   D

Findings: (**A**) Axial CT scan at the level of T8-T9. The T8 vertebral body is translated forward over the T9 vertebra and the posterior elements of T8 are fractured. Extensive pleural and pulmonary disease is present. (**B**) Sagittal reformatted CT scan through the midline. The extent of the forward translation of T8 over T9 is clearly shown. There are tension fractures of the posterior elements of T8 and an anterior wedging deformity of T9. Fragments of bone have been displaced into the spinal canal. (**C**) Sagittal T2-weighted MRI through the midline. Edema and hemorrhage involve the spinal cord extensively. Disruption of the posterior longitudinal ligament and the posterior elements at T8 is visible, along with the T8 translation and the T9 fractures. (**D**) Lateral radiograph following reduction and internal fixation of the injury. The fusion construct involves multiple levels above and below the lesion.

Differential Diagnosis: None.

Diagnosis: Hyperflexion fractures, thoracic spine.

Discussion: The typical initial emergency trauma series of radiographs in patients with polytrauma is a lateral cervical spine, an AP chest, and an AP pelvis, all obtained without moving the patient for positioning. Injuries to the spine should be recognized from these limited radiographs before the patient is moved. In this case, the diagnosis of thoracic spine injury was difficult to make from the AP radiograph of the chest because of the extensive pleural and pulmonary disease and limiting technical factors. Key radiographic features of thoracic spine injuries would include focal soft tissue swelling of the paravertebral region, misalignment of the vertebral bodies or posterior elements, and loss of vertebral height. CT is considered the imaging method of choice for identifying and characterizing traumatic injuries of the thoracic and lumbar spine. Reformatted images from CT of the chest, abdomen, and pelvis using protocols designed to identify blunt injuries of the viscera have been shown to be superior to radiographs in screening for thoracic and lumbar spine injuries [45].

The thoracic spine is supported by the rib cage and intercostal muscles and therefore is not very mobile. Fractures are uncommon and require at least four times the force necessary to cause a fracture elsewhere in the spine. Acute traumatic compression fractures are most common at the T6-7 levels. The vast majority of these injuries are anterior wedge fractures or lateral wedge fractures. Patients complain of localized pain and may have increased kyphosis. On imaging, paraspinal hematoma (lasting up to one month), disruption of the cortical surface, and loss of height is present. Severe trauma may cause burst fractures, but these are much more common in the thoracolumbar region. Hyperflexion injuries, uncommon in the mid-thoracic region, are characterized radiologically by narrowing of the anterior structures, including wedging fractures of the vertebral bodies, narrowing of the disc space, and widening of the posterior structures, including distraction or vertical subluxation of the facet joints and tension fractures of the posterior elements. In this mechanism of injury, the anterior portion is loaded under compression, while the posterior portion is loaded under tension.

Clinical History: 12-year-old girl with back pain.

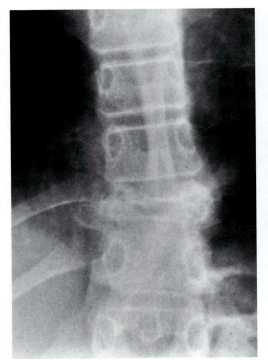

Figure 3-21   A   Figure 3-21   B

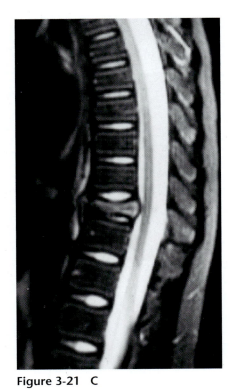

Figure 3-21   C

Findings: (A, B) AP and lateral radiographs of the thoracic spine. There is collapse and flattening of T10 with focal kyphosis. (C) Sagittal T2-weighted MRI. There is loss of the normal marrow signal from the flattened body and effacement of the anterior spinal cord.

Differential Diagnosis: Eosinophilic granuloma, leukemia, metastasis.

Diagnosis: Eosinophilic granuloma.

Discussion: Pathologic vertebral body collapse in a child is most commonly due to eosinophilic granuloma [46]. The term *vertebra plana* is used to designate an extremely flat vertebra, as is often the result.

Eosinophilic granuloma is a granulomatous lesion characterized by a focal proliferation of macrophages, eosinophils, and a specific histiocyte (Langerhans cells, which contain diagnostic cytoplasmic inclusion bodies). Langerhans cell histiocytosis is a process of uncertain etiology that includes Letterer-Siwe disease, Hand-Schuller-Christian disease, and multiple and solitary eosinophilic granuloma of bone. Eosinophilic granuloma of bone presents with skeletal rather than systemic manifestations. Destruction and replacement of bone by eosinophilic granuloma produces a lytic, aggressive-appearing geographic lesion early in the clinical course, sometimes with periosteal reaction. In the spine, asymmetric and symmetric vertebra plana are equally likely to occur. The clinical presentation of eosinophilic granuloma involving the spine is usually localized pain, but lesions may cause neurologic syndromes. The clinical course of both solitary and multiple eosinophilic granuloma of bone is benign, since lesions may regress spontaneously. Therapy is curettage, steroid injection, low-dose radiotherapy, and, rarely, chemotherapy. Lesions heal with sclerosis. After regression of lesions, regrowth of flattened vertebral bodies with reconstitution of vertical height may occur. There is no metastatic potential.

Clinical History: 15-year-old girl with increased thoracic kyphosis.

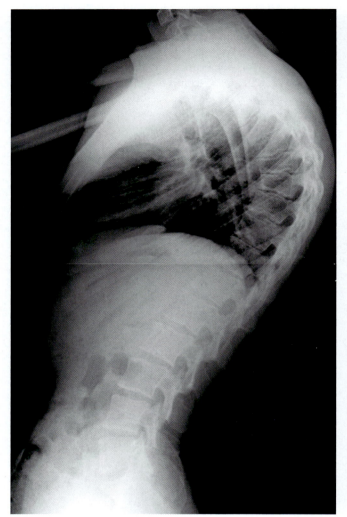

Figure 3-22   A

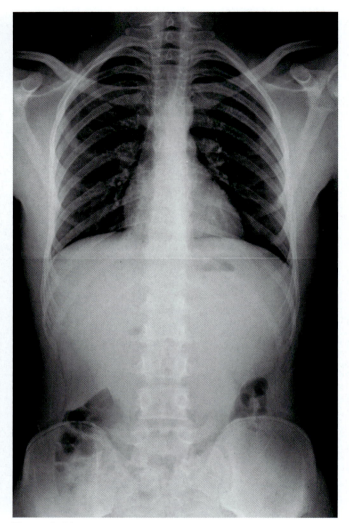

Figure 3-22   B

Findings: (A) Standing lateral of the entire spine. The thoracic kyphosis is increased. There are wedging deformities of multiple lower thoracic vertebral bodies with irregular sclerosis at the endplates. (B) Standing AP of the entire spine. Alignment is straight, without scoliosis.

Differential Diagnosis: Scheuermann's disease, postural kyphosis, histiocytosis X, osteogenesis imperfecta, trauma.

Diagnosis: Scheuermann's disease.

Discussion: The normal range of thoracic kyphosis is about 20 to 40 degrees in adolescents, as measured from the superior endplate of T3 or T4 to the inferior endplate of T12 [47]. Most cases of kyphosis in adolescents are postural kyphosis, and may simply represent the extremes of normal variation. On radiographs, the morphology of the vertebral bodies is normal and the kyphosis is reduced with hyperextension.

Scheuermann's disease is a condition with a strong familial tendency [48], which may be diagnosed on standing lateral thoracic spine radiographs when there is increased kyphosis with anterior wedging that involves three or more consecutive vertebrae, by at least 5 degrees each. Additional radiographic features, all demonstrated in this case, include decreased disc space heights, increased AP dimension, endplate irregularity and flattening, and Schmorl's nodes. The underlying abnormality is thought to be mechanical, with increased stress on the anterior portion of the vertebral bodies resulting in abnormal remodeling of the vertebrae during growth. These wedged vertebral bodies are not compression fractures. The kyphosis is accompanied by a scoliosis in up to 75% of patients, usually in the thoracic spine, either at the same level or a higher or lower compensatory level.

Clinical History: 67-year-old woman with back pain.

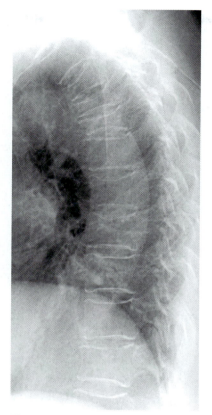

Figure 3-23

Findings: Lateral radiograph of the thoracic spine. The bones are severely osteoporotic. Prominent anterior wedge compression fractures are present with 50% vertebral body height loss at T4, T5, and T6. There is a mild anterior wedge compression fracture of T12, and slight superior end plate compression of T7 through T11.

Differential Diagnosis: Involutional osteoporosis, osteomalacia, multiple myeloma.

Diagnosis: Involutional osteoporosis (type I—postmenopausal).

Discussion: Osteopenia, compression fractures, and a resultant kyphosis are typical of this disease. Osteoporosis is characterized by generalized loss of mass from otherwise normal bone [49]. More than 95% of adults with osteoporosis have involutional osteoporosis (also called idiopathic or primary osteoporosis). There are two main clinical types: postmenopausal (also called type I) and senile (type II). Type I involutional osteoporosis is characterized by accelerated bone loss, mainly trabecular, and is caused by factors related to menopause. Type II involutional osteoporosis is characterized by slowly progressive trabecular and cortical bone loss, and is caused by factors related to aging. The pathogenesis of osteoporosis is incompletely understood, but it seems to involve not only excessive bone resorption but also impaired bone formation. Deteriorating bone strength results in increased vulnerability to traumatic and fatigue fractures. Most fractures of the spine, proximal femur, and distal radius in adults older than 50 are associated with osteoporosis. In type I involutional osteoporosis, vertebral crush fractures and distal radius fractures are the most common. In type II, multiple vertebral wedge fractures and hip fractures are the most common. Fractures are the major cause of morbidity and mortality in osteoporosis.

The radiographic hallmark of osteoporosis is osteopenia, the increased radiolucency of bone. Osteopenia may not be recognizable on plain films until 30% to 50% of the bone mineral has been lost. A coarsened trabecular pattern results from loss of the smaller trabeculae, making the remaining trabeculae more prominent. Cortical thinning is a generalized, uniform, slowly progressive process. Vertebral deformities are related to insufficiency fractures of the endplates. These can have the form of biconcave depressions of contiguous superior and inferior endplates (so-called fish or codfish vertebrae, named for their resemblance to vertebrae in codfish), anterior wedge fractures, crush fractures of entire vertebral bodies, and increased thoracic kyphosis (dowager's hump). The net result is progressive loss of stature.

Clinical History: 52-year-old woman with neck pain, and a companion case.

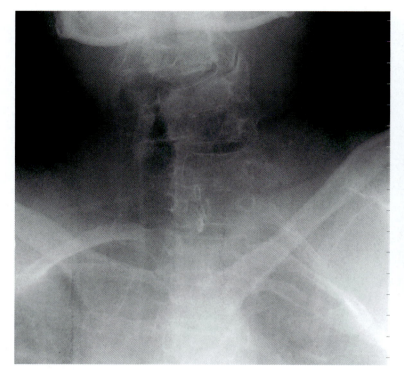

Figure 3-24   A

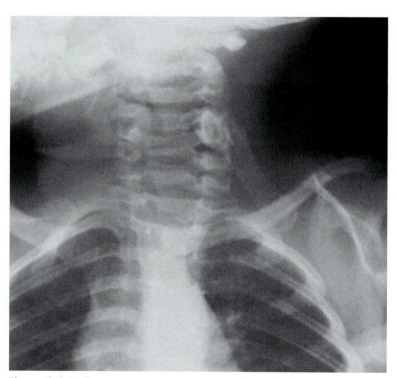

Figure 3-24   B

Figure 3-24   C

Findings: (A, B) AP and lateral cervical spine. Congenital fusion of C2–3, C4–5, and C6–7 with decreased AP dimension of the fused lower cervical vertebral bodies. An omovertebral bone is present on the left. The upper left ribs are dysplastic. Elevation of the left scapula.(C) Companion case: 2-year-old girl. AP view of the cervical spine showing dysplasia of the cervical vertebral bodies and an omovertebral bone.

Differential Diagnosis: Klippel-Feil Syndrome, juvenile chronic arthritis.

Diagnosis: Klippel-Feil Syndrome.

Discussion: Klippel-Feil is a congenital syndrome of unknown cause [50]. It can be associated with many other anomalies and is not clearly genetic, but likely results from an insult to the circulatory system in the 6th week of embryologic development. Common findings are fusion of the cervical spine vertebral bodies and congenital scoliosis. Deformities of the craniocervical junction can cause severe neurologic impairment. Approximately one third of patients will have an elevated and rotated scapula, known as a Sprengel deformity. An accessory bone extending from the medial border of the scapula to the spine—an omovertebral bone—is also commonly seen [51].

Clinical History: 11-year-old girl with short stature, macrocephaly, and dysmorphic features, and a companion case.

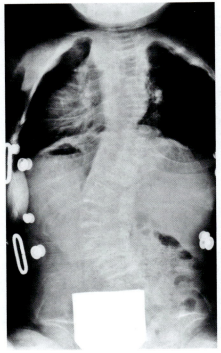

Figure 3-25 A

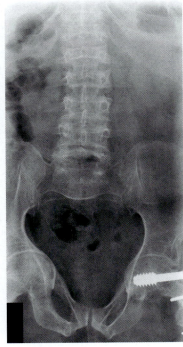

Figure 3-25 B

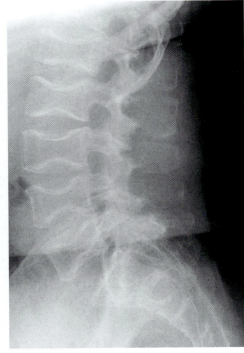

Figure 3-25 C

Findings: (A) Posteroanterior (PA) radiograph of the thoracolumbar spine. There is generalized osteopenia, multiple vertebral body compression fractures, and mild S-shaped scoliosis. The pelvis is symmetrically distorted, with marked protrusio acetabuli. (**B, C**) Companion case: 39-year-old woman. PA and lateral views of the lumbar spine showing multi-level compression deformities and bilateral protrusio acetabuli.

Differential Diagnosis: Osteogenesis imperfecta, fibrous dysplasia, juvenile idiopathic arthritis, Cushing's syndrome, homocystinuria, idiopathic juvenile osteoporosis, renal osteodystrophy, hypophosphatasia.

Diagnosis: Osteogenesis imperfecta.

Discussion: Severe osteoporosis and insufficiency compression fractures of the vertebral bodies in a pediatric patient are uncommon. The diffuse distribution of disease in this case, including the pelvis, would exclude conditions that may cause vertebral compression fractures at multiple (but not all) levels, such as eosinophilic granuloma and leukemia. Congenital conditions, endocrinopathies, systemic diseases,

and iatrogenic forms of osteoporosis (as from treatment with heparin or steroids) may also cause osteoporosis, with resultant compression fractures. In this case, the severity of the changes and the diffuseness of its distribution (all bones) are most consistent with osteogenesis imperfecta. Osteogenesis imperfecta is a generalized connective tissue disorder affecting both collagen and osteoid production [52]. In addition to gracile, osteoporotic, fragile bones, ligamentous laxity and vascular and platelet abnormalities may be seen. Disproportion in stature is caused predominantly by spinal involvement, with a greater decrease in body height than leg length [53]. Platyspondyly, progressive kyphosis, and progressive scoliosis contribute to progressive spinal deformities. Several different specific errors in collagen synthesis may cause osteogenesis imperfecta. Cyclic administration of bisphosphonates, drugs known to reduce bone turnover, have been reported to improve clinical outcomes in patients with severe osteogenesis imperfecta, apparently by reducing bone resorption and increasing bone density [54].

Clinical History: 56-year-old man with kidney problems.

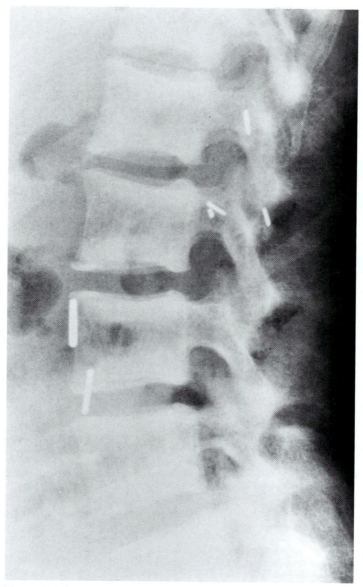

Figure 3-26

Findings: Lateral radiograph of the lumbar spine. There are sclerotic bonds following the superior and inferior vertebral body end plates. The endosteal margins of these bonds are irregular. The overall size and shape of the vertebral bodies is preserved and surgical clips are present.

Differential Diagnosis: None.

Diagnosis: Renal osteodystrophy with rugger jersey spine.

Discussion: The alternating bands of sclerosis and osteoporosis are characteristic of the rugger jersey appearance in the spine, so called because of the thick horizontal stripes [55]. The surgical clips remain from nephrectomies in this patient on chronic hemodialysis. In renal osteodystrophy, the combination of osteoporosis and osteomalacia is due to secondary hyperparathyroidism, abnormal vitamin D metabolism, and aluminum toxicity (if the patient is on hemodialysis). Osteosclerosis is a common finding that results from an increased volume of abnormal osteoid. The classic site for this finding is in the subchondral location in the spine, giving the rugger jersey appearance with a smudgy transition between normal and dense bone [56]. Other common areas of increased sclerosis in renal osteodystrophy include the pelvis and metaphyses of long bones.

Clinical History: 45-year-old man with back pain and other medical problems.

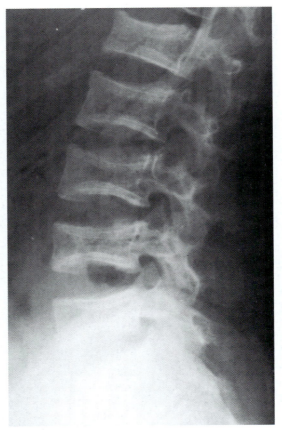

Figure 3-27

Findings: Lateral radiograph of the lumbar spine. The spine is profoundly osteoporotic, with insufficiency fractures of the superior endplates of T12 through L3.

Differential Diagnosis: Osteoporosis (from any cause), osteomalacia, multiple myeloma.

Diagnosis: Cushing's disease.

Discussion: A severely osteoporotic lumbar spine in a man of middle age is distinctly unusual. The presence of shortening of the vertebral body height with uniform biconcave deformities of the endplates at every level suggests a chronic process of gradual onset. The most common cause is iatrogenic, in particular, chronic systemic corticosteroid use. Hypercortisolism, or Cushing's disease, is the clinical manifestation of excessive amounts of glucocorticoids from any cause [57]. Cushing's disease refers to endogenous, spontaneous hypercortisolism caused by an autonomously functioning pituitary or adrenal lesion, or by nonendocrine adrenocorticotropic hormone-producing tumors. Demineralization of bone is almost always present if hypercortisolism has been present for a sufficient period of time. Glucocorticoids inhibit the absorption of calcium from the intestine and increase renal calcium loss, leading to secondary hyperparathyroidism. Glucocorticoids also exert a direct stimulatory effect on osteoclasts. At the same time, glucocorticoids inhibit osteoblastic activity by suppressing the collagen synthesis necessary for the formation of osseous matrix. The net result is continued generalized loss of bone that is prominent in the spine, pelvis, ribs, and cranial vault. In addition to osteopenia, there may be thinning of the cortex, loss of trabecular structure, intracortical tunneling, vertebral central endplate depressions, and insufficiency fractures. Insufficiency fractures characteristically heal with exuberant callus formation. The vertebral endplates may have a sclerotic appearance, resulting from a combination of insufficiency compressive microfractures and subsequent healing. The osteoporosis of hypercortisolism is virtually indistinguishable from involutional osteoporosis. Osteoporosis may persist long after cortisol metabolism has been restored to normal, or synthetic corticosteroid treatment has ended. Patients who chronically take even low doses of systemic corticosteroids are at increased risk for osteoporosis and should undergo routine screening with bone mineral density measurements.

Clinical History: 20-year-old man with recurrent bone pain, and two companion cases.

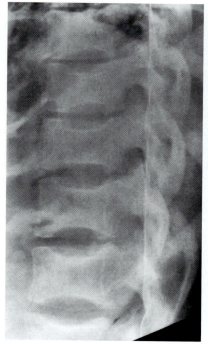

Figure 3-28 A

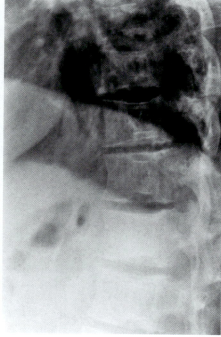

Figure 3-28 B

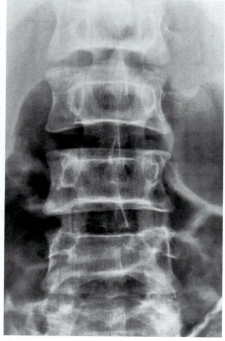

Figure 3-28 C

Findings: (A) Lateral radiograph of the thoracic spine shows H-shaped or "Lincoln log" vertebral bodies. (B) Companion case 1. Lateral thoracic spine radiograph shows vertebral bodies with more subtle H-shapes. (C) Companion case 2. AP radiograph of the thoracic spine shows H-shaped vertebral bodies.

Differential Diagnosis: Sickle cell disease, Gaucher's disease, spherocytosis, thalassemia, osteogenesis imperfecta.

Diagnosis: Sickle cell disease.

Discussion: The H-shaped or "Lincoln log" vertebrae are classically described from the AP radiograph, but are also seen on the lateral film. They are thought to result from infarction of the central growth plate, which then collapses in a squared-off pattern, but they actually represent a central, focal depression in the endplate [58]. H-shaped vertebrae have been described in thalassemia, osteoporosis, Gaucher's disease, and congenital hereditary spherocytosis, but they are much more common in sickle cell anemia.

The radiographic appearance is that of squared-off defects in the superior and inferior endplates, unlike the biconcave codfish vertebrae seen in osteoporosis.

The additional radiographic features reflect vascular infarctions and marrow hyperplasia in other areas. The marrow hyperplasia results in generalized granular-appearing radiolucency of bone, cortical thinning, and trabecular prominence. Vascular infarction tends to result in dactylitis between the ages of 6 months and 2 years; diaphyseal infarctions of larger, more commonly than smaller, tubular bones; epiphyseal infarction (typically in the hip); and growth disturbances. In addition, the patients are more susceptible to fractures, osteomyelitis, septic arthritis, hemarthrosis, joint effusions, and uric acid deposition.

Companion case 1 is a more subtle case of the H-shaped vertebrae that are classic for sickle cell disease. Companion case 2 is an AP radiograph showing the three-dimensional nature of the vertebral body abnormality.

Clinical History: 46-year-old man with spine motion limitation in flexion.

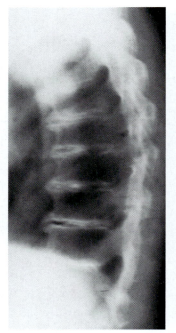 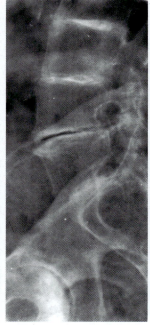 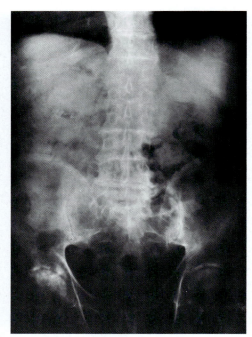

Figure 3-29 A   Figure 3-29 B   Figure 3-29 C

Findings: (A) Lateral radiograph of the thoracic spine shows marked narrowing of the disc space with ossification. Small marginal disc osteophytes are noted. Diffuse osteopenia is noted. (B) Lateral radiograph of the lumbar spine shows narrowing and ossification of the disc spaces without significant osteophyte formation. (C) AP radiograph of the abdomen demonstrates subchondral sclerosis of the sacroiliac joints, without the erosive changes that would be expected in ankylosing spondylitis. Severe subchondral sclerosis and narrowing of the right hip is noted, without osteophyte formation.

Differential Diagnosis: Degenerative disc disease, ochronosis, calcium pyrophosphate dihydrate (CPPD) deposition disease, hemochromatosis, hyperparathyroidism, acromegaly, poliomyelitis, amyloidosis.

Diagnosis: Ochronosis.

Discussion: Calcification of intervertebral discs may be idiopathic or may be associated with CPPD deposition disease, hemochromatosis, hyperparathyroidism, acromegaly, poliomyelitis, amyloidosis, and spinal fusion. In addition to history, morphology may be useful in making the distinction. The calcification is usually "wafer-like" or dystrophic in ochronosis, and there is marked joint space narrowing [59].

Ochronosis arthropathy results from an absence of the enzyme homogentisic acid oxidase, with resultant accumulation of homogentisic acid in the joints and disc spaces. This is usually inherited as an autosomal recessive trait. Clinical symptoms become evident in patients in their 30s and are usually more severe in men. The clinical presentation is usually similar to rheumatoid arthritis or ankylosing spondylitis.

The basic pathophysiology involves deposition in the articular cartilage, which stiffens it and eventually leads to fragmentation. Secondary osteoarthritic changes then ensue. In the spine, involvement of the hyaline cartilage separating the disc and vertebral body, as well as of the annulus fibrosis, results in premature degeneration. Dystrophic discal calcification thus begins at the margin of the vertebral body, rather than in the center of the disc as seen in idiopathic thoracic disc calcification. The tendency toward collapse of the disc space is more pronounced than in other processes, and may result in a loss of the lumbar lordosis. Ossification of the anterior longitudinal ligament can mimic the syndesmophyte formation seen in ankylosing spondylitis. Osteoporosis quickly ensues after fusion.

Extraspinal involvement is manifest as articular space narrowing with resultant secondary fragmentation (hence, intraarticular loose bodies) and subchondral sclerosis.

Osteophytes are not a major finding in this disease. Ligaments and tendons can calcify or ossify, predisposing them to rupture. Involvement is limited largely to the large joints, sacroiliac joints, and symphysis pubis. The peripheral joints are spared. Other organ systems commonly involved by the pigment include the cardiovascular and genitourinary systems, and the upper respiratory tracts.

In large joints, ochronosis looks like degenerative joint disease, but the articular sites are unusual (e.g., shoulder), have an abnormal distribution (e.g., isolated lateral compartment disease in the knee), and are more severe, with more ossified loose bodies and less osteophytosis than is typically seen. Diagnostic considerations include CPPD deposition disease (although the findings are not as marked as seen in ochronosis), calcium hydroxyapatite deposition disease (periarticular calcification may distinguish this), acromegaly (heel pad thickening and widened joints are characteristic), epiphyseal and spondyloepiphyseal dysplasia (history and survey films can distinguish), and neuropathic joints (history distinguishes).

Clinical History: 39-year-old immigrant with chronic cough and worsening back pain.

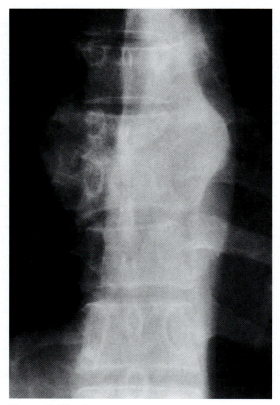

Figure 3-30 A

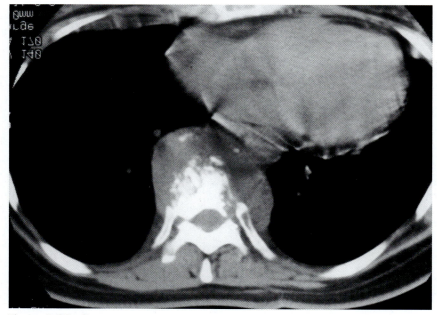

Figure 3-30 B

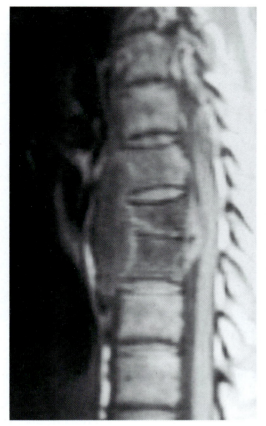

Figure 3-30   C

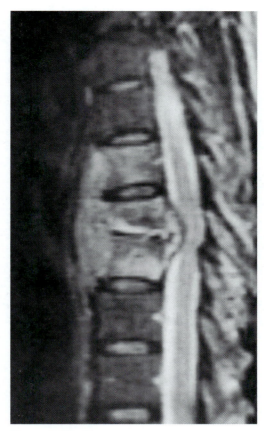

Figure 3-30   D

Findings: (**A**) AP radiograph of the thoracic spine. There is destruction of the T9–10 intervertebral disc space and adjacent portions of the T9 and T10 vertebral bodies, with prominent paraspinal soft tissue swelling. (**B**) CT through T9. There is destruction and fragmentation of the T9 vertebral body, with paraspinal soft tissue swelling. (**C, D**) Sagittal proton density and T2-weighted MRI through the midline shows involvement of three contiguous vertebrae. There is an extensive anterior soft tissue inflammatory mass and a smaller, posterior, epidural mass. The posterior mass impinges on the spinal cord.

Differential Diagnosis: Pyrogenic infection, tuberculosis, multiple myeloma, metastasis, lymphoma, chordoma.

Diagnosis: Tuberculous spondylitis (Pott's disease).

Discussion: The features distinguishing tuberculosis from other infectious agents are:

- Involvement of more than one spinal segment.
- Delay in disc destruction.
- Absence of reparative bone.
- Large calcified paravertebral mass.

It may be difficult to distinguish tuberculosis from tumors such as metastases, multiple myeloma, and lymphoma, which may have all of these features. Similarly, sarcoid should be included in the differential.

Tuberculous spondylitis is most common at L1 and the contiguous levels [60]. Multilevel (usually three levels) contiguous involvement is characteristic, but separate lesions can be detected in 1% to 4% of cases. Posterior element involvement is seen in 40% of cases, epidural disease in 53% of cases, and disc disease in 73% of cases.

As in pyogenic cases, the lesion begins in the subchondral bone and secondarily spreads to a contiguous vertebral disc, but the process is far more indolent. It also burrows under the anterior longitudinal ligament, allowing spread to additional levels. A kyphosis or scoliosis often results from partial vertebral body collapse. Tuberculosis is unique in that it frequently spills over into the soft tissue and contiguous structures before presentation. Psoas abscesses can develop faint amorphous calcifications or teardrop-shaped calcifications; other soft tissue abscesses typically do not calcify.

Unusual presentations include isolated posterior element involvement, solitary vertebral involvement, "bone within bone" appearance due to growth recovery lines, bony ankylosis, ivory vertebrae, atlantoaxial destruction, and intramedullary involvement.

Clinical History: 10-year-old girl undergoing treatment for an extremity tumor.

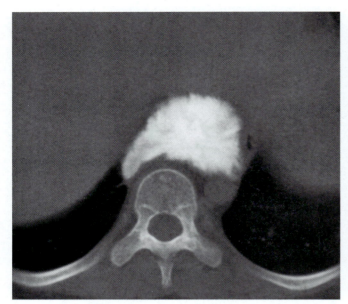

Figure 3-31 A

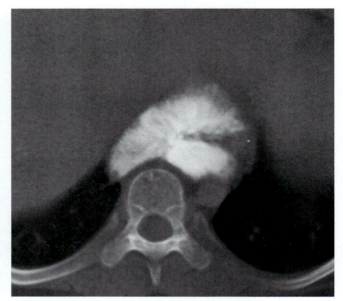

Figure 3-31 B

Findings: (A, B) Axial CT images demonstrate an ossified mass anterior to T10, but separate from it, with a spiculated, sunburst appearance.

Differential Diagnosis: Osteosarcoma, treated Ewing's sarcoma (or other round cell tumor), treated lymphoma, metastasis.

Diagnosis: Metastatic osteosarcoma.

Discussion: This lesion has the cloudlike, spiculated matrix typical of osteosarcoma, but it is located in the soft tissues anterior to the spine. Differential considerations include metastasis, metachronous osteosarcomas, or extraosseous osteosarcoma. Metastases are more common than the latter lesions.

Metachronous osteosarcomas are subtyped into osteosarcomatosis, multiple metachronous osteosarcomas, and unicentric osteosarcoma with metastasis [61]. Osteosarcomatosis is a rare form that occurs in children. All of the lesions are similar in size and radiographic and histologic appearance; this patient had a dominant lesion in her extremity before this lesion was identified. Similarly, this would not fall into the multiple, metachronous subtype because of the short period of time between the treatment of the original tumor and this site's identification. A unicentric osteosarcoma with a subsequent metastasis is most common if the primary is in a long bone, or a recurrence occurs in the spine or pelvis. Extraosseous primary osteosarcomas are rare.

Conventional osteosarcomas are currently treated with preoperative chemotherapy, followed by resection and prosthetic or allograft placement. Metastasis can appear as ossified or calcified lesions in the lymph nodes, soft tissues, and viscera; these are likewise treated with surgery, chemotherapy, and/or irradiation. Metastases to the lungs can appear quite dense and have a high association with spontaneous pneumothoraces.

Clinical History: 63-year-old woman with back pain, and a companion case.

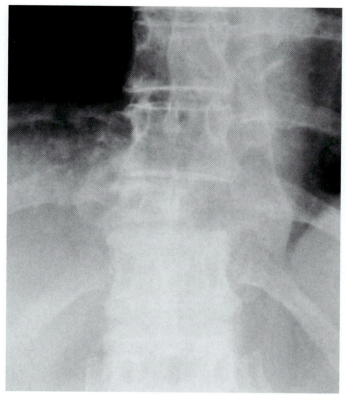

Figure 3-32 A

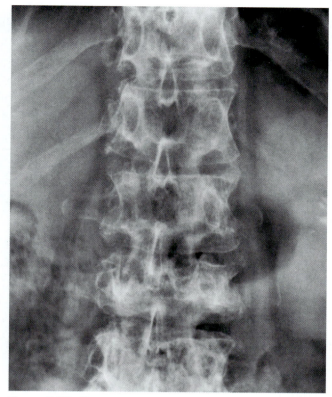

Figure 3-32 B

Findings: (A) AP radiograph of the thoracolumbar spine. There is an absent left T11 pedicle and compression of the T11 vertebral body. Widening of the paravertebral soft tissues is evidence of a large associated soft tissue mass. (B) Companion case. AP radiograph of the thoracolumbar spine. The bones are osteopenic. There is loss of the medial aspect of the left pedicle at T12. The right L1 pedicle is absent. The L2 body is compressed.

Differential Diagnosis: Metastasis, multiple myeloma, lymphoma, leukemia.

Diagnosis: Breast cancer metastasis.

Discussion: Destruction of the pedicle is a classic sign of metastatic disease that differentiates it from multiple myeloma [62]. Usually a large bulk of the vertebral body is involved before extension into the pedicle is demonstrated.

Osteosclerosis of the pedicle can occur in metastatic disease, but it can also be seen in Paget's disease or as a stress reaction to contralateral spondylolysis. Metastasis to the thoracic or lumbar spine vertebral bodies is common. Contiguous tumor extension would be most common in prostate, breast, lymphoma, and multiple myeloma.

Osteolysis is an insensitive clue to metastatic disease, which explains our reliance on bone scan or MRI for early detection. Extraosseous extension can usually be distinguished from infectious etiologies by the lack of disc involvement.

Surgical management of metastases includes intramedullary rods for long bones, and joint reconstruction for acetabular lesion. The success rate for reducing pain is 96% for long bones, 84% for acetabuli, and 82% for vertebrae. At least 32% survived 2 years after spinal decompression for epidural metastases or extension.

Clinical History: Young child with abnormal spinal curvature, and a companion case.

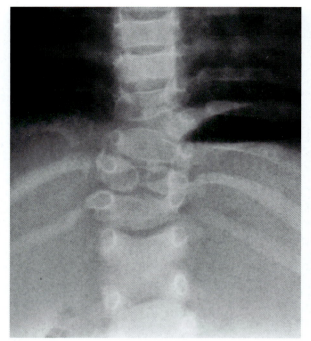

Figure 3-33   A

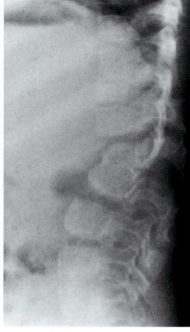

Figure 3-33   B

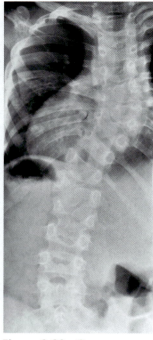

Figure 3-33   C

Findings: (A, B) Standing PA and lateral scoliosis study. Multiple segmentation anomalies are present in the lower thoracic and upper lumbar spine, including butterfly vertebrae at T11 and on the left between T9 and T10. (C) Companion case. Standing PA scoliosis study showing multiple anomalies in the thoracic and lumbar spine, with S-shaped scoliosis.

Differential Diagnosis: None.

Diagnosis: Congenital scoliosis.

Discussion: The presence of fusion or segmentation anomalies in combination with scoliosis makes this a congenital scoliosis.

The obvious causes of congenital scoliosis relate to failure of normal formation of individual vertebrae [63]. During the embryonic conversion of mesenchymal vertebrae to cartilaginous vertebrae before week 9 of development, each vertebral body becomes chondrified from two centers of chondrification on either side of the midline. If chondrification fails on only one side, an isolated hemivertebra results. If the centers of chondrification do not fuse at the same level (as they should), but instead fuse across levels, a block vertebra results. Similarly, a pediculate bar or neural arch fusion can result from fusion anomalies. Rarely, a supernumerary hemivertebra can result from partial reduplication. The most common vertebral anomalies causing congenital scoliosis include hemivertebrae, trapezoidal vertebrae, and unilateral neural arch fusions. Combinations of anomalies and multilevel involvement are frequent.

Patients with congenital scoliosis must be carefully examined for the VACTERL syndrome (Vertebral, Anal, Cardiac, Tracheal, Esophageal, Renal, and Limb anomalies). At a minimum beyond physical examination, evaluation of the genitourinary tract is recommended.

Clinical History: 24-year-old woman with painful scoliosis.

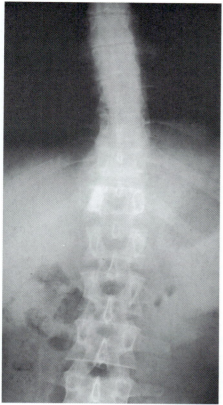

Figure 3-34 A

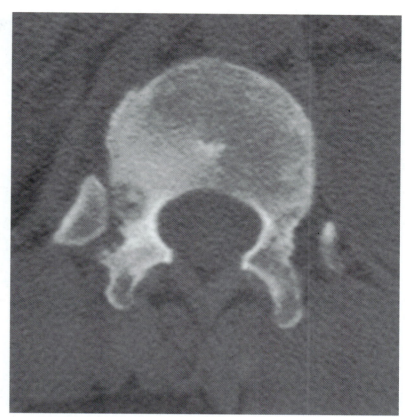

Figure 3-34 B

Findings: (A) Standing PA radiograph shows a mild left thoracolumbar scoliosis. The right side of the T12 vertebra is densely sclerotic. (B) CT through T12 shows a 1-cm rounded lesion within the right lateral portion of the vertebral body adjacent to the costovertebral joint. The lesion has a sclerotic central focus, and a zone of surrounding sclerosis that extends well into the vertebral body and right pedicle.

Differential Diagnosis: Osteoid osteoma, osteoblastoma, bone island, Brodie's abscess.

Diagnosis: Osteoid osteoma.

Discussion: Osteoid osteoma is a benign neoplasm of bone that is distinguished from osteoblastoma principally by size: osteoid osteoma is typically 1 cm or smaller, while osteoblastoma is typically 2 cm or larger. The pain syndrome associated with osteoid osteoma can be highly suggestive, often as night pain relieved by aspirin. A painful scoliosis may develop due to reflexive splinting in the spine.

This case demonstrates the classic appearance on CT of an osteoid osteoma. Features include the round shape, the dense, central sclerosis, and the surrounding reactive bone formation. The lucent portion of the lesion consists of fibrovascular tissue but is also mineralized, although less so than the central sclerosis. On MRI, osteoid osteomas have high signal on T2-weighted images and enhance following gadolinium injection. They may be less conspicuous than on CT. Bone islands may develop in the vertebral column, but they are painless and are not associated with scoliosis. On CT, they tend to be homogeneously dense, with a spiculated margin where they blend into the surrounding trabecular bone. Although a Brodie's abscess could be expected to be painful, have extensive surrounding sclerosis, and possibly have a round shape, it should not contain mineralization. Current standard treatment of osteoid osteoma is radiofrequency ablation performed under CT guidance [64].

Clinical History: 70-year-old man with prostate cancer, and a companion case.

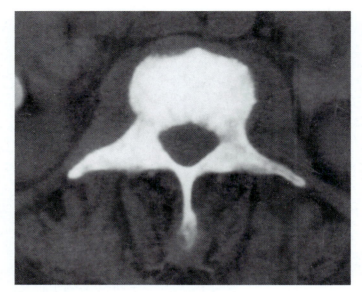

Figure 3-35   A

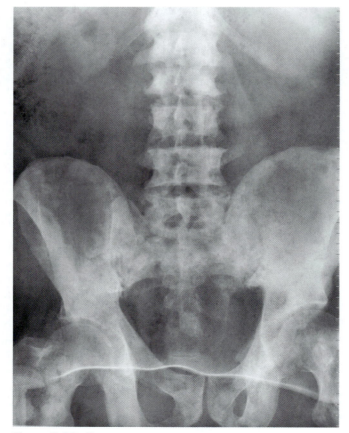

Figure 3-35   B

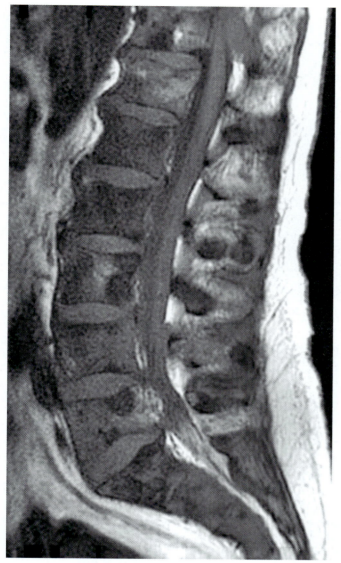

Figure 3-35 C

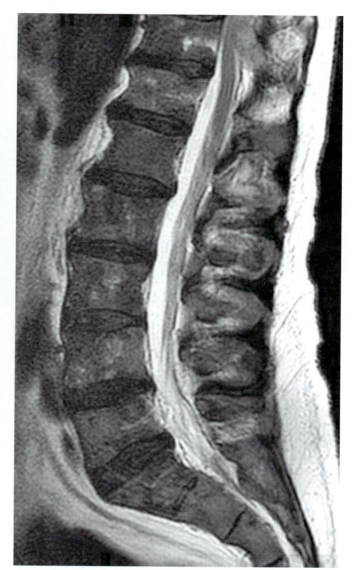

Figure 3-35 D

Findings: (A) Axial CT shows increased sclerosis of a lumbar vertebra, with no increase in the size of the bone. (B) Companion case: 67-year-old man with prostate cancer. AP view of the lumbar spine and pelvis demonstrates sclerotic lesions throughout the thoracic and lumbar spine, pelvis, and proximal femora. (C, D) Sagittal T1-weighted and T2-weighted MRI of the lumbar spine reveals multiple bone marrow obliterating masses within the vertebral bodies. A T11 epidural mass extending from the left lamina compresses the adjacent spinal cord.

Differential Diagnosis: Metastasis, Paget's disease, lymphoma, chordoma, mastocytosis.

Diagnosis: Ivory vertebrae from sclerotic prostate metastasis.

Discussion: Sclerosis of the vertebral body in an elderly man is suggestive of prostate carcinoma, but it can also be seen in other metastases, myeloma, Paget's disease, lymphoma, and chordomas [65]. Additional etiologies of an "ivory vertebrae" include sclerosing osteomyelitis (but disc involvement can be documented), mastocytosis, tuberous sclerosis, myelofibrosis, and osteosarcoma.

Lesions that can cause differential vertebral sclerosis include the hemangioma (accentuated vertical striations), renal osteodystrophy ("rugger jersey," horizontal radiodense stripes on the bottom and top of the vertebral body), Paget's disease (coarsened trabecular pattern with "picture frame" thickening along the margins of the vertebral body), and osteopetrosis (horizontal, thick, densities along both endplates).

Clinical History: 70-year-old man with prostate cancer.

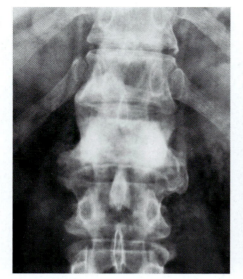

Figure 3-36 A

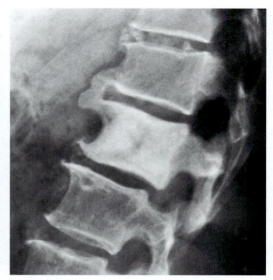

Figure 3-36 B

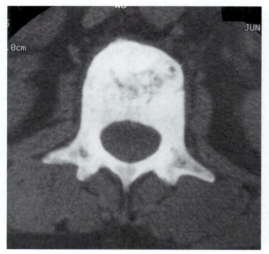

Figure 3-36 C

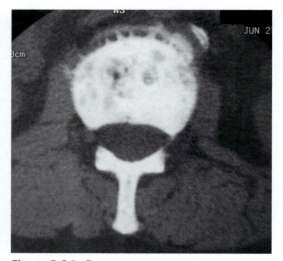

Figure 3-36 D

Findings: (A, B) AP and lateral radiographs of the thoracolumbar spine show increased sclerosis of the L1 vertebral body with subtle overall enlargement relative to the vertebra below. (C, D) CT axial slices show definite increase in the anterior to posterior dimension.

Differential Diagnosis: Metastasis, Paget's disease, lymphoma, chordoma, mastocytosis.

Diagnosis: Ivory vertebrae from Paget's disease.

Discussion: Paget's disease is another etiology for an Ivory vertebra. The radiologic findings include a coarsened trabecular pattern and an overall increase in density [66]. However, it is the vertebral enlargement that distinguishes this from other causes of Ivory vertebrae. The picture frame appearance secondary to condensation of mineralization at the margins of the vertebral body is another appearance that is diagnostic.

Paget's disease most commonly involves the lumbar spine and sacrum. Sacral abnormalities can be detected by a subtle thickening of the arcuate lines, as seen on the AP radiograph. Usually sacral abnormalities are seen in conjunction with other pelvic findings, such as thickening of the iliopectineal or iliopubic lines. Neurologic symptoms can result from canal or neural foramen mechanical narrowing secondary to ligamentous ossification, vertebral enlargement or collapse, or a vascular steal phenomenon.

Clinical History: 19-year-old woman in automobile accident.

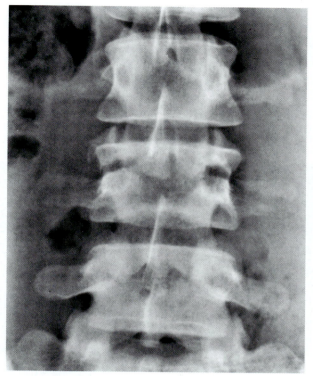

Figure 3-37 A

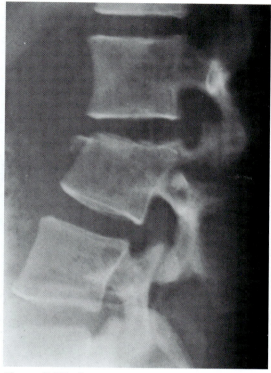

Figure 3-37 B

Findings: (A) AP radiograph of the lumbar spine shows horizontal lucent clefts through both L1 pedicles and transverse processes. (B) Lateral radiograph demonstrates a compression deformity of the L1 vertebral body, with a horizontal extension through the pedicles. Marked distraction is present at the pedicle fracture site. The facets still articulate normally.

Differential Diagnosis: None.

Diagnosis: Chance fracture.

Discussion: A "seat belt" injury refers to the osseous and ligamentous hyperflexion injuries that commonly occur at the thoracolumbar or upper lumbar levels in adult passengers, or at the midlumbar levels in child passengers.

Because the ligamentous structures withstand the distraction forces better than the vertebral bodies, a horizontal fracture that begins in the posterior elements and propagates anteriorly can result [68]. People with combination shoulder-lap belts incur different types of injuries (compression fractures of the cervicothoracic spine and anterolateral wedge compressions of the thoracolumbar vertebrae on the side opposite the shoulder strap) that have a lower incidence of neurologic sequelae, and therefore better prognosis.

There are four subtypes of Chance fractures:

- Type A (47%) is the original description of a horizontal fracture involving all three columns.

- Type B (11%) is restricted to disruption of the ligaments and intervertebral disc.
- Type C (26%) involves the posterior and middle columns, extending into the anterior disc.
- Type D (16%) involves the posterior column, extending then into the disc.

The radiographic features include a preserved to decreased anterior vertebral body height with a preserved to increased posterior vertebral body height, with a characteristic rounding of the superior posterior vertebral body on the lateral. The AP radiograph may be quite useful (as in this case) in defining the extension of the fracture into the pedicles, or widening of the posterior disc space as the damage propagates anteriorly. The findings can be quite subtle on a transaxial CT; therefore, two-dimensional coronal and sagittal reconstructions are mandatory.

Pure posterior ligament disruption results in interspinous widening with subluxation, perching, or distraction of the facets. If there is more than 20 degrees of flexion or 10% lateral bending in the upper lumbar levels (without a fracture), ligamentous disruption must be present.

Clinical History: 68-year-old woman with newly discovered breast cancer.

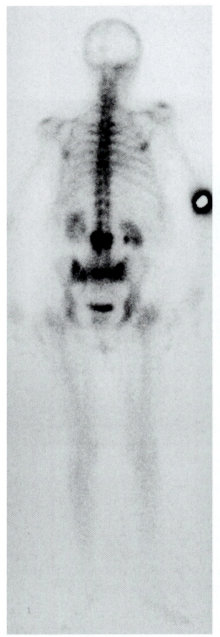

Figure 3-38   A

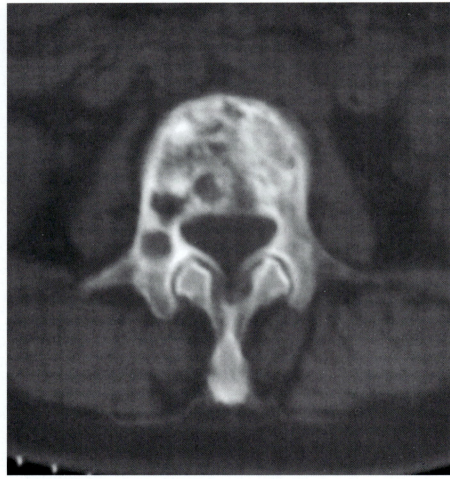

Figure 3-38   B

Findings: (A) Radionuclide bone scan. Posterior whole-body view shows intense accumulation of activity in L3. (B) Axial CT image through the L3 vertebra shows diffuse enlargement. The bone is a mosaic of sclerosis and lucent regions, with a disordered trabecular bone pattern.

Differential Diagnosis: Metastasis, Paget's disease, lymphoma, chordoma, mastocytosis.

Diagnosis: Paget's disease.

Discussion: The coarsened trabecular pattern is a prominent feature in this case. However, it is sometimes difficult to arrive at the diagnosis quickly on CT images, because each level is read in isolation. Two-dimensional sagittal reconstructions can be helpful in identifying a subtle increase in vertebral body size.

Because Paget's disease leads to weakened bone, biconcave vertebrae can sometimes result, with secondary degenerative changes in the disc. Occasionally, posterior element involvement may be seen in isolation or in conjunction with vertebral body abnormalities. In these cases, sclerosis of the pedicle will usually be accompanied by a subtle, overall increase in interpediculate distance.

Differential considerations of a dense vertebra include blastic metastases, myelofibrosis, fluorosis, mastocytosis, renal osteodystrophy, fibrous dysplasia, and tuberous sclerosis. Two other entities that can be seen in elderly patients include axial osteomalacia and fibrogenesis imperfecta ossium, both of which can be distinguished pathologically. A juvenile form of Paget's disease, called familial idiopathic hyperphosphatasia, is recognized as having similar features, except there is sparing of the epiphyses.

Clinical History: 56-year-old man with chronic back pain, and a companion case.

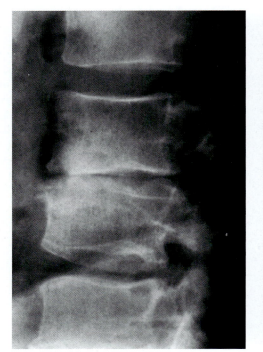

Figure 3-39   A

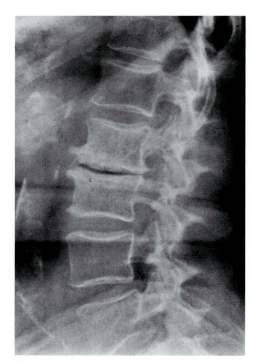

Figure 3-39   B

Figure 3-39   C

Findings: (A, B) Lateral and detail radiographs at the L3–4 level demonstrate a vacuum phenomenon in a narrowed disc with adjacent endplate sclerosis. (C) Companion case. Lateral radiograph of the lumbar spine shows narrowing, osteophytes, and sclerosis.

Differential Diagnosis: Degenerative disc disease, infection, posttraumatic deformity.

Diagnosis: Degenerative disc disease.

Discussion: Degenerative disease of the spine can be subcategorized into intervertebral osteochondrosis, spondylosis deformans, and osteoarthritis. The primary abnormality in intervertebral osteochondrosis is in the nucleus pulposus, the shock absorber of the spine. Radiographic manifestations include decreased disc height, vacuum phenomenon, and sclerosis of the endplates. In spondylosis deformans, the annulus fibrosis has decreased elasticity and results in osteophytosis with a normal to slightly decreased disc space. Osteoarthritis is a disease of the facet joints alone, and is manifest by joint space narrowing and sclerosis.

These entities must be differentiated from other processes that cause disc space narrowing [67]. Diskitis will typically show poorly defined endplate sclerosis that graduates into distinct erosive changes, with an associated soft tissue mass. Trauma with herniation of the nucleus pulposus will usually have a visible fracture or secondary signs of ligamentous instability with the appropriate clinical history. In neuropathic osteoarthropathy, the disc space narrowing, sclerosis, and osteophytosis are more pronounced and associated with debris and disorganization. Rheumatoid arthritis is typically seen in the cervical spine, and shows additional evidence of subluxations resulting from apophyseal and ligamentous involvement. The changes of CPPD deposition disease can include fragmentation, subluxation, and calcification, in addition to disc space narrowing and endplate sclerosis. Ochronosis can be suggested if there is prominent disc calcification and osteoporosis.

CASE 3-40

Clinical History: 35-year-old woman with back pain.

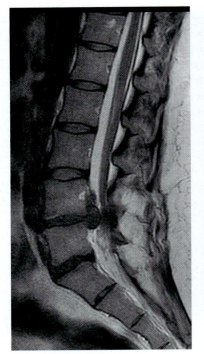

Figure 3-40   A

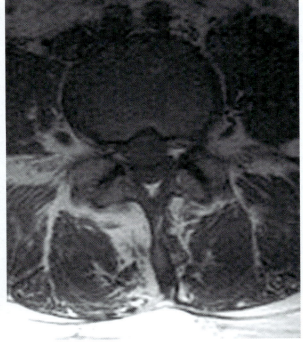

Figure 3-40   B

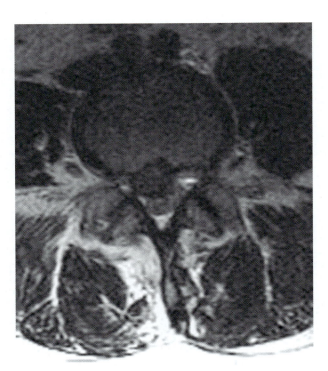

Figure 3-40   C

Findings: Sagittal T2-weighted (A), axial T1-weighted (B), and axial T2-weighted (C) MRI demonstrates a bilobed disc extrusion, with a large fragment migrated superiorly lying in the lateral recess behind the L4 vertebral body. The fragment in the lateral recess behind L4 may impinge the right L4 nerve root. There is severe central canal stenosis present due to this lesion. The involved disc space is reduced in height and low in signal.

Differential Diagnosis: None.

Diagnosis: Herniated nucleus pulposus.

Discussion: The presence of a low signal mass extending from a flattened, degenerated disc into the spinal canal is diagnostic of a herniated nucleus pulposus. Mechanical impingement of the herniated fragment on nerve roots may cause disabling back pain with radiation to the lower limbs. Low back pain in adults is exceedingly common, affecting the majority of adults at some time during their lives, and it is the most common cause of disability under the age of 45 years. MRI is the study of choice in the setting of acute low back pain complicated by radicular symptoms. Sometimes the distinction between infection and degenerative disc disease can be particularly challenging. However, in discogenic sclerosis, the endplates tend to be uniformly sclerotic, without the focal erosions seen in infection. Defects in the endplates can result from herniated Schmorl's nodes. The presence of a vacuum phenomenon is suggestive of degenerative disc disease; even in the setting of infection superimposed on degenerative disc disease, the bacteria commonly consume the available nitrogen before the patient is imaged.

Other entities that can cause disc space narrowing associated with subchondral sclerosis include the seronegative spondyloarthropathies, CPPD deposition disease, ochronosis, neuropathic disease, and sarcoidosis.

Clinical History: 52-year-old man with back pain for 3 months, and a companion case.

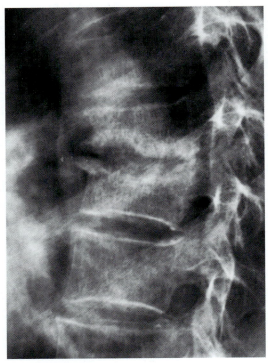

Figure 3-41   A

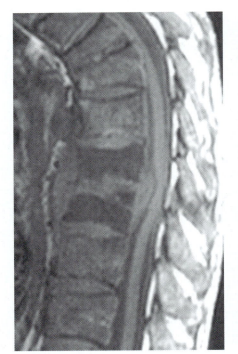

Figure 3-41   B

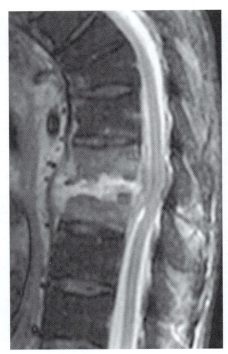

Figure 3-41   C

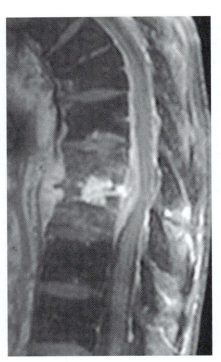

Figure 3-41   D

Findings: (A) Lateral radiograph of the thoracic spine shows apparent widening of a lower intervertebral disc space with erosions and sclerosis of the adjacent vertebral endplates. (B, C, D) Companion case: 58-year-old renal transplant patient with back pain. (B) Sagittal T1-weighted MRI shows low signal centered at the T8–9 interspace, extending into the adjacent vertebral bodies. (C) Sagittal inversion recovery MRI shows the abnormal disc space-centered fluid collection, which causes irregularity of the adjacent end plates and impinges on the epidural space underneath the posterior longitudinal ligament, displacing the thecal sac and cord posteriorly. Abnormal fluid-signal intensity extends anteriorly and tracks cephalad and caudal along the anterior longitudinal ligament. (D) Gadolinium-enhanced sagittal T1-weighted MRI shows enhancement in the central portion of the disc space, as well as in the subligamentous collections anterior and posterior to the disc space.

Differential Diagnosis: Pyrogenic diskitis, myeloma, metastasis, tuberculosis.

Diagnosis: Pyrogenic diskitis.

Discussion: This is an aggressive process centered at the disc space, with narrowing and destruction of the facing vertebral endplates. As the process evolves, increasing reactive sclerosis occurs. Bony ankylosis is one eventual outcome. The clinical presentation is fever, back pain, and stiffness.

Diagnosis is often delayed, and radiographic findings may not be apparent until 2 to 8 weeks after onset. A causative organism is often difficult to culture from the patient. In 60% of cases where the agent is recovered, the recovered organism is *Staphylococcus aureus*, and in 30% of cases the organisms are species of *Enterobacteriaceae*. In 40% of cases, a remote source of infection will be known—usually genitourinary tract, skin, or respiratory tract. In the absence of an identified organism, antibiotics are chosen empirically.

Pyogenic vertebral osteomyelitis [69,70] occurs in elderly adults with genitourinary tract infections, patients who are immunocompromised, and intravenous drug abusers. The thoracic spine (50%) is involved more commonly than the lumbar (35%) or cervical spine (15%). Organisms from genitourinary tract infections ascend the vertebral column by way of the vertebral plexus of Batson, a valveless venous bed that allows retrograde blood flow. The initial site of infection is the subcortical bone of the vertebral body, adjacent to the intervertebral disc. The infection typically extends through the endplate, involving the disc and the adjacent vertebral body. Multiple levels of involvement are not uncommon, particularly among immunocompromised or debilitated patients, and the levels may be contiguous or noncontiguous. Lateral extension causes a paraspinal abscess; posterior extension can result in epidural abscess, cord compression, and meningitis.

Clinical History: 58-year-old man with paraplegia after a car accident.

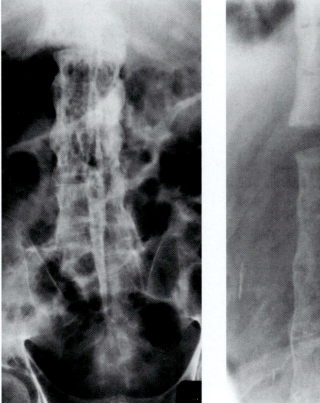

Figure 3-42 A

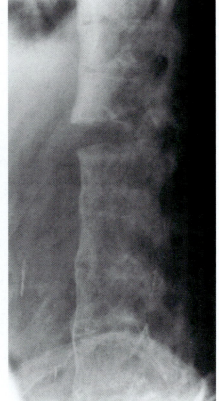

Figure 3-42 B

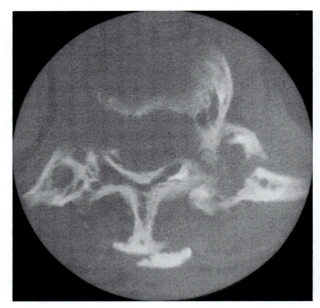

Figure 3-42 C

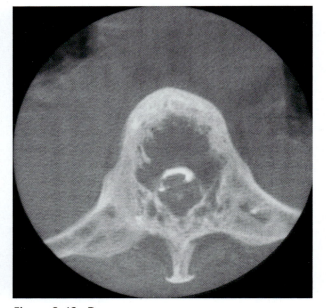

Figure 3-42 D

Findings: (A, B) AP and lateral radiographs of the lumbar spine reveal a lateral distraction-dislocation at L1–2, with an increase in the disc space. Syndesmophyte formation is noted, fusing all other levels. The sacroiliac joints are ankylosed. (C, D) Axial CT images demonstrate marked narrowing of the spinal canal, with no myelographic contrast seen at the most severe level. The "double spinous process" sign at this level is due to avulsion of the ossification along the spinous process. A second fracture site is noted through the left facet.

Differential Diagnosis: Fracture-dislocation in ankylosing spondylitis, DISH (diffuse idiopathic skeletal hyperostosis), or juvenile idiopathic arthritis.

Diagnosis: Ankylosing spondylitis with fracture-dislocation.

Discussion: A fracture-dislocation is one of the most devastating complications of ankylosing spondylitis. The fused spine in ankylosing spondylitis is much weaker than a normal spine, because its rigidity does not allow it to absorb and dissipate the forces of traumatic loading. In the normal spine, the intervertebral discs, endplates, ligaments, and paravertebral musculature absorb most of these forces. The function of these structures is nullified by ankylosis. In addition, the bone in ankylosing spondylitis is osteoporotic. Relatively minor traumatic loading may cause fractures through syndesmophytes [71]. With greater force, fractures extend through the posterior elements, and the entire spine becomes unstable and may displace. Cord contusion or transection is a significant risk in these patients, a risk made greater by preexisting spinal stenosis that is associated with ossification of the posterior ligamentous complex. In addition to the immediate risk of neurologic catastrophe or even death, delayed neurologic deterioration is a well-recognized complication. Surgical stabilization is the preferred treatment, but the underlying vulnerability of the spine will remain.

Clinical History: 28-year-old man with short stature, and a companion case.

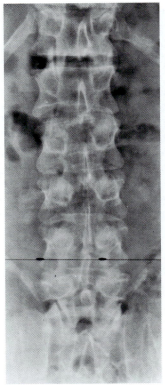

Figure 3-43   A

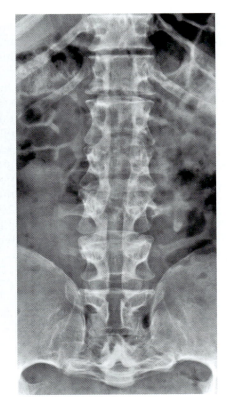

Figure 3-43   B

Findings: (A) AP radiograph of the lumbar spine. There is severe developmental spinal stenosis in the lumbar region, with progressive narrowing of the interpediculate distances caudally. (B) Companion case. AP radiograph of the lumbar spine in a patient with similar findings, but who had laminectomies at multiple levels.

Differential Diagnosis: None.

Diagnosis: Achondroplasia.

Discussion: Progressive narrowing of the interpediculate distance as one proceeds caudally is seen only in achondroplasia and thanatophoric dwarfism [72]. In an adult, it is only seen in achondroplasia. Achondroplasia is the most common type of dwarfism, and has a classic radiologic appearance. It is the result of a generalized defect in enchondral bone formation, leading to underdevelopment of the portions of bones that grow by this mechanism. The result is a symmetric, short-limbed dwarfism in which the proximal segments of the extremities are disproportionately short (rhizomelic micromelia). Because periosteal bone growth is unaffected, the shafts of the long bones are of normal diameter, but there is metaphyseal flaring. The fingers are short and stubby. The skull base, formed by enchondral bone formation, is abnormally short and has a small foramen magnum. The calvarium, formed by intramembranous bone formation, is appropriately large for the intracranial contents, giving the head a characteristic brachycephaly with frontal bossing and a small face. The spinal canal is narrow in both anteroposterior and lateral dimensions, but the trunk length is nearly normal. This becomes most prominent in the lumbar area, where there is narrowing in the distance between pedicles, as opposed to the maintained or increased distance noted in normal patients as one progresses caudally. There is an exaggerated lumbar lordosis with prominent buttocks. The ribs are likewise shortened, leading to a decrease in intrathoracic volume. These abnormalities are usually evident at birth and become more apparent with age.

Achondroplasia has autosomal dominant genetic transmission, but most cases are sporadic. The classic form is heterozygous, has no associated congenital defects, and may be compatible with a normal life expectancy. Complications of congenital spinal stenosis are common in adulthood. The homozygous condition is lethal in infancy and has a radiologic appearance identical to thanatophoric dwarfism. Thanatophoric ("death bringing") dwarfism is the most common lethal bone dysplasia. The chromosomal distinction between homozygous achondroplasia and thanatophoric dwarfism is important for genetic counseling of the parents.

CASE 3-44

Clinical History: 40-year-old woman with back pain, and a companion case.

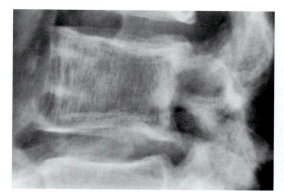

Figure 3-44   A

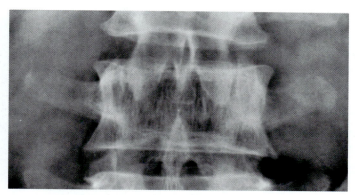

Figure 3-44   B

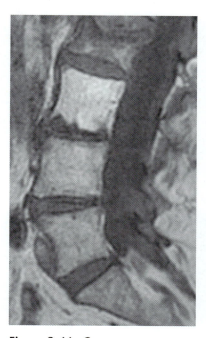

Figure 3-44   C

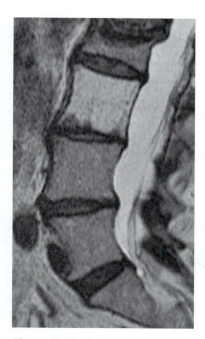

Figure 3-44   D

Findings: (A, B) AP and lateral detail radiographs of L2. There are thick vertical striations of the vertebral body. The posterior elements are not affected. The overall vertebral body size is normal. The cortex is of normal thickness. (C, D) Companion case. Sagittal T1-weighted and T2-weighted MRI of the lumbar spine shows diffusely high signal in the L3 vertebral body. A benign compression fracture of L2 is also present.

Differential Diagnosis: Hemangioma, metastasis, lymphoma, myeloma, chordoma, Paget's disease, osteoporosis.

Diagnosis: Hemangioma.

Discussion: Radiographic features of hemangioma include a coarse reinforcement of the vertical trabecular pattern in response to the horizontal trabeculae that are lost [73]. This "corduroy" pattern is usually identified in the vertebral body, but can extend into the posterior elements. It is more typical to have a focal osseous lesion with a "cartwheel" pattern than involvement of the entire vertebral body. There is usually increased uptake of the radiopharmaceutical on bone scan. T1 hyperintensity results from the fat content, and T2 hyperintensity results from the blood content. Gadolinium enhancement is expected.

Differential considerations include metastatic disease, lymphoma, myeloma, or chordoma, when the lesion extends into the soft tissues. The lesions can usually be differentiated from Paget's disease by the lack of cortical thickening.

Clinical History: 23-year-old woman whose back pain became much worse during pregnancy.

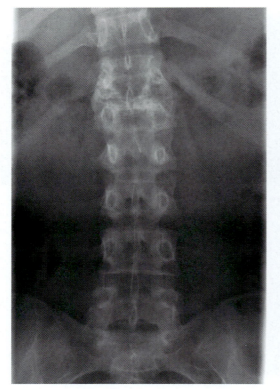

Figure 3-45   A

Figure 3-45   B

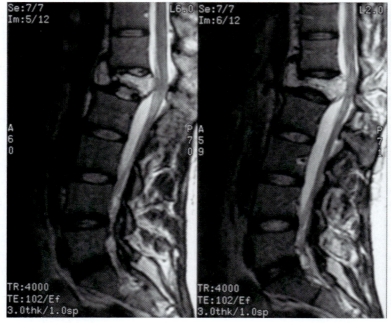

Figure 3-45   C

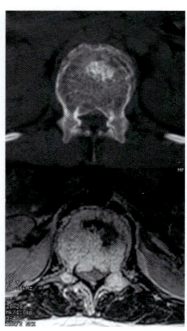

Figure 3-45   D

Findings: (**A, B**) AP and lateral radiographs of the lumbar spine. The L2 vertebral body is compressed and expanded outward circumferentially. (**C**) Sagittal T2-weighted MRI shows high signal intensity in the L2 body. Posterior expansion impinges on the thecal sac. There is no paravertebral edema, and the cortex appears intact. (**D**) Axial CT and T2-weighted MRI shows expansion with sparse, but thick, reinforced trabecular bone.

Differential Diagnosis: Hemangioma with collapse, metastasis with collapse, eosinophilic granuloma with collapse.

Diagnosis: Hemangioma with vertebral collapse.

Discussion: Hemangioma is a benign lesion proliferation of vascular channels that can occur in the bone or soft tissues. Typical asymptomatic osseous lesions are often discovered incidentally in adults, and there is a female predominance. Autopsy data suggest that the prevalence of spinal involvement is approximately 10%, but far fewer lesions are of sufficient size to be detected radiographically. Both CT and MRI are more sensitive than radiographs, but the radionuclide bone scan is typically negative. The thoracic spine is involved more frequently than the lumber spine, and the cervical spine is not commonly involved. Malignant degeneration does not occur.

Vertebral hemangiomas enlarge during pregnancy and often become symptomatic. The vascular and hemodynamic changes that occur during pregnancy act to enlarge a preexisting hemangioma [74,75]. The average increase in circulatory volume during pregnancy is 40%, with a concomitant increase in venous capacitance. As the gravid uterus enlarges sufficiently to fill the pelvis and begins to extend into the abdominal cavity, its bulk interferes with venous return from the lower extremities into the inferior vena cava. As a collateral pathway, blood engorges the valveless Batson's plexus and flows retrograde in large volume into a preexisting vertebral hemangioma to produce progressive enlargement. Hormonal changes during pregnancy may also produce structural changes. Progesterone increases venous distensibility, and estrogen promotes endothelial growth. Most patients whose vertebral hemangiomas become symptomatic during pregnancy do so in the third trimester, when the gravid uterus begins to redirect blood flow into Batson's plexus. Many patients show spontaneous remission after delivery, but many do not.

Clinical History: 43-year-old man with rash and low back pain for 2 weeks.

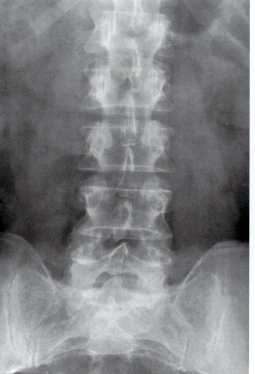
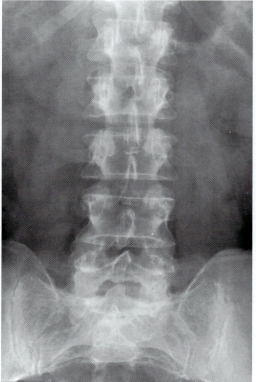

Figure 3-46   A

Figure 3-46   B

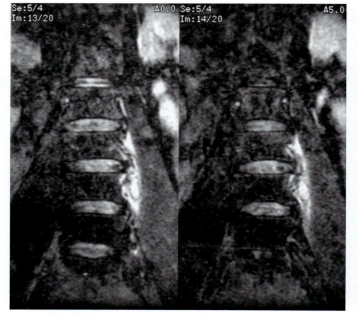

Figure 3-46   C

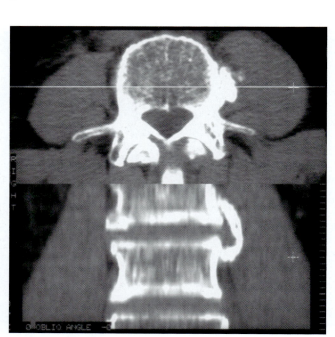

Figure 3-46   D

Findings: (A) AP radiograph of the lumbar spine taken at presentation is normal. (**B, C, D**) Six weeks later. AP radiograph of the lumbar spine taken at 6-week follow-up shows paravertebral ossification along the left lateral aspect at the L3–4 level. (**C**) Coronal short-tau inversion recovery MRI shows high signal in the left L3–4 paravertebral soft tissues. The intervertebral disc spaces are normal in height and hydration. (**D**) Axial CT with coronal reconstruction shows the paravertebral ossification bridging the lateral aspects of the L3–4 vertebral bodies.

Differential Diagnosis: Ankylosing spondylitis, psoriatic arthritis, Reiter's disease, DISH, fluorosis.

Diagnosis: Psoriatic spondyloarthropathy.

Discussion: The radiographs demonstrate paravertebral ossification becoming visible after 6 weeks, which is a typical length of time for bone formation to occur. The MRI shows inflammatory changes surrounding the site of ossification, and the coronal CT reconstruction shows the particular morphology of the bony bridge in relation to the involved vertebral bodies. Paravertebral ossification that bridges adjacent vertebral bodies is a classic radiographic feature of psoriatic arthritis and Reiter's syndrome. The ossification is typically present at only a few levels—at one level in this case—and extends from the lateral cortex of one vertebral body to the lateral cortex of the next with a curvilinear shape. This particular form of vertebral hyperostosis is distinguishable from spondylosis deformans, in which the bony growth is oriented horizontally from the endplate (osteophytes); from DISH, in which the bony growth flows over multiple contiguous vertebral bodies (ligamentous ossification); and from ankylosing spondylitis, in which the bony growth is vertically oriented from the margins of the vertebral endplates (syndesmophytes). Paravertebral ossification is an early skeletal manifestation of psoriatic arthritis, typically preceding changes in the sacroiliac joints or in the peripheral joints [76]. This patient was not previously known to have psoriatic arthritis.

SOURCES AND READINGS

1. Crawford NR, Duggal N, Chamberlain RH, Park SC, Sonntag VK, Dickman CA. Unilateral cervical facet dislocation: injury mechanism and biomechanical consequences. *Spine*. 2002;27(17):1858–1864.

2. Daffner SD, Daffner RH. Computed tomography diagnosis of facet dislocations: the "hamburger bun" and "reverse hamburger bun" signs. *J Emerg Med*. 2002;23(4):387–394.

3. Vaccaro AR, Madigan L, Schweitzer ME, Flanders AE, Hilibrand AS, Albert TJ. Magnetic resonance imaging analysis of soft tissue disruption after flexion-distraction injuries of the subaxial cervical spine. *Spine*. 2001;26(17):1866–1872.

4. Vandemark RM. Subtle malalignments resulting in diagnoses of occult severe cervical spine hyperextension or flexion injuries. *AJR Am J Roentgenol*. 1997;168:1378.

5. Tehranzadeh J, Palmer S. Imaging of cervical spine trauma. *Semin Ultrasound CT MR*. 1996;17:93–104.

6. Taylor JR, Twomey LT. Acute injuries to cervical joints. An autopsy study of neck sprain. *Spine*. 1993;18:1115–1122.

7. Barquet A, Dubra A. Occult severe hyperflexion sprain of the lower cervical spine. *Can Assoc Radiol J*. 1993;44:446–449.

8. Braakman M, Braakman R. Hyperflexion sprain of the cervical spine. Follow-up of 45 cases. *Acta Orthop Scand*. 1987;58:388–393.

9. Matsui H, Imada K, Tsuji H. Radiographic classification of os odontoideum and its clinical significance. *Spine*. 1997;22:1706–1709.

10. Schatzker J, Rorabeck CH, Waddell JP. Fractures of the dens (odontoid process): an analysis of 37 cases. *J Bone Joint Surg Br*. 1971:53-B:392–405.

11. Leite CC, Escobar BE, Bazan C III, Jinkins JR. MRI of cervical facet dislocation. *Neuroradiology*. 1997;39:583–588.

12. Holmes JF, Mirvis SE, Panacek EA, Hoffman JR, Mower WR, Velmahos GC. For the NEXUS Group. Variability in computed tomography and magnetic resonance imaging in patients with cervical spine injuries. *J Trauma*. 2002;53:524–529.

13. Jackson RS, Banit DM, Rhyne AL 3rd, Darden BV 2nd. Upper cervical spine injuries. *J Am Acad Orthop Surg*. 2002;10(4):271–280.

14. Quencer RM, Nunez D, Green BA. Controversies in imaging acute cervical spine trauma. *AJNR Am J Neuroradiol*. 1997;18:1866–1868.

15. Kim KS, Chen HH, Russell EJ, Rogers LF. Flexion tear-drop fracture of the cervical spine: radiographic characteristics. *AJR Am J Roentgenol*. 1989:152:319–326.

16. Kathol MH. Cervical spine trauma. What is new? *Radiol Clin North Am*. 1997;35:507–532.

17. Kinoshita H. Pathology of hyperextension injury of the cervical spine: a case report. *Spinal Cord*. 1997;35:857–858.

18. Harris JH Jr, Edeiken-Monroe B. *The Radiology of Acute Cervical Spine Trauma*. 2nd ed. New York: Williams and Wilkins; 1987:65–91.

19. Weller SJ, Malek AM, Rossitch E Jr. Cervical spine fractures in the elderly. *Surg Neurol*. 1997;47:274–280.

20. Ryan MD, Henderson JJ. The epidemiology of fractures and fracture-dislocations of the cervical spine. *Injury*. 1992;23:38–40.

21. Lieberman IH, Webb JK. Cervical spine injuries in the elderly. *J Bone Joint Surg Br*. 1994;76:877–881.

22. Nischal K, Chumas P, Sparrow O. Prolonged survival after atlanto-occipital dislocation: two case reports and review. *Br J Neurosurg*. 1993;7:677–682.

23. Harmanli O, Koyfman Y. Traumatic atlanto-occipital dislocation with survival: a case report and review of the literature. *Surg Neurol*. 1993;39:324–330.

24. Ferrera PC, Bartfield JM. Traumatic atlanto-occipital dislocation: a potentially survivable injury. *Am J Emerg Med*. 1996;14:291–296.

25. Henry MB, Angelastrao DB, Gillen JP. Unrecognized traumatic atlanto-occipital dislocation. *Am J Emerg Med*. 1998;16:406–408.

26. Guigui P, Milaire M, Morvan G, Lassale B, Deburge A. Traumatic atlantooccipital dislocation with survival: case report and review of the literature. *Eur Spine J*. 1995;4(4):242–247.

27. Rawlins BA, Girardi FP, Boachie-Adjei O. Rheumatoid arthritis of the cervical spine. *Rheum Dis Clin North Am*. 1998;24:55–65.

28. Azouz EM. Arthritis in children: conventional and advanced imaging. *Semin Musculoskelet Radiol*. 2003;7(2):95–102.

29. Flemming DJ, Murphey MD, Carmichael BB, Bernard SA. Primary tumors of the spine. *Semin Musculoskelet Radiol*. 2000;4(3):299–320.

30. Unni KK. *Dahlin's Bone Tumors. General Aspects and Data on 11,087 Cases*. 5th ed. Philadelphia: Lippincott-Raven Publishers; 1996:131–142.

31. Lucas DR, Unni KK, McLeod RA, O'Connor MI, Sim FH. Osteoblastoma: clinicopathologic study of 306 cases. *Hum Pathol*. 1994;25:117–134.

32. Zambelli P, Lechevallier J, Bracq H, Carlioz H. Osteoid osteoma or osteoblastoma of the cervical spine in relation to the vertebral artery. *J Pediatr Orthop*. 1994;14:788–792.

33. Andronikou S, Jadwat S, Douis H. Patterns of disease on MRI in 53 children with tuberculous spondylitis and the role of gadolinium. *Pediatr Radiol*. 2002;32(11):798–805.

34. Jain AK. Treatment of tuberculosis of the spine with neurologic complications. *Clin Orthop*. 2002;(398):75–84.

35. Taybi H, Lachman RS. *Radiology of Syndromes, Metabolic Disorders, and Skeletal Dysplasias*. 4th ed. St. Louis: Mosby; 1996:677–679.

36. Mikles M, Stanton RP. A review of Morquio syndrome. *Am J Orthop*. 1997;26:533–540.

37. Ruiz-Maldonado R, Tamayo-Sanchez L, Orozco-Covarrubias ML. The use of retinoids in the pediatric patient. *Dermatol Clin*. 1998;16:553–569.

38. DiGiovanna JJ. Isotretinoin effects on bone. *J Am Acad Dermatol*. 2001;45(5):S176–S182.

39. David M, Hodak E, Lowe NJ. Adverse effects of retinoids. *Med Toxicol Adverse Drug Exp*. 1988;3:273–288.

40. Torok L, Galuska L, Kasa M, Kada L. Bone-scintigraphic examinations in patients treated with retinoids: a prospective study. *Br J Dermatol*. 1989;120:31–36.

41. McAlister WH, Herman TE. Osteochondrodysplasias, dysostoses, chromosomal aberrations, mucopolysaccharidoses, and mucolipodoses. In: Resnick D, ed. *Diagnosis of Bone and Joint Disorders*. 4th ed. Philadelphia: WB Saunders; 2001:4489–4491.

42. Kovanlikaya A, Loro ML, Gilsanz V. Pathogenesis of osteosclerosis in autosomal dominant osteopetrosis. *AJR Am J Roentgenol*. 1997;168:929–932.

43. Lim MR, Yoon SC, Green DW. Symptomatic spondylolysis: diagnosis and treatment. *Curr Opin Pediatr*. 2004;16(1):37–46.

44. Fujii K, Katoh S, Sairyo K, Ikata T, Yasui N. Union of defects in the pars interarticularis of the lumbar spine in children and adolescents. The radiological outcome after conservative treatment. *J Bone Joint Surg Br*. 2004;86(2):225–231.

45. Sheridan R, Peralta R, Rhea J, Ptak T, Novelline R. Reformatted visceral protocol helical computed tomographic scanning allows conventional radiographs of the thoracic and lumbar spine to be eliminated in the evaluation of blunt trauma patients. *J Trauma*. 2003 Oct;55(4):665–669.

46. Floman Y, Bar-On E, Mosheiff R, Mirovsky Y, Robin GC, Ramu N. Eosinophilic granuloma of the spine. *J Pediatr Orthop B*. 1997;6:260–265.

47. Harreby M, Neergaard K, Hesselsoe G, Kjer J. Are radiologic changes in the thoracic and lumbar spine of adolescents risk factors for low back pain in adults? A 25-year prospective cohort study of 640 school children. *Spine*. 1995;20:2298–2302.

48. Gustavel M, Beals RK. Scheuermann's disease of the lumbar spine in identical twins. *AJR Am J Roentgenol*. 2002;179(4):1078–1079.

49. Andersson GB, Bostrom MP, Eyre DR, et al. Consensus summary on the diagnosis and treatment of osteoporosis. *Spine*. 1997;22:63S–65S.

50. Tracy MR, Dormans JP, Kusumi K. Klippel-Feil syndrome: clinical features and current understanding of etiology. *Clin Orthop*. 2004;(424):183–190.

51. Ogden JA, Conlogue GJ, Phillips MS, Bronson ML. Sprengel's deformity. Radiology of the pathologic deformation. *Skeletal Radiol.* 1979;4(4):204–211.

52. Rauch F, Glorieux FH. Osteogenesis imperfecta. *Lancet.* 2004;363 (9418):1377–1385.

53. Engelbert RH, Gerver WJ, Breslau-Siderius LJ, et al. Spinal complications in ostegenesis imperta: 47 patients 1–16 years of age. *Acta Orthop Scand.* 1998;69:283–286.

54. Arikoski P, Silverwood B, Tillmann V, Bishop NJ. Intravenous pamidronate treatment in children with moderate to severe osteogenesis imperfecta: assessment of indices of dual-energy x-ray absorptiometry and bone metabolic markers during the first year of therapy. *Bone.* 2004;34(3):539–546.

55. Resnick D. The "rugger jersey" vertebral body. *Arthritis Rheum.* 1981;24: 1191–1194.

56. Mulligan ME. *Classic Radiologic Signs. An Atlas and History.* New York: Parthenon; 1997:138–139.

57. Khanine V, Fournier JJ, Requeda E, Luton JP, Simon F, Crouzet J. Osteoporotic fractures at presentation of Cushing's disease: two case reports and a literature review. *Joint Bone Spine.* 2000;67(4):341–345.

58. Kooy A, de Heide LJ, ten Tiji AJ, et al. Vertebral bone destruction in sickle cell disease: infection, infarction, or both. *Neth J Med.* 1996;48:227–231.

59. Mannoni A, Selvi E, Lorenzini S, et al. Alkaptonuria, ochronosis, and ochronotic arthropathy. *Semin Arthritis Rheum.* 2004;33(4):239–248.

60. Loke TK, Ma HT, Chan CS. Magnetic resonance imaging of tuberculous spinal infection. *Australas Radiol.* 1997;41:7–12.

61. Murphey MD, Robbin MR, McRae GA, Flemming DJ, Temple HT, Kransdorf MJ. The many faces of osteosarcoma. *Radiographics.* 1997;17:1205–1231.

62. Resnick, D. Skeletal mestastases. In: Resnick D, ed. *Diagnosis of Bone and Joint Disorders.* 4th ed. Philadelphia: WB Saunders; 2001:4295.

63. Arlet V, Odent T, Aebi M. Congenital scoliosis. *Eur Spine J.* 2003;12(5): 456–463.

64. Rosenthal DI, Hornicek FJ, Torriani M, Gebhardt MC, Mankin HJ. Osteoid osteoma: percutaneous treatment with radiofrequency energy. *Radiology.* 2003;229:171–175.

65. Carpineta L, Gagne M. The ivory vertebra: an approach to investigation and management based on two case studies. *Spine.* 2002;27(9):E242–E247.

66. Whitten CR, Saifuddin A. MRI of Paget's disease of bone. *Clin Radiol.* 2003;58(10):763–769.

67. Carragee EJ, Hannibal M. Diagnostic evaluation of low back pain. *Orthop Clin North Am.* 2004;35(1):7–16.

68. Saifuddin A, Noordeen H, Taylor BA, Bayley I. The role of imaging in the diagnosis and management of thoracolumbar burst fractures: current concepts and a review of the literature. *Skeletal Radiol.* 1996;25(7):603–613.

69. Honan M, White GW, Eisenberg GM. Spontaneous infectious discitis in adults. *Am J Med.* 1996;100:85–89.

70. Fouquet B, Goupille P, Gobert F, Cotty P, Roulot B, Valat JP. Infectious discitis diagnostic contribution of laboratory tests and percutaneous discovertebral biopsy. *Rev Rhum Engl Ed.* 1996;63:24–29.

71. Hitchon PW, From AM, Brenton MD, Glaser JA, Torner JC. Fractures of the thoracolumbar spine complicating ankylosing spondylitis. *J Neurosurg.* 2002;97(suppl):218–222.

72. Lachman RS. Neurologic abnormalities in the skeletal dysplasias: a clinical and radiological perspective. *Am J Med Genet.* 1997;69: 33–43.

73. Friedman DP. Symptomatic vertebral hemangiomas: MR findings. *AJR Am J Roentgenol.* 1996;167:359–364.

74. Redekop GJ, Del Maestro RF. Vertebral hemangioma causing spinal cord compression during pregnancy. *Surg Neurol.* 1992;38:210–215.

75. Tekkok IH, Acikgoz B, Saglam S, Onol B. Vertebral hemangioma symptomatic during pregnancy—report of a case and review of the literature. *Neurosurgery.* 1993;32:302–306.

76. Sundaram M, Patton JT. Paravertebral ossification in psoriasis and Reiter's disease. *Br J Radiol.* 1975;48:628–633.

CHAPTER FOUR
PELVIS

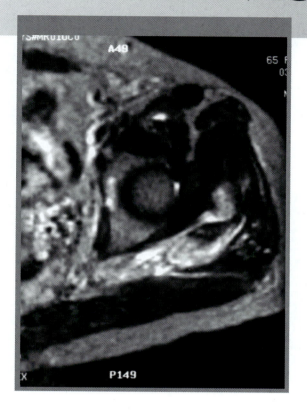

CASE 4-1

Clinical History: 40-year-old man with sacral pain for several months.

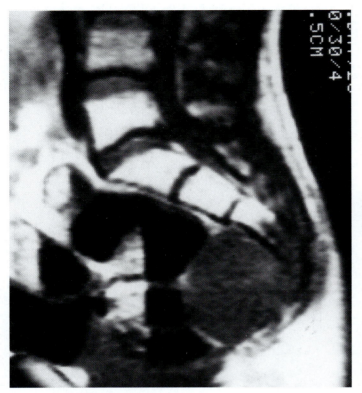

Figure 4-1 A

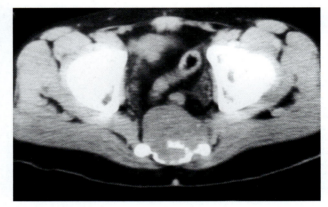

Figure 4-1 B

Findings: (A) Sagittal T1-weighted magnetic resonance image (MRI) demonstrates a low signal intensity mass replacing the distal sacrum, and extending anteriorly into the pelvis as a well-defined mass. (B) Axial computed tomography (CT) shows a midline mass creating moth-eaten destruction of the sacrum and exophytic anterior extension of the mass, extending to (but not involving pathologically) the rectum.

Differential Diagnosis: Chordoma, chondrosarcoma, giant cell tumor, plasmacytoma, metastasis.

Diagnosis: Chordoma.

Discussion: The diagnosis is made from the characteristic location in the midline of the sacrococcygeal region, with asymmetric expansion from the bone into the anterior soft tissues. The radiologic features typical of chordoma in this location are irregular osteolysis and expansion with an associated anterior soft tissue mass. Fifty percent to 70% of cases may show amorphous calcification, usually in the periphery of the tumor; some lesions present with sclerosis instead of osteolysis. On T2-weighted MRI, the lesions are typically as bright as hydrated intervertebral discs. Differential considerations include giant cell tumor, plasmacytoma, chondrosarcoma, neurogenic tumor, meningocele, and metastasis. Chordoma is a locally aggressive lesion of notochordal origin [1]. Chordomas are most common in the sacrococcygeal region (50% to 60% of lesions), in men (2:1 predilection), and between the ages of 40 and 70. Sphenooccipital lesions account for almost all of the remainder of lesions (25% to 40%). Low lumbar and high occipital lesions are the next most common, followed by the remainder of the vertebrae. Sphenooccipital involvement is more typical in children. Sacrococcygeal lesions typically present with pain and perineal numbness. The lesions usually arise from the vertebral body, but they can extend into the posterior elements.

Clinical History: 50-year-old man after treatment for prostate carcinoma.

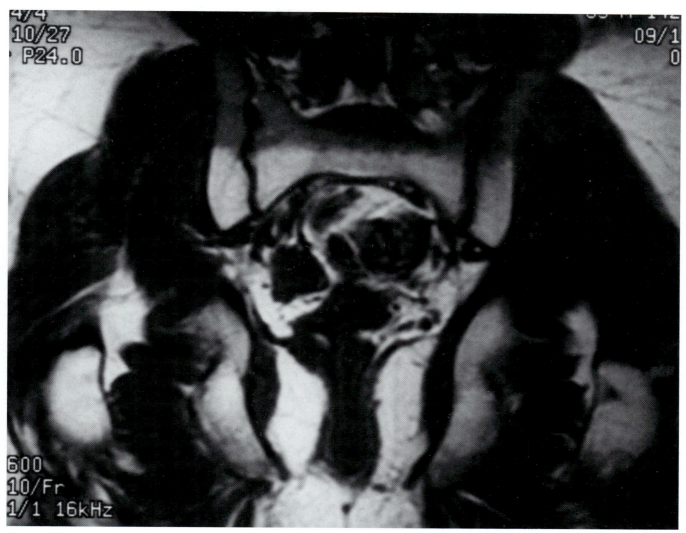

Figure 4-2

Findings: Coronal T1-weighted MRI of the pelvis demonstrates a band of increased signal in the inferior sacrum, with a well-defined horizontal border.

Differential Diagnosis: Radiation changes, insufficiency fracture, imaging artifact.

Diagnosis: Radiation changes.

Discussion: MRI is commonly used to study the spine after therapeutic irradiation. On T1-weighted MRI, there is an increased signal in the involved bone due to replacement of the hematopoietic marrow with fat. This alteration can be seen 3 months after initiation of therapy, and may remain indefinitely [2]. Insufficiency fractures of the sacrum may result after as little as 53 Gy is introduced, with an incidence of 20% [3]. Radiation can also give rise to fibrosis. Fibrosis should have low signal intensity on both T1-weighted and T2-weighted MRI, whereas tumor typically has increased signal on T2-weighted MRI due to the increased water content. Other effects of radiation therapy can include inhibition of bone growth, slipped capital epiphyses in children, scoliosis, avascular necrosis, and radiation-induced neoplasms.

CASE 4-3

Clinical History: 43-year-old man with posterior left thigh pain.

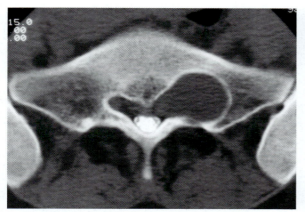

Figure 4-3   A

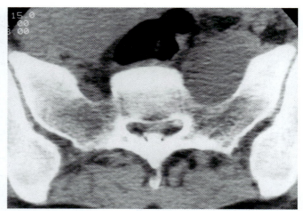

Figure 4-3   B

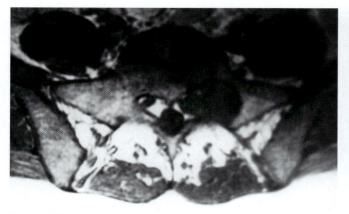

Figure 4-3   C

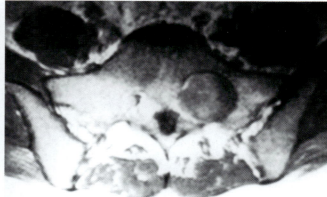

Figure 4-3   D

Findings: (A, B) Oblique axial CT scan after injection of myelographic contrast material shows a large S1 nerve root mass, with a remodeled and enlarged S1 neural foramen. There is no actual bone destruction. The uncalcified mass protrudes anteriorly into the pelvis. (C) Axial T1-weighted MRI shows the mass has intermediate signal. (D) Axial T1-weighted MRI after gadolinium injection shows slight enhancement of the mass.

Differential Diagnosis: Neurofibroma, schwannoma, sarcoma.

Diagnosis: Neurofibroma.

Discussion: The particular location and morphology of this lesion suggests the diagnosis of a nerve sheath tumor. The remodeling of the bone around the enlarging tumor indicates very slow growth. This patient was not previously suspected of having neurofibromatosis. Neurofibromas are benign fibroblastic neoplasms of peripheral nerves, whose consistency and histologic appearance vary from myxoid to fibrous according to the differentiation of the neoplastic elements [4]. The bulk of the tumor volume consists of intercellular collagen fibrils in an unorganized myxoid matrix. Their imaging characteristics depend on the relative balance of fibrous and myxoid material. On MRI, neurofibromas tend to be isointense to muscle on T1-weighted images and hyperintense on T2-weighted images, and can be inhomogeneous [5].

CASE 4-4

Clinical History: 75-year-old man with back pain and history of chronic lymphocytic leukemia (CLL).

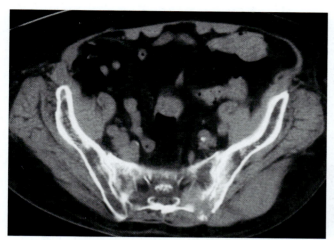

Figure 4-4   A

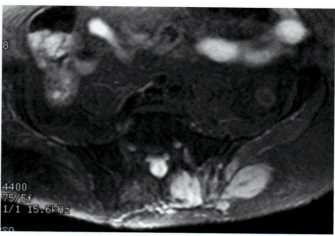

Figure 4-4   B

Findings: (**A**) Axial CT scan shows lytic bone destruction of the sacrum and ilium. The soft tissue masses have no calcification, and there is no reactive bone formation. (**B**) Axial T2-weighted MRI with fat saturation at the level of S1 shows masses in the paraspinal musculature and superficial to the gluteus maximus. The lesions have homogeneous high signal, and there is contiguous involvement of the ilium and sacrum.

Differential Diagnosis: Lymphoma, leukemia, metastases, infection.

Diagnosis: Lymphoma (Richter's syndrome).

Discussion: The images show soft tissue masses involving the paraspinal and gluteus musculature, an appearance that raises the differential diagnosis of lymphoma, leukemia, metastases, and infection. The presence of bone destruction eliminates hematoma as a possibility, and the lack of a single dominant mass lesion is very uncharacteristic of a connective tissue sarcoma.

The specific diagnosis depends on the clinical situation and must be confirmed by biopsy. Secondary malignancies develop in approximately 5% of patients with CLL, the most common of which is non-Hodgkin's lymphoma, followed by Hodgkin's lymphoma and multiple myeloma [7,8]. The development of non-Hodgkin's lymphoma in CLL is called Richter's syndrome. These lymphomas are high-grade malignancies of B-cell origin, associated with abrupt onset of constitutional symptoms, rapidly progressive lymphadenopathy, and rapid clinical deterioration to a fatal outcome. They are resistant to current therapies and may develop while the CLL is in remission. In approximately 60% of cases, the lymphoma evolves from the original leukemic cell clone, but in the remainder it has a different clonal evolution.

Clinical History: 40-year-old man with low back pain.

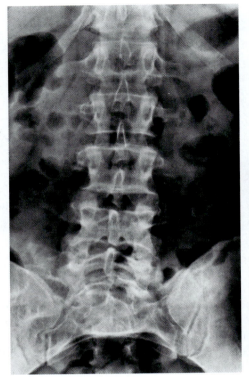

Figure 4-5 A

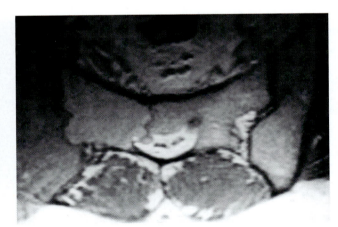

Figure 4-5 B

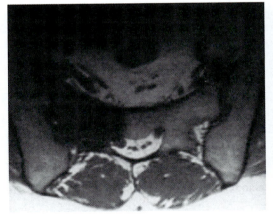

Figure 4-5 C

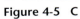

Figure 4-5 D

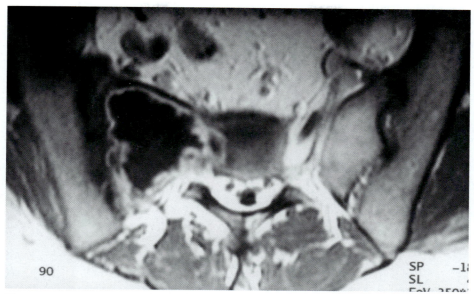

Figure 4-5   E

Findings: (**A**) Anteroposterior (AP) radiograph of the lumbar spine reveals expansile lucent lesion in the right sacral wing, extending to the sacroiliac joint. (**B**) Axial CT image shows replacement of the right sacral wing by a mass of soft tissue density that has engulfed the S1 and S2 neural foramen. No mineralization is seen within the mass. (**C–E**) T1-weighted, T2-weighted, and enhanced T1-weighted MRI shows T1 hypointensity, T2 hyperintensity, and peripheral enhancement of the sacral lesion.

Differential   Diagnosis: Chondrosarcoma, chordoma, giant cell tumor, plasmacytoma, metastasis, lymphoma, infection.

Diagnosis: Chondrosarcoma.

Discussion: Differential considerations for a large osteolytic lesion in a flat bone, with or without an associated soft tissue mass, include chondrosarcoma, metastases, lymphoma, plasmacytoma or multiple myeloma, or infection. Additional benign possibilities might include giant cell tumor, hemophiliac pseudotumor (if history of a bleeding dyscrasia), brown tumor (if other evidence of hyperparathyroidism), or aneurysmal bone cysts (if more expansile). Most of the aforementioned lesions will show more than

peripheral enhancement. The lack of reactive bone is ominous for an aggressive, malignant process. Without the characteristic calcification and lobular structure, the diagnosis of chondrosarcoma cannot be made prospectively, and a biopsy is required.

Chondrosarcomas are malignant, cartilage-containing tumors that arise de novo in preexisting cartilage lesions or rests. They are the third most common primary malignant bone tumor [6]. Chondrosarcomas tend to present in patients between the ages of 30 to 60. Lesions in the axial skeleton tend to present in an older age group than lesions in the peripheral skeleton.

This patient presented with the usual clinical scenario: slowly progressive back pain over a 2-year period that did not improve with chiropractic manipulations. This case illustrates how subtle the findings can be on plain radiography—mild expansion of the superior sacral cortex, loss of the arcuate lines, and a relative hyperlucency may be the only evidence for the diagnosis. Chondrosarcomas follow a slow clinical evolution. They tend to metastasize late in the clinical course, and although the lesions are often large, patients rarely present with metastatic disease.

Clinical History: Newborn baby girl.

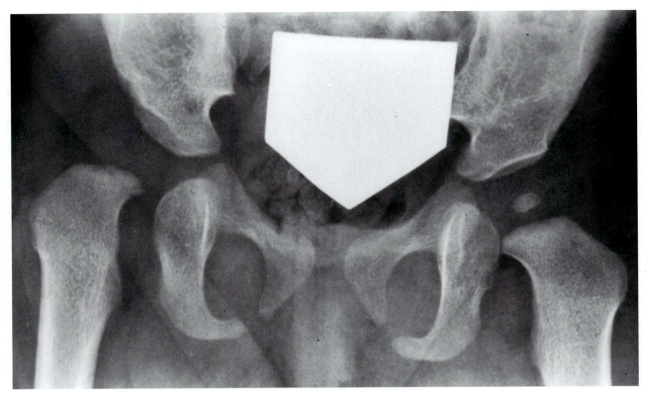

Figure 4-6

Findings: AP pelvis radiograph shows a dysplastic, dislocated right hip. The capital femoral ossification is not yet present, unlike the contralateral side. The acetabular angle is steep and shallow.

Differential Diagnosis: None.

Diagnosis: Developmental dysplasia of the hip (DDH).

Discussion: In DDH, an abnormally lax joint capsule allows the femoral head to fall out of the acetabulum shortly before or after birth, leading to congenital or postnatal deformation of an initially normal structure. The causes are multifactorial and appear to be related to the effects of restricted intrauterine movement and maternal hormones. Restricted fetal movement during the third trimester may result from conditions such as breech presentation or oligohydramnios, and may partially or completely dislocate the hip. Maternal hormones (such as estrogen) that relax the pelvic ligaments to facilitate childbirth also increase the laxity of the fetal ligaments and joint capsules. This effect is particularly evident in female fetuses and may account for the 6:1 female preponderance of DDH. DDH also has a familial tendency, which is possibly related to an inherited abnormality in estrogen metabolism. Although sonography is the imaging examination of choice in the neonate and has the advantage of immediate correlation with physical examination, results vary with technical and interpretive factors [9]. In older infants, the AP radiograph becomes more reliable as the capital femoral epiphysis becomes ossified.

Each hip can be divided into quadrants by drawing a horizontal baseline through the triradiate cartilages (Hilgenreiner's horizontal line) and a perpendicular line through the most lateral ossified margin of the roof of the acetabulum (Perkins' line). The normal location of the femoral head is in the lower inner quadrant (down and in). A dislocated femoral head will be in the upper outer quadrant (up and out), and a subluxated femoral head will be in the lower outer quadrant (down and out). The angle between the acetabulum and the horizontal baseline should be less than 40 degrees in a newborn, 33 degrees in a 6 month old, and 30 degrees in a 1 year old. In the normal hip, a smooth curve can be drawn along the inferior margin of the superior pubic ramus and the medial femoral cortex (Shenton's line). Other findings include a shallow acetabulum, development of a false acetabulum, and delayed ossification of the involved capital femoral epiphysis. CT scanning may be necessary to confirm anatomic relocation of the hips once the patient has been placed in a cast [10]. MRI may be used to evaluate problematic cases.

CASE 4-7

Clinical History: 21-year-old woman with mild hip pain.

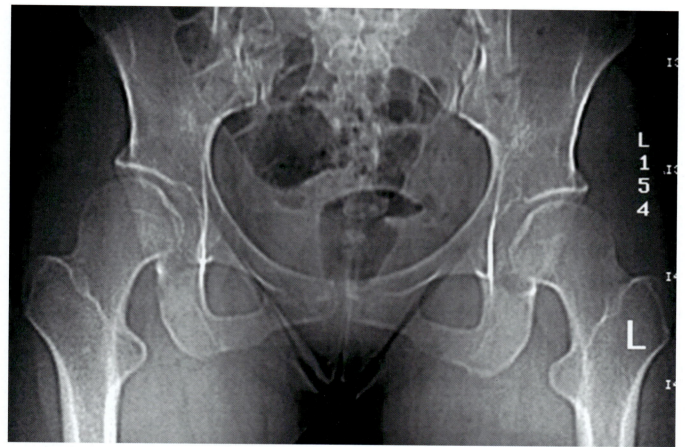

Figure 4-7

Findings: Radiograph of the pelvis shows shallow, minimally dysplastic acetabuli. Both femoral heads are normally formed and located.

Differential Diagnosis: None.

Diagnosis: Acetabular dysplasia.

Discussion: Acetabular dysplasia is a common cause of early osteoarthritis in adults [13]. The normal acetabulum is nearly a full hemisphere, forming the socket for the femoral head. The dysplastic acetabulum is like a shallow bowl, normally oriented but forming only a shallow socket for the femoral head. As a consequence, both the anterior and posterior articular surfaces are reduced in area, and a smaller proportion of the femoral head is covered by bone. On the radiograph, the roof of the acetabulum normally covers the top of the femoral head and inclines downward at its lateral margin. In acetabular dysplasia, the roof often fails to reach a horizontal orientation at its lateral margin, with much less incline downward. Patients are usually moderately symptomatic when they present at 30 or 40 years old, but will progress inevitably to end-stage osteoarthritis if untreated. An acetabular osteotomy provides more complete bony coverage of the femoral head and can prevent accelerated osteoarthritis [14].

Clinical History: 62-year-old woman with pelvic mass referred to the orthopedist by the gynecologist.

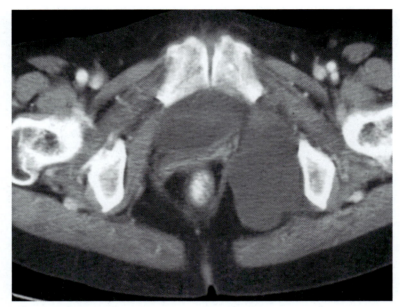

Figure 4-8   A

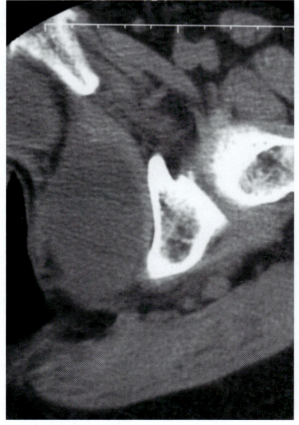

Figure 4-8   B

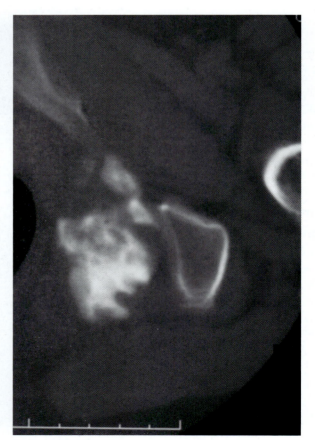

Figure 4-8   C

Findings: (A) CT scan through the pelvis shows an ovoid, well-marginated, low-attenuation, soft tissue mass occupying the left side of the true pelvis. The visceral structures have been displaced. (B) High-resolution CT image shows the lesion is located within the obturator internus muscle. There is no involvement of the adjacent bone. (C) CT image after aspiration biopsy and injection of radiographic contrast shows the cystic nature of the lesion.

Differential Diagnosis: Soft tissue sarcoma, intramuscular myxoma, nerve sheath tumor.

Diagnosis: Intramuscular myxoma.

Discussion: The location of the mass is within the obturator internus muscle, eliminating genitourinary or gastrointestinal lesions from consideration. The possibility of soft tissue sarcoma, particularly sarcomas with myxoid components, can only be definitively excluded by biopsy. Intramuscular myxoma is a benign, soft tissue tumor that presents as a deep mass within skeletal muscle [11]. It is a hypocellular and hypovascular lesion with a gelatinous consistency. On CT, the lesion is spherical or ovoid and is sharply marginated, but with no discernible capsule. Attenuation is typically 10 to 30 Hounsfield units, the lesions are homogeneous, and they do not exhibit enhancement. On MRI, the lesions have low signal intensity on T1-weighted images and high signal intensity on T2-weighted images. Typical size at presentation is 6 cm, and the most common location is in the thigh musculature. CT-guided biopsy may be nondiagnostic if only fine-needle aspiration is used; usually aspiration with a large-bore needle (larger than 20 gauge) is required to sample the gelatinous material. Surgical excision is virtually always curative. The lesion is more common in women (2:1) and is found in adults (mean age 52 years). The association of intramuscular myxomas with fibrous dysplasia of bone is called Mazabraud's syndrome [12].

CASE 4-9

Clinical History: 28-year-old man with hip pain and poor muscle development.

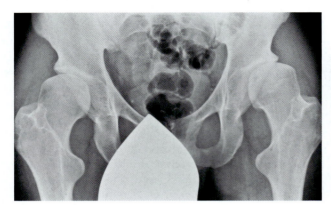

Figure 4-9   A

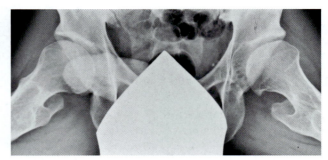

Figure 4-9   B

Findings: (A, B) AP radiograph of the hips. The acetabuli are shallow and the proximal femurs are dysplastic but normally located. Asymmetric joint space narrowing, subchondral sclerosis, and early osteophyte formation are present in the left hip.

Differential Diagnosis: DDH, neuromuscular syndrome, epiphyseal dysplasia, acetabular dysplasia.

Diagnosis: Muscular dystrophy.

Discussion: The dysplastic changes involve the acetabulum as well as the femoral head and neck, but the hip is normally located. The changes are bilaterally symmetric, an observation that narrows the range of possibilities. Early osteoarthritis in the hip is typically the result of abnormal anatomic development. Common underlying conditions include developmental dysplasias, neuromuscular syndromes,

Legg-Calve-Perthes disease, slipped capital femoral epiphysis, and trauma.

Muscular dystrophy describes a heterogeneous group of genetic diseases in which there is generalized or focal neuromuscular disease that may cause secondary bone changes. These changes are the result of abnormal stresses on the growing skeleton from muscular spasm, weakness, atrophy, and imbalance. When the normal skeleton remodels in response to abnormal stress, dysplastic changes in the bones and joints may result. Long bones often appear overtubulated (narrow shaft, broad epiphysis). Hip dysplasia secondary to chronic spastic dislocation is common. Scoliosis, soft tissue atrophy, and flexion or extension contractures may be found. Similar developmental changes are seen in conditions such as arthrogryposis, cerebral palsy, peripheral nerve palsy, and polio.

Clinical History: 17-year-old girl with progressive stiffness involving the hip and other joints.

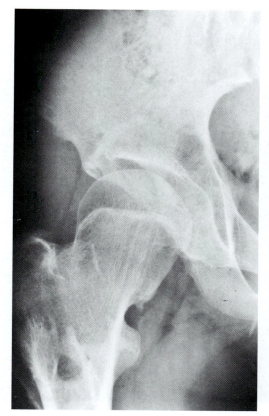

Figure 4-10   A

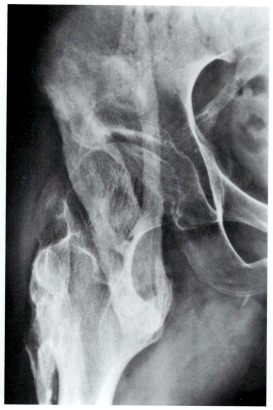

Figure 4-10   B

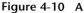

Findings: (A) AP radiograph at presentation reveals a deformity of the femoral neck, with broadening and a small medial inferior protuberance. (B) Two years later, AP radiograph shows ossification of the sacrotuberous ligament, as well as ossification of a small band from the medial femoral neck to the high iliac crest, and a larger band from the mid femoral neck to the supraacetabular region.

Differential Diagnosis: Burns, trauma, paralysis, diffuse idiopathic skeletal hyperostosis, fibrodysplasia ossificans progressiva.

Diagnosis: Fibrodysplasia ossificans progressiva.

Discussion: Ossification in the soft tissues can be recognized and distinguished from calcification by the presence of a cortical and trabecular structure. The most commonly seen soft tissue ossification is that occurring after trauma, not only in the form of myositis ossificans, but more frequently at sites of ligamentous sprains. Burns and paralysis may also be associated with focal or periarticular soft tissue ossification. Diffuse idiopathic skeletal hyperostosis is a condition of soft tissue ossification, but in this condition it is always enthesal (at the attachment of ligaments, capsules, and tendons to bone).

Fibrodysplasia ossificans progressiva (also called myositis ossificans progressiva) is a rare hereditary connective tissue disorder characterized by progressive ossification of striated muscle, tendons, ligaments, and fascia associated with congenital skeletal anomalies [15]. The process of ossification is associated with pain and disability, and involvement of the spine, hips, and extremities leads to extraarticular ankylosis, the so-called "stone man." Congenital malformations of the hands and feet, particularly the great toes, are also associated. The condition is transmitted as an autosomal dominant defect [16]. Soft tissue swelling may progress to heterotopic ossification within 3 to 4 weeks, with edema and fibroblasts incited by local trauma, surgery, or injections [17]. Severe disability results from progressive immobilization of the limbs, jaw, and chest wall. Life-threatening complications include restrictive chest wall disease [17,18] and falls [19]. Falls can be particularly catastrophic, and frequently they initiate a painful flare-up that leads to the permanent loss of movement. Intracranial injuries are common and may be severe, probably the result of deficiencies in coordinated gait and protective reflexes. Most patients die of pneumonia.

CASE 4-11

Clinical History: 25-year-old man in a high-speed motor vehicle crash.

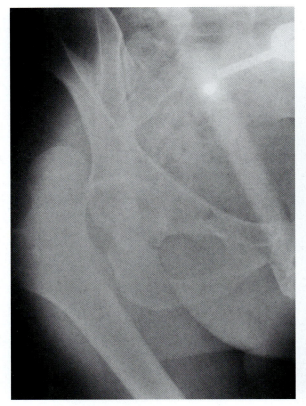

Figure 4-11 A

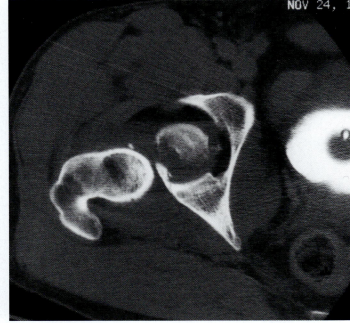

Figure 4-11 B

Findings: (A) AP detail of the right hip shows superior and lateral dislocation of the femoral head. (B) CT scan of the right hip shows fracture-dislocation of the right femoral head, with the head coming to rest posterior to the iliac wing. There is a fat-fluid level in the hip joint and a single bubble of intracapsular gas.

Differential Diagnosis: Anterior hip dislocation, posterior hip dislocation.

Diagnosis: Posterior hip dislocation.

Discussion: Hip dislocations result from severe trauma such as motor vehicle accidents. Posterior dislocations, with or without acetabular fractures, account for 85% to 90% of traumatic hip dislocations. The mechanism of injury is a blow along the axis of the femoral shaft with the hip flexed (e.g., hitting the dashboard with the knee). The posterior wall or column of the acetabulum is often fractured, and the femoral shaft or knee may also be injured. Associated fractures of the femoral head occur occasionally, and intraarticular fragments may be particularly problematic for reduction.

The thigh is characteristically adducted after a posterior dislocation. CT can identify intraarticular fragments and confirm relocation of the hip after reduction. The presence of gas bubbles in the hip joint capsule after trauma, in the absence of penetrating injury, is a reliable indicator of recent hip dislocation [20]. Most bubbles are located anterior to the femoral neck, but bubbles may also be found posteriorly.

If hip dislocation is unsuspected because of spontaneous relocation or reduction at the scene, the presence of gas should alert the clinician to the possibility of complications. Complications of hip dislocation include avascular necrosis of the femoral head, transient or permanent sciatic nerve palsy, myositis ossificans, and posttraumatic degenerative arthrosis. A posteriorly dislocated hip stretches and twists the external iliac, common femoral, and circumflex arteries, resulting in changes in extraosseous blood flow. Although collateral circulation from gluteal vessels may preserve intraosseous blood flow, delayed relocation may produce a progressive and delayed form of arterial damage that leads to osteonecrosis [21].

Clinical History: 31-year-old woman hit by a car while biking.

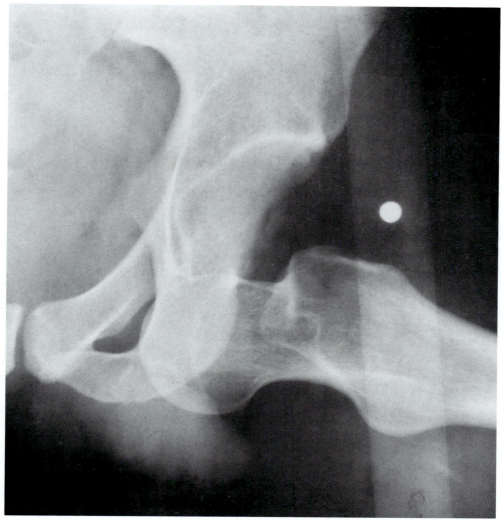

Figure 4-12

Findings: AP radiograph of the left hip shows dislocation. The femoral head overlies the obturator foramen and is inferior to the empty acetabulum. The femur is severely abducted. No fracture is seen.

Differential Diagnosis: Anterior hip dislocation, posterior hip dislocation.

Diagnosis: Anterior hip dislocation.

Discussion: This case illustrates an obviously dislocated hip, but where has the femoral head come to rest? About 11% of traumatic hip dislocations are anterior [22], with the femoral head in most cases resting inferiorly over the obturator foramen, as in this case. The mechanism of injury is forced abduction, external rotation, and flexion of the hip, causing the femoral head to slip anteriorly and medially through the hip capsule, but beneath the strong pubofemoral ligament. The pubofemoral ligament runs from the base of the superior pubic ramus to the lesser trochanter. In approximately 10% of anterior hip dislocations, forced abduction, external rotation, and extension of the hip causes the femoral head to rupture the anterior hip capsule above the pubofemoral ligament, with the femoral head resting superiorly, above the level of the anterior pubic ramus, over the anterior abdominal wall. The iliofemoral ligament may be torn or avulsed from its insertion at the anterior inferior iliac spine. Associated with anterior hip dislocations may be an impaction fracture of the superolateral aspect of the femoral head where it impinges on the anterior inferior rim of the acetabulum after it dislocates. Long-term sequelae include arthritis and osteonecrosis.

Clinical History: 43-year-old woman with bone pain and muscle weakness.

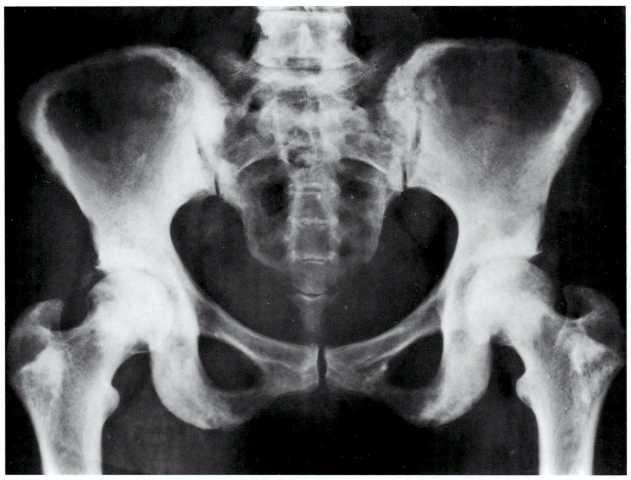

Figure 4-13

Findings: AP radiograph of the pelvis shows symmetrically dense bones, involving principally the cortices. The medullary space is present, and the trabecular pattern is normal. There are degenerative changes in the hips, sacroiliac joints, and lumbar spine.

Differential Diagnosis: Osteopetrosis, fluorosis, hypervitaminosis A, renal osteodystrophy, sickle cell anemia, other causes of diffuse sclerosis.

Diagnosis: Fluorosis.

Discussion: Generalized osteosclerosis and hyperostosis can be seen in a variety of metabolic and systemic conditions. Fluorosis may be related to chronic ingestion of drinking water with endemic, excessive levels of fluoride (four parts or more per million), occupational exposure, or fluoride-containing medication. Endemic regions with large populations include parts of India and China [23,24]. In some circumstances, endemic fluorosis has been described even when fluoride levels in drinking water are not excessive. Tea plants may concentrate the fluoride found in the water and soil. The fluoride content of leaves from these tea plants is related to the length of time they have been growing, resulting in high fluoride levels in tea that is brewed from old leaves and stems, but not in tea brewed from tender leaves and buds [25]. Among occupational exposures, aluminum workers are at particular risk of fluorosis.

The definitive diagnosis is from direct measurements of bone fluoride content. Bone fluoride content is related to exposure, and radiographic findings are found more frequently among those with higher bone fluoride content [26,27]. Radiographic findings include osteopenia, osteosclerosis and hyperostosis involving the axial skeleton, periostitis and enthesopathy in the appendicular skeleton, and dental abnormalities. Early degenerative arthropathy may also be seen. Clinically, there may be decreasing range of motion in the limbs that often progresses to rigidity.

Clinical History: 8-year-old girl with sacroiliac joint pain and chronic disease.

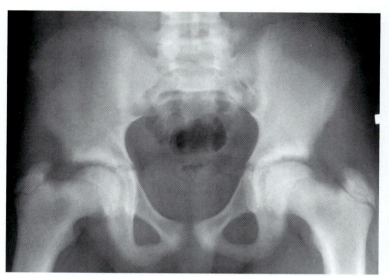

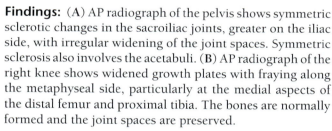

Figure 4-14   A

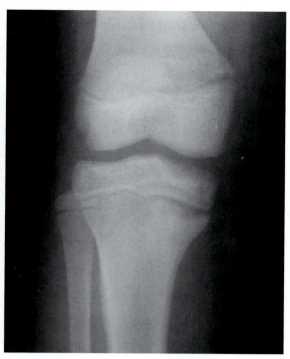

Figure 4-14   B

Findings: (A) AP radiograph of the pelvis shows symmetric sclerotic changes in the sacroiliac joints, greater on the iliac side, with irregular widening of the joint spaces. Symmetric sclerosis also involves the acetabuli. (B) AP radiograph of the right knee shows widened growth plates with fraying along the metaphyseal side, particularly at the medial aspects of the distal femur and proximal tibia. The bones are normally formed and the joint spaces are preserved.

Differential Diagnosis: Rickets, juvenile idiopathic arthritis.

Diagnosis: Rickets.

Discussion: The history indicates chronic, systemic disease, and the changes in the growth plates at the knee are classic for rickets in an older child. Sacroiliac disease may also occur in childhood onsets of spondyloarthropathy, particularly ankylosing spondylitis. In this case, the patient has vitamin-D-resistant rickets. Rickets can manifest with a wide variety of symptoms, including symptoms that suggest sacroiliitis [30]. It has been suggested that secondary hyperparathyroidism with subchondral bone resorption may result in subchondral insufficiency fractures or microfractures at the sacroiliac joints, causing the symptoms. On MRI, the changes in the physeal regions can be striking, with high T2-weighted signal in the broad region of unossified cartilage [31].

Clinical History: 65-year-old woman with progressive left buttock pain, now unable to walk.

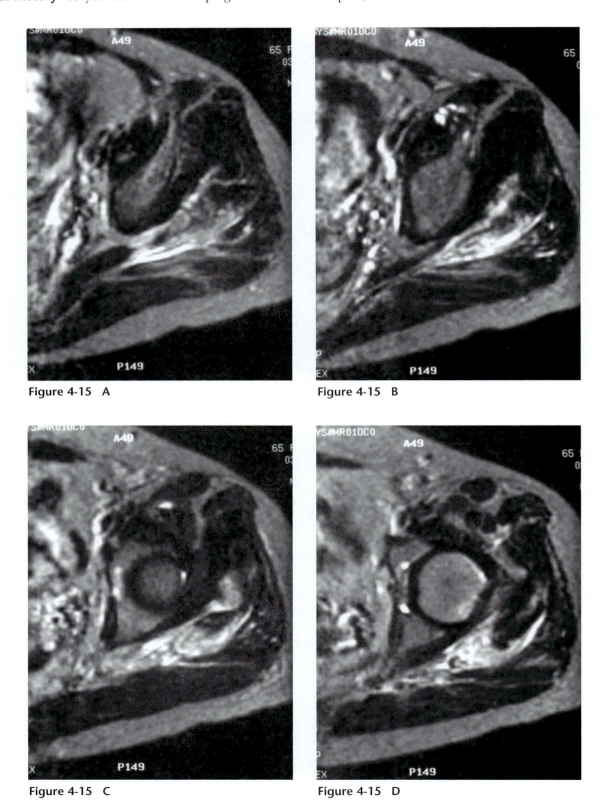

Figure 4-15   A

Figure 4-15   B

Figure 4-15   C

Figure 4-15   D

Findings: (A–D) Axial T2-weighted fast spin-echo images with fat saturation through the left hip region show abnormal high signal in the region of the gluteus medius. There is no mass effect, and the bone marrow signal is normal. The curled, retracted stump of the gluteus medius tendon may be seen at its insertion along the greater trochanter of the femur.

Differential Diagnosis: None.

Diagnosis: Gluteus medius tendon tear.

Discussion: The lack of mass effect in this soft tissue abnormality suggests a nonneoplastic process. The particular location and appearance are diagnostic of an injury to the gluteus medius muscle-tendon unit. An injury to a muscle-tendon unit from indirect loading is called a strain or tear. The injury is most common in muscles with eccentric rather than concentric activation, and typically occurs at or near the myotendinous junction [28]. Fluid collects at the site of disruption and dissects along the sheath of connective tissue that invests the muscle (epimysium). Subcutaneous edema may also be present if the muscle is superficial in location. The muscle belly may show marked high signal on MRI, with edema and inflammation. If the tear is complete, the tendon will be retracted away from the muscle belly and is typically surrounded by fluid. Gluteus medius tears, or tendinopathy, are a common finding on MRI in patients with buttock, hip, or groin pain [29]. Follow-up imaging may show atrophy, fibrosis, and calcification.

Clinical History: 63-year-old woman with increasing pelvic pain on the right side.

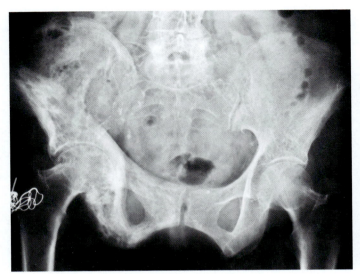

Figure 4-16 A

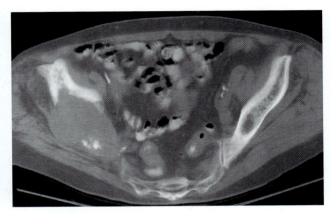

Figure 4-16 B

Findings: (A) AP radiograph of the pelvis shows typical findings of Paget's disease in the right hemipelvis and hip. There is also a medial region of destruction adjacent to the sacroiliac joint. (B) Axial CT (bone windows) shows a destructive mass in the right hemipelvis extending to the sacroiliac joint and the hip. Typical changes of Paget's disease are seen in the adjacent bone, with enlargement of the bone, thickening of the cortex, and coarsening of the trabecular pattern.

Differential Diagnosis: Paget's disease, sarcoma.

Diagnosis: Sarcoma arising in Paget's disease.

Discussion: Paget's disease (osteitis deformans) is a bone disease seen in middle-aged and elderly individuals. It is characterized by excessive and abnormal remodeling of bone. Usually asymptomatic, Paget's disease has a prevalence of 3% in the adult population older than 40 years. In most cases, involvement is polyostotic. Although any bone may be involved, the preponderance of cases involves the pelvis, spine, skull, femur, or tibia. The incidence of sarcoma arising in symptomatic Paget's disease has been estimated at less than 1% [32,33], with the most common lesions being malignant fibrous histiocytoma and osteosarcoma. The prognosis for patients with sarcomas arising in Paget's disease is poor. Involvement of pagetoid bone by metastases is very unusual.

Clinical History: 46-year-old man with back stiffness and skin disease.

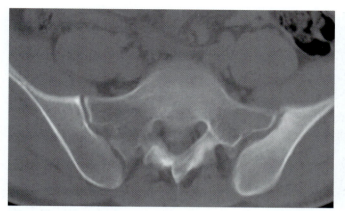

Figure 4-17   A

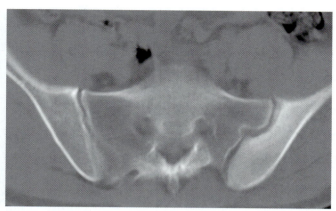

Figure 4-17   B

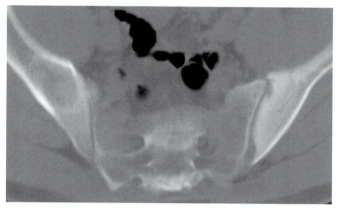

Figure 4-17   C

Findings: Axial CT scans (superior to inferior) show erosions of the left sacroiliac joint. Sclerosis is present on the iliac side, and early ankylosis is present anteriorly.

Differential Diagnosis: Ankylosing spondylitis, psoriatic arthritis, Reiter's disease, rheumatoid arthritis, septic arthritis, degenerative arthritis.

Diagnosis: Psoriatic arthritis.

Discussion: Combined with the presence of skin disease, the asymmetry of involvement is the key to the diagnosis. Bilateral, symmetric involvement of the sacroiliac joints in psoriatic arthritis is more common than unilateral, asymmetric involvement. However, when unilateral involvement is present, psoriatic arthritis or Reiter's disease are much more likely diagnoses than ankylosing spondylitis. The presence of ankylosis is common in psoriatic arthritis but uncommon in Reiter's disease. Unlike degenerative arthritis, where the subchondral sclerosis is well-defined, in psoriatic sacroiliitis the zone of subchondral sclerosis is wide and poorly defined. The lack of sacral involvement rules out septic arthritis, which involves the subchondral bone on both sides of the joint. The prevalence of sacroiliitis in patients with moderate-to-severe psoriatic skin disease is approximately 10% to 25%. Radiographic changes include erosions, sclerosis (predominantly of the ilium), and widening of the joint space. Ankylosis is less common than in ankylosing spondylitis. Other findings about the pelvis include enthesal calcification and ossification.

Clinical History: 29-year-old man with history of intravenous drug abuse.

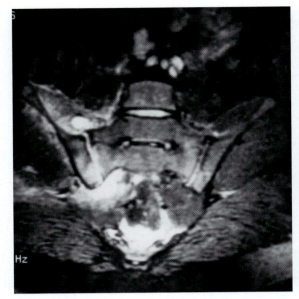

Figure 4-18 A   **Figure 4-18 B**

Findings: (A, B) Coronal and axial T2-weighted MRI demonstrates fluid within the right sacroiliac joint, spreading anteriorly under the iliopsoas and posteriorly along the gluteal fascial plane.

Differential Diagnosis: Ankylosing spondylitis, psoriatic arthritis, Reiter's disease, inflammatory bowel disease, rheumatoid arthritis, septic arthritis.

Diagnosis: Septic sacroiliitis.

Discussion: Increased signal intensity on T2-weighted MRI in the sacroiliac joint area, with fluid in the joint space, is characteristic of sacroiliitis. The inflammatory changes in the adjacent muscle are characteristic of acute infection, but not for the HLA-B27 spondyloarthropathies [34,35]. The findings and history of intravenous drug abuse further support the diagnosis of septic sacroiliitis.

The sacroiliac joint may become infected through the hematogenous route, by direct extension from contiguous infection, and by direct implantation from surgery or trauma. Blood flow in the iliac subchondral bone is slow, and this is a favored site for hematogenous implantation; the sacroiliac joint becomes involved by contiguous extension. Gram-negative bacteria are frequently implicated in the population testing positive for HIV, whereas intravenous drug abuse itself is more commonly associated with staphylococcal infections. Pelvic abscesses and decubitus ulcers may extend to the sacroiliac joint, and infection may occur as a complication of trauma, surgery, or instrumentation, including injections and acupuncture [36].

Clinical History: 24-year-old man with hip pain.

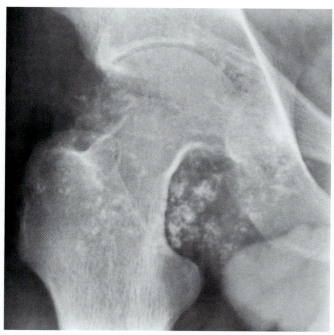

Figure 4-19   A

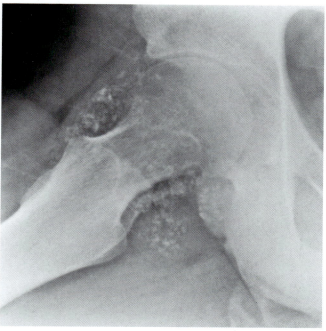

Figure 4-19   B

Findings: (A) AP and (B) frog lateral radiographs show multiple small calcifications in the right hip, with secondary erosive changes of the femoral neck. The calcifications are dense and punctate and do not have a cortical or trabecular structure. The erosions are shallow and well-marginated, and degenerative arthritis is not evident. The morphology of the underlying bone is otherwise normal.

Differential Diagnosis: Synovial osteochondromatosis, synovial hemangiomatosis, synovial sarcoma.

Diagnosis: Synovial osteochondromatosis.

Discussion: The presence of innumerable calcifications in the joint or synovium, with shallow, well-marginated erosions, is virtually diagnostic of primary synovial osteochondromatosis. Synovial hemangiomatosis with multiple phleboliths would be an extremely rare mimic, as would be synovial sarcoma [38]. Pigmented villonodular synovitis (PVNS) causes erosions similar to synovial osteochondromatosis, but PVNS does not calcify. However, in one case report, it has been described coexisting in the same joint as synovial osteochondromatosis [39].

Synovial osteochondromatosis is a condition in which there are multiple intracapsular cartilaginous nodules whose presence results in swelling, effusion, superficial erosions of bone, and degenerative arthritis. The nodules may be attached to the synovium or loose within the joint. Highly cellular nodules tend to be poorly calcified, whereas nodules with low cellularity tend to be heavily calcified. The pathogenesis of synovial osteochondromatosis is uncertain, but there is increasing evidence that the process is neoplastic rather than reactive [40]. The lesion occurs in adults, with the average age of presentation in the 50s. There is a male predominance of nearly 2:1. The most common sites are the knee (70%) and the hip (20%), and the condition is monarticular. No relationship between the extent of calcification and ossification and the age of the patient has been shown. Well-established degenerative disease appears in only a few cases at presentation, and the malignant risk has been estimated at 5% [41]. Malignant lesions arising in synovial osteochondromatosis include chondrosarcoma [42].

Clinical History: 38-year-old man with history of back pain and ulcerative colitis. Radiographs are 5 years apart.

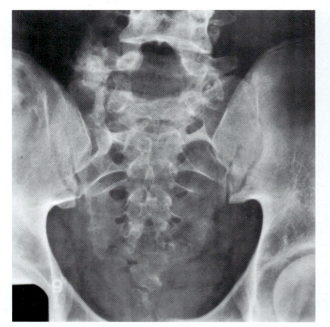

Figure 4-20   A

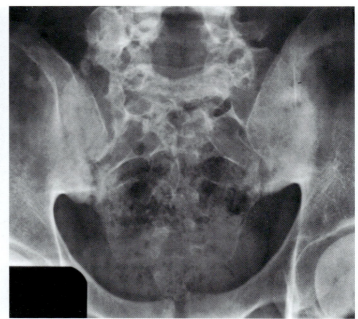

Figure 4-20   B

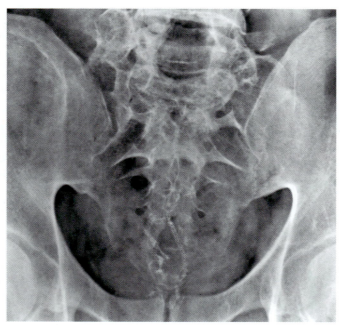

Figure 4-20   C

Findings: (A) AP radiograph from 10 years earlier demonstrates normal sacroiliac joints. Note laminectomy defect and surgical fusion at L4–5. (B) AP radiograph from 5 years earlier demonstrates bilaterally symmetric erosions of both sacroiliac joints, with surrounding sclerosis. (C) Current AP radiograph demonstrates complete ankylosis of both sacroiliac joints. Colectomy has been performed.

Differential Diagnosis: Ankylosing spondylitis, psoriatic arthritis, Reiter's disease, rheumatoid arthritis, septic arthritis.

Diagnosis: Ankylosing spondylitis.

Discussion: Ankylosing spondylitis is a chronic inflammatory disease with predominant manifestations in the spine and sacroiliac joints [37]. The etiology is unknown, but there is a genetic component; 90% to 95% of caucasian patients with classic ankylosing spondylitis have human leukocyte antigen (HLA-B27) (compared with 9% of all caucasians). Symptomatic disease affects about 1% of the general population; the prevalence of severe disease is about 0.1%. Therefore, the disease is much less common than rheumatoid arthritis.

Inflammatory bowel diseases associated with ankylosing spondylitis include ulcerative colitis, Crohn's disease, and Whipple's disease. The causal relationship of the bowel disease and the ankylosing spondylitis has not been proven definitively, but it is thought that the diseases are incidentally coexistent in some patients (those with HLA-B27), and that the spondylitis may be secondary to the bowel disease in the others (those without HLA-B27). The disease activity in the bowel does not appear to be correlated with the disease activity in the sacroiliac joints or spine.

Ankylosing spondylitis typically begins in the lumbosacral region and ascends to the cervical spine. Local pain and tenderness over the sacroiliac joints in the early phases of the disease are common, and may dominate the initial clinical presentation. Initial involvement of the sacroiliac joints may be asymmetric or unilateral, although ultimately, bilaterally symmetric involvement is virtually invariable. Inflammatory involvement of the synovial portion of the sacroiliac joints can manifest as patchy periarticular osteoporosis, erosions of the subchondral bone leading to fraying of the osseous surface and widening of the joint space, and sclerosis of the subchondral bone. These changes predominate on the iliac side of the joint, although in advanced disease both sides are involved. Calcification and ossification of the ligamentous portion of the sacroiliac joint will accompany changes in the synovial portion of the joint. The sacroiliac joints may ultimately become blurred, sclerotic, and fused.

Clinical History: 35-year-old woman with chronic right hip pain.

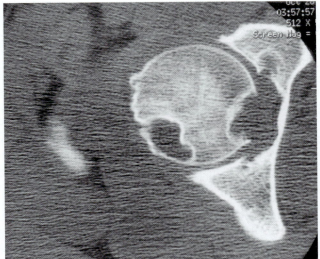

Figure 4-21   A

Figure 4-21   B

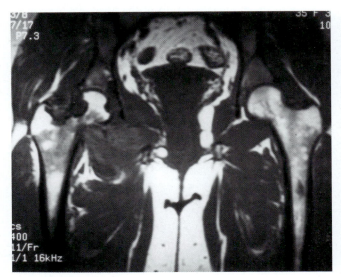

Figure 4-21   C

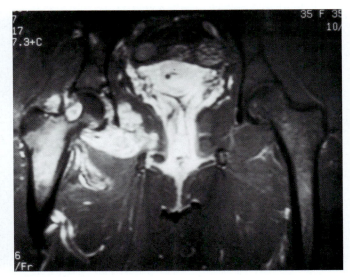

Figure 4-21   D

Findings: (A, B) CT scan of the right hip shows scalloped erosions of the femoral head, femoral neck, greater trochanter, and acetabulum. The erosions have well-defined sclerotic margins. (C) Coronal T1-weighted MRI shows lobulated, low signal intensity, soft tissue masses about the right hip involving the proximal femur and pelvis. The masses have eroded the bones. Marrow changes are also present in the proximal femur. (D) Coronal T1-weighted MRI with fat saturation after intravenous gadolinium administration shows marked enhancement of the soft tissue masses about the right hip.

Differential Diagnosis: Pigmented villonodular synovitis (PVNS), tuberculosis, synovial chondromatosis, amyloid arthropathy, rheumatoid arthritis.

Diagnosis: Pigmented villonodular synovitis.

Discussion: Although tuberculosis of the hip and synovial cysts in rheumatoid arthritis may result in erosions and lobulated masses about the joint, the MRI findings are not that of simple, fluid-filled structures. Synovial chondromatosis would typically demonstrate calcifications, which are not present in this case. PVNS is a benign neoplasm (rather than an inflammatory condition) of the synovium that usually presents in adults as recurrent monarticular hemorrhagic effusions. Common locations include the knee or hip, but any synovial tissue may be involved. Involvement of the synovium may be focal or diffuse. Chronic, erosive changes from thickened, nodular, synovial proliferation may be seen on radiographs. Localized osteoporosis is common. Arthritic changes such as joint space narrowing and osteophytes are generally absent. MRI shows effusion and multiple low signal intensity synovial masses on T1-weighted and T2-weighted images that typically enhance after gadolinium injection [43]. Amyloid deposition may have a similar pattern, but would generally involve multiple joints. The lesion in PVNS is pigmented on gross examination because of hemosiderin deposits from repeated bleeding. The presence of hemosiderin causes the lesion to have low signal intensity on all MRI pulse sequences. Treatment of PVNS is surgical. Although there is no metastatic potential, the lesion may recur locally if synovectomy is incomplete.

Clinical History: 50-year-old woman with progressive hip pain.

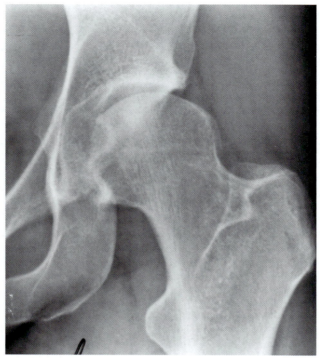

Figure 4-22   A

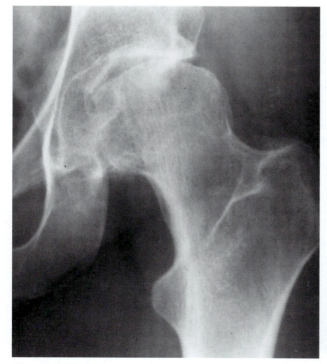

Figure 4-22   B

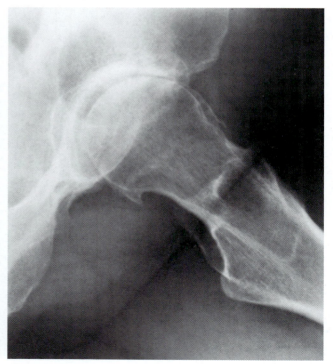

Figure 4-22   C

Findings: (A) AP radiograph of the left hip shows minimal superior lateral cartilage space narrowing, with associated osteophyte formation and subchondral sclerosis. (**B, C**) Six years later. AP and frog lateral radiographs of the left hip show the findings have progressed, including medial femoral osteophyte formation and further cartilage space narrowing.

Differential   Diagnosis: Osteoarthritis,   inflammatory arthritis.

Diagnosis: Osteoarthritis.

Discussion: Osteoarthritis of the hip is one of the most common conditions in adults leading to the continuing use of medication, elective surgery, or both. In young adults, there is usually an underlying abnormality of the hip, such as previous trauma, previous hip disease, or acetabular dysplasia. In older adults, no underlying abnormality may be obvious, but a genetic basis for development of osteoarthritis is becoming apparent [44]. Radiographic findings of osteoarthritis in the hip are those of osteoarthritis in other joints, including cartilage space narrowing, subchondral sclerosis, osteophyte formation, and preservation of bone mineralization. Erosions are notably absent, but subchondral cyst formation is common. Serial radiographs may document the progress of hip osteoarthritis. In a retrospective study of adult patients with osteoarthritis of the hip who ultimately received total hip replacements, the progression of cartilage space narrowing ranged from 0 mm to 2.6 mm per year, with a mean progression of 0.4 mm per year. Progression was slower in patients with hypertrophic bony changes [45].

Intraarticular injection of local anesthetic has been advocated as a diagnostic test to determine whether an osteoarthritic hip is the source of clinical symptoms, thus aiding in the clarification of the cause of pain. In one study, patients who had relief after administration of the intraarticular anesthetic were treated successfully by joint replacement, whereas those who did not obtain relief proved to be unsuitable candidates for joint replacement [46].

Clinical History: 39-year-old woman with chronic hip and hand pain.

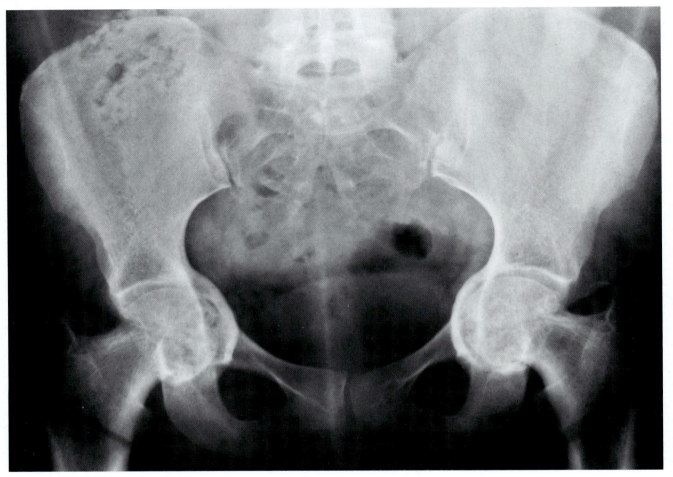

Figure 4-23

Findings: Bilateral acetabuli protrusio is noted with axial migration of both hips symmetrically. No osteophytes are noted. The sacroiliac joints are normal. Bone structure appears normal.

Differential Diagnosis: Rheumatoid arthritis, osteoarthritis, spondyloarthropathy.

Diagnosis: Rheumatoid arthritis.

Discussion: Protrusio acetabuli is defined radiographically and is present when the medial acetabular wall protrudes medially by 3 mm or more in men, or 6 mm or more in women [47]. It is a complication seen primarily in rheumatoid arthritis, but it may also be present in seronegative spondyloarthropathy, osteoarthritis, juvenile chronic arthritis, and other hip conditions. Its presence does not appear to be correlated with disease duration, clinical severity of hip involvement, or previous medication. In this case, the lack of sacroiliac joint or spine abnormality and the lack of hypertrophic bone formation favors rheumatoid arthritis.

Any condition that causes weakening of the bone may cause protrusio, including entities such as Paget's disease, osteomalacia, polyostotic fibrous dysplasia, therapeutic irradiation, and osteogenesis imperfecta. Prior fractures of the acetabulum, particularly with medial displacement from lateral compression, may produce this deformity. Protrusio may also occur on a familial or idiopathic basis. Protrusio acetabuli is a classic finding in rheumatoid arthritis of the hip and, as a rule, the changes are bilateral and symmetric. Subchondral cystic lesions, subchondral collapse of the acetabulum and femoral head, and osteoporosis may be associated findings. When sclerosis is present, it is a sign of reparative response and secondary osteoarthritis. Typical progression of the protrusion in rheumatoid arthritis is 2 mm to 3 mm per year, but a small subset may have rapid progression (7.5 mm over 6 weeks) occurring at the same time as a marked increase in symptoms and disability [48].

CASE 4-24

Clinical History: 10-year-old boy with joint stiffness.

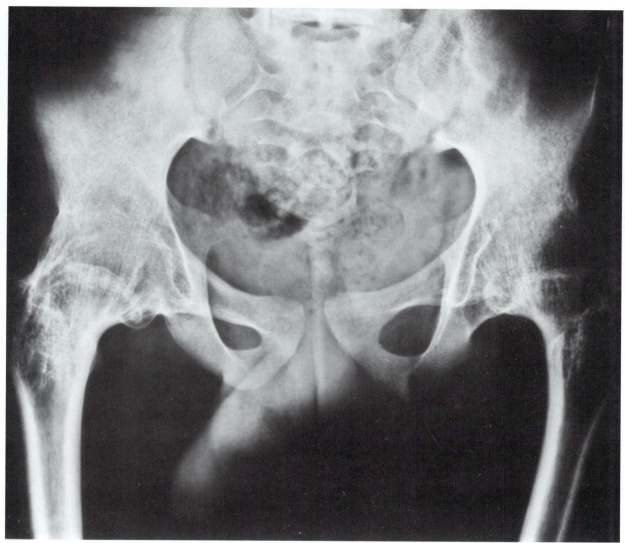

Figure 4-24

Findings: Both femoral heads are enlarged and flattened on top. The hip joints are ankylosed. The sacroiliac joints are normal.

Differential Diagnosis: Juvenile idiopathic arthritis, septic arthritis.

Diagnosis: Juvenile idiopathic arthritis (juvenile chronic arthritis).

Discussion: Childhood arthritis has been combined into a single classification of juvenile idiopathic arthritis [49,50]. Although ankylosis may occur after septic arthritis, the finding of bilaterally symmetric ankylosis of the hips suggests juvenile idiopathic arthritis rather than infection. The dysplastic overgrowth of the femoral heads suggests chronic disease. Similar dysplastic changes may be seen in a variety of other conditions, including neuromuscular syndromes, hemophilia, and Legg-Calve-Perthes disease, but the presence of ankylosis excludes them. Of the various forms of juvenile idiopathic arthritis, Still's disease would be the most likely because of the lack of sacroiliac joint involvement, although ankylosis of the hips occurs in juvenile-onset seronegative spondyloarthropathy. Adult-form rheumatoid arthritis typically does not produce ankylosis of large synovial joints.

Clinical History: 24-year-old man with hard inguinal mass.

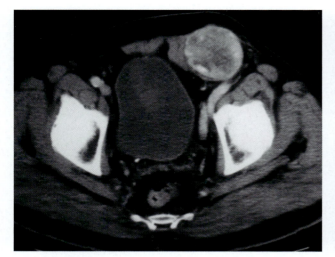

Figure 4-25   A

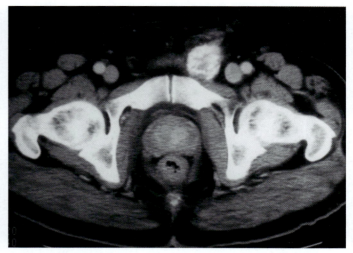

Figure 4-25   B

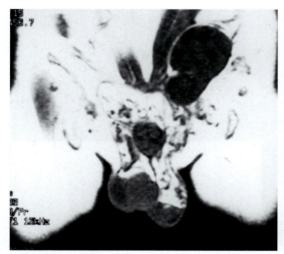

Figure 4-25   C

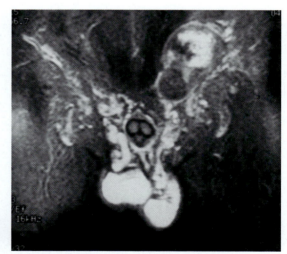

Figure 4-25   D

Findings: (**A**, **B**) Axial CT demonstrates a well-defined ossified mass, originating from the left rectus sheath, medial to the femoral vessels. Some muscle fibers have been displaced medially by the mass. (**C**) Coronal T1-weighted MRI shows heterogeneous low signal within the mass. (**D**) Coronal T2-weighted MRI shows heterogeneous high signal in the lesion (corresponding to the soft tissue component), with regions of low signal (corresponding to the areas of heavy calcification).

Differential Diagnosis: Myositis ossificans, extraskeletal osteosarcoma, extraskeletal chondrosarcoma, metastasis, synovial cell sarcoma, leiomyoma.

Diagnosis: Extraskeletal osteosarcoma.

Discussion: Myositis ossificans in the rectus sheath would by far be the most common calcifying soft tissue mass in this location, but the rounded, lobular morphology of the lesion and the finding that it has displaced rather than infiltrated muscle fibers within the rectus sheath eliminates that diagnosis. The diagnosis of myositis ossificans is also unlikely because of the central rather than peripheral location of the calcifications. A rare bone-producing or cartilage-producing tumor such as extraskeletal osteosarcoma or extraskeletal chondrosarcoma is a consideration. Chondroid lesions tend to produce a distinct chondroid type of calcification in a pattern of rings and arcs, although they can become more disorganized and more difficult to characterize in malignant chondroid lesions. Tumors with a prominent component of hemorrhage or necrosis, such as leiomyoma or leiomyosarcoma, may calcify. The calcifications in leiomyoma have been described as a mulberry pattern, similar to that seen in degenerated fibroids in the uterus. Synovial sarcoma, on occasion, may show dense calcification with osteoid and bone formation [51]. The well-encapsulated appearance of this lesion does not ensure benignity, because sarcomas may often be well demarcated on CT and MRI owing to a pseudocapsule.

Extraskeletal osteosarcomas are rare lesions that generally occur at a later age (60s and 70s) than conventional osteosarcoma. They have a predilection for the lower extremity, especially the thigh, and as many as 6% of patients may have a history of previous radiation therapy [52]. Prognostically, they are not unlike their counterparts in bone. These lesions are high-grade tumors and display metastases in 65% of patients, most often to the lungs. The 5-year survival rate is about 40%; however, patients with the chondroblastic rather than the osteoblastic variety of the tumor survive longer [53]. Although osteosarcomas, in general, show calcified tumor, these soft tissue lesions often do not demonstrate any visible calcific component [54]. As with many soft tissue sarcomas, the imaging features are usually nonspecific and the diagnosis must be obtained by biopsy.

Clinical History: 42-year-old man with small fingernails.

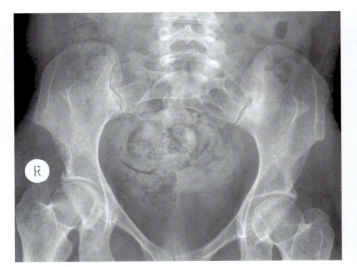

Figure 4-26   A

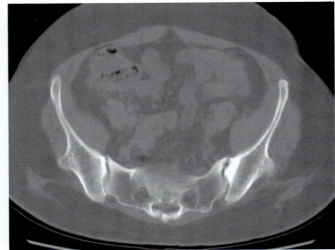

Figure 4-26   B

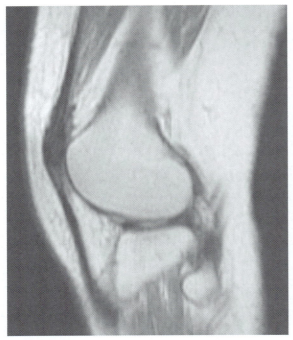

Figure 4-26   C

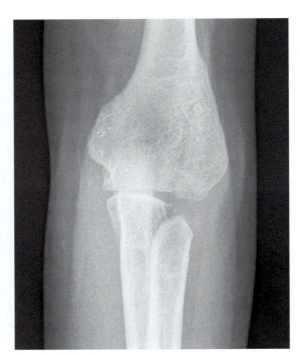

Figure 4-26   D

Findings: (**A**) AP view of the pelvis shows small horns on each iliac body. (**B**) CT scan through the pelvis shows small horns projecting posteriorly. (**C**) Sagittal T1-weighted MRI of the knee shows a hypoplastic patella. (**D**) AP view of the elbow shows hypoplasia of the proximal radius with absent radial head.

Differential Diagnosis: None.

Diagnosis: Nail-patella syndrome (osteoonychodysostosis, Fong's syndrome).

Discussion: Posteriorly located iliac horns are pathognomonic of nail-patella syndrome. These bony outgrowths are located at the origin of the gluteus medius muscles [55]. The iliac horns are present in 80% of patients with this syndrome, and may be unilateral. Eighty percent to 90% of patients have absent or hypoplastic finger nails and toenails. Other skeletal anomalies are often present, including hypoplastic patellae, hypoplastic capitella, and hypoplastic, dislocated radial heads. This disorder is autosomal dominant, but about 20% of cases are sporadic, with no family history. Nail-patella syndrome has multiple extraskeletal associations, the most common of which are renal disease (50%) and eye disorders, such as glaucoma and cataracts.

Clinical History: 57-year-old man with progressive anemia.

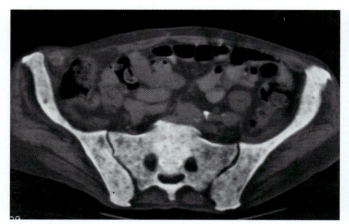

Figure 4-27 A

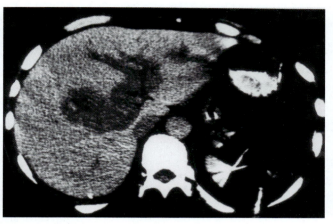

Figure 4-27 B

Findings: (A) Axial CT scan of the pelvis shows mottled sclerosis of the sacrum and both iliac wings, without cortical destruction or bone expansion. The cortex itself is not thickened, and the trabecular bone pattern is obscured. (B) Axial CT scan of the upper abdomen shows surgical clips from a prior splenectomy. A low-attenuation lesion in the center of the liver was proved by biopsy to represent extramedullary hematopoiesis.

Differential Diagnosis: Paget's disease, lymphoma, leukemia, metastases, myelofibrosis, mastofibrosis.

Diagnosis: Myelofibrosis.

Discussion: Paget's disease would be the most common benign cause of sclerosis in the pelvis in an older adult, but the distinctive pattern of cortical thickening and trabecular coarsening is absent. Other differential considerations include mastocytosis, leukemia, and lymphoma. The degree of sclerosis is usually less marked in leukemia and lymphoma patients, and often there are lytic regions, cortical destruction, and soft tissue involvement. Metastases would typically have more asymmetric distribution, as well as cortical involvement. The absence of proliferative hyperostosis would argue against fluorosis or retinoid intoxication.

Myelofibrosis is a replacement of the bone marrow with fibrosis, necessitating extramedullary hematopoiesis [56]. It can be primary (idiopathic) or secondary to exposure to environmental toxins, such as benzene, or in association with a chronic blood dyscrasia, such as polycythemia vera, chronic myelocytic leukemia, and miscellaneous anemias. One hypothesis [56] regarding the etiology of the marrow fibrosis postulates exposure to an excessive quantity of platelet-derived growth factor from altered megakaryocytes. The population typically affected includes patients in their 60s and 70s.

The onset is commonly insidious and prognosis is variable. The fibrosis initially involves sites of active marrow production including the vertebrae, ribs, and pelvis. Intramedullary hematopoiesis then shifts to the proximal and distal ends of the femora, humeri, and tibiae. These are the secondary sites to undergo osteosclerosis, and then the marrow production will shift to tertiary osseous or extraosseous sites. The radiographic findings include sclerosis in 40% to 50% of cases, and cortical thickening (most marked on the endosteal surface rather than periosteal surface). Extramedullary hematopoiesis may be located in the paravertebral location or within the liver or spleen, as seen in this case. Polymyalgia and polyarthralgia may be related to an immunologic etiology, as seen in rheumatoid arthritis, or may result from secondary hyperuricemia or recurrent hemarthrosis from low platelet counts. MRI shows replacement of the normal fatty marrow with hypointense fibrosis on T1-weighted MRI. The apophyses are more resistant to reconversion than epiphyses.

Clinical History: 24-year-old woman with pelvic pain.

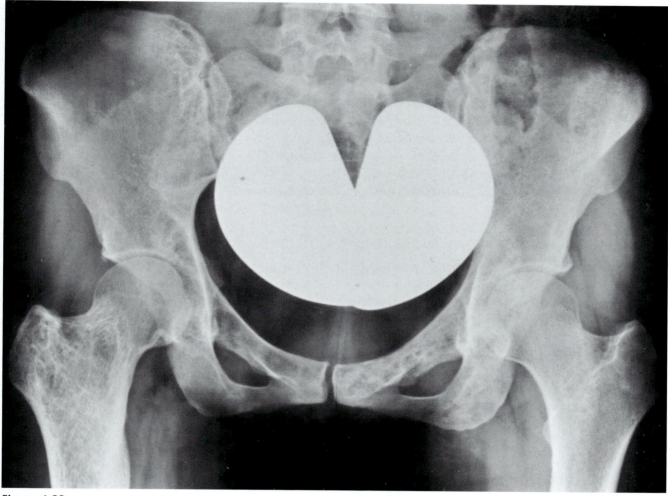

Figure 4-28

Findings: AP radiograph of the pelvis. There are cystic changes with sclerotic borders involving the left pubis and ischium, right ilium adjacent to the sacroiliac joint, and right pubis. A lace-like pattern is noted in the right femoral neck and shaft, with a widening of the bone.

Differential Diagnosis: Hemangiomatosis, metastases, lymphoma, eosinophilic granuloma, osteomyelitis, tuberculosis.

Diagnosis: Hemangiomatosis.

Discussion: The lesions are multifocal, and although they have both lucent and sclerotic components, the impression should be more of a multifocally abnormal trabecular pattern, rather than multiple lesions with bone destruction and reactive bone formation. Hemangioma of bone is one of the few benign bone lesions with a female predominance (the others are giant cell tumor and aneurysmal bone cyst). The lesions consist of abnormal vascular spaces and fat, and they may enlarge slowly in a permeative fashion, allowing the trabecular bone to remodel. Common sites of involvement include the axial skeleton, femur, and pelvis, but any bone may be involved. Contiguous involvement of multiple bones is not uncommon. The lesions may occur in a synchronous or metachronous fashion. Lymphangiomatosis and cystic angiomatosis are related multifocal vascular lesions of bone with a virtually indistinguishable appearance [57].

Clinical History: 34-year-old man with low back pain.

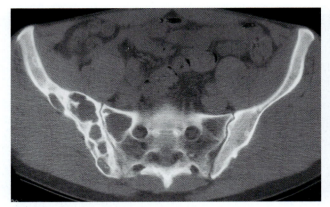

Figure 4-29   A

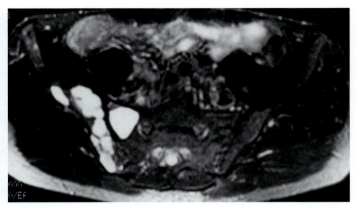

Figure 4-29   B

Findings: (A) Axial CT of the pelvis with soft tissue window shows multiple lytic lesions on both sides of the right sacroiliac joint. The lesions have soft tissue attenuation. The bone is moderately expanded. There is no cortical destruction or soft tissue component. (B) Axial T2-weighted MRI with fat saturation through the pelvis demonstrates high signal intensity in the lytic lesions, with no soft tissue involvement.

Differential Diagnosis: Metastases, lymphoma, multiple myeloma, angiomatosis, tuberculosis, fungal osteomyelitis.

Diagnosis: Cystic angiomatosis.

Discussion: The presence of multiple lucent lesions in contiguous bones of the pelvis, with remodeled, sclerotic margins, suggests an indolent process. The MRI is suggestive of fluid signal intensity, favoring some form of angiomatosis, including lymphangiomatosis or hemangiomatosis. Cystic angiomatosis shows multiple cystic areas in bone, with or without involvement of other organ systems. Occasionally, the lesions may be sclerotic [58]. Other multifocal vascular lesions, such as multifocal hemangioma, hemangioendothelioma, and angiosarcoma, may have a similar radiographic appearance. Indolent or atypical infections, such as caused by tuberculosis, atypical mycobacteria, or fungal pathogens, may have a similar appearance, but soft tissue extension, or at least edema, would be expected. The lack of cortical destruction makes metastases, lymphoma, and myeloma less likely.

Clinical History: 21-year-old woman.

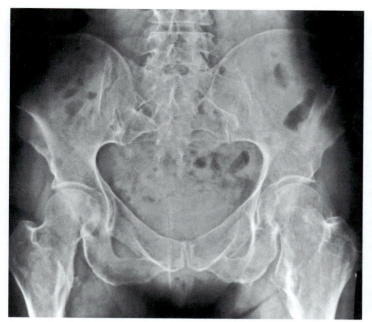

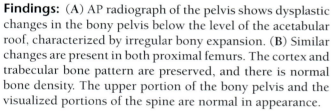

Figure 4-30   A

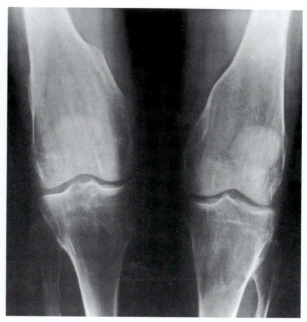

Figure 4-30   B

Findings: (A) AP radiograph of the pelvis shows dysplastic changes in the bony pelvis below the level of the acetabular roof, characterized by irregular bony expansion. (B) Similar changes are present in both proximal femurs. The cortex and trabecular bone pattern are preserved, and there is normal bone density. The upper portion of the bony pelvis and the visualized portions of the spine are normal in appearance.

Differential Diagnosis: None.

Diagnosis: Multiple hereditary exostoses (osteochondromatosis).

Discussion: Multiple hereditary exostoses (osteochondromatosis, multiple osteochondromas, diaphyseal aclasis) is one of the most common skeletal dysplasias. The condition is inherited with autosomal dominant transmission and incomplete penetrance. The expression is variable, with more severe manifestations in males. In one large series, 62% of cases were inherited, and 38% of cases were sporadic [59]. The skeleton is involved symmetrically, and the limbs are affected more than the spine. Forty percent are about the knee.

These lesions, like other cartilaginous tumors, form in bones that undergo enchondral ossification as opposed to intramembranous ossification. The number of exostoses varies. Deformities of the tubular bones are present and cause disproportionately short limbs, but the degree of shortness appears to be unrelated to the number of exostoses. Growth of the lesions slows as the skeleton matures, and new lesions do not appear in adulthood. The exostoses are radiologically and histologically indistinguishable from solitary ones. They may appear sessile or pedunculated, with the sessile variety showing a greater propensity for malignant transformation. Secondary development of chondrosarcoma in a solitary exostosis or in one of the multiple exostoses is a small but definite risk, probably on the order of 0.5% to 3% [60]; the onset of pain or of growth in an adult suggests the possibility. The radiologic distinction between a benign exostosis and an exostotic chondrosarcoma is difficult, unless growth and change in appearance can be demonstrated on serial imaging.

Clinical History: 39-year-old woman with acute onset of left pelvic pain.

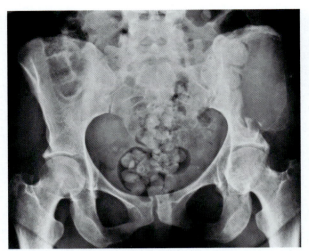

Figure 4-31 A

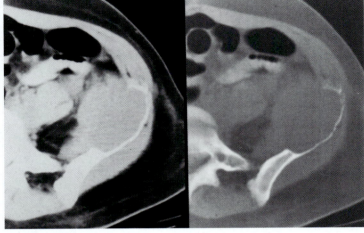

Figure 4-31 B

Findings: (A) AP radiograph of the pelvis shows an expansile, lytic lesion in the left iliac wing. A pathologic fracture is present at the inferior margin of the lesion. (B) Axial CT scan with soft tissue and bone windows shows destruction of the anterior cortex with soft tissue mass. There is no mineralization within the mass.

Differential Diagnosis: Plasmacytoma, lymphoma, desmoplastic fibroma, bone cyst, metastasis, giant cell tumor.

Diagnosis: Plasmacytoma.

Discussion: The imaging features in this case are nonspecific but alarming, because of the cortical breakthrough. A biopsy is necessary for diagnosis.

Plasmacytoma (also called solitary myeloma) is a malignant neoplasm arising from a single clone of plasma cells that has a solitary focus in the marrow; when multiple foci of disease are present, the condition is called multiple myeloma. Serum protein electrophoresis may show a monoclonal spike of immunoglobulins, corresponding to the products of the neoplastic clone, but sometimes both the findings from serum protein electrophoresis and the findings from blind iliac crest bone marrow aspiration are negative in plasmacytoma. Regardless of whether the initial lesion is resected, virtually all patients with plasmacytoma ultimately develop multiple myeloma. However, 10 years or more may pass before the progression of disease becomes apparent. Plasmacytoma commonly presents as an expansile lesion in the spine, a rib, the pelvis, or the sacrum, with pathologic fracture.

Clinical History: 78-year-old woman with progressive bilateral groin pain and inability to walk, and two companion cases.

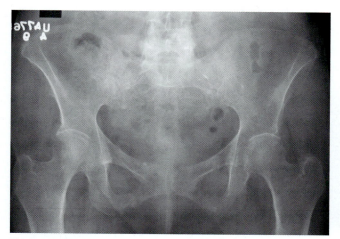

Figure 4-32   A

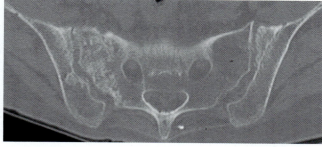

Figure 4-32   B

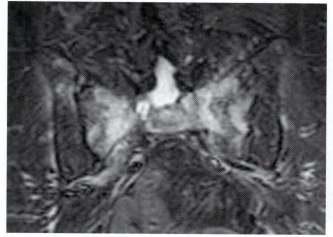

Figure 4-32   C

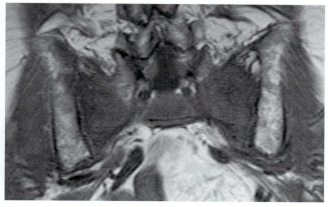

Figure 4-32   D

Findings: (A) AP radiograph of the pelvis shows healing fractures of the inferior and superior pubic rami, bilaterally. The bones are osteopenic. (B) Companion case 1: 81-year-old woman with low back pain. Axial CT through sacrum demonstrating sclerosis of the right sacral ala. (C, D) Companion case 2: 72-year-old woman with low back pain. Coronal short tau inversion recovery (STIR) and T1-weighted MRI showing marked edema in each side of the sacrum.

Differential Diagnosis: None.

Diagnosis: Insufficiency fractures.

Discussion: Insufficiency fractures in elderly women may present with progressive inguinal or back pain, limping, and inability to walk. Predisposing conditions include osteoporosis, osteomalacia, rheumatoid arthritis, pelvic irradiation, prolonged corticosteroid treatment, and mechanical changes following hip replacement surgery [61]. Initial radiographs at the time of presentation may not necessarily show the fracture, and radionuclide bone scan, CT, or MRI may be required for the diagnosis. MRI would appear to have the greatest sensitivity and specificity for occult fractures such as these in the elderly [62]. Most patients improve with nonsurgical treatment of the fracture and the underlying cause. Similar appearing stress fractures (as opposed to insufficiency fractures) in the inferior pubic rami have been described in young, healthy female military recruits, an injury that appears to result from increased stride length when marching during basic training in mixed-sex groups [63]. Sacral and pubic rami stress fractures have also been described in long-distance runners.

Clinical History: 57-year-old woman with bone pain and history of mastectomy for breast cancer 10 years earlier.

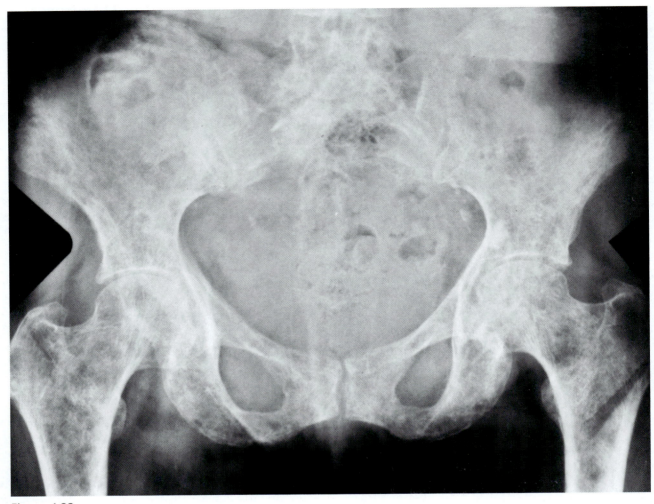

Figure 4-33

Findings: AP radiograph of the pelvis demonstrates a diffuse, mixed lytic and sclerotic process without distortion of the cortical surface or pathologic fracture. Radiographs of the thoracic and lumbar spine (not shown) are similar.

Differential Diagnosis: Metastases, multiple myeloma, osteomalacia.

Diagnosis: Diffuse breast carcinoma metastases.

Discussion: The diffuse distribution of mixed osteolytic and osteoblastic changes is characteristic of disseminated cancer. The skeleton is the most common site of metastatic disease in the body, particularly from primary tumors arising in the prostate, breast, thyroid, lung, and kidney [64]. Metastatic breast carcinoma commonly spreads to bone without visceral involvement. Median survival in breast cancer patients with only bone metastases is approximately 2 to 3 years. Complications from bone metastases and their treatment are frequently the principle cause of morbidity and proximal cause of death in breast cancer patients. The most common symptom is bone pain from structural damage, periosteal irritation, and nerve involvement. Increased bone resorption leading to hypercalcemia may also cause bone pain, and this pain is often ameliorated by treatment with bisphosphonates. Pathologic fractures are a late complication. Intensive screening for metastatic disease in breast cancer patients without bone symptoms has been found to have no effect on the 5-year survival rate, even though more metastases can be detected earlier [65].

CASE 4-34

Clinical History: 17-year-old girl with episodic bone and joint pain.

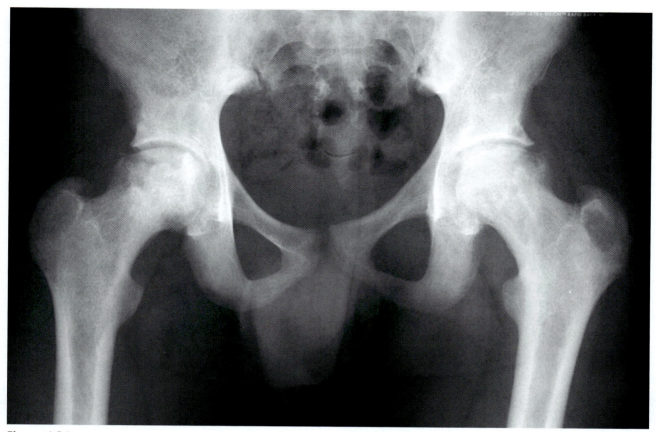

Figure 4-34

Findings: AP radiograph of the pelvis reveals patchy osteosclerosis of all visualized bones. Dense sclerosis of both femoral heads is noted, with subchondral collapse.

Differential Diagnosis: Sickle cell disease, osteopetrosis, Gaucher's disease, trauma, systemic lupus erythematosus, renal osteodystrophy, endogenous or exogenous corticosteroid excess.

Diagnosis: Sickle cell disease.

Discussion: Patchy osteosclerosis combined with bilateral osteonecrosis of the femoral heads suggests a systemic disease leading to diffuse bone infarcts. Sickle cell anemia is an autosomal dominant anemia characterized by sickle-shaped erythrocytes and accelerated hemolysis. A single amino acid substitution in the beta hemoglobin chain is responsible. Episodes of microvascular occlusion ("crises") result in severe bone pain, bone infarcts, and other effects. Bone infarcts manifest radiographically as regions of sclerosis, where new bone is apposed to infarcted bone when the site becomes revascularized. The process of creeping substitution may replace some infarcted bone, but if the repair is interrupted by repeated episodes of infarction, the bone simply becomes more and more dense. Osteonecrosis of the femoral head is a common complication of sickle cell disease. In one study, 10% of patients with sickle cell disease demonstrated radiographic evidence of unilateral or bilateral osteonecrosis of the femoral head [66]. Collapse of the necrotic femoral head may lead to degenerative arthrosis. Treatment may be accomplished with conventional hip replacement arthroplasty [67]. Due to the increased risk of surgical complications, such as high-output congestive failure, intraoperative femoral fracture, infection, blood loss, transfusion reaction, and loosening of prosthesis, alternative methods of treatment have been performed with some success. These include core decompression and acrylic cement injection [68,69].

Clinical History: 29-year-old man with bone pain and right inguinal mass.

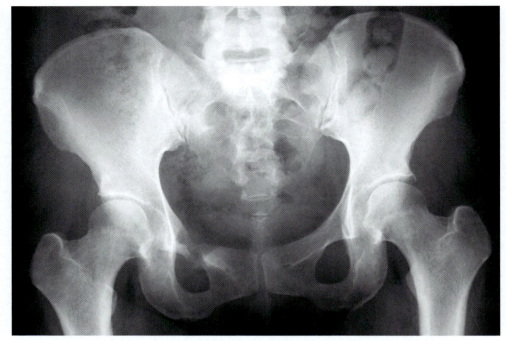

Figure 4-35   A

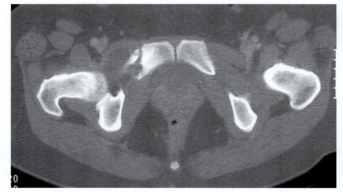

Figure 4-35   B

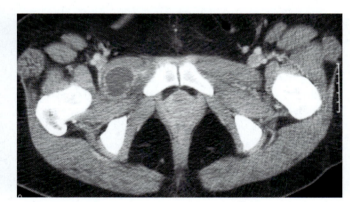

Figure 4-35   C

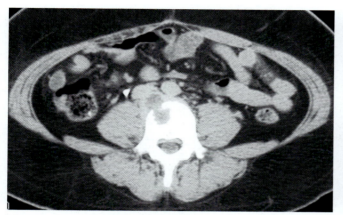

Figure 4-35 D

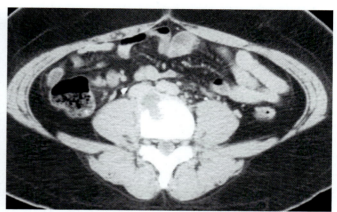

Figure 4-35 E

Findings: (**A**) AP radiograph of the pelvis. A lytic process involves the right superior pubic ramus. Some reactive sclerosis is present. Contrast-enhanced axial CT scans at two levels through the superior pubic rami viewed with bone settings (**B**) and soft tissue settings (**C**) show bone destruction on the right, with reactive sclerosis and low-attenuation soft tissue mass. The soft tissue mass has an enhancing rim. (**D, E**) Contrast-enhanced axial CT scan at the L5 level shows a destructive bone lesion involving the anterior aspect of the vertebral body, with extension into the anterior soft tissues. The lesion has low attenuation and an enhancing rim.

Differential Diagnosis: Metastases, multiple myeloma, tuberculosis, osteomyelitis, lymphoma, leukemia.

Diagnosis: Tuberculosis.

Discussion: Differential considerations include other fungal or pyogenic types of osteomyelitis, as well as metastatic or multifocal neoplasms. The presence of reactive bone formation is much more common in infections than in tumors. The morphology of the bone involvement and the large size of the soft tissue lesions relative to the bone lesions suggest a nonpyogenic infectious agent, beginning in bone but causing abscess formation. Factors that suggest the specific diagnosis include a positive chest radiograph or tuberculin skin test, low frequency of neurologic symptoms in the presence of severe spine involvement, normal erythrocyte sedimentation rate, and indolent symptoms disproportionate to a destructive radiographic appearance.

The prevalence of tuberculosis has been rising in North America after notable successes from public health measures earlier in the twentieth century. It is seen most commonly in immunocompromised patients and among immigrant populations [70]. Skeletal involvement is the result of hematogenous spread, typically from the lungs. Between 25% and 60% of cases concerning bone involve the spine. The body of L1 is the most commonly affected site in the spine, but involvement of multiple contiguous levels (classically three levels) is frequent. Involvement of the upper cervical levels, thoracolumbar junction, posterior elements, and sacroiliac joints is also known to occur. Paravertebral abscesses are common and may extend into the groin or thigh. MRI can be very helpful in differentiating pyogenic spondylitis from tuberculous spondylitis [71]. Tuberculosis may also spread to the joints [72], resulting in a granulomatous synovial infection that requires synovial biopsy or joint aspiration for diagnosis. In the typical situation, the process is monarticular, and there is osteomyelitis adjacent to the involved joint.

Clinical History: 32-year-old woman with pelvic pain.

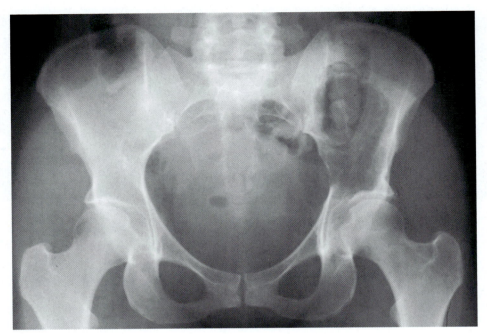

Figure 4-36   A

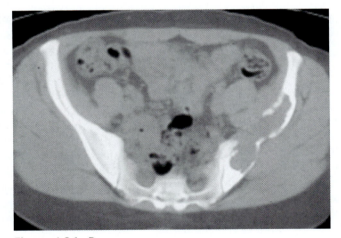

Figure 4-36   B

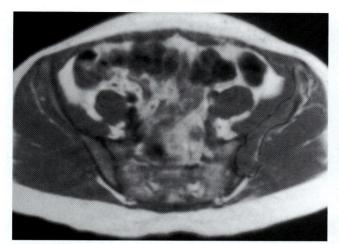

Figure 4-36   C

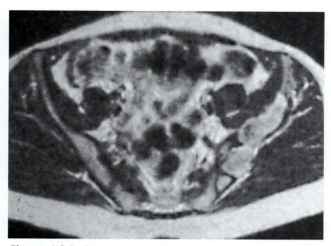

Figure 4-36   D

Findings: (**A**) AP radiograph of the pelvis shows a large destructive lesion in the left iliac wing, with loss of the iliopectineal line. The lesion appears to have no internal matrix mineralization. Some surrounding reactive bone formation may be present. (**B**) CT scan shows a lucent lesion in the ilium with thinning of the cortex. A break in the mineralized cortex is present anteriorly. The lesion is mildly expansile, with no evident soft tissue mass. There is no mineralization within the lesion. (**C**) Axial proton-density MRI shows intermediate signal within the lesion, with apparently intact periosteum. No extension into the soft tissues is present. (**D**) Axial T2-weighted MRI shows heterogeneous high signal within the lesion. There is no surrounding soft tissue or marrow edema.

Differential Diagnosis: Plasmacytoma, lymphoma, chondrosarcoma, osteosarcoma, bone cyst, fibroma, giant cell tumor, fibrous dysplasia, metastasis.

Diagnosis: Desmoplastic fibroma.

Discussion: Desmoplastic fibroma is a rare, benign, primary bone tumor that is the osseous counterpart of the extraabdominal desmoid tumor of soft tissues (fibromatosis). There is a male predominance, and most patients are 20 to 30 years old at presentation. The most frequently affected sites are the pelvis and femur. Although soft tissue extension may be present in desmoplastic fibroma, the radiographic features are typically those of nonaggressive lesions: geographic pattern of destruction, sharply defined margins, and reactive bone formation at the margins [73,74].

The imaging features in this case are not specific, but the lack of mineralization decreases the likelihood of fibrous dysplasia and the bone-forming or cartilage-forming tumors. The MRI appearance is variable, but foci of low to intermediate signal on T2-weighted images, which are not due to calcification, can aid diagnosis [75]. Plasmacytoma, lymphoma, and metastasis might be expected to have a more aggressive appearance, with cortical penetration, soft tissue mass, and soft tissue edema, but the appearance is not specific enough to obviate the need for biopsy. There is a high incidence of local recurrence after treatment of desmoplastic fibroma by intralesional curettage [76], but no metastatic potential has been documented.

Clinical History: 67-year-old woman with total hip replacement who is unable to walk.

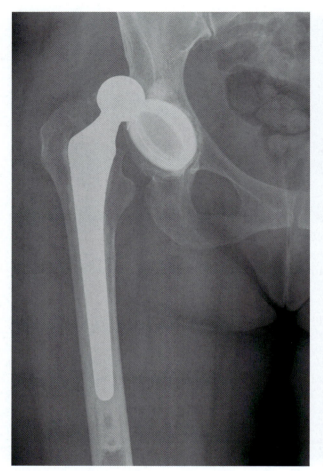

Figure 4-37   A

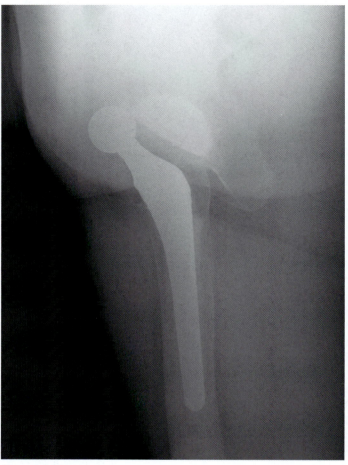

Figure 4-37   B

Findings: (A) AP radiograph of the right hip shows a total hip replacement, with superior and lateral dislocation of the prosthetic femoral head. (B) True lateral radiograph shows the anterior position of the prosthetic femoral head. The prosthesis has cemented acetabular and femoral components.

Differential Diagnosis: None.

Diagnosis: Dislocated total hip replacement.

Discussion: Lateral hip dislocation is a common complication of total hip replacement, with an overall incidence of 2% to 3%. It is associated with significant cost and morbidity. An increased incidence of dislocation has been observed in women, in the elderly, in patients with cerebral dysfunction, with small femoral head components, and after revision procedures [77–79]. Approximately one-third of dislocations will occur within a few weeks of surgery. Most cases can be treated successfully by closed reduction, but sometimes surgery is required, particularly in cases of recurrent dislocation.

The principal causes of recurrent dislocation are component malposition and separation, and nonunion of the greater trochanter [80]. Separation of the greater trochanter results in failure of the abductor mechanism, so that the unopposed adductor muscles tend to pull the hip out of its socket.

Total hip replacement and total knee replacement are the most common elective orthopedic operations in the United States. Osteoarthritis is the most common indication for total hip replacement. The cost effectiveness of total hip replacement compares favorably with nonsurgical treatments for advanced arthritis [81]. Even in elderly patients, dramatic improvements in pain and function can be achieved consistently with low complication rates and length of hospital stays comparable to younger patients [82].

Clinical History: 73-year-old man with painful total hip prosthesis.

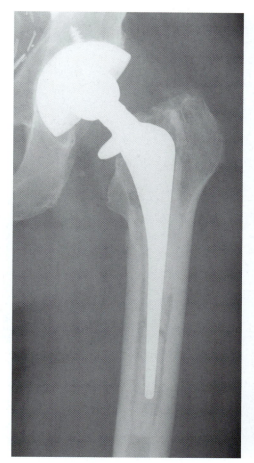

Figure 4-38 A

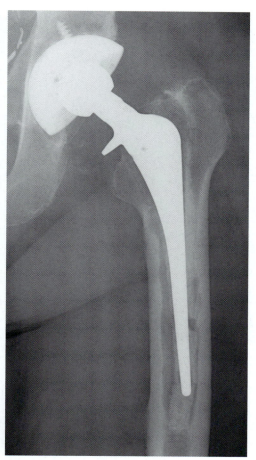

Figure 4-38 B

Findings: (A) AP radiograph of the left hip shows a hybrid total hip prosthesis with a partially cemented femoral component. There is a lucent zone at the prosthesis-to-bone interface of the proximal medial and lateral portions of the femoral component. (B) Three months later, AP radiograph shows that regions of lucency at the prosthesis-to-bone interface have enlarged, and new lucent zones have developed more distally at the femoral prosthesis-to-bone interface. The femoral stem has also detached from the bone cement along its lateral aspect.

Differential Diagnosis: Total hip replacement failure caused by osteolysis or infection.

Diagnosis: Total hip replacement failure caused by osteolysis.

Discussion: Loss of bone at the interface with a prosthetic joint replacement may cause catastrophic failure from loosening of components. Radiographic findings [83] that suggest loosening of prosthetic components include widening of the lucent zone at the prosthesis-to-bone interface or metal-to-bone interfaces to greater than 2 mm, migration of

components from their original positions, development of a lucent gap between metal and cement, cement fracture, periosteal reactive bone, and osteolysis. Osteolysis in total joint replacements is usually caused by foreign body granulomatous reaction. The mechanical friction on polyethylene components abrades microscopic particles of the plastic, which then incite an osteolytic granulomatous foreign body reaction. Migration of polyethylene debris and its accompanying reaction along cement-to-bone or metal-to-bone interfaces, often in the form of a thin membrane, may eventually cause gross loosening. Massive localized osteolysis may also occur; these lesions are filled with the same polyethylene foreign body reaction that causes component loosening.

Polyethylene osteolysis usually progresses slowly over many years. Debris may pass through lymphatics to regional lymph nodes. Because the radiolucent polyethylene liners of total joint replacements are responsible for the joint space on radiographs, thinning or gross failure of the polyethylene is evident on radiographs as narrowing of the joint space. Many polyethylene components have embedded metal markers that indicate their position on radiographs.

Clinical History: 56-year-old man with left hip pain. Other history withheld.

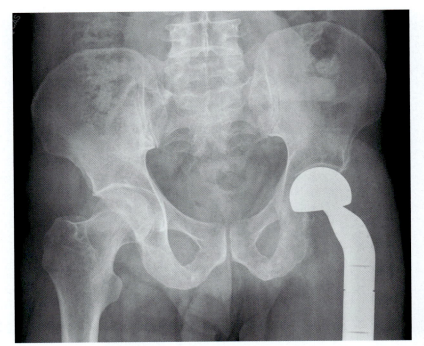

Figure 4-39   A

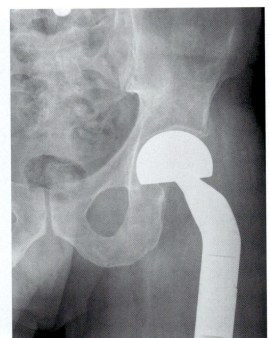

Figure 4-39   B

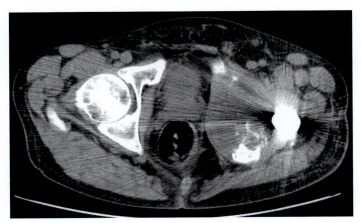

Figure 4-39   C

Findings: (A) AP radiograph of the pelvis shows a left modular bipolar femoral endoprothesis. Compared with the contralateral side, the left periacetabular region is osteopenic. Loss of cortex at the lateral aspect of the left ischium suggests a destructive process. (B) AP radiograph of the left hip obtained 4 months earlier shows no bone loss and intact cortex. (C) CT scan of the pelvis obtained 2 months later shows advanced destructive changes around the acetabulum.

Differential Diagnosis: Metastasis, infection, primary bone sarcoma, complex regional pain syndrome, osteolysis.

Diagnosis: Metastasis (from lung carcinoma).

Discussion: Comparison to previous imaging is a key strategy for the radiologist, particularly in the area of post-surgical imaging. Modular prosthetic hip components are used exclusively for reconstruction of large portions of the proximal femur. Bipolar and other hemiarthroplasties are used exclusively for proximal femoral disease, as opposed to hip disease. These two factors suggest that this patient may have had previous resection of a proximal femur for malignant neoplasm. Indeed, this patient was known to have lung carcinoma with previous resection of a metastasis for palliation, following a pathologic fracture of the subtrochanteric portion of the femur. Infection and primary bone sarcoma could also result in destructive changes in the bone, but are much less likely in the clinical circumstance.

Complex regional pain syndrome has been well described following total knee arthroplasty [84], but may also occur following total hip arthroplasty [85]. One might then hypothesize that the bone loss was the result of regional osteoporosis. Osteolysis is a common event in total hip replacement, but is less of an issue in hemiarthroplasties. Although many hemiarthroplasties do not have polyethylene components, bipolar prosthesis have a polyethylene liner between the prosthetic head and neck that allows motion between these two components (hence the name bipolar). Motion may also occur between the prosthetic head and the native acetabulum, reducing the potential wear on the polyethylene.

Clinical History: 68-year old man with left hip pain and bilateral total hip replacements.

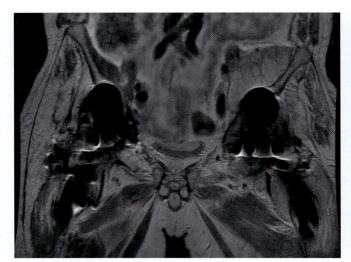

Figure 4-40 A

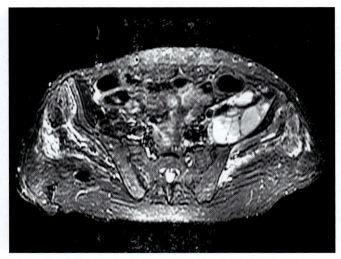

Figure 4-40 B

Findings: (A) Coronal proton density MRI demonstrates low signal and artifact from the metallic hip prosthesis. A lobulated fluid collection is seen adjacent to the supraacetabular region of the iliac bone on the left side, displacing the iliacus muscle superiorly. (B) Axial short tau inversion recovery (STIR) MRI above the level of the prostheses shows septations in the fluid collection. Abnormal high signal is also seen posterior to the left iliac wing.

Differential Diagnosis: Abscess, synovial cyst, hematoma.

Diagnosis: Abscess from septic hip.

Discussion: Fluid collections surrounding a total hip replacement may indicate infection. In this case, percutaneous needle aspiration of the collection produced pus. The use of cross-sectional imaging in the evaluation of complications of total hip replacement has been gaining popularity as techniques for reducing artifacts have improved. In one study, MRI was able to visualize the periprosthetic soft tissues around total hip replacements, including the prosthetic-bone interface, and provided substantially more diagnostic information about osteolysis than radiographs [86]. The prosthesis itself cannot be evaluated by MRI, and because a relatively large metallic object may result in spatial distortion, other means of imaging guidance should be used if percutaneous needle sampling is to be performed. CT also has a role in the assessment of osteolysis and other complications after total hip replacement [87].

Clinical History: 32-year old woman who crashed her bicycle 1 week prior to imaging.

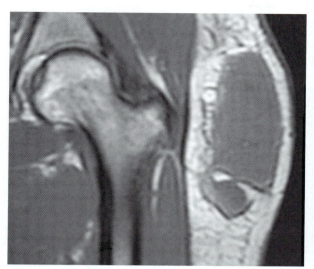

Figure 4-41   A

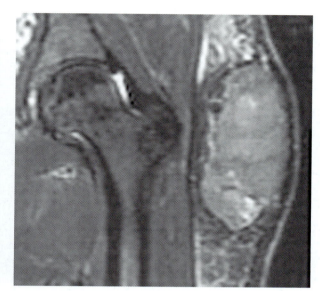

Figure 4-41   B

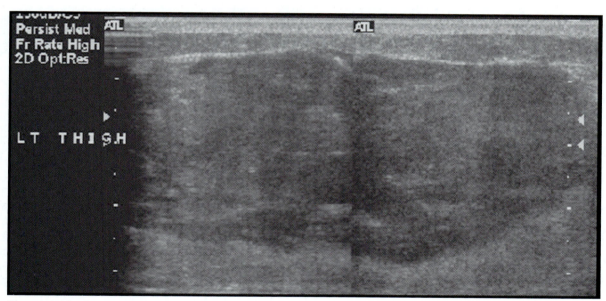

Figure 4-41   C

Findings: (A) Coronal T1-weighted MRI demonstrates a subcutaneous mass of intermediate signal intensity. (B) The coronal inversion recovery shows the mass to have heterogeneous increased signal intensity. (C) An ultrasound shows mixed echogenicity.

Differential Diagnosis: Hematoma, malignant fibrous histiocytoma, soft tissue neoplasm, abscess.

Diagnosis: Hematoma.

Discussion: In the clinical context of trauma in a young patient, a hematoma would be the most likely diagnosis. However, sarcomas and benign soft tissue neoplasms can have a similar appearance to the case above, and can present after trauma [88,89]. Features that would indicate malignancy include enhancement after contrast administration, internal blood flow on Doppler exam, and failure to decrease in size over time. An abscess would typically have an enhancing rim, complex internal fluid and debris, and surrounding inflammatory change in a patient with systemic symptoms. If the etiology of a mass is unclear, either short-term follow-up or needle biopsy should be performed.

CASE 4-42

Clinical History: 7-year-old girl with right hip pain.

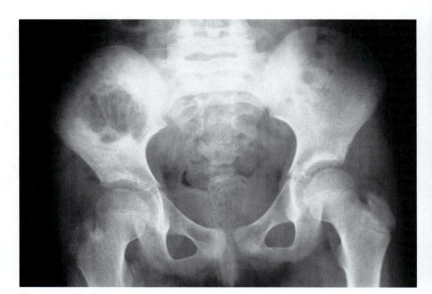

Figure 4-42 A

Figure 4-42 B

Findings: (A) AP radiograph of the pelvis shows a large, focal lytic lesion in the right iliac wing. The zone of transition appears to be relatively sharp, and there may be trabeculations within the lesion. (B) Representative CT scan images show a lucent lesion centered in the cortex. The posterior cortex has been largely destroyed, and the anterior cortex has been expanded. No mineralization is present within the lesion. There are no fluid-fluid levels. Edema gives the adjacent soft tissues lower attenuation than the normal contralateral side.

Differential Diagnosis: Ewings sarcoma, osteosarcoma, eosinophilic granuloma, lymphoma, aneurysmal bone cyst, osteomyelitis.

Diagnosis: Eosinophilic granuloma.

Discussion: The lesion has aggressive features, particularly on the CT scan. Cortical destruction, expansion into the soft tissues, and peritumoral edema represent a combination of features that is frequently seen in Ewings sarcoma and lymphoma. The lack of mineralization makes osteosarcoma less likely, and the location is not typical; however, fibroblastic and telangiectatic variants of osteosarcoma may not have much visible mineralization. The expansile nature of the lesion fits well with aneurysmal bone cyst. MRI would be helpful to determine whether the lesion is cystic or solid. Rapidly growing aneurysmal bone cysts may expand the periosteum faster than it can make bone, sometimes making it appear as if it has been destroyed, even though it may still be present. Finally, infection can be considered. The paucity of reactive bone formation relative to the extent of the destruction makes this less likely. This lesion requires a tissue diagnosis, and biopsy should be recommended. A CT-guided approach parallel to the anterior aspect of the iliac wing would preserve most surgical options should the lesion prove malignant.

SOURCES AND READINGS

1. Unni KK. *Dahlin's Bone Tumors: General Aspects and Data on 11,087 Cases*. 5th ed. Philadelphia: Lippincott-Raven; 1996:291–305.

2. Mitchell MJ, Logan PM. Radiation-induced changes in bone. *Radiographics*. 1998;18:1125–1136.

3. Mammone JF, Schweitzer ME. MR imaging of occult sacral insufficiency fractures following radiotherapy. *Skeletal Radiol*. 1995;24:101–104.

4. Harkin JC, Reed RJ. *Tumors of the Peripheral Nervous System*. Washington, D.C.: Armed Forces Institute of Pathology; 1969:51–97.

5. Siegel MJ. Magnetic resonance imaging of musculoskeletal soft tissue masses. *Radiol Clin North Am*. 2001;39(4):701–720.

6. Murphey MD, Walker EA, Wilson AJ, Kransdorf MJ, Temple HT, Gannon FH. From the archives of the AFIP: imaging of primary chondrosarcoma: radiologic-pathologic correlation. *Radiographics*. 2003;23(5):1245–1278.

7. Giles FJ, O'Brien SM, Keating MJ. Chronic lymphocytic leukemia in (Richter's) transformation. *Semin Oncol*. 1998;25:117–125.

8. Bessudo A, Kipps TJ. Origin of high-grade lymphomas in Richter syndrome. *Leuk Lymphoma*. 1995;18:367–372.

9. Roovers EA, Boere-Boonekamp MM, Geertsma TS, Zielhuis GA, Kerkhoff AH. Ultrasonographic screening for developmental dysplasia of the hip in infants. Reproducibility of assessments made by radiographers. *J Bone Joint Surg Br*. 2003;85(5):726–730.

10. Mandel DM, Loder RT, Hensinger RN. The predictive value of computed tomography in the treatment of developmental dysplasia of the hip. *J Pediatr Orthop*. 1998;18:794–798.

11. Nielsen GP, O'Connell JX, Rosenberg AE. Intramuscular myxoma: a clinicopathologic study of 51 cases with emphasis on hypercellular and hypervascular variants. *Am J Surg Pathol*. 1998;22:1222–1227.

12. Iwasko N, Steinbach LS, Disler D, et al. Imaging findings in Mazabraud's syndrome: seven new cases. *Skeletal Radiol*. 2002;31(2):81–87.

13. Murphy SB, Kijewski PK, Millis MB, Harless A. Acetabular dysplasia in the adolescent and young adult. *Clin Orthop*. 1990;261:214–223.

14. Yasunaga Y, Takahashi K, Ochi M, et al. Rotational acetabular osteotomy in patients forty-six years of age or older: comparison with younger patients. *J Bone Joint Surg Am*. 2003;85-A(2):266–272.

15. Hagiwara H, Aida N, Machida J, Fujita K, Okuzumi S, Nishimura G. Contrast-enhanced MRI of an early preosseous lesion of fibrodysplasia ossificans progressiva in a 21-month-old boy. *Am J Roentgenol*. 2003;181(4):1145–1147.

16. Semonin O, Fontaine K, Daviaud C, Ayuso C, Lucotte G. Identification of three novel mutations of the noggin gene in patients with fibrodysplasia ossificans progressiva. *Am J Med Genet*. 2001;102(4):314–317.

17. Kocyigit H, Hizli N, Memis A, Sabah D, Memis A. A severely disabling disorder: fibrodysplasia ossificans progressiva. *Clin Rheumatol*. 2001;20(4):273–275.

18. Kussmaul WG, Esmail AN, Sgar Y, Ross J, Gregory S, Kaplan FS. Pulmonary and cardiac function in advanced fibrodysplasia ossificans progressiva. *Clin Orthop*. 1998;346:104–109.

19. Glaser DL, Rocke DM, Kaplan FS. Catastrophic falls in patients who have fibrodysplasia ossificans progressiva. *Clin Orthop*. 1998;356:110–116.

20. Fairbairn KJ, Mulligan ME, Murphey MD, Resnik CS. Gas bubbles in the hip joint on CT: an indication of recent dislocation. *AJR Am J Roentgenol*. 1995;164:931–934.

21. Yue JJ, Wilber JH, Lipuma JP, et al. Posterior hip dislocations: a cadaveric angiographic study. *J Orthop Trauma*. 1996;10:447–454.

22. Erb RE, Steele JR, Nance EP Jr, Edwards JR. Traumatic anterior dislocation of the hip: spectrum of plain film and CT findings. *AJR Am J Roentgenol*. 1995;165:1215–1219.

23. Mithal A, Trivedi N, Gupta SK, Kumar S, Gupta RK. Radiological spectrum of endemic fluorosis: relationship with calcium intake. *Skeletal Radiol*. 1993;22:257–261.

24. Lian ZC, Wu EH. Osteoporosis—an early radiographic sign of endemic fluorosis. *Skeletal Radiol*. 1986;15:350–353.

25. Cao J, Bai X, Zhao Y, et al. The relationship of fluorosis and brick tea drinking in Chinese Tibetans. *Environ Health Perspect*. 1996;104:1340–1343.

26. Boillat MA, Garcia J, Velebit L. Radiological criteria of industrial fluorosis. *Skeletal Radiol*. 1980;5:161–165.

27. Czerwinski E, Nowak J, Dabrowska D, Skolarczyk A, Kita B, Ksiezyk M. Bone and joint pathology in fluoride-exposed workers. *Arch Environ Health*. 1988;43:340–343.

28. El-Khoury GY, Brandser EA, Kathol MH, Tearse DS, Callaghan JJ. Imaging of muscle injuries. *Skeletal Radiol*. 1996;25:3–11.

29. Kingzett-Taylor A, Tirman PF, Feller J, et al. Tendinosis and tears of gluteus medius and minimus muscles as a cause of hip pain: MR imaging findings. *Am J Roentgenol*. 1999;173(4):1123–1126.

30. Onur O, Celiker R, Cetin A, Alikasifoglu A, Ugur O, Basgoze O. Hypophosphatemic rickets with sacroiliitis-like presentation in an adolescent. *Scand J Rheumatol*. 1997;26:332–335.

31. Ecklund K, Doria AS, Jaramillo D. Rickets on MR images. *Pediatr Radiol*. 1999;29(9):673–675.

32. Wick MR, Siegal GP, Unni KK, McLeod RA, Greditzer HC 3rd. Sarcomas of bone complicating osteitis deformans (Paget's disease): fifty years' experience. *Am J Surg Pathol*. 1981;5:47–59.

33. Lopez C, Thomas DV, Davies AM. Neoplastic transformation and tumour-like lesions in Paget's disease of bone: a pictorial review. *Eur Radiol*. 2003;13(suppl 4):L151–L163.

34. Braun J, Sieper J, Bollow M. Imaging of sacroiliitis. *Clin Rheumatol*. 2000;19(1):51–57.

35. Sturzenbecher A, Braun J, Paris S, Biedermann T, Hamm B, Bollow M. MR imaging of septic sacroiliitis. *Skeletal Radiol*. 2000;29(8):439–446.

36. Lau SM, Chou CT, Huang CM. Unilateral sacroiliitis as an unusual complication of acupuncture. *Clin Rheumatol*. 1998;17(4):357–358.

37. Levine DS, Forbat SM, Saifuddin A. MRI of the axial skeletal manifestations of ankylosing spondylitis. *Clin Radiol*. 2004;59(5):400–413.

38. Ishida T, Iijima T, Moriyama S, Nakamura C, Katagawa T, Machinami R. Intra-articular calcifying synovial sarcoma mimicking synovial chondromatosis. *Skeletal Radiol*. 1996;25:766–769.

39. Ekman EF, Cory JW, Poehling GG. Pigmented villonodular synovitis and synovial chondromatosis arthroscopically diagnosed and treated in the same elbow. *Arthroscopy*. 1997;13:114–116.

40. Sciot R, Dal Cin P, Bellemans J, Samson I, Van den Berghe H, Van Damme B. Synovial chondromatosis: clonal chromosome changes provide further evidence for a neoplastic disorder. *Virchows Arch*. 1998;433:189–191.

41. Davis RI, Hamilton A, Biggart JD. Primary synovial chondromatosis: a clinicopathologic review and assessment of malignant potential. *Hum Pathol*. 1998;29:683–688.

42. Hermann G, Klein MJ, Abdelwahab IF, Kenan S. Synovial chondrosarcoma arising in synovial chondromatosis of the right hip. *Skeletal Radiol*. 1997;26:366–369.

43. Al-Nakshabandi NA, Ryan AG, Choudur H, et al. Pigmented villonodular synovitis. *Clin Radiol*. 2004;59(5):414–420.

44. Loughlin J, Dowling B, Chapman K, et al. Functional variants within the secreted frizzled-related protein 3 gene are associated with hip osteoarthritis in females. *Proc Natl Acad Sci USA*. 2004;101(26):9757–9762.

45. Conrozier T, Jousseaume CA, Mathieu P, et al. Quantitative measurement of joint space narrowing progression in hip osteoarthritis: a longitudinal retrospective study of patients treated by total hip arthroplasty. *Br J Rheumatol*. 1998;37:961–968.

46. Crawford RW, Gie GA, Ling RS, Murray DW. Diagnostic value of intra-articular anaesthetic in primary osteoarthritis of the hip. *J Bone Joint Surg Br*. 1998;80:279–281.

47. Resnick D. Anatomy of individual joints. In: Resnick D, ed. *Diagnosis of Bone and Joint Disorders*. 4th ed. Philadelphia: Saunders; 2002;708–792.

48. Damron TA, Heiner JP. Rapidly progressive protrusio acetabuli in patients with rheumatoid arthritis. *Clin Orthop*. 1993;289:186–194.

49. Johnson K, Gardner-Medwin J. Childhood arthritis: classification and radiology. *Clin Radiol.* 2002;57(1):47–58.

50. Cohen PA, Job-Deslandre CH, Lalande G, Adamsbaum C. Overview of the radiology of juvenile idiopathic arthritis (JIA). *Eur J Radiol.* 2000;33(2):94–101.

51. Milchgrub S, Ghander-Manaymneh L, Dorfman HD, Albores-Saavedra J. Synovial sarcoma with extensive osteoid and bone formation. *Am J Surg Pathol.* 1993;17:357–363.

52. Chung EB, Enzinger FM. Extraskeletal osteosarcoma. *Cancer.* 1987; 60:1132–1142.

53. Lee JS, Fetsch JF, Wasdhal DA, Lee BP, Pritchard DJ, Nascimento AG. A review of 40 patients with extraskeletal osteosarcoma. *Cancer.* 1995;76:2253–2259.

54. Varma DG, Ayala AG, Guo SQ, Moulopoulos LA, Kim EE, Charnsangavej C. MRI of extraskeletal osteosarcoma. *J Comput Asst Tomogr.* 1993;17:414–417.

55. Goshen E, Schwartz A, Zilka LR, Zwas ST. Bilateral accessory iliac horns: pathognomonic findings in nail-patella syndrome. Scintigraphic evidence on bone scan. *Clin Nucl Med.* 2000;25(6):476–477.

56. Guermazi A, de Kerviler E, Cazals-Hatem D, Zagdanski AM, Frija J. Imaging findings in patients with myelofibrosis. *Eur Radiol.* 1999;9(7):1366–1375.

57. Lomansey LM, Martinez S, Demos TC, Harrelson JM. Multifocal vascular lesions of bone: imaging characteristics. *Skeletal Radiol.* 1996; 25:255–261.

58. Ishida T, Dorfman HD, Steiner GC, Norman A. Cystic angiomatosis of bone with sclerotic changes mimicking osteoblastic metastases. *Skeletal Radiol.* 1994;23:247–252.

59. Legeai-Mallet L, Munnich A, Maroteaux P, Le Merrer M. Incomplete penetrance and expressivity skewing in hereditary multiple exostoses. *Clin Genet.* 1997;52:12–16.

60. Gordon SL, Buchanan JR, Ladda RL. Hereditary multiple exostoses: report of a kindred. *J Med Genet.* 1981;18:428–430.

61. Schapira D, Militeanu D, Israel O, Scharf Y. Insufficiency fractures of the pubic ramus. *Semin Arthritis Rheum.* 1996;25:373–382.

62. Pandley R, McNally E, Ali A, Bulstrode C. The role of MRI in the diagnosis of acute hip fractures. *Injury.* 1998;29:61–63.

63. Hill PF, Chatterji S, Chambers D, Keeling JD. Stress fracture of the pubic ramus in female recruits. *J Bone Joint Surg Br.* 1996;78:383–386.

64. Roodman GD. Mechanisms of bone metastasis. *N Engl J Med.* 2004; 350(16):1655–1664.

65. Roselli Del Turco M, Palli D, Cariddi A, Ciatto S, Pacini P, Distante V. The efficacy of intensive follow-up testing in breast cancer cases. *Ann Oncol.* 1995;6(suppl 2):37–39.

66. Milner PF, Kraus AP, Sebes JI, et al. Sickle cell disease as a cause of osteonecrosis of the femoral head. *N Engl J Med.* 1991;325:1476–1481.

67. Al-Mousawi F, Malki A, Al-Aradi A, Al-Bagali M, Al-Sadadi A, Booz MM. Total hip replacement in sickle cell disease. *Int Orthop.* 2002;26(3):157–161.

68. Styles LA, Vichinsky EP. Core decompression in avascular necrosis of the hip in sickle-cell disease. *Am J Hematol.* 1996;52:103–107.

69. Hernigou P, Bachir D, Galacteros F. Avascular necrosis of the femoral head in sickle cell disease. Treatment of collapse by injection of acrylic cement. *J Bone Joint Surg Br.* 1993;75:875–880.

70. Vohra R, Kang HS, Dogra S, Saggar RR, Sharma R. Tuberculous osteomyelitis. *J Bone Joint Surg Br.* 1997;79:562–566.

71. Jung NY, Jee WH, Ha KY, Park CK, Byun JY. Discrimination of tuberculous spondylitis from pyogenic spondylitis on MRI. *Am J Roentgenol.* 2004;182(6):1405–1410.

72. Sawlani V, Chandra T, Mishra RN, Aggarwal A, Jain UK, Gujral RB. MRI features of tuberculosis of peripheral joints. *Clin Radiol.* 2003;58(10):755–762.

73. Taconis WK, Schutte HE, van der Heul RO. Desmoplastic fibroma of bone: a report of 18 cases. *Skeletal Radiol.* 1994;23(4):283–288.

74. Bohm P, Krober S, Greschniok A, Laniado M, Kaiserling E. Desmoplastic fibroma of the bone. A report of two patients, review of the literature, and therapeutic implications. *Cancer.* 1996;78:1011–1123.

75. Vanhoenacker FM, Hauben E, De Beuckeleer LH, Willemen D, Van Marck E, De Schepper AM. Desmoplastic fibroma of bone: MRI features. *Skeletal Radiol.* 2000;29(3):171–175.

76. Inwards CY, Unni KK, Beabout JW, Sim FH. Desmoplastic fibroma of bone. *Cancer.* 1991;68:1978–1983.

77. Mahoney CR, Pellicci PM. Complications in primary total hip arthroplasty: avoidance and management of dislocations. *Instr Course Lect.* 2003;52:247–255.

78. Woolson ST, Rahimtoola ZO. Risk factors for dislocation during the first 3 months after primary total hip replacement. *J Arthroplasty.* 1999;14(6):662–668.

79. Yuan L, Shih C. Dislocation after total hip arthroplasty. *Arch Orthop Trauma Surg.* 1999;119(5–6):263–266.

80. Joshi A, Lee CM, Markovic L, Vlatis G, Murphy JC. Prognosis of dislocation after total hip arthroplasty. *J Arthroplasty.* 1998;13:17–21.

81. Hirsch HS. Total joint replacement: a cost-effective procedure for the 1990s. *Med Health R I.* 1998;81:162–164.

82. Brander VA, Malhotra S, Jet J, Heinemann AW, Stulberg SD. Outcome of hip and knee arthroplasty in persons aged 80 years and older. *Clin Orthop.* 1997;345:67–78.

83. Weissman BN. Imaging of total hip replacement. *Radiology.* 1997; 202:611–623.

84. Katz MM, Hungerford DS, Krackow KA, Lennox DW. Reflex sympathetic dystrophy as a cause of poor results after total knee arthroplasty. *J Arthroplasty.* 1986;1:117–124.

85. Robbins GM, Masri BA, Garbuz DS, Duncan CP. Evaluation of pain in patients with apparently solidly fixed total hip arthroplasty components. *J Am Acad Orthop Surg.* 2002;10:86–94.

86. Potter HG, Nestor BJ, Sofka CM, Ho ST, Peters LE, Salvati EA. Magnetic resonance imaging after total hip arthroplasty: evaluation of eriprosthetic soft tissue. *J Bone Joint Surg Am.* 2004;86-A:1947–1954.

87. Puri L, Wixson RL, Stern SH, Kohli J, Hendrix RW, Stulberg SD. Use of helical computed tomography for the assessment of acetabular osteolysis after total hip arthroplasty. *J Bone Joint Surg Am.* 2002;84-A:609–614.

88. Kassenoff TL, Tabaee A, Kacker A. Myofibroma of the cheek: a case report. *Ear Nose Throat J.* 2004;83(6):404–407.

89. Torok L, Kirschner A, Ocsai H, Olasz K. Hematoma-like metastasis in melanoma. *J Am Acad Dermatol.* 2003;49(5):912–913.

CHAPTER FIVE
PROXIMAL FEMUR AND THIGH

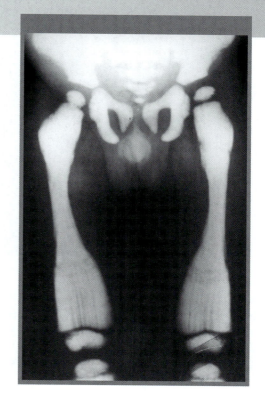

Clinical History: 54-year-old alcoholic man with worsening bilateral hip pain.

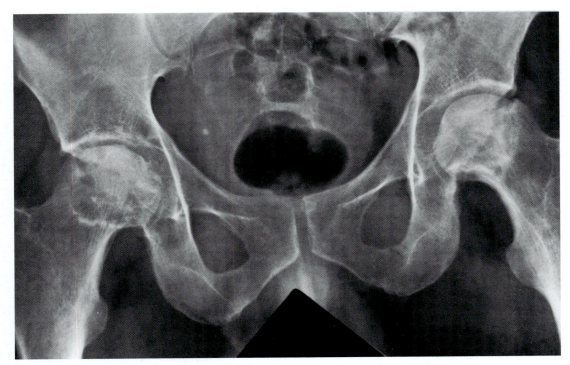

Figure 5-1

Findings: Anteroposterior (AP) radiograph of both hips. Both femoral heads are sclerotic and show subchondral fractures of the weight-bearing superior quadrants. Step-off at the lateral margins of both articular surfaces indicates the amount of collapse—a few millimeters in this case. There is relatively little acetabular disease.

Differential Diagnosis: Osteonecrosis, osteoarthritis.

Diagnosis: Osteonecrosis.

Discussion: The principal differential diagnostic consideration is osteoarthritis. The severity of the femoral head involvement with the relative sparing of the acetabulum indicates that the primary process is in the femoral head rather than the hip joint. Secondary osteoarthritis develops soon after femoral head collapse in osteonecrosis, but that is not yet seen in this case. Some patients with osteonecrosis present with the abrupt onset of hip pain, but femoral neck fracture is generally not a consideration without a history of falling or trauma. Most bones have a dual blood supply through the rich network of vessels that supply the periosteum and the ramifications of the nutrient arteries that supply the endosteum. Portions of bone that are covered with articular cartilage, or that are enclosed within joint capsules, have no periosteum and therefore have only an endosteal blood supply, leaving them more vulnerable to ischemic infarction. The femoral head is the most important clinical site of osteonecrosis because of its critical weight-bearing function.

Men are affected by osteonecrosis of the femoral head more often than women by a 4:1 ratio, and the usual age range of patients at presentation is 30 to 70 years. Known causes of osteonecrosis include sickle cell disease, Gaucher's disease, corticosteroids, trauma, alcoholism, collagen vascular diseases, renal transplantation, and pancreatitis, but many cases are idiopathic. The typical clinical complaint is abrupt onset of hip pain without trauma. In 50% of cases, bilateral involvement is present; bilateral disease is usually asymmetric. After the ischemic event, the infarcted, avascular region becomes revascularized from the periphery, and creeping substitution of devitalized bone occurs. When repair begins, plain films may show an increase in bony density around the periphery of the infarction. This increased peripheral density may slowly progress centrally as repair proceeds. Sometimes the dead bone is incompletely resorbed, and a sclerotic zone remains indefinitely. Because this repair process involves both resorption and replacement of bone, the mechanical strength may decrease transiently, and subchondral insufficiency fractures may result. Insufficiency fractures of the subchondral bone may be recognized by a crescentic lucent zone that separates the fragment. This late segmental collapse of the femoral head may rapidly lead to deformity and secondary osteoarthrosis of the hip.

Clinical History: 3-year-old girl with limb-length discrepancy and gait disturbance.

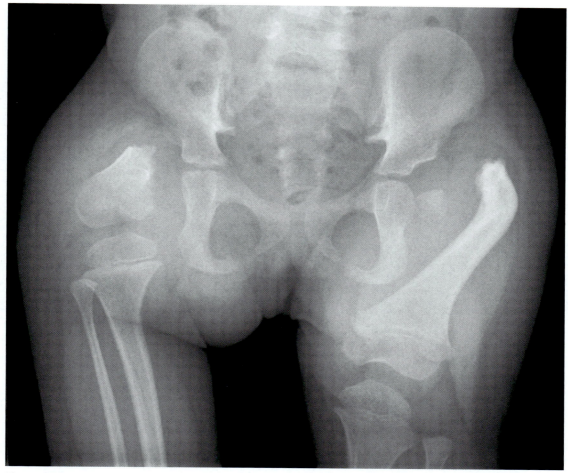

Figure 5-2

Findings: AP radiograph of the pelvis shows bilateral deficiency of the proximal femurs. On the right side, the femur is very short, with presence of only the distal portion. The acetabulum has not developed. On the left side, a small femoral head is present within a shallow acetabulum. The femoral neck and proximal shaft are absent, and the portion of shaft that is present is dysplastic.

Differential Diagnosis: Developmental dysplasia of the hip, proximal focal femoral deficiency (PFFD), postsurgical state.

Diagnosis: Proximal focal femoral deficiency.

Discussion: Aplasia, present in this case on the right, is not an aspect of developmental dysplasia of the hip. There is no normal development of the acetabulum or the portions of the femur present, suggesting the abnormality is not postsurgical or otherwise acquired.

PFFD designates a spectrum of developmental deficiencies of the proximal femur, ranging from shortening and varus deformity of the shaft, to aplasia of the femoral head, neck, and proximal shaft. Dysplastic changes in the acetabulum correlate with the degree of femoral head deformity or hypoplasia, and they represent the secondary effects of growth in the absence of a normal femoral head and normal weight-bearing stresses. The superior femoral epiphysis is typically mobile within the acetabulum, but in some cases it may be fixed and fused as part of the anomaly [6]. Congenital but not heritable, the cause of PFFD is unknown. The condition is unilateral more frequently than bilateral. When bilateral, it is usually asymmetric.

Clinical History: 38-year-old woman with right hip pain.

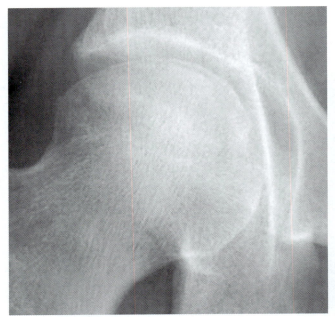

Figure 5-3   A

Figure 5-3   B

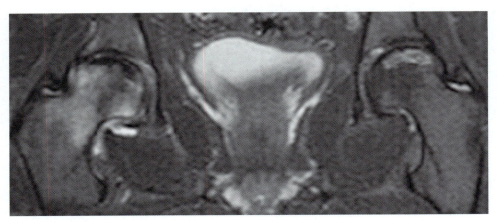

Figure 5-3   C

Findings: (A) AP view of the right femoral head showing a crescentic subchondral lucency. (B) Anterior nuclear medicine blood pool image demonstrating increased radiotracer uptake at the right hip. (C) Coronal T2-weighted fat-suppressed magnetic resonance imaging (MRI) through both hips shows bilateral abnormalities. On the right side, the normally low-signal fatty marrow of the femoral head and neck shows extensive marrow edema. The very low signal crescentic line along the weight-bearing surface corresponds to the subchondral fracture seen on the radiograph. There is a small right hip effusion. On the left side, there is a serpiginous high-signal line along the weight-bearing portion of the femoral head, with normal low signal from the fatty marrow on both sides of the line.

Differential Diagnosis: Osteonecrosis, fracture, septic joint, osteomyelitis, transient osteoporosis.

Diagnosis: Osteonecrosis.

Discussion: In this case, the left femoral head shows a region of previous osteonecrosis with repair. The right femoral head is acutely osteonecrotic, with extensive marrow edema. Osteonecrosis begins with interruption of the blood supply to the femoral head. The precise event that initiates the loss of circulation may be unknown, although a large number of clinical conditions appear to be associated with it. One possible event is an increase in intraosseous pressure within the femoral head; when this pressure exceeds the perfusion pressure, blood flow stops. Ischemic necrosis of the marrow and bone follows with the onset of pain, but radiographs will be normal. Intramedullary pressure measurements of the proximal femur will be elevated. The typical distribution of infarction is a wedge-shaped region under the weight-bearing surface of the femoral head. The articular cartilage itself remains viable, because its nutrition is derived from the synovial fluid. MRI best demonstrates early osteonecrosis [1]. The region of infarction is evident as a loss of the normal bright marrow signal on T1-weighted images. The radionuclide bone scan may show changes of initial loss of radionuclide accumulation in the avascular stage, with subsequent variable increases in accumulation in the reparative stage. The nuclear scan is less sensitive than MRI and gives poor anatomic detail. The frequent asymmetric bilaterality of osteonecrosis of the femoral head may complicate interpretation of the bone scan.

Initial treatment of osteonecrosis is controversial. The treatment of osteonecrosis of the femoral head focuses on preserving the normal articular surface, typically by core decompression of the neck and head, or placement of a vascularized fibular graft [2]. As one might expect, the earlier the stage at which osteonecrosis is treated, the better the long-term outcome [3].

Clinical History: 44-year-old woman with severe right hip pain.

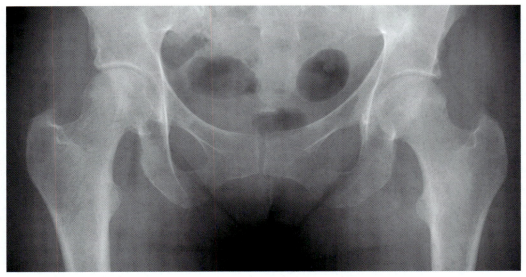

Figure 5-4   A

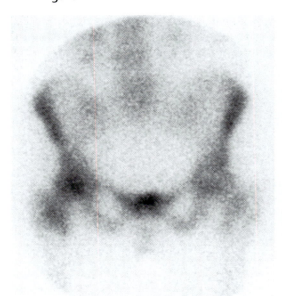

Figure 5-4   B

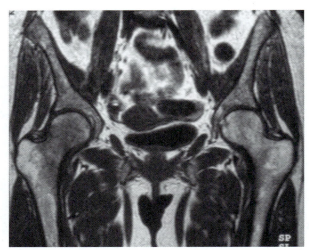

Figure 5-4   C

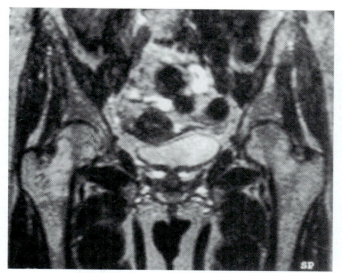

Figure 5-4 D

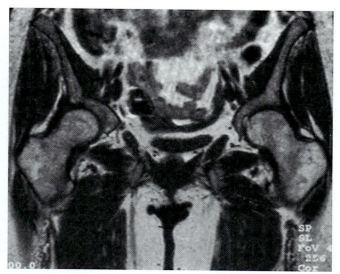

Figure 5-4 E

Findings: (**A**) AP radiograph of the pelvis is normal. (**B**) Bone scan shows increased radiotracer uptake in the right femoral head and neck. (**C**) Coronal T1-weighted MRI of the hips shows loss of the normal bright marrow signal in the right proximal femur, including the entire head and neck. (**D**) Coronal T2-weighted MRI shows edema in the marrow of the entire right proximal femur. There is no effusion in the right hip. (**E**) Coronal T1-weighted MRI taken 6 weeks later demonstrates near-complete normalization of marrow signal, indicating resolution of the edema.

Differential Diagnosis: Osteonecrosis, transient bone marrow edema, reflex sympathetic dystrophy, osteomyelitis, fracture.

Diagnosis: Transient bone marrow edema.

Discussion: In the absence of fracture, the key clinical and radiologic differential diagnosis is between osteonecrosis, which would typically require surgical intervention, and transient bone marrow edema or reflex sympathetic dystrophy, either of which would not. The distinction is clear from the MRI. Transient bone marrow edema is a condition characterized by a rapidly developing bone marrow edema and osteoporosis, affecting periarticular bone that is self-limited, reversible, and has no clear-cut inciting event. It affects previously healthy middle-aged men, and women in the third trimester of pregnancy. Its etiology is still unclear, but in view of similarities to regional migratory osteoporosis and reflex sympathetic dystrophy, vascular and neurologic disturbances have been proposed as the possible pathogenetic mechanisms.

Pain in the hip area and functional disability of the affected limb are the main clinical signs. Diagnosis is supported by local radiologic osteopenia whose gradual disappearance parallels the spontaneous recovery. Transient bone marrow edema usually presents with monoarticular joint pain [4]. It typically involves either hip in men, or the left hip in women. Self-limited but aggravated by activity, the pain regresses in 2 to 6 months without permanent sequelae. Radiographs are often normal, but they may show a rapidly developing periarticular osteoporosis, particularly in the femoral head, which returns to normal after resolution of symptoms. MRI shows diffuse edema and hip effusion, but no infarction [5]. Bone scans demonstrate increased activity consistent with the bone marrow edema. The initial site of involvement in regional migratory osteoporosis may be the hip, in which case the initial presentation may have been called transient bone marrow edema (osteoporosis) of the hip.

Clinical History: 14-year-old girl with gait problems.

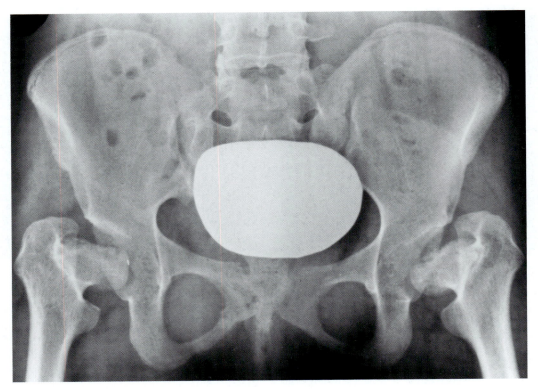

Figure 5-5

Findings: AP radiograph of the pelvis shows bilaterally small femoral heads with a flattened morphology. Both hips are normally located, but the acetabulae are shallow, steep, and dysplastic, to accommodate the abnormal shape of the femoral heads. The femoral necks assume a horizontal orientation but do not appear particularly abnormal in size or shape, given the deformity of the heads. The bones otherwise appear relatively normal.

Differential Diagnosis: Multiple epiphyseal dysplasia, spondyloepiphyseal dysplasia, Legg-Calvé-Perthes disease, developmental dysplasia of the hip, slipped capital femoral epiphysis (SCFE), achondroplasia, juvenile chronic arthritis, mucopolysaccharidosis.

Diagnosis: Multiple epiphyseal dysplasia (dysplasia epiphysealis multiplex).

Discussion: Bilateral hip disease during childhood may encompass all of the entities in the differential diagnosis. Legg-Calvé-Perthes disease is associated with dysplastic enlargement and flattening of the femoral heads, and juvenile chronic arthritis is associated with epiphyseal overgrowth, cartilage loss, and ankylosis. The hips are normally located, eliminating developmental dysplasia of the hip from further consideration, and although the patient's age would be typical for SCFE, the radiologic appearance is not. Skeletal changes in the mucopolysaccharidoses may include irregular epiphyses, but biochemical abnormalities will be present clinically, and there is frequent involvement of the thorax and skull, sites that are not affected in multiple epiphyseal dysplasia. The femoral heads in achondroplasia are typically small and dysplastic, with short and disproportionately broad necks, but the absence of bony abnormalities in the pelvis and lumbar spine excludes achondroplasia as a diagnosis in this case. Multiple epiphyseal dysplasia and spondyloepiphyseal dysplasia may be indistinguishable radiographically, except for the absence or presence of spinal column dysplasia. Radiographs of the spine are not included for this case, because they were normal.

Multiple epiphyseal dysplasia is a term used to designate a heterogeneous group of disorders that appear to have an abnormality of the epiphyseal chondrocyte in common [7]. Chondrocytes in the growth plates appear to be defective in morphology and organization and deficient in number, with abnormal production of matrix, leading to delayed and disorderly growth and ossification of the ends of the bones. When the hips are involved, the profound loss of growth of the femoral heads results in a markedly decreased range of motion and a waddling gait.

Clinical History: 34-year-old woman with crippling joint disease.

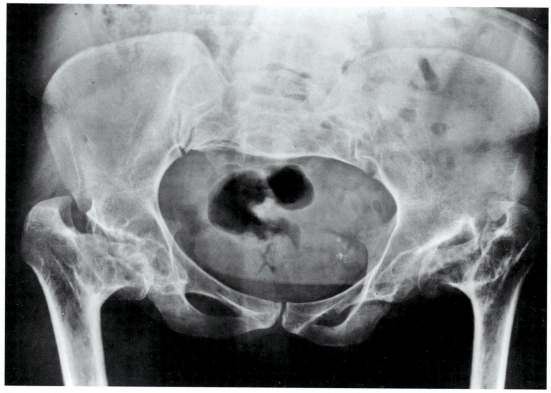

Figure 5-6

Findings: AP radiograph of the hips shows small, dysplastic femoral heads, with adaptive changes in acetabular morphology and secondary degenerative changes.

Differential Diagnosis: Secondary osteoarthritis caused by multiple epiphyseal dysplasia, spondyloepiphyseal dysplasia, Legg-Calvé-Perthes disease, developmental dysplasia of the hip, SCFE, achondroplasia, mucopolysaccharidosis, juvenile chronic arthritis.

Diagnosis: Secondary osteoarthritis resulting from multiple epiphyseal dysplasia.

Discussion: This case should be compared with the previous case. The major cause of long-term morbidity in multiple epiphyseal dysplasia is the early development of secondary osteoarthritis [8,9], which is a result of the joint incongruity caused by defective growth of the ends of the bones in this condition. Degenerative changes in weight-bearing joints are frequently present before the third decade of life. The condition is often inherited, with most families having an autosomal dominant gene with high penetrance; sporadic cases and families with autosomal recessive inheritance have also been described [10]. There is an equal sex incidence in multiple epiphyseal dysplasia, and osseous involvement is bilateral and symmetric, but the number of joints involved and the severity of involvement is highly variable. The most frequent sites of involvement are the hips, knees, shoulders, ankles, and wrists. Short stature or even dwarfism may be present, a condition sometimes called pseudoachondroplasia. Degenerative joint disease in the hip is treated by total hip replacement.

Clinical History: Infant boy with bone dysplasia.

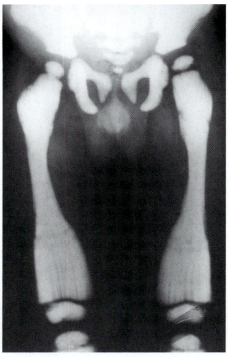

Figure 5-7

Findings: AP radiographs of the pelvis and thigh show symmetric increased density involving all the bones. There is no cortical or trabecular structure, and there are prominent transverse and vertical striations. The shapes of the metaphyses are undertubulated—they are shaped like a juggling club.

Differential Diagnosis: None.

Diagnosis: Osteopetrosis.

Discussion: The diffuse disease is indicative of a systemic process, and the radiologic features are distinctive enough to be pathognomonic. Osteopetrosis is a group of heritable diseases characterized by reduced bone resorption from osteoclast failure [11]. Many genetic defects may cause osteoclast failure, each having different underlying biochemical and histopathologic abnormalities. One form is associated with renal tubular acidosis and rickets. The common final effect is that bone remodels incompletely or not at all.

There are three major clinical groups:

- Infantile malignant autosomal recessive, which is fatal within the first few years of life (in the absence of effective therapy).
- Intermediate autosomal recessive, which appears during the first decade of life but does not follow a malignant course.

- Autosomal dominant (Albers-Schoenberg disease or marble bones), with normal life expectancy but many orthopedic problems.

The infantile variant has clinical manifestations that correlate with the lack of marrow development (anemia and thrombocytopenia), and the lack of enlargement of bony remodeling (small cranial foramina result in cranial nerve dysfunction, hydrocephalus, convulsions, and mental retardation).

Radiographs show uniformly dense bones with no medullary space, broadened metaphyses (Erlenmeyer flask deformity), and bone-within-a-bone appearance at the tarsals, carpals, phalanges, vertebrae, and iliac wings. Transverse insufficiency fractures occur frequently. Medical treatments involve high-dose calcitriol to stimulate osteoclast differentiation, and bone marrow transplantation to provide monocytic osteoclast precursors. The intermediate and autosomal dominant forms have mild manifestations that include anemia, cranial nerve palsies, and orthopedic problems. The fragility of osteopetrotic bone, and its inability to remodel in response to stress, results in repeated insufficiency fractures. Coxa vara, long-bone bowing, hip and knee degenerative arthritis, and mandibular and long-bone osteomyelitis may occur. Milder forms of osteopetrosis may be asymptomatic and discovered incidentally on radiographs.

Clinical History: 21-year-old man with limb deformity.

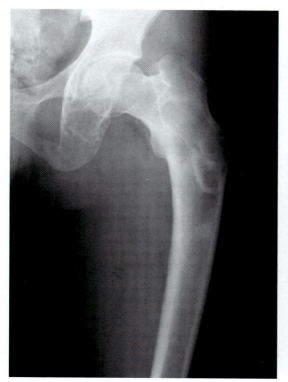

Figure 5-8   A

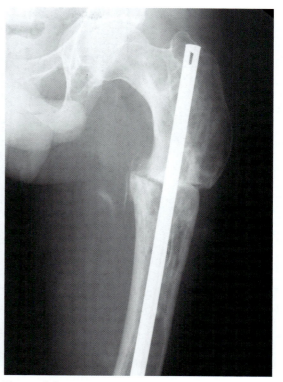

Figure 5-8   B

Findings: (A) AP radiograph of the left hip. There are expansile lesions in the ischium. There are dysplastic changes in the left proximal femur, with mild expansion and mineralization. The mineralization has a ground-glass appearance; some portions are curvilinear and densely sclerotic. There is a bowing deformity of the proximal femur. (B) Follow-up AP radiograph of the left hip after treatment shows osteotomy of the proximal femoral shaft, with intramedullary rod fixation. The bowing deformity has been corrected.

Differential Diagnosis: Fibrous dysplasia, Paget's disease, osteogenesis imperfecta, osteomalacia.

Diagnosis: Fibrous dysplasia (with shepherd's crook deformity).

Discussion: Bowing deformities of the proximal femur in adults include the items in the differential diagnosis. Paget's disease can be eliminated because of the young age of the patient, and the lack of cortical thickening and bony enlargement. Osteogenesis imperfecta would affect all bones and would include osteoporosis as a feature. Osteomalacia, particularly in the setting of renal osteodystrophy, could result in bowing deformity, but other radiologic features should be present. Fibrous dysplasia, both monostotic and polyostotic, commonly involves the proximal femur, and the distinctive shepherd's crook bowing deformity of fibrous dysplasia is illustrated by this case.

Fibrous dysplasia is a benign fibroosseous lesion that is neither familial nor hereditary, but appears to be a developmental abnormality involving the proliferation and maturation of fibroblasts [12]. Bowing deformities result from biomechanically insufficient bone, and from malunion of pathologic fractures. Orthopedic management is typically restricted to treatment of complications. The results of curettage, bone grafting, and mechanical realignment of proximal femoral lesions are much better in monostotic forms of the disease [13]. Long-term follow-up has shown that bone graft is resorbed and remodeled in fibrous dysplasia.

Malignant transformation has been documented, but it is rare and, in some cases, may have occurred due to previous radiation treatment. Its occurrence has been documented in both polyostotic and monostotic varieties of fibrous dysplasia [14]. These reported secondary sarcomas have been mostly osteosarcomas, but fibrosarcoma, chondrosarcoma, and giant cell sarcoma has also been reported.

Clinical History: 3-year-old boy with mild hip pain.

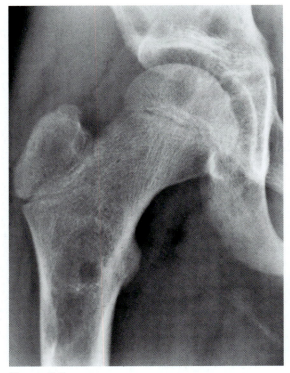

Figure 5-9

Findings: AP radiograph of the right hip shows multiple lucent lesions in the acetabulum, femoral head and neck, and subtrochanteric region. These are well-defined, ovoid lesions, some of which have partial sclerotic margins. The lesions have no internal mineralization. There is no reactive bone formation in the periosteum. There is no cortical breakthrough or cortical expansion.

Differential Diagnosis: Eosinophilic granuloma, metastatic disease, osteomyelitis, enchondromatosis, multiple nonossifying fibromas, hemangiomatosis, lymphangiomatosis.

Diagnosis: Lymphangiomatosis.

Discussion: The differential diagnosis revolves primarily around the number and distribution of lesions. The single radiograph demonstrates involvement of two contiguous bones. There is epiphyseal, metaphyseal, and diaphyseal involvement. Although eosinophilic granuloma would be the most common entity in this circumstance, the lack of reactive bone formation would be unusual, because eosinophilic granuloma provokes an inflammatory response. The lack of internal calcification and bony expansion would argue against enchondromatosis, and an epiphyseal lesion would be very odd. The epiphyseal involvement also eliminates multiple nonossifying fibromas from consideration. Skeletal metastatic disease is virtually unheard of in children.

Lymphangiomatosis is a rare congenital entity that can involve bone, soft tissue, or viscera in a diffuse fashion [15]. It is typically composed of the following triad of traits: bone lesions, lymphedema, and chylous effusions. The radiographic appearance of the bony lesions is typically lytic, with a lace-like pattern and sclerotic margins of variable thickness. Individual lesions may simulate a wide array of benign and malignant entities, but their multiplicity significantly narrows the differential diagnosis. These lesions demonstrate no metastatic potential. When there is extensive visceral involvement and chylothorax, the prognosis is poor, but lesions limited to the extremities have a good prognosis [16].

CASE 5-10

Clinical History: Young boy with hip problems.

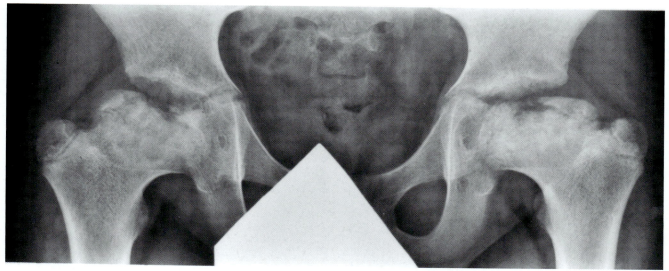

Figure 5-10

Findings: AP radiograph of both hips shows large femoral heads with short broad necks (coxa magna). The femoral heads are too large to fit fully into the acetabulae. The capital femoral epiphyses are enlarged and ossifying from multiple centers.

Differential Diagnosis: Developmental dysplasia of the hip, epiphyseal dysplasia, Legg-Calvé-Perthes disease, SCFE, juvenile idiopathic arthritis.

Diagnosis: Legg-Calvé-Perthes disease.

Discussion: The abnormalities are bilateral and nearly symmetric, and characterized by enlarged, deformed femoral heads. The relatively mild changes in the acetabulae suggest the disease is primarily in the femoral heads. Overgrowth of the femoral heads may occur in juvenile idiopathic arthritis, but there is no apparent joint disease seen in this case. Developmental dysplasia of the hip usually presents in infancy, whereas SCFE usually presents in adolescence.

Legg-Calvé-Perthes disease is idiopathic osteonecrosis of the capital femoral epiphysis in a skeletally immature child. Boys are affected more often than girls by a 4:1 ratio. The mean age of onset is 7 years, and the range is 2 to 13 years. In 20% of cases the condition is bilateral. The bone age of affected children is usually 1 to 3 years behind their chronologic age. Interruption of the blood supply to the femoral head leads to partial or total osteonecrosis. Enchondral ossification of the capital femoral epiphysis and activity at the growth plate both stop. The articular cartilage, nourished by synovial fluid, continues to grow. If the disease is detected at this stage, the ossific nucleus of the capital femoral epiphysis will be smaller than normal, and overgrowth of the articular cartilage will be apparent as joint space widening. The patient may be asymptomatic.

Revascularization of the femoral head leads to centripetal ossification, usually from multiple sites that are not contiguous with the original ossific nucleus, resulting in an appearance often described as fragmentation of ossification. Apposition of new bone to the dead bone may increase the radiographic density of the head. Resorption of subchondral bone may lead to subchondral fracture and the onset of clinical symptoms: hip pain and limp. The severity of the clinical findings is highly variable and does not necessarily correlate with the radiographic findings. The end result is a short, thick femoral neck and an enlarged femoral head (coxa magna). Premature closure of the growth plate accentuates the deformity. Secondary osteoarthritis is a complication in early adult life.

Clinical History: 65-year-old man with newly diagnosed prostate cancer.

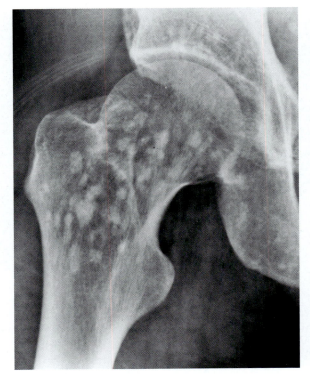

Figure 5-11   A

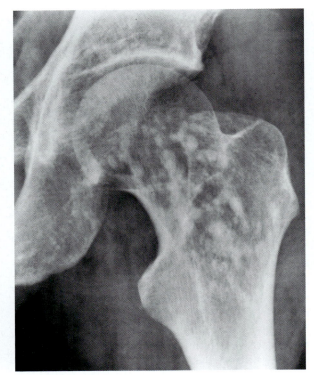

Figure 5-11   B

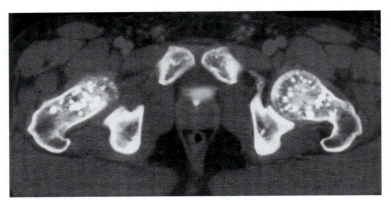

Figure 5-11   C

Findings: (A, B) AP radiographs of the hips show multiple oval sclerotic foci present in the femoral head, neck, and intertrochanteric region. A few are noted in the acetabulum. (C) Axial computed tomography (CT) (bone windows) obtained after intravenous contrasts enhancement. There are multiple focal bone densities in the acetabulae and proximal femurs on both sides.

Differential Diagnosis: Osteopoikilosis, metastatic disease.

Diagnosis: Osteopoikilosis.

Discussion: Multiple sclerotic lesions may be seen with metastatic disease, mastocytosis, and occasionally lymphoma. However, the symmetric periarticular distribution of the sclerotic lesions, their well-defined borders, their uniform size, their oval shape, and their orientation to the long axis of the bone supports the diagnosis of osteopoikilosis. Osteopoikilosis (spotted bones, osteopathia condensans disseminata) is an uncommon osteosclerotic dysplasia with sporadic and familial occurrence. The lesions may increase or decrease in size or number. Symptoms are generally absent or mild, and its discovery is frequently incidental. Histologically identical to bone islands, the lesions have no clinical significance beyond their confusion with osseous metastatic disease [17]. Osteopoikilosis can show increased activity on bone scan [18].

CASE 5-12

Clinical History: 15-year-old boy with right hip pain.

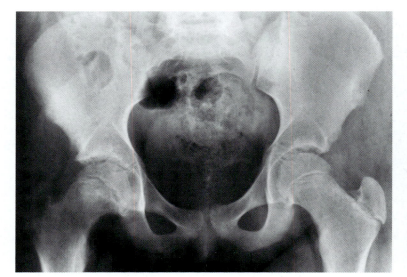

Figure 5-12   A

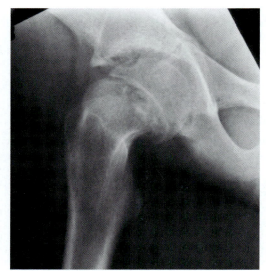

Figure 5-12   B

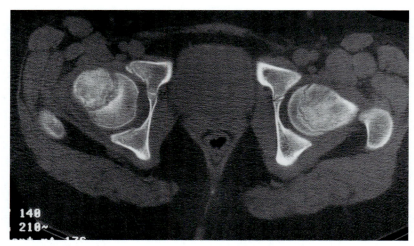

Figure 5-12   C

Findings: (A) AP pelvis radiograph shows abnormal right proximal femur. The growth plate appears widened, with irregularity of the metaphyseal margin. The femoral neck appears slightly displaced laterally compared with the capital femoral epiphysis, and an imaginary line drawn along the superior cortex of the femoral neck would not intersect the femoral head (as it would on the normal left side). (B) Frog lateral radiograph better shows the abnormal displacement and angulation of the femoral neck relative to the femoral head. An imaginary line drawn along the anterior cortex of the neck would completely miss the head, rather than intersect its margin. (C) Axial CT shows the widened, abnormal growth plate, and abnormal alignment of neck and shaft. The growth plate has a rounded contour.

Differential Diagnosis: SCFE, healing Salter type I fracture.

Diagnosis: Slipped capital femoral epiphysis.

Discussion: SCFE is displacement of the femoral head relative to the femoral neck through the open growth plate in an adolescent. The head remains in the acetabulum as the neck progressively displaces anteriorly and superiorly (the head goes inferiorly and posteriorly). SCFE occurs in boys and girls of approximately the same skeletal age shortly before closure of the growth plate (chronologic age of about 11 years in girls and 14 years in boys). Boys are affected more often than girls by a ratio of 2.5:1. Many patients are overweight and have mildly delayed skeletal ages. Bilateral involvement is present in about half of the patients, and some cases are familial. The etiology is not known; the pathophysiology may be related to an endocrine process or a biomechanical problem.

The slippage between the femoral head and neck occurs between the proliferative and hypertrophic zones of the growth cartilage, and early abnormalities of the growth plate may be seen on MRI before changes on radiographs [19]. SCFE is different from a Salter type I fracture, which occurs between the hypertrophic and provisional calcification zones of the cartilage. SCFE may be a chronic, slow process that allows bony remodeling of both head and neck as the deformity progresses, or it may be a relatively acute process (usually lasting less than 3 weeks) whose presentation is not unlike that of a stress fracture. SCFE is treated by stabilization of the head without attempt at anatomic reduction. Pins may be used to fix the position of the head and promote closure of the growth plate. Dysplasia of the hip and early osteoarthritis may develop, and osteonecrosis is a devastating complication that is more common in acute slips.

Clinical History: 5-year-old boy with hip pain and limp.

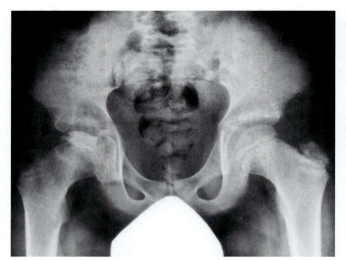

Figure 5-13   A

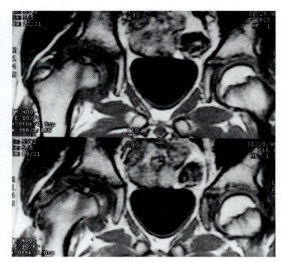

Figure 5-13   B

Findings: (A) AP radiograph of both hips. The right femoral head is sclerotic and diminutive. Periarticular osteoporosis is present. (B) T1-weighted MRI shows a low signal intensity, small, flattened head. Associated marrow edema (dark on T1-weighted MRI) extends into the femoral neck. The opposite hip is normal.

Differential Diagnosis: Legg-Calvé-Perthes disease, other cause of femoral head osteonecrosis.

Diagnosis: Legg-Calvé-Perthes disease.

Discussion: The therapy goal for Legg-Calvé-Perthes disease is to prevent the development of femoral head deformity and subsequent osteoarthritis. Centering of the femoral head within the acetabulum during the revascularization and ossification stages of healing presumably allows the acetabulum to act as a mold for the healing femoral head, averting the development of deformity. Acetabular coverage for the femoral head may be obtained by abduction of the femoral head relative to the acetabulum with a brace, varus osteotomy of the proximal femur, or osteotomy of the pelvis. MRI of the hip may be helpful for estimating the extent of epiphyseal necrosis and delineating the morphology of the uncovered, unossified portion of the femoral head for treatment planning [20,21]. The amount of ultimate deformity depends on the age at onset and the remaining growth potential of the femur. The degree of synovitis accompanying Legg-Calvé-Perthes disease appears to correlate with the extent of epiphyseal necrosis and the clinical outcome [22]. Osteonecrosis of the femoral head and other growing epiphyses may occur as a result of trauma, infection, sickle disease, or other conditions. The pathophysiology and the gamut of radiologic findings are similar to that of Legg-Calvé-Perthes disease.

Clinical History: 45-year-old woman with muscle weakness.

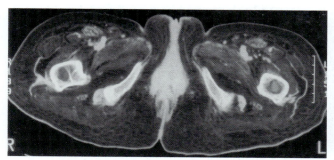

Figure 5-14   A

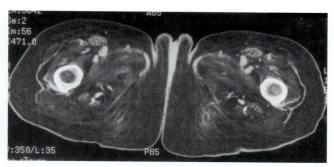

Figure 5-14   B

Findings: (A, B) Axial CT through the proximal thigh demonstrates marked fatty replacement of all the visualized musculature. The bones are normal, with hematopoietic marrow in the proximal femurs.

Differential Diagnosis: Polymyositis, paralysis, corticosteroid excess, arthrogryposis, muscular dystrophy.

Diagnosis: Polymyositis.

Discussion: Fatty replacement of the musculature may occur on a neuropathic basis or a myopathic basis. In this particular case, the diagnosis is polymyositis and there are no specific distinguishing features. There is a lack of the dysplastic bone and joint changes common in arthrogryposis and muscular dystrophy, suggesting a disease process acquired in adulthood. The presence of soft tissue calcification would strongly implicate dermatomyositis or polymyositis, but none is present on these images.

Clinically, patients with polymyositis demonstrate proximal muscle weakness and pain, which may be progressive or self-limited. This entity may occur with a skin rash (dermatomyositis), Raynaud's phenomenon, other connective tissue diseases (overlap syndromes), and cancers. The latter association is noted more often in elderly men; however, in general, polymyositis is encountered more frequently in women.

Polymyositis is marked by muscle inflammation followed by atrophy and fibrosis. Soft tissue calcifications may occur in the subcutaneous and deep tissues and, when present, may help distinguish this entity from other causes of muscle atrophy. There is progressive atrophy with fatty replacement, as seen here, which may be demonstrated on CT or MRI [34,35]. The soft tissue changes are best assessed with MRI, which shows increased signal intensity on T2-weighted images within the muscle in the acute setting, and fatty replacement in the chronic setting. Although bony changes are not a feature, arthralgias, contractures, and juxtaarticular osteoporosis may develop. When bony findings such as erosive changes occur, an overlap syndrome or other connective tissue disorders should be considered. Although the primary target of this entity is skeletal muscle, pulmonary fibrosis, pericarditis, and dysphasia may also be present.

Clinical History: Acute hip distress in an infant girl with fever.

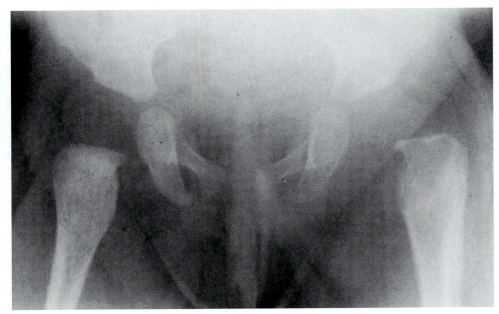

Figure 5-15 A

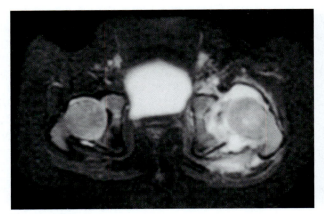

Figure 5-15 B

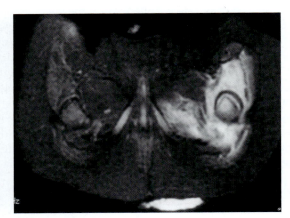

Figure 5-15 C

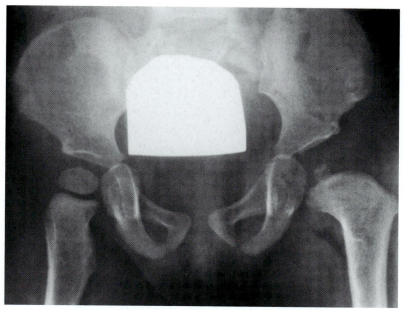

Figure 5-15   D

Findings: (**A**) AP radiographs of the pelvis and femurs show lateral subluxation of left hip and periosteal reaction in the femur. (**B, C**) Axial T2-weighted MRI demonstrates marked high-signal fluid in the left hip joint, mixed with low-signal debris. This is causing a secondary lateral subluxation of the left hip. Edema is seen in the musculature and soft tissues surrounding the hip. (**D**) AP radiograph taken 6 months later shows delayed ossification of the capital femoral epiphysis, with associated underdeveloped concavity of the acetabulum and broadening of the femoral neck.

Differential Diagnosis: Septic arthritis, developmental dysplasia of the hip, Legg-Calvé-Perthes disease.

Diagnosis: Septic arthritis, with secondary osteonecrosis of the capital femoral epiphysis.

Discussion: The historical facts in this case make the etiology clear. Lateral subluxation of the hip can be the result of mild developmental dysplasia of the hip, but the clinical presentation and the periosteal reaction along the proximal femur is indicative of infection. In the follow-up radiograph, the left proximal femur shows the characteristic changes of osteonecrosis of the growing capital femoral epiphysis: delayed ossification (to be followed by ossification from

multiple separate centers), dysplastic enlargement, and a short, broad neck. Sometimes distinction of this entity from Legg-Calvé-Perthes or juvenile idiopathic arthritis can be difficult, and additional imaging should be directed by each child's clinical presentation [23,24].

Septic arthritis in young children can result from seeding of the joint through hematogenous spread from a remote source, contiguous spread from osteomyelitis, or direct introduction by penetrating trauma. The knee and hip are the most commonly affected sites, and *S. aureus* is the most common organism. The most common presenting sign is that of joint effusion. On sonography, the surrounding capsular structures can be edematous. Juxtaarticular osteoporosis quickly ensues due to the aggressive hyperemia. The elicited pannus quickly erodes the cartilage and then bone, leading to joint space loss and associated erosions.

Complications of septic arthritis can include fibrous or osseous ankylosis, synovial cysts, cellulitis or abscesses of the surrounding tissues, osteomyelitis, avascular necrosis, and secondary degenerative joint disease. In this case, the avascular necrosis was presumably a result of an increase in capsular pressure combined with the septic capillary thrombosis.

CASE 5-16

Clinical History: 75-year-old man with left hip pain after a fall.

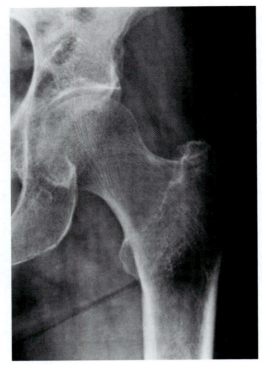

Figure 5-16   A

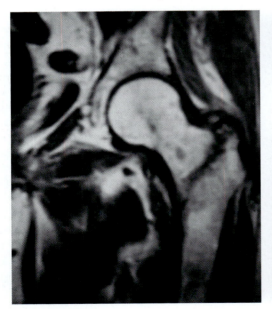

Figure 5-16   B

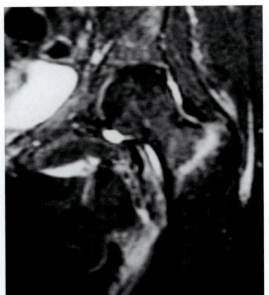

Figure 5-16   C

Findings: (A) AP radiograph of the left hip is well positioned (the hip is not externally rotated). The presence of a faint zone of sclerosis in the intertrochanteric region is equivocal and was not prospectively identified as a fracture. (B) Coronal T1-weighted MRI shows a line of hypointensity extending in the sagittal plane between the greater and lesser trochanters. (C) Coronal T2-weighted, fat-suppressed MRI shows a line of hyperintensity in the intertrochanteric region, thicker superiorly, and not quite reaching the medial cortex.

Differential Diagnosis: None.

Diagnosis: Intertrochanteric hip fracture.

Discussion: The major fracture line of intertrochanteric fractures extends diagonally from superolateral (greater trochanter) to inferomedial (lesser trochanter). Biomechanical analysis of the fracture suggests a bending movement with the lesser trochanter as the fulcrum, as might occur when stumbling off a curb or falling onto the knee. Most intertrochanteric fractures are comminuted, with the greater and lesser trochanters sometimes present as separate fragments; the lesser trochanter fragment would be the equivalent of a butterfly fragment. Unlike intracapsular femoral neck fractures, these injuries tend to heal promptly and without complication. The incidence of avascular necrosis of the femoral head is about 1%.

Intertrochanteric fractures occur with almost equal frequency in males and females. They occur most frequently in elderly patients older than 75, although they can occur in any age group as a result of massive trauma, such as automobile accidents. Nondisplaced fractures, as seen in this case, are usually two-part in nature and may not be evident on radiographs; even true lateral or oblique views may not show the fracture. MRI is exquisitely sensitive and highly specific in identifying radiographically occult intertrochanteric fractures, and the risk of avascular necrosis as a complication may sometimes be estimated [25,26]. The radionuclide bone scan may not be positive for as many as 4 days [27,28] and is no longer considered an appropriate option in this clinical setting. Treatment consists of open reduction and internal fixation with a dynamic hip screw.

Clinical History: Young boy with right distal thigh pain for 2 weeks.

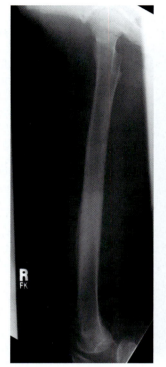
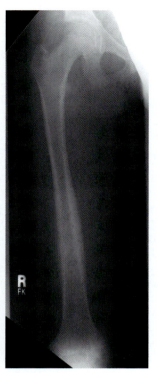

Figure 5-17   A   Figure 5-17   B

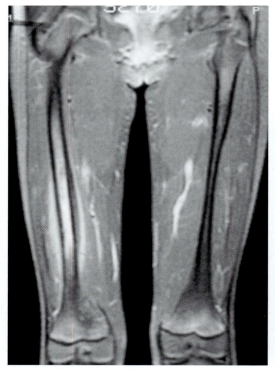

Figure 5-17   C

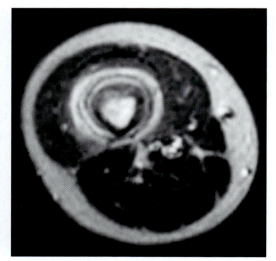

Figure 5-17   D

Findings: (A, B) Lateral and AP radiographs of the right femur show a region of cortical thickening and sclerosis involving the middle third of the shaft. Smooth periosteal elevation is present in a single layer. (C) Coronal inversion recovery MRI of both femurs shows a high-signal-intensity abnormality in the right femoral shaft and surrounding edema. The marrow abnormality has a diffuse margin, with the normal marrow in the proximal and distal shaft. The soft tissue abnormality has tapered margins proximally and distally. It appears symmetric and fusiform in morphology. (D) Axial T2-weighted MRI through the middle of the lesion shows high signal intensity in the medullary space, in the anterior femoral cortex, and in the surrounding soft tissues. The femur is surrounded by a couple of layers of dark periosteal new bone.

Differential Diagnosis: Ewing's sarcoma, osteosarcoma, lymphoma, osteomyelitis, stress fracture.

Diagnosis: Stress fracture.

Discussion: The exquisite sensitivity of MRI to changes in the bone marrow and soft tissues may lead to an overestimation of the aggressiveness and extent of some benign bone lesions, particularly in children [29,30]. Such lesions include chondroblastoma, osteoid osteoma, eosinophilic granuloma, and stress fractures. Commonly seen potentially misleading MRI features include prominent marrow edema, soft tissue edema, and apparent mass effect adjacent to the bone lesion. Features that these lesions have in common that may explain the MRI findings include associated inflammatory reactions caused by the lesions, and their occurrence in childhood, when the periosteum is attached more loosely.

CASE 5-18

Clinical History: 58-year-old man with recurrent episodes of thigh pain and drainage, separated by decades of good health after a fracture at age 22.

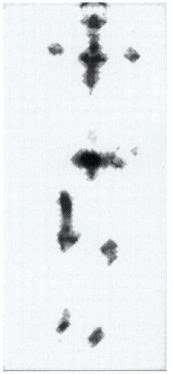

Figure 5-18 A

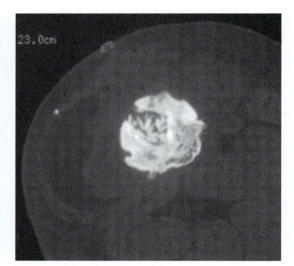

Figure 5-18   B

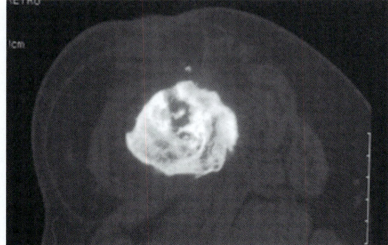

Figure 5-18   C

Figure 5-18   D

Findings: (A) Radionuclide bone scan shows intense radionuclide accumulation at the distal femoral shaft on the right. (B) CT through the femur shows a healed fracture with a central remodeled medullary space that lacks the normal fatty marrow. (C) Nearby CT slice shows a small opening in the femoral cortex with smooth, remodeled, corticated margins. A sinus tract leading to the skin surface extends from the opening in the cortex. (D) CT after treatment shows debridement of the femoral cavity and packing with bone chips.

Differential diagnosis: Chronic osteomyelitis, squamous cell carcinoma.

Diagnosis: Chronic osteomyelitis.

Discussion: Chronic osteomyelitis is exceedingly difficult to eradicate, and quiescent, minimally symptomatic periods of many years are not unusual between episodes of sinus tract formation and purulent drainage. Pathogens may persist indefinitely within the interstices of sequestra, inaccessible to systemically administered antibiotics, so the treatment of chronic osteomyelitis is therefore surgical. The main implication of a chronic sinus tract is the potential complication of squamous cell carcinoma [31,32]. Epithelialization of the sinus tract lining may be the initial event, and malignant transformation of this process may lead ultimately to squamous cell carcinoma [33]. The lower extremity is a favored site for chronic osteomyelitis with sinus tract formation.

Clinical History: 56-year-old woman with metabolic disease.

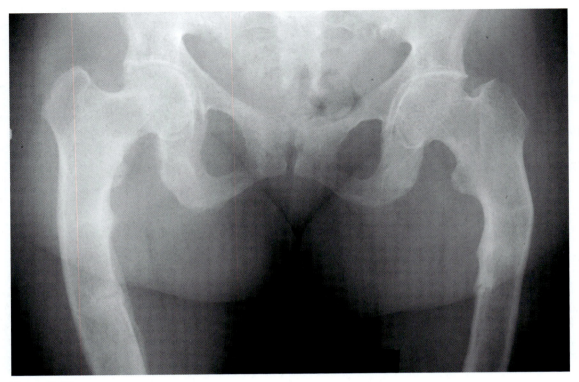

Figure 5-19

Findings: AP radiograph of the pelvis shows osteopenia. The femoral shafts have bowing deformities, and there are horizontal lines with periosteal reactive bone along the medial aspects.

Differential Diagnosis: Osteomalacia, osteoporosis, insufficiency fractures.

Diagnosis: Osteomalacia, with Looser's zones.

Discussion: Osteomalacia is the adult manifestation of a systemic disease in which the calcification of osteoid is deficient; the childhood counterpart is rickets. The common final pathway in both conditions is the lack of available calcium or phosphorus (or both) for mineralization of osteoid. In rickets, the predominant effect is on the growth plates; in osteomalacia, the predominant effect is on remodeling of mature bone. Dietary deficiency of vitamin D, usually coupled with inadequate exposure to sunlight so that photochemical synthesis of vitamin D in the skin does not occur, results in reduced gastrointestinal calcium absorption, hypocalcemia, and secondary hyperparathyroidism to mobilize calcium from the skeleton.

Pure vitamin D deficiency-induced rickets and osteomalacia is relatively rare in the United States, except among immigrants, food faddists, the institutionalized elderly, and patients on total parenteral nutrition. Other causes include failure of enzymatic conversion of 25-hydroxyvitamin D to its physiologically more active metabolite 1,25-dihydroxyvitamin D, end-organ insensitivity to 1,25-dihydroxyvitamin D, genetic and acquired renal tubular reabsorptive defects, and gastrointestinal malabsorption of dietary calcium or phosphorus.

In the United States, gastrointestinal malabsorption from a variety of etiologies is the most common cause of osteomalacia. It may also be caused by chronic use of anticonvulsant medications or of aluminum-containing antacids. In osteomalacia, the radiologic findings are more subtle than in rickets, because the adult skeleton is less metabolically active. Osteopenia is the predominant appearance, and it may be indistinguishable from osteoporosis unless Looser's zones or bowing deformities are present. Occasionally, the bone texture may be recognized as subtly coarsened. As in osteoporosis, the risk of fractures from trauma escalates with deteriorating bone strength.

Clinical History: 54-year-old woman on chronic hemodialysis for renal failure.

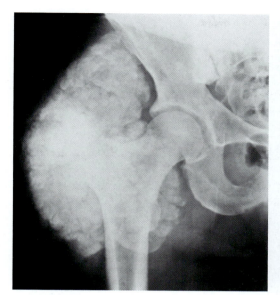

Figure 5-20 A

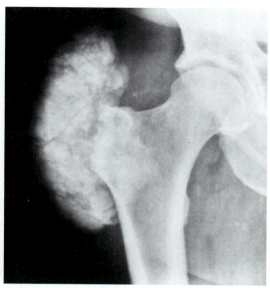

Figure 5-20 B

Findings: (A) AP hip radiograph shows an amorphous calcific mass overlying the greater trochanter. (B) Follow-up radiograph taken after 2 weeks of treatment.

Differential Diagnosis: Tumoral calcinosis, chondrosarcoma, synovial sarcoma, osteosarcoma, myositis ossificans, synovial osteochondromatosis.

Diagnosis: Periarticular calcinosis (tumoral calcinosis, metastatic calcification).

Discussion: If we consider only the initial radiograph and ignore the clinical history, the radiologic differential diagnosis is that of a densely mineralized soft tissue lesion surrounding the proximal femur. The underlying bone is intact, and the morphology of the calcifications is not that of osteoid (which would be very dense and cloud-like), cartilage (rings and arcs), myositis ossificans (peripheral), or sarcoma (dystrophic). Rather, the calcifications in aggregate have a multilocular structure like a bunch of grapes, and the individual clumps have a cystic appearance, like milk of calcium. The clinical history and the rapid improvement with treatment (by modification of the dialysate) clinches the diagnosis. Metastatic soft tissue deposits of calcium found around joints in patients on dialysis for chronic renal failure is in the form of hydroxyapatite. Because the crystals are often aqueous suspensions (milk of calcium), CT and upright radiographs may demonstrate fluid-sediment levels.

Clinical History: 15-year-old girl with leg pain.

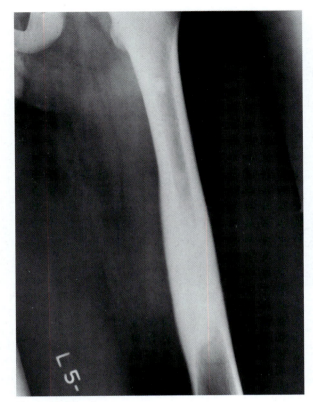

Figure 5-21 A

Figure 5-21 B

Findings: (A) AP radiograph of the femur. The middle third of the femoral shaft is involved by a densely mineralized lesion that fills the medullary cavity. More proximally, there is a second, similar lesion in the femoral metaphysis. There is no evidence of cortical expansion or breakthrough, and no periosteal reaction. (B) Detail of anterior whole-body radionuclide bone scan. There is markedly increased uptake of the radiotracer in these two areas, relative to normal cortex and medullary space.

Differential Diagnosis: Osteosarcoma, Ewing's sarcoma, lymphoma.

Diagnosis: Osteosarcoma with skip metastasis.

Discussion: Any blastic bone lesion in the femur of a child or adolescent should raise concern for osteosarcoma. Although osteosarcomas are relatively uncommon, they may have a range of different radiologic appearances that may be mistaken for a variety of benign lesions, and vice versa. The presence of a small, proximal satellite lesion in the same bone raises the differential diagnosis of blastic lesions in children that may produce skip metastases. In addition to osteosarcoma, the differential diagnosis includes Ewing's sarcoma and lymphoma. Both Ewing's sarcoma and lymphoma tend to cause permeated bone destruction and raise successive layers of periosteum as they penetrate the cortex to form soft tissue masses, features that are absent in this case. In addition, the dense, blastic appearance of this lesion would be unusual for either Ewing's sarcoma or lymphoma.

Osteosarcoma is the most common primary malignant bone-forming neoplasm. Metaphyseal sites about the knee are the most common location, but diaphyseal or epiphyseal involvement is seen in approximately 20% to 30% of cases, and diaphyseal or epiphyseal tumor without metaphyseal involvement may be seen in 10% to 20% of cases. This tumor demonstrates avid uptake of radionuclide on conventional bone scanning, even in metastatic foci outside of bone. Skip lesions are not considered metastatic per se, but represent intramedullary spread of tumor. The frequency of skip lesions has been reported from less than 2% to about 20% [36]. Skip metastases may also occur in Ewing's sarcoma [37]. The extent of tumor involvement is best assessed with MRI [38].

Clinical History: 64-year-old woman with fatigue and weight loss.

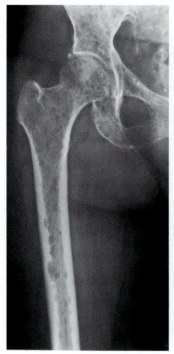 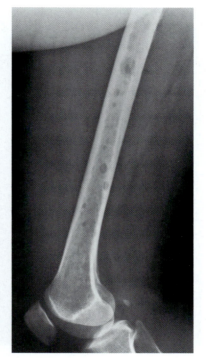

Figure 5-22   A   **Figure 5-22   B**

Findings: AP and lateral femur radiographs show multiple lytic lesions of varying size.

Differential Diagnosis: Multiple myeloma, metastases, lymphoma.

Diagnosis: Multiple myeloma.

Discussion: Multiple myeloma is a malignant neoplasm of plasmacytes, the cells of the bone marrow that make immunoglobulins. Myeloma arises in the bone marrow and involves it diffusely. Bony abnormalities usually occur at multiple sites, including the vertebrae in 66% of patients, the ribs in 45%, the skull in 40%, the shoulder girdle in 40%, the pelvis in 30%, and the long bones in 25% of patients. Myeloma lesions are sharply defined, purely lytic areas of bone destruction with no reactive bone formation. The pattern of destruction may be geographic, moth-eaten, or permeated; involvement may be so diffuse that the bones will be simply osteopenic or even normal in radiographic appearance. The lesions may be expansile, may penetrate the cortex, and may form large extraosseous soft tissue masses. Pathologic fractures are common. The plain film skeletal survey is a better method for disclosing sites of bone destruction than the radionuclide bone scan, but MRI shows the replacement of the normal marrow by myeloma tissue in a diffuse or multifocal pattern, and is currently the most sensitive study for detection of multiple myeloma lesions in bone [39,40].

Several differential points may help distinguish between multiple myeloma and osseous metastases in a patient with multiple destructive bone lesions. Myeloma tissue produces a number of osteoclast-stimulating factors resulting in bone destruction that is cleanly marginated and purely lytic. Although metastases also produce osteoclast-stimulating factors, they tend to provoke reactive bone, frequently resulting in a more ragged and irregular appearance. Myeloma may involve the intervertebral discs and the mandible, but metastases rarely do. Metastases often involve the vertebral pedicles, but myeloma rarely does. A large soft tissue mass is more likely to be present with myeloma than with metastases. The bone scan is usually positive in the presence of bone metastases and often negative in myeloma. Bisphosphonates have been advocated for reducing the incidence of pathologic fractures and skeletal pain in patients with multiple myeloma [41]. Bisphosphonates stabilize the hydroxyapatite crystalline structure of newly formed bone and interfere with osteoclastic resorption.

Clinical History: 10-year-old girl with thigh swelling and pain.

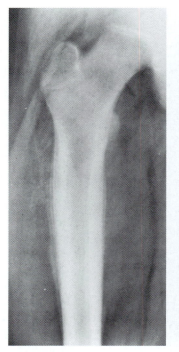 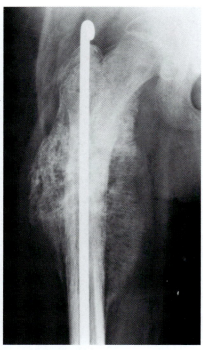

Figure 5-23   A   Figure 5-23   B

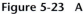

Findings: (A) AP femur radiograph at presentation shows layered periosteal reaction and thickening of the femoral cortex. A soft tissue mass surrounds the femur. (B) AP radiograph of the femur after treatment shows an intramedullary rod in place. A large fusiform bony mass surrounds the femur, with both layered and sunburst periosteal reaction.

Differential Diagnosis: Ewing's sarcoma, osteosarcoma, lymphoma, osteomyelitis, stress fracture.

Diagnosis: Ewing's sarcoma.

Discussion: The aggressive appearance of this lesion suggests a malignant lesion such as round cell tumor, osteosarcoma, or lymphoma, or a benign lesion with aggressive features such as acute osteomyelitis. Stress fractures of the long bones in children heal with periosteal callus that may be mistaken for the periosteal reaction to tumor or infection. Hematogenous osteomyelitis spreads through bone in a fashion similar to Ewing's sarcoma, leading to a superficially similar radiologic appearance, but the diaphyseal rather than metaphyseal location strongly favors tumor rather than infection. Both may occur in the same age group and have similar clinical presentations.

Ewing's sarcoma is a tumor consisting of small, round, undifferentiated cells, probably of neuroectodermal histogenesis. Although 75% of Ewing's sarcomas occur in patients less than 20 years old, these lesions may develop at any age. They are the most common primary bone tumor in the first decade of life, and the second most common (behind osteosarcoma) in the second decade. Patients present with local pain and swelling, fever, anemia, and elevated erythrocyte sedimentation rate; the clinical impression is often that of osteomyelitis. Up to 30% of patients will have metastases at presentation. Ewing's sarcoma may develop in practically any bone, although the majority of cases involve the sacrum, innominate bone, and long bones of the lower extremities. Only 3% of tumors affect the hands and feet. Most Ewing's sarcomas are found in the metadiaphysis of long bones, mostly the femur, but they also occur in the diaphysis and metaphysis. In the long bones, the typical radiographic appearance is that of permeated intramedullary bone destruction with periosteal reactive bone. Treatment is typically radiotherapy, often combined with surgery and chemotherapy. After treatment, response to radiotherapy can be followed by enhanced MRI and positron emission tomography (PET) [42], although, the role of PET is still under investigation [43].

Clinical History: 22-year-old man with increasing left thigh mass.

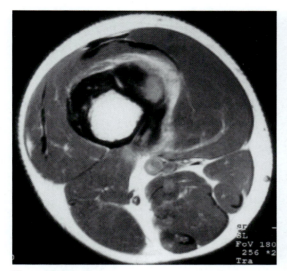

Figure 5-24 A

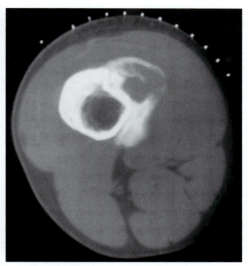

Figure 5-24 B

Findings: (**A**) Axial T1-weighted MRI shows a mass on the anteromedial surface of the femoral shaft. The mass has regions of signal void as well as regions of intermediate signal. The interface of the lesion with the surrounding tissue is irregular. The marrow space has not become involved. (**B**) Axial CT shows a densely ossified mass on the surface of the bone with a broad pedicle. The mass has a cleavage plane posteriorly, but a significant nonmineralized region. There is no involvement of the medullary space.

Differential Diagnosis: Aneurysmal bone cyst, periosteal chondroma, parosteal osteosarcoma or other surface variant, Ewing's sarcoma, lymphoma, osteochondroma.

Diagnosis: High-grade surface osteosarcoma.

Discussion: The imaging shows a bone-forming lesion on the cortical surface, making the primary consideration a surface variant of osteosarcoma. The other items in the differential diagnosis, although they may occur on the cortical surface, would not be expected to form bone. The amorphous mineralization wrapping partially around the cortex is distinguishable from periosteal reaction or cortical expansion. The lack of involvement of the medullary space indicates that this is not a lesion penetrating the cortex from the inside to form a soft tissue mass.

Several variants of osteosarcomas arising on the surface of bone have been recognized, with distinctive radiologic and pathologic features [48,49]. Parosteal osteosarcomas are densely ossified surface masses that may have unossified portions. Periosteal osteosarcomas are chondroblastic lesions, and high-grade surface osteosarcomas are like classic high-grade intramedullary osteosarcomas except that they arise on the surface. Histologically, parosteal osteosarcomas are usually low grade, whereas periosteal and high-grade surface osteosarcomas are generally high-grade tumors. The densely ossified mass wrapping partially around the cortex with a cleavage plane is characteristic of parosteal osteosarcoma, but the infiltrative margin and the significant unmineralized proportion should be considered aggressive features.

Clinical History: 41-year-old man with thigh mass.

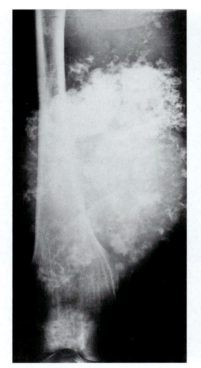

Figure 5-25   A

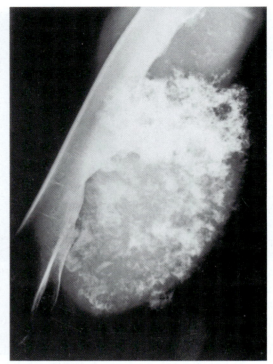

Figure 5-25   B

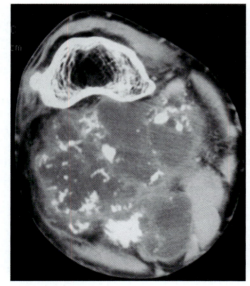

Figure 5-25   C

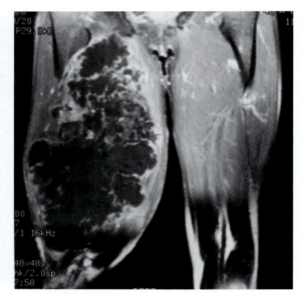

Figure 5-25   D

Findings: (A, B) AP and lateral radiographs of the distal thigh show a mass along the posterior aspect of the distal femur, with mineralization in the form of rings and arcs. (C) CT shows lobular regions of the lesion with low-attenuation matrix and peripheral calcifications. These peripheral calcifications superimposed over the lobular structure result in the radiographic rings-and-arcs appearance. The lesion is exostotic. (D) Coronal T1-weighted MRI with contrast shows a low-signal-intensity soft tissue mass with peripheral enhancement in a lobular configuration.

Differential Diagnosis: Chondrosarcoma, osteochondroma.

Diagnosis: Chondrosarcoma.

Discussion: The morphology and specific features of this lesion leave no doubt that it represents an exostotic cartilage lesion. The large size and relatively sparse calcification suggests that it is malignant and, in this circumstance, the lesion should be treated as a sarcoma until proven otherwise. Needle biopsy may be misleading because of sampling error in such a large lesion; in general, the biologic behavior of a sarcoma is that of its highest-grade part, regardless of how large or small that part is in relation to the remainder of the lesion.

Calcified rings and arcs, dense punctate calcifications, or flocculent calcifications (small, loosely aggregated masses) are patterns of mineralization of chondroid matrix, formed by benign and malignant cartilage-forming lesions. The rings-and-arcs configuration of mineralization corresponds to calcification and ossification around the periphery of cartilaginous lobules. Chondroid matrix that is not mineralized typically has attenuation on CT that is lower than muscle but greater than water. On MRI, chondroid matrix has low signal on T1-weighted images and high signal on T2-weighted MRI, similar to hyaline cartilage [44].

Clinical History: 18-year-old man with sudden, severe left hip pain.

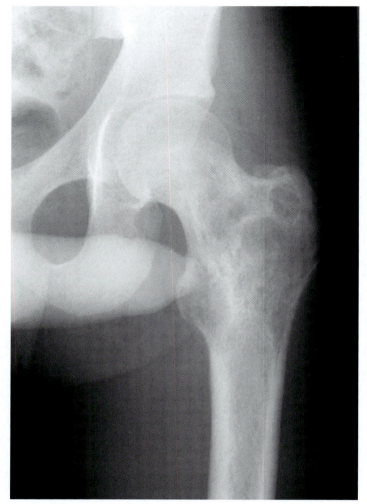

Figure 5-26   A

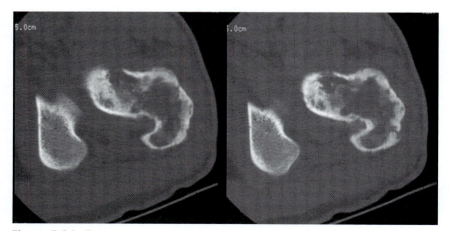

Figure 5-26   B

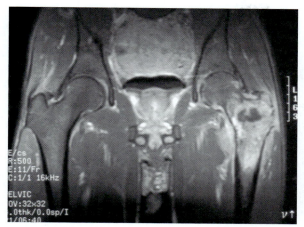

Figure 5-26   C

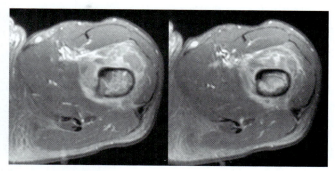

Figure 5-26   D

Findings: (A) AP radiograph of the left hip shows permeated destruction of bone involving the femoral neck and intertrochanteric region. (B) Consecutive axial CT shows permeated bone destruction with pathologic fracture seen best in the lateral aspect of the lesser trochanter, but extending laterally through the greater trochanter. Irregular mineralization within the intramedullary lesion may represent reactive bone or residual trabecular bone. There is no mineralization in the soft tissues. (C, D). Coronal and axial T1-weighted MRI with fat saturation after intravenous gadolinium injection shows high signal in the soft tissues immediately surrounding the proximal femur, with circumferential mass effect and heterogeneous enhancement within the femoral lesion with interior portions that are nonenhancing.

Differential Diagnosis: Osteosarcoma, lymphoma, Ewing's sarcoma, osteomyelitis.

Diagnosis: Non-Hodgkin's B-cell lymphoma, involving bone secondarily.

Discussion: Non-Hodgkin's lymphoma involving the bone usually occurs in the setting of disseminated disease, typically presenting first in the abdomen. Non-Hodgkin's lymphoma is more likely to involve bone than Hodgkin's lymphoma, and the axial skeleton is the predominant site of occurrence. The undifferentiated and histiocytic forms more commonly involve bone, and large lesions frequently have necrotic portions. Involvement of the bone and bone marrow is frequently occult and is best demonstrated by MRI [45].

The mechanism of bone destruction in lymphoma is similar to that of multiple myeloma, with lymphoma cells producing osteoclast-activating factors that mediate the bone destruction [46]. The lesions are therefore lytic, and may have a moth-eaten or permeated appearance. A soft tissue component is not uncommon. Periosteal reaction and sclerosis are seen more commonly in Hodgkin's lymphoma, but may also be a feature in non-Hodgkin's lymphoma. Pathologic fracture is noted in as many as 25% of cases. It has been suggested that 18F-fluorodeoxyglucose-positron emission tomography (FDG-PET) may be more accurate than 67Ga scanning in staging the extent of disease [47].

Clinical History: 2-year-old boy with failure to thrive.

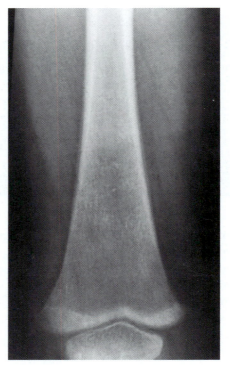

Figure 5-27   A

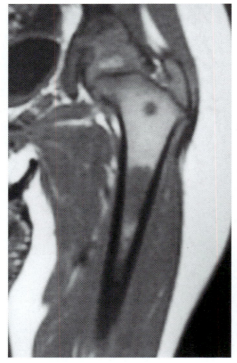

Figure 5-27   B

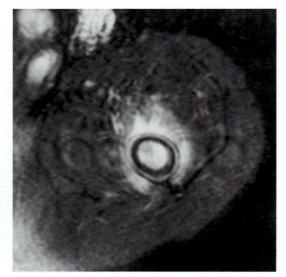

Figure 5-27   C

Findings: (A) AP radiograph demonstrates a faint lucency in the distal femoral metadiaphysis, with a thin rim of smooth diaphyseal periosteal reaction. (B) Coronal T1-weighted MRI of the proximal femur demonstrates replacement of the normal marrow hyperintensity with geographic areas of low signal intensity. (C) Axial T2-weighted MRI shows high signal of the involved marrow. Associated edematous changes are noted in the adjacent soft tissues. The periosteal reaction is evident as a thin, well-defined, low-signal-intensity circle surrounding the bone.

Differential Diagnosis: Osteomyelitis, lymphoma, leukemia, metastases, stress fracture, eosinophilic granuloma.

Diagnosis: Leukemia.

Discussion: The patchy involvement of the medullary space eliminates osteomyelitis and stress fracture as considerations, although either may cause subtle periosteal reaction. Leukemia is a neoplasm of leukocytes that may involve bone secondarily, and it is the most common malignancy in children. Leukemic infiltration of many organs and tissues, including the marrow spaces, will be present and may have a diffuse or nodular character. Packing of the marrow spaces with leukemic cells causes pressure atrophy of cancellous trabeculae, and is seen radiographically as diffuse osteopenia. In children, lucent metaphyseal bands may occur, reflecting zones of trabeculae that are thinner and sparser than normal in areas of rapid bone growth. Nodular collections of leukemic cells cause focal areas of medullary, cortical, or subperiosteal bone destruction. Leukemic infiltration can extend through the cortex by way of the haversian systems, enlarging them by eroding the bone. This causes the cortex to appear fuzzy and osteopenic, often with lucent streaks. Infiltration of subperiosteal spaces lifts the periosteum and stimulates bone formation. Widespread marrow space involvement is the rule, and can be confirmed by MRI or bone marrow aspiration [50,51]. In patients who have been treated successfully for leukemia with chemotherapy, it may be difficult to distinguish fibrosis from residual lesions in the bone marrow by any imaging method other than biopsy [52].

CASE 5-28

Clinical History: 19-year-old man with increasing thigh girth over 6 months.

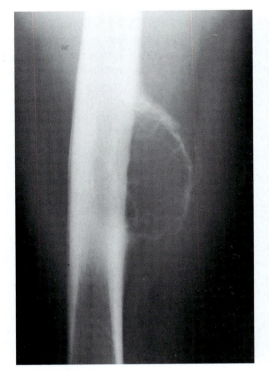

Figure 5-28   A

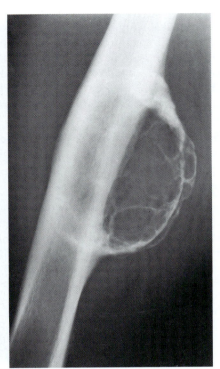

Figure 5-28   B

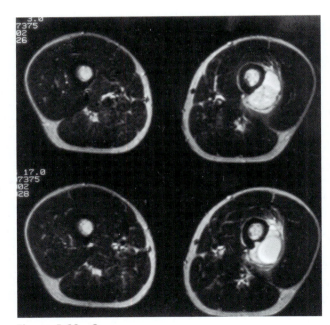

Figure 5-28   C

Findings: (A) Lateral radiograph of the femur demonstrates an expansile, eccentric diaphyseal lesion with thin septations. (B) Six months later. Follow-up lateral radiographs. The lesion has increased dramatically in size, with apparent maturation of the peripheral shell of bone. (C) Axial T2-weighted MRI shows there are several compartments within the lesion that contain fluid. A sedimentation effect is suggested in the lower right image. The periosteal margin is well defined, and reactive edema in the soft tissues is virtually absent.

Differential Diagnosis: Aneurysmal bone cyst, osteosarcoma, Ewing's sarcoma, lymphoma.

Diagnosis: Aneurysmal bone cyst.

Discussion: Aneurysmal bone cysts are lytic, eccentric, expansile, blood-filled lesions with incomplete septations that allow for communicating compartments. Their peak age of occurrence is in children and young adults. Choice locations are metaphyses of long bones and posterior elements of the spine.

Primary aneurysmal bone cysts are believed to form on the basis of trauma. One hypothesis postulates that arteriovenous fistulae form as a sequela to trauma and give rise to this nonneoplastic lesion [53]. Aneurysmal bone cysts may simulate aggressive malignant lesions by expanding rapidly and demonstrating cortical breakthrough of the soft tissue component. Secondary aneurysmal bone cysts may comprise fully one-third of these lesions and occur in association with the following lesions: chondroblastoma, chondromyxoid fibroma, fibrous dysplasia, giant cell tumor, osteoblastoma, solitary bone cyst, brown tumor, angiosarcoma, nonossifying fibroma, giant cell reparative granuloma, malignant fibrous histiocytoma (MFH), and telangiectatic osteosarcoma [54,55]. Fluid levels, reflecting their hemorrhagic constituents, may be seen with CT or MRI, but they are not pathognomonic, because fluid levels may also be seen in giant cell tumor, solitary bone cyst, chondroblastoma, MFH, soft tissue hemangioma, synovial sarcoma, and telangiectatic osteosarcoma. Unlike giant cell and chondroblastoma, these lesions rarely involve the end of the bone. Solid fibrous components may be seen on histologic examination.

Clinical History: 41-year-old man with hip pain.

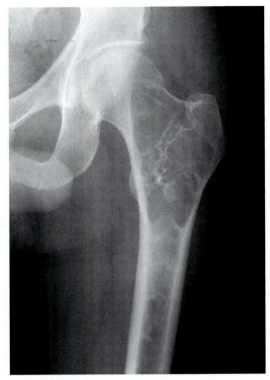

Figure 5-29   A

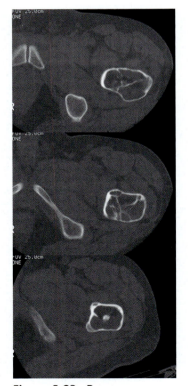

Figure 5-29   B

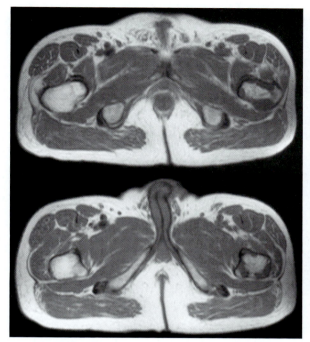

Figure 5-29   C

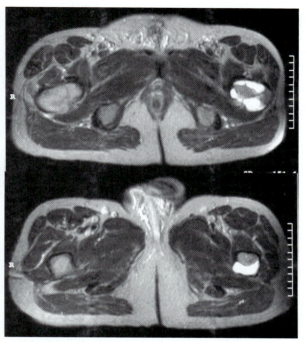

Figure 5-29   D

Findings: (**A**) AP radiograph of the proximal femur shows thickened septa in a geographic lesion in the femoral neck, extending down to the proximal diaphysis. No periostitis is noted, but portions of the lesion appear sclerotic. There is no apparent cortical break or soft tissue mass. (**B**) CT axial cut better defines the thickened septa. The loculations contain fluid density and are not expansile. Distribution is again noted in the femoral neck and proximal femoral diaphysis. (**C, D**) Axial proton density and T2-weighted MRI demonstrates heterogenous regions of signal intensity within the lesion, including fat and fluid or myxoid tissue.

Differential Diagnosis: Fibrous dysplasia, unicameral bone cyst, intraosseous lipoma, nonossifying fibroma, osteoblastoma, desmoplastic fibroma, posttraumatic deformity, bone infarct, Paget's disease, liposclerosing myxofibrous tumor.

Diagnosis: Liposclerosing myxofibrous tumor of bone.

Discussion: The lesion has benign radiologic characteristics and, from a clinical management perspective, is straightforward. From an imaging perspective, the multiple different constituents of the lesion suggest a variety of possibilities, none of which is completely satisfactory in explaining all of the features.

Atypical fibroosseous lesions like this one, almost always in the proximal femur, are a common consultative diagnostic problem. The presence of a variety of patterns individually reminiscent of fibrous dysplasia, fibroxanthoma (nonossifying fibroma), myxofibroma, lipoma, cyst, bone infarct, Paget's disease, and, occasionally, chondroma, indicates a benign process, but one that is difficult to label. The same variety of patterns is also evident on histologic examination, and the term liposclerosing myxofibrous tumor has been applied to these heterogenous lesions with consistent clinical, radiologic, and histologic features [56,57].

Discovered incidentally in most cases, liposclerosing myxofibrous tumors occur in a broad adult age range, but it is believed they represent hamartomas in childhood, rather than true neoplasms, and that gradual changes in their appearance as the body ages may account in part for their variability. In the majority of instances, asymptomatic discovery, lack of distortion of bone outline, and sclerotic borders are indications of stability over many years. There does not appear to be a particular predilection for pathologic fracture, and it is evident from imaging that bone has remodeled around these lesions to accommodate normal weight-bearing stresses. Malignant transformation has been reported to range from 10% to 16% [58].

Clinical History: 15-year-old boy with thigh pain that is worse at night and is relieved by aspirin and nonsteroidal anti-inflammatory drugs.

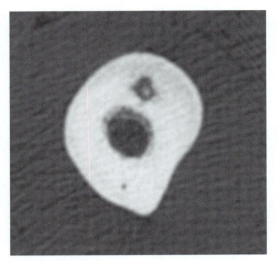

Figure 5-30   A

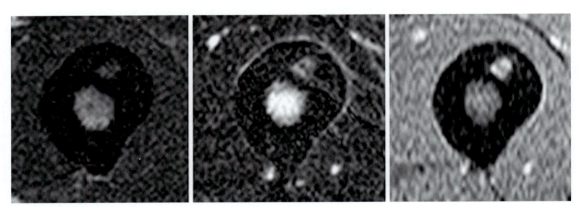

Figure 5-30   B

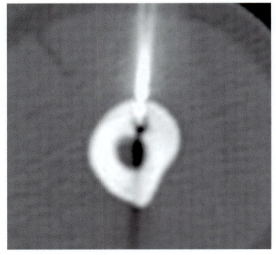

Figure 5-30   C

Findings: (A) Axial CT shows a round lesion in the femoral cortex surrounded by dense cortical bone. There is a dense, punctate, central calcification in the nidus. (B) MRI (axial T1-weighted, T2-weighted fat-suppressed, and gadolinium enhanced T1-weighted fat-suppressed sequences) demonstrates the nidus to have low T1 signal, high T2 signal, and intense arterial enhancement. Prominent marrow edema is also seen on the T2-weighted sequence. (C) CT fluoroscopic image during radiofrequency ablation.

Differential Diagnosis: Osteoid osteoma, stress fracture, osteosarcoma, Brodie's abscess.

Diagnosis: Osteoid osteoma.

Discussion: Although any bone-forming lesion in the femur of an adolescent should trigger some consideration of osteosarcoma, however brief, the history and radiologic appearance of this lesion is virtually diagnostic of osteoid osteoma. Stress fractures may also occur at this particular location and may be evident as cortical thickening, but there should not be a focal lesion at the center of the cortical reaction, and pain would be relieved at night but worse with activity during the daytime. Osteoid osteomas are relatively common bone-forming neoplasms that consist of a circumscribed nodule of woven bone and osteoid (called the nidus), and a surrounding reactive zone of thickened cortical or trabecular bone and loose fibrovascular tissue. Patients complain of a peculiar pain syndrome that is virtually unique among bone tumors: nocturnal pain that is relieved by aspirin and other prostaglandin inhibitors. Unlike other bone tumors, osteoid osteomas have abundant nerve fibers, particularly in the reactive zone, and this innervation appears to correlate with the pain syndrome [59]. The reactive zone results in a flare of bone and soft tissue edema on MRI, and there is typically an intense, reactive periosteal response that is disproportionate to the small size of the nidus (1 cm or less). Osteoid osteomas show intense arterial phase enhancement with washout on delayed phase MRI [60]. Treatment of osteoid osteoma is ablation, either percutaneously [61] or by surgery. Cost and morbidity are both lower using CT-guided percutaneous ablation rather than open surgery.

Clinical History: 63-year-old woman with an enlarging thigh mass.

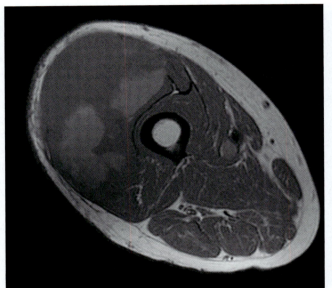

Figure 5-31   A

Figure 5-31   B

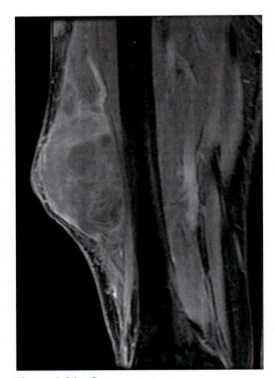

Figure 5-31   C

Findings: (A, B) Axial T1-weighted and T2-weighted fat-suppressed MRI shows a large soft tissue mass in the anterolateral right thigh. The lesion has an ovoid shape with heterogeneous signal intensity. Regions of high T1-weighted signal intensity within the mass suggest hemorrhage. (C) Coronal gadolinium-enhanced, T1-weighted, fat-suppressed MRI shows the lesion to have inhomogeneous enhancement.

Differential Diagnosis: Soft tissue sarcoma, extraskeletal osteosarcoma, extraskeletal chondrosarcoma, myositis ossificans, lymphoma.

Diagnosis: Malignant fibrous histiocytoma, soft tissue sarcoma.

Discussion: A large, necrotic mass in the deep soft tissues of an extremity, particularly the thigh, should be considered malignant until proven otherwise. The vast majority of soft tissue sarcomas present in adults. Patients typically complain of a slowly enlarging, palpable mass of long duration, and pain or tenderness of insidious onset. Patients may delay seeking medical attention, and this long chronicity may falsely suggest an indolent process. The patient shown above completed 6 months of acupuncture therapy before having a physician evaluate the mass. Soft tissue sarcomas metastasize to lung, liver, or bone. They have nonspecific appearances on imaging, and there are no reliable criteria for distinguishing among them.

Once benign soft tissue masses with specific features, such as lipoma, myositis ossificans, aneurysm, bursitis, and hematoma, have been eliminated as possibilities, factors that suggest sarcoma include older age, location in the thigh, large size, round or ovoid shape, and involvement of adjacent bone. Malignant soft tissue masses usually have areas of inhomogeneity and lower density on CT or high signal intensity on T2-weighted MRI that correspond to regions of necrosis and hemorrhage. Sarcomas that calcify or ossify include synovial sarcoma, extraskeletal osteosarcoma, extraskeletal chondrosarcoma, rhabdomyosarcoma, MFH, and liposarcoma. Enhancement with intravenous contrast can be expected on both CT and MRI. The treatment of soft tissue sarcomas is surgical, sometimes with neoadjuvant and/or adjuvant radiation therapy and/or chemotherapy. Five-year survival rates of 25% to 60% have been reported. MFH is a pleomorphic sarcoma that arises most frequently in the deep soft tissues of the extremities, and less commonly in bone. MFH is the most common soft tissue sarcoma of late adult life. Cortical involvement by a primary soft tissue MFH is more common than with other sarcomas [62].

Clinical History: 19-year-old man with muscle weakness.

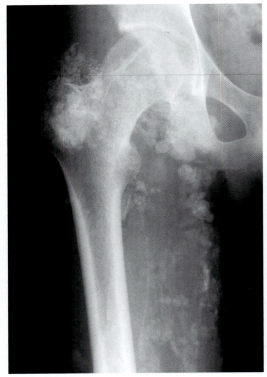

Figure 5-32 A

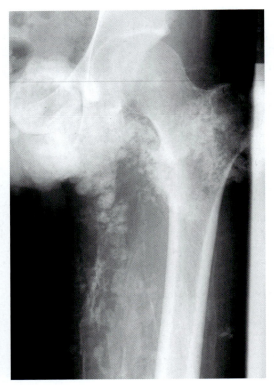

Figure 5-32 B

Findings: AP radiographs of the hips show extensive soft tissue calcification about the hips and thighs. The calcifications are mostly rounded, dense, and amorphous, but some of the calcifications in the medial thighs appear sheet-like. The bones appear relatively normal.

Differential Diagnosis: Dermatomyositis, polymyositis, scleroderma, parasitic infestation, mixed connective tissue disease, fibrodysplasia ossificans progressiva, burns, calcific myonecrosis, hemangiomatosis, tumoral calcinosis.

Diagnosis: Mixed connective tissue disease (calcinosis universalis).

Discussion: The differential diagnosis is that of extensive soft tissue calcification. Many of these possibilities can be discarded on the basis of clinical history, and the morphology and distribution of the calcifications may be helpful. Calcinosis universalis refers to a widespread distribution of soft tissue calcifications. It is a nonspecific, descriptive term, not a disease entity. In considering the morphology of soft tissue calcifications as a means of narrowing the differential diagnosis, some general patterns may be applicable.

- Central lucency would be typical of phleboliths.
- Osseous masses with cortex and medullary space would be typical of fibrodysplasia ossificans progressiva and burns.

- Peripheral calcifications around soft tissue masses would be typical of posttraumatic myositis ossificans.
- Calcifications of uniform size and shape would be typical of parasitic infestation.
- Cystic calcifications would be typical of tumoral calcinosis.
- Reticulated or linear soft tissue calcifications would be typical of dermatomyositis or collagen vascular disease.

Periarticular calcifications are associated with hypercalcemic states and collagen vascular disease. The bilateral distribution of the calcifications favors a systemic disease rather than a localized process. The clinical history may be used to eliminate additional diagnostic possibilities, particularly tumoral calcinosis (no history of hemodialysis for renal failure), calcific myonecrosis (no history of compartment syndrome), and myositis ossificans (no history of trauma). Mixed connective tissue disease refers to syndromes of rheumatic disease with features that overlap those of more well-defined disease, including rheumatoid arthritis, scleroderma, systemic lupus erythematosus, and dermatomyositis.

Clinical History: 22-year-old hockey player with posterior thigh mass and previous history of anterior thigh mass on the contralateral side.

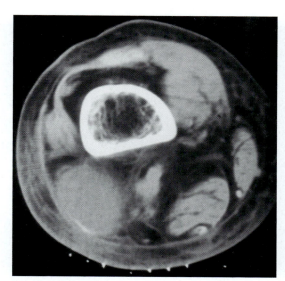

Figure 5-33   A

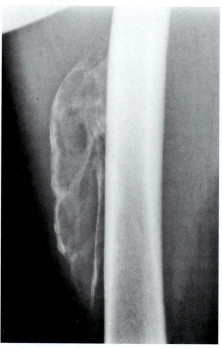

Figure 5-33   B

Findings: (A) Axial CT through the right distal thigh shows edema in the lateral subcutaneous tissues, with swelling of the biceps femoris and stranding of the adjacent fat. A thin rim of calcification lies along the posterolateral aspect of this muscle. (B) Lateral radiograph of the left thigh shows an ossified mass in the anterior soft tissues that appears to be attached to bone. The soft tissue ossification appears mature, with a cortex and trabecular pattern. The underlying femur is intact.

Differential Diagnosis: Myositis ossificans, soft tissue sarcoma, surface osteosarcoma, osteochondroma.

Diagnosis: Myositis ossificans.

Discussion: The radiologic appearance of the right side may raise soft tissue sarcoma as a possibility, and the most common soft tissue sarcoma in this age group tends to calcify (synovial sarcoma). However, the peripheral calcification (rather than central) and the clinical history (contusion in hockey player) provides the correct diagnosis. On the left side, a bony mass in the soft tissues adjacent to the femur may initially raise the question of osteosarcoma. However, the lack of destruction and the well-formed cortex indicates

a benign process. Osteochondromas would not typically be located in the diaphysis of a long bone.

Myositis ossificans commonly refers to posttraumatic heterotopic ossification in the muscles and other soft tissues after blunt trauma and hemorrhage. Most common in the quadriceps muscles or around the elbow, it progresses over a few weeks from hematoma to ill-defined calcification to well-organized cortical and trabecular bone. The process is similar to the formation and maturation of fracture callus, and may initially be confused with sarcoma. However, myositis ossificans evolves over a period of weeks into an organized, peripherally calcified mass that begins to ossify. The ectopic bone may ultimately blend with underlying bone, sometimes causing mechanical problems. Myositis ossificans may complicate acute or chronic bony or soft tissue trauma. It may occur in association with neurologic diseases of a wide variety, including paralysis and coma. A localized form that occurs without a history of significant trauma is called myositis ossificans circumscripta. Myositis ossificans may be mistaken for sarcoma on MRI [63], but the presence of an ossific rim on CT or radiography is diagnostic. The appearance on MRI depends on the stage of maturation [64].

Clinical History: 35-year-old woman with painless soft tissue mass in the medial thigh.

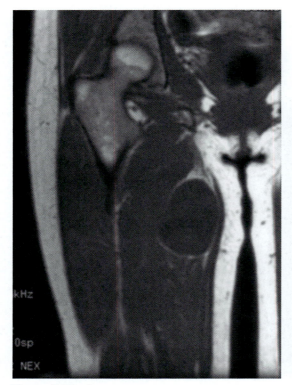

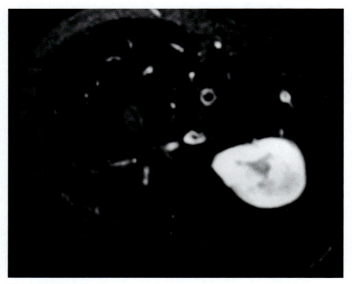

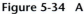

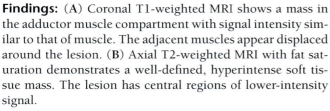

Figure 5-34 A

Figure 5-34 B

Findings: (A) Coronal T1-weighted MRI shows a mass in the adductor muscle compartment with signal intensity similar to that of muscle. The adjacent muscles appear displaced around the lesion. (B) Axial T2-weighted MRI with fat saturation demonstrates a well-defined, hyperintense soft tissue mass. The lesion has central regions of lower-intensity signal.

Differential Diagnosis: Soft tissue sarcoma, nerve sheath tumor (neurofibroma or schwannoma), myxoma.

Diagnosis: Neurofibroma.

Discussion: The imaging findings in this case are fairly nonspecific, and both benign and malignant soft tissue masses must be considered. Both malignant and benign soft tissue tumors tend to have a well-encapsulated appearance. Soft tissue sarcomas tend to be quite large at the time of presentation, and when they are heterogeneous on MRI, the central portion tends to have high intensity (from liquefactive necrosis) rather than the periphery. The appearance on the T2-weighted MRI thus provides a clue to the diagnosis in this case.

Neurofibromas are seen most commonly around the spine, but they may occur in any peripheral nerve and favor the flexor compartments when present in the extremities. Radiographically, they may show erosion of the adjacent bone, but in this case, the lesion is not adjacent to bone. On MRI, a well-defined lesion is usually seen with increased signal intensity on T2-weighted images, and often a decreased-signal-intensity center, or target appearance, which is somewhat specific for these lesions [65]. Enhancement with contrast is usually noted. When the presence of neurofibromatosis is already established, the diagnosis of these lesions is fairly straightforward, although the possibility of malignant degeneration of a neurofibroma to neurofibrosarcoma should always be considered.

Clinical History: 33-year-old woman with posterior thigh pain.

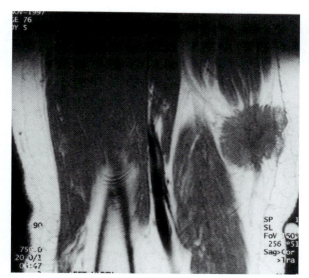

Figure 5-35 A

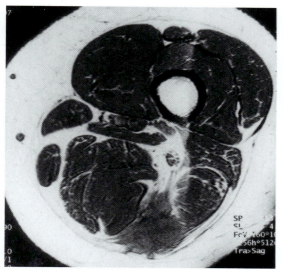

Figure 5-35 B

Findings: Sagittal and axial T1-weighted MRI through the distal thigh shows an ill-defined mass, slightly hyperintense to muscle, situated between the long head of the biceps muscle and the semitendinosus muscle. The margins of the lesion are feathered and irregular, with stranding, and the lesion appears to have grown between the adjacent structures rather than displacing them.

Differential Diagnosis: Lymphoma, leukemia, infection, hematoma, desmoid, soft tissue sarcoma, nerve sheath tumor.

Diagnosis: Granular cell tumor.

Discussion: The imaging findings are nonspecific, but unlike most soft tissue masses in the extremities, this lesion is not ovoid in shape and does not have well-defined margins. Its shape suggests an infiltrating process without encapsulation or stroma. In addition, although the lesion is within the posterior thigh muscle compartment, it is not intramuscular. Both benign and malignant soft tissue tumors can display this appearance, but it would be unusual.

Granular cell tumor is also known as myoblastoma, due to the previously maintained erroneous belief that these lesions were of myogenic origin. Granular cell tumors are now believed to be of Schwann cell derivation. Common locations for these lesions are the breast, chest wall, skin, and subcutaneous tissue. Occurrence in the lower extremities is unusual. MRI may show a lesion that is isointense or nearly isointense to muscle on the T1-weighted MRI [66]. Granular cell tumors are generally benign lesions, but malignant granular cell tumors are rarely seen and are typically larger, with a more variable histologic appearance demonstrating large numbers of mitotic figures [67]. In one study of granular cell tumors, the correct diagnosis was made prospectively in only 3 of 110 patients [68].

Clinical History: 43-year-old man with painless soft tissue mass in the medial thigh.

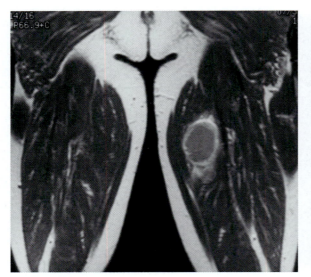

Figure 5-36   A

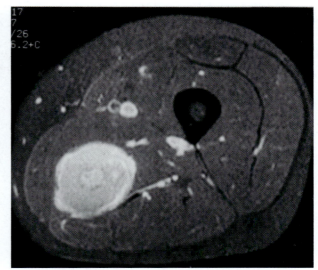

Figure 5-36   B

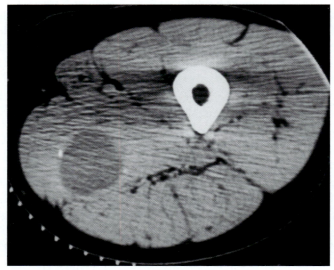

Figure 5-36   C

Findings: (A) Coronal T1-weighted MRI after gadolinium injection shows an ovoid mass in the adductor magnus muscle with rim enhancement. (B) Axial T1-weighted MRI with fat saturation after gadolinium injection shows enhancement and a target appearance. (C) CT scan shows a well-defined mass with low attenuation coefficients and a fleck of dystrophic border calcification.

Differential Diagnosis: Soft tissue sarcoma, benign mesenchymal tumor, nerve sheath tumor.

Diagnosis: Glomus tumor.

Discussion: The imaging features of this case are not specific, and a biopsy is mandatory. Glomus tumors are benign neoplasms whose cell of origin appears to be the neuromyoarterial glomus; they are considered to be a subtype of benign hemangiopericytoma. These lesions occur in males and females with equal incidence, and principally involve the soft tissues. Bony involvement usually occurs as a result of infiltration from the adjacent soft tissues, with the most common location being the subungual aspect of the distal phalanges of the hands. Primary bone lesions are unusual [69]. Other soft tissue sites are the palms, wrist, chest wall, foot, and eyelid. Multiple lesions are more common in children than in adults. The treatment is surgical excision; there is no metastatic or malignant potential.

Clinical History: 18-year-old man with marked soft tissue swelling of the thigh.

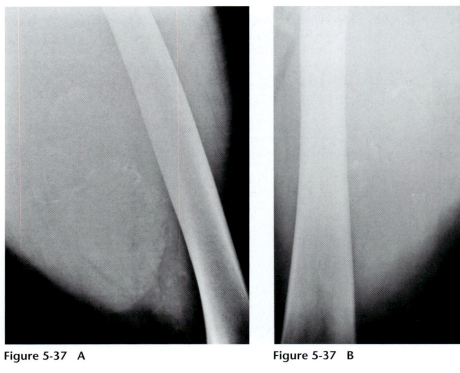

Figure 5-37   A   Figure 5-37   B

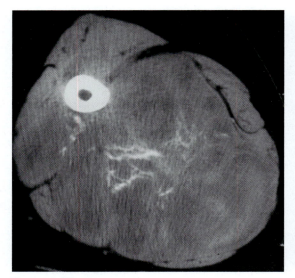

Figure 5-37   C

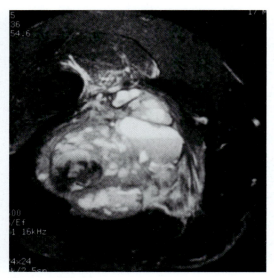

Figure 5-37   D

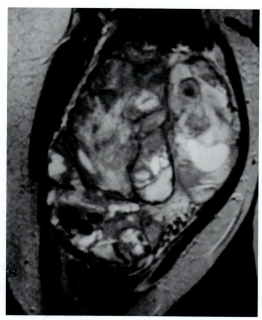

Figure 5-37 E

Findings: (A, B) Lateral and AP radiographs demonstrate ill-defined calcification in an enormous posterior thigh soft tissue mass. The underlying femur appears normal. (C) CT without contrast injection shows that the posterior compartment mass is predominantly low attenuation, but it has calcified septations. It has replaced most of the muscles and may extend into the anterior and adductor compartments. The underlying femur appears intact. (D, E) Axial and coronal T2-weighted MRI with fat saturation demonstrates marked heterogeneity with compartmentalized fluid-fluid levels suggesting a hemorrhagic component.

Differential Diagnosis: Soft tissue sarcoma, myositis ossificans, extraskeletal osteosarcoma, tumoral calcinosis.

Diagnosis: Synovial sarcoma.

Discussion: This huge, heterogeneous soft tissue is very suspicious for malignancy and should be considered to be a sarcoma unless proven otherwise. Biopsy is necessary. The most common primary malignancy of the musculoskeletal soft tissues is MFH, but in the young adult, synovial sarcoma is more common. Synovial sarcomas are more likely to be calcified than other types of mesenchymal sarcomas (synovial sarcomas have an approximately 30% incidence of radiographic calcification). Other malignant sarcomas that may calcify include extraskeletal chondrosarcoma and osteosarcoma, as well as the occasional soft tissue sarcoma. The MRI features of these lesions are protean and not specific [70], and calcification is difficult to recognize on MRI. Synovial sarcomas bear a superficial resemblance to synovial cells on light microscopy, but they are not actually thought to arise from the synovium. Although synovial sarcomas frequently arise within a few centimeters of joints, actual involvement of the synovium by a synovial sarcoma is rare. The age of peak incidence is 20 to 49 years. Synovial sarcomas are slow-growing lesions, but local recurrence and metastases may occur. Treatment is by wide resection.

Clinical History: 39-year-old man with painless posterior thigh mass.

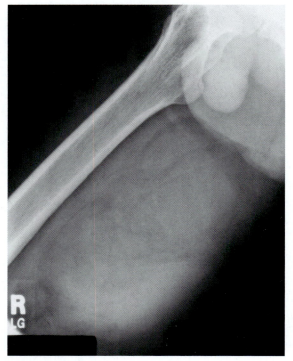

Figure 5-38   A

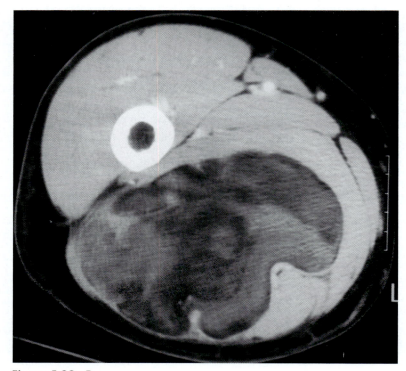

Figure 5-38   B

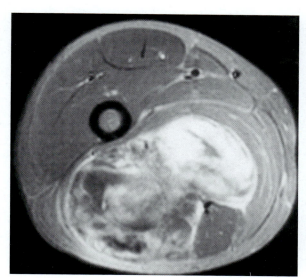

Figure 5-38 C

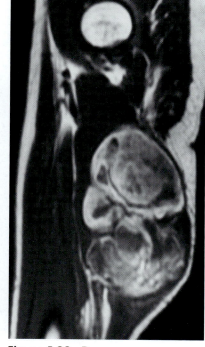

Figure 5-38 D

Findings: (A) Lateral radiograph of the thigh shows a large, fat-containing soft tissue lesion in the posterior thigh musculature. (B) CT through the midportion of the lesion shows a heterogeneous lesion, with some regions of fat attenuation. The lesion occupies the posterior muscular compartment and does not involve the bone. (C) Axial T2-weighted MRI with fat saturation shows that some portions of the image have high signal whereas other portions have low signal, which is consistent with fat. (D) Sagittal T1-weighted MRI shows a heterogenous lobular lesion containing fat.

Differential Diagnosis: Soft tissue sarcoma, lipoma, nerve sheath tumor, myositis ossificans.

Diagnosis: Liposarcoma.

Discussion: A large mass in the deep soft tissues of the thigh is always worrisome. The specific imaging features of this lesion suggest a sarcoma containing fat, but biopsy is necessary. Benign lipomas would be bland and nearly homogeneously fat, reflecting a paucity of cellular components. Myositis ossificans would be expected to calcify around the periphery and should not contain fat. Nerve sheath tumors often contain lipid but would typically present at a much smaller size because of early nerve impingement.

Liposarcoma is the most common soft tissue sarcoma of the lower extremities in adults between the ages of 26 and 45; however, most liposarcomas are found in patients in their 50s and 60s [71]. Liposarcoma usually arises in the deep soft tissues, and patients present with a large, painless mass. Liposarcoma originates from a primitive mesenchymal cell (not from mature fat), and there are several morphologic subtypes, all with histologic evidence of fat differentiation. The well-differentiated and myxoid subtypes are low or intermediate grade. They typically have large amounts of gross fat or extracellular myxoid material, whereas the round cell, pleomorphic, and dedifferentiated subtypes are considered high grade and are typically very cellular, with little if any gross fat.

Radiographs usually show a nonspecific soft tissue mass, but on CT and MRI, the appearance of liposarcoma tends to reflect the degree of fat differentiation. The lower-grade lesions generally appear fat-like, with low attenuation on CT and signal characteristics similar to subcutaneous fat on MRI. The higher-grade lesions frequently have no radiologically evident fat [72]. Large size, lobular shape, circumscription, heterogeneity, enhancement, hemorrhage, and necrosis are common features of liposarcomas. Soft tissue sarcomas of other histologic types may also contain fat as the result of engulfment, especially in recurrent lesions. Liposarcomas are treated operatively with wide margins. Most patients are candidates for limb-sparing surgery [73].

Clinical History: 33-year-old woman with bone pain and muscle weakness.

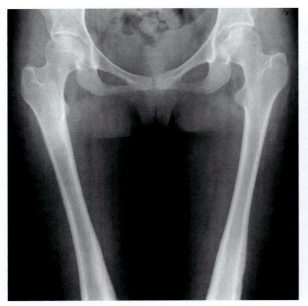

Figure 5-39 A

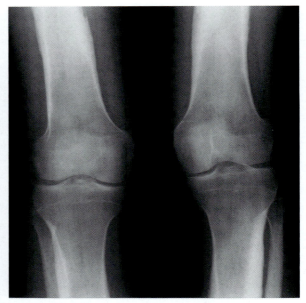

Figure 5-39 B

Findings: AP radiographs of the femurs and knees show marked cortical thickening is present along the distal femoral shafts and the proximal tibial and fibular shafts bilaterally. The thickening includes both periosteal and endosteal surfaces. There are no associated soft tissue or joint abnormalities.

Differential Diagnosis: Healed fractures, stress fracture, chronic infection, melorheostosis, Paget's disease, hypertrophic osteoarthropathy, osteopetrosis, Camurati-Engelmann disease.

Diagnosis: Camurati-Engelmann disease (progressive diaphyseal dysplasia).

Discussion: The absolute symmetry of the findings suggests a systemic disease, eliminating most of the items from the differential diagnosis, all of which could result in cortical thickening. Hypertrophic osteoarthropathy would not result in narrowing of the medullary cavity, and Paget's disease would begin at the ends of the bones rather than in the diaphyses. Osteopetrosis should involve all portions of all the bones.

Camurati-Engelmann disease is a dysplastic condition characterized radiographically by fusiform cortical thickening of the diaphyses of the long bones, resulting from endosteal and periosteal bone deposition. The medullary cavity is narrowed, and the hyperostosis is bilaterally symmetric. On histology, the thickened bone shows intense, simultaneous increases in both osteoblastic and osteoclastic activity. The increased bone turnover may be reflected in increased activity on radionuclide bone scan and in biochemical markers [74]. Although the causation and pathogenesis is uncertain, it has been proposed that the disease is the result of defective haversian bone formation or deficient cortical vascular supply. In the latter case, localized cortical hypoxia would be the stimulus for bone formation. The condition may occur sporadically or as an autosomal dominant heritable condition with variable expressivity [75].

Clinical History: 32-year-old woman with pulmonary symptoms.

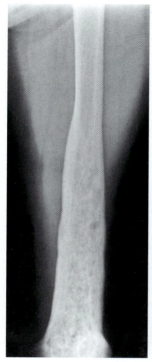
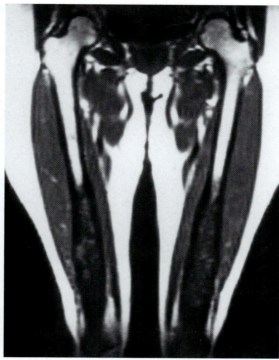

Figure 5-40 A   **Figure 5-40 B**

Findings: (A) AP radiograph of the distal femur shows abnormality involving the distal half of the femur. The bone is mildly expanded, and the medullary space is irregularly sclerotic with some lucent lesions. There is no layered periosteal reaction or soft tissue mass. The morphology of the proximal femur appears normal. (B) Coronal T1-weighted MRI of both femurs shows normal bone and marrow signal proximally. The distal halves of the femurs, including the condyles, show expanded but not thinned cortex, and low signal replacing the normal high fatty-marrow signal. The surrounding musculature appears normal. The lesions demonstrate heterogeneous high signal on T2-weighted images (not shown).

Differential Diagnosis: Osteonecrosis, eosinophilic granuloma, metastatic disease, multifocal chronic osteomyelitis, enchondromatosis, Camurati-Engelmann disease, healed trauma, radiation change, Paget's disease, Gaucher's disease, Erdheim-Chester disease.

Diagnosis: Erdheim-Chester disease.

Discussion: Patchy areas of sclerosis with intramedullary component may be seen with infarcts, but the typical lacy pattern of calcification is not noted in this case, and the cortical expansion would be unexplained. Paget's disease may demonstrate sclerosis and bone enlargement, but usually in a cortical distribution. Radiation changes may show patchy areas of sclerosis, similar to bone infarcts, and the expansion of the cortex might be explained by whatever underlying process was treated by radiation, but we have no history of radiation, and the bilateral distribution would be puzzling. Gaucher's disease may produce cortical expansion and infarcts, but not cortical thickening. Chronic osteomyelitis, metastatic disease, enchondromatosis, and eosinophilic granuloma could have some similar radiologic features, but the symmetric distribution would be unusual. Other systemic diseases that result in hyperostosis or multiple osteosclerotic lesions would tend to be more widely distributed.

Lipid granulomatosis, or Erdheim-Chester disease, is an exceedingly rare condition that demonstrates patchy areas of sclerosis with or without focal osteolytic regions [76,77]. Predominant changes occur at diametaphyseal sites and involve corticomedullary sclerosis. There is increased uptake of radionuclide on bone scan and gallium scan. Cholesterol deposition in foam cells, fibrosis, lipid granulomas, and lymphocyte and plasma cell infiltration are histologic findings. A relationship to Langerhans histiocytosis has been suggested [78]. Extraskeletal manifestations may affect the cardiopulmonary system and kidneys.

Clinical History: 50-year-old man with knee pain.

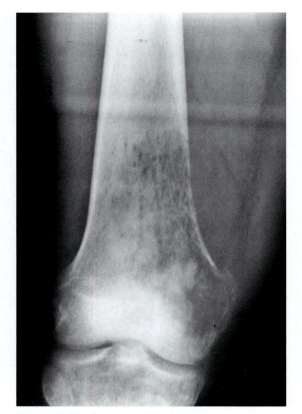

Figure 5-41   A

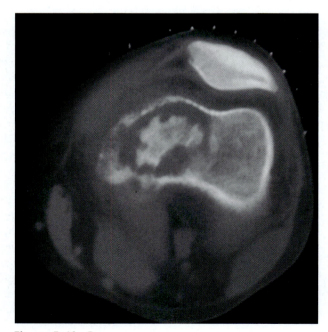

Figure 5-41   B

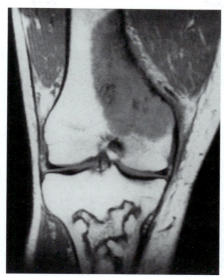

Figure 5-41   C

Findings: (**A**) AP radiograph of the distal femur shows permeated bone destruction without reactive bone formation or mineralization. (**B**) Axial CT shows replacement of the medial femur with a lucent lesion. The cortex is violated in multiple areas, with associated extraosseous soft tissue extension and joint effusion. A giant sequestrum of medullary bone with irregular margins is present centrally. (**C**) Coronal T1-weighted MRI shows a lesion of intermediate signal intensity in the medial femoral metadiaphysis with cortical penetration. Several irregularly shaped signal voids are present within the lesion. Marrow infarcts are present in the tibia.

Differential Diagnosis: Osteosarcoma, malignant fibrous histiocytoma, osteomyelitis, metastases, lymphoma.

Diagnosis: Malignant fibrous histiocytoma, arising in bone infarct.

Discussion: The cortical destruction here implies an aggressive process. The central sequestration may represent dystrophic or matrix calcification or a remnant from a pre-existing process, such as malignant degeneration in a pre-existing bone infarct with a bony sequestrum, now engulfed by tumor. The latter is most likely, due to the focal nature of the calcific component and its irregular shape. MFH may occur as primary lesions or secondary to dedifferentiation of chondrosarcoma or malignant degeneration in an infarct, radiation, or Paget's disease. Fifteen percent of primary lesions may demonstrate dystrophic calcification or sequestration. Lesions arising from bone infarcts may show retained calcification in the underlying infarct. Typical radiographic features include bony lysis with a permeative pattern. Diametaphyseal sites in long bones are favored locations. They tend to be sizable lesions with a broad zone of transition. Periosteal reaction may or may not accompany these

findings. These lesions have a higher incidence in males. The age range is broad, with a peak at approximately 50 years old. These lesions carry a poor prognosis, with metastases occurring to lung, bone, and lymph nodes.

MFH of bone is a rare entity [81,82]. As in this case, it is typically seen in men between 40 and 60 years old. Approximately one-half of patients will present with a pathologic fracture. MFH may develop in a preexisting bone infarct, lipoma, Paget's disease, or radiation therapy. The distribution is the metaphyses of long bones, usually in the lower extremity. The radiographic presentation is that of an aggressive lesion, usually osteolytic, with limited reactive periostitis and an associated soft tissue mass. The appearance is difficult to distinguish from a fibrosarcoma; MFH tends to have a more aggressive appearance, whereas fibrosarcoma is more likely to have a sequestrum. Other considerations include a nonexpansile osteolytic metastasis (such as lung or breast), multiple myeloma, lymphoma, and osteosarcoma. Infection should always be mentioned whenever a small cell tumor is included.

Pathologically, MFH is characterized by a storiform appearance that distinguishes it from the herringbone appearance seen in fibrosarcoma. The osseous form of this disease has local recurrences in up to 80% of patients in the early experience, but is comparable to primary osteosarcoma of bone at this time. Metastases occur hematogenously as well as to lymphatics. Sarcoma associated with bone infarct is rare, with most reported cases being MFH, fibrosarcoma, or osteosarcoma [83,84]. The pathogenesis of sarcoma arising in bone infarct is unknown, but the most common sites are the tibia, femur, and humerus. Most patients have multiple infarcts of unknown cause with large medullary components. The prognosis for patients with these sarcomas is poor [85].

Clinical History: 72-year-old woman with right groin pain referred from an outside institution for removal of a "tumor." She is 5 years status post right total hip arthroplasty.

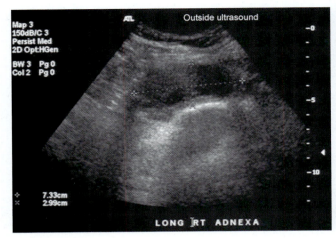

Figure 5-42　A

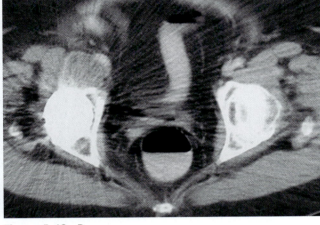

Figure 5-42　B

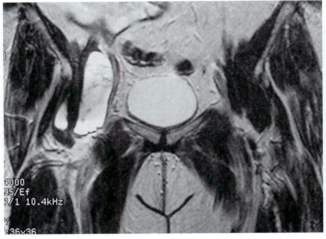

Figure 5-42　C

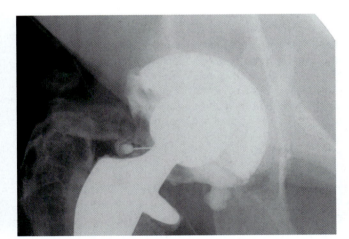

Figure 5-42　D

Findings: (**A**) An ultrasound demonstrates a complex cystic mass, which was misinterpreted by an outside institution as being adnexal in location. (**B, C**) On axial CT and coronal T2-weighted MRI, an elongated cystic structure extends along the anterior border of the iliopsoas muscle to the level of the hip arthroplasty distally. The mass displaces the right external iliac artery and vein medially. (**D**) A conventional hip arthrogram demonstrates flow of contrast from the hip joint superiorly and medially into the cystic mass.

Differential Diagnosis: Distended iliopsoas bursa, inguinal hernia, abscess, sarcoma.

Diagnosis: Iliopsoas bursitis.

Discussion: The iliopsoas bursa is the largest bursa in the body. This bursa communicates with the hip joint in 15% of normal adults. Bursal communication with the hip is more commonly seen after hip arthroplasty, possibly due to surgical disruption of the bursal wall or increased intraarticular pressure from excess joint fluid. The iliopsoas bursa may become distended due to any condition that causes excess joint fluid or bursal synovial proliferation. Distended iliopsoas bursae have been associated with hip arthroplasties, arthritis (inflammatory and degenerative), trauma, overuse, osteomyelitis, and metastatic disease. A joint effusion is commonly, but not always, seen at presentation.

The diagnosis of a distended iliopsoas bursa can typically be made with standard CT or MRI, with attention to the anatomic location and communication with the hip joint [86–88]. On ultrasonography, the location and joint communication can be harder to assess [89]. However, ultrasound best evaluates for mass effect on adjacent structures [90]. In cases where an outside institution has labeled the mass as suspicious for a neoplasm, or when the bursal contents are complex in nature, it may be helpful to do an enhanced study to exclude a solid neoplasm. Alternatively, a conventional hip arthrogram can be performed to prove that the bursa communicates with the hip joint. Treatment is usually only necessary if the distended bursa is painful or is impinging adjacent structures. Therapeutic options include treatment of the underlying cause of excess joint fluid (loose prosthesis replacement, anti inflammatory medication), the use of sclerosing agents, and surgical bursectomy.

Clinical History: 63-year-old man with hyperviscosity syndrome and monoclonal macroglobulinemia.

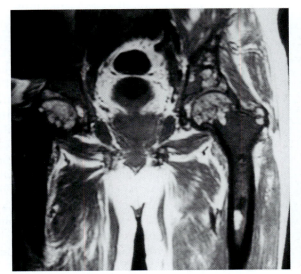

Figure 5-43 A

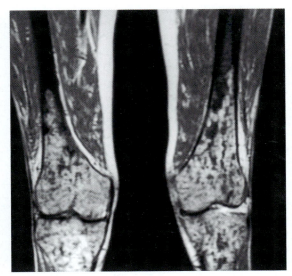

Figure 5-43 B

Findings: Coronal T1-weighted MRI of the hips and knees demonstrates replacement of the normal hyperintense marrow fat with multiple deposits of diffuse low signal. Fatty marrow in the epiphyses is mainly preserved. The bony cortex is intact, and there is no periosteal reaction or surrounding edema.

Differential Diagnosis: Lymphoma, multiple myeloma, Waldenstrom's macroglobulinemia, leukemia, metastases.

Diagnosis: Waldenstrom's macroglobulinemia.

Discussion: These images demonstrate diffuse infiltration of the marrow by a systemic process, which is a nonspecific finding. Correlating the clinical history makes the diagnosis in this case. Waldenstrom's macroglobulinemia is a low-grade, small cell lymphoma with monoclonal IgM production [79,80]. The entity comprises approximately 2% of hematologic cancers. The median age at diagnosis is 63 years. There is a slight male predominance, and family clusters have been described. Manifestations of disease are related to tumor infiltration, circulating monoclonal proteins, and tissue-bound monoclonal proteins. Approximately 90% of patients with Waldenstrom's macroglobulinemia will have overt lymphoma involving the bone marrow, although lytic lesions demonstrable by radiographs do occur. When present, the appearance is similar to multiple myeloma. Approximately one-third of patients will have involvement of lymph nodes or the spleen. Circulating monoclonal macroglobulins may cause hyperviscosity, cryoglobulinemia, and cold agglutinin anemia. Tissue deposition of these proteins may cause peripheral neuropathy, glomerular disease, and amyloidosis. Hyperviscosity can lead to capillary sludging and marrow infarction.

SOURCES AND READINGS

1. Watson RM, Roach NA, Dalinka MK. Avascular necrosis and bone marrow edema syndrome. *Radiol Clin North Am.* 2004;42(1):207–219.

2. Scully SP, Aaron RK, Urbaniak JR. Survival analysis of hips treated with core decompression or vascularized fibular grafting because of avascular necrosis. *J Bone Joint Surg Am.* 1998;80:1270–1275.

3. Iorio R, Healy WL, Abramowitz AJ, Pfeifer BA. Clinical outcome and survivorship analysis of core decompression for early osteonecrosis of the femoral head. *J Arthroplasty.* 1998;13:34–41.

4. Schapira D. Transient osteoporosis of the hip. *Semin Arthritis Rheum.* 1992;22:98–105.

5. Froberg PK, Braunstein EM, Buckwalter KA. Osteonecrosis, transient osteoporosis, and transient bone marrow edema: current concepts. *Radiol Clin North Am.* 1996;34(2):273–291.

6. Court C, Carlioz H. Radiological study of severe proximal femoral focal deficiency. *J Pediatr Orthop.* 1997;17:520–524.

7. Goldman AB. Heritable diseases of connective tissue, epiphyseal dysplasias, and related conditions. In: Resnick D, ed. *Diagnosis of Bone and Joint Disorders.* 4th ed. Philadelphia: WB Saunders; 2002:4382–4448.

8. Williams CJ, Jimenez SA. Skeletal dysplasias and the osteoarthritic phenotype. *Best Pract Res Clin Rheumatol.* 2003;17(6):1005–1018.

9. Chapman KL, Briggs MD, Mortier GR. Review: clinical variability and genetic heterogeneity in multiple epiphyseal dysplasia. *Pediatr Pathol Mol Med.* 2003;22(1):53–75.

10. Goldman AB. Heritable diseases of connective tissue, epiphyseal dysplasias, and related conditions. In: Resnick D, ed. *Diagnosis of Bone and Joint Disorders.* 4th ed. Philadelphia: WB Saunders; 2002:4382–4448.

11. Stoker DJ. Osteopetrosis. *Semin Musculoskelet Radiol.* 2002;6(4):299–305.

12. Smith SE, Kransdorf MJ. Primary musculoskeletal tumors of fibrous origin. *Semin Musculoskelet Radiol.* 2000;4(1):73–88.

13. Guille JT, Kumar SJ, MacEwen GD. Fibrous dysplasia of the proximal part of the femur. Long-term results of curettage and bone-grafting and mechanical realignment. *J Bone Joint Surg Am.* 1998;80:648–658.

14. Kaushik S, Smoker WR, Frable WJ. Malignant transformation of fibrous dysplasia into chondroblastic osteosarcoma. *Skeletal Radiol.* 2002;31(2):103–106.

15. Wunderbaldinger P, Paya K, Partik B, et al. CT and MR imaging of generalized cystic lymphangiomatosis in pediatric patients. *Am J Roentgenol.* 2000;174(3):827–832.

16. Gomez CS, Calonje E, Ferrar DW, Browse NL, Fletcher CD. Lymphangiomatosis of the limbs. Clinicopathologic analysis of a series with a good prognosis. *Am J Surg Pathol.* 1995;19:125–133.

17. Ghandur-Mnaymneh L, Broder LE, Mnaymneh W. Lobular carcinoma of the breast metastatic to bone with unusual clinical, radiologic, and pathologic features mimicking osteopoikilosis. *Cancer.* 1984;53:1801–1803.

18. Mungovan JA, Tung GA, Lambiase RE, Noto RB, Davis RP. Tc-99m MDP uptake in osteopoikilosis. *Clin Nucl Med.* 1994;19(1):6–8.

19. Umans H, Liebling MS, Moy L, Haramati N, Macy NJ, Pritzker HA. Slipped capital femoral epiphysis: a physeal lesion diagnosed by MRI, with radiographic and CT correlation. *Skeletal Radiol.* 1998;27:139–144.

20. Lahdes-Vasama T, Lamminen A, Merikanto J, Marttinen E. The value of MRI in early Perthes' disease: an MRI study with a 2-year follow-up. *Pediatr Radiol.* 1997;27:517–522.

21. Lamer S, Dorgeret S, Khairouni A, et al. Femoral head vascularisation in Legg-Calvé-Perthes disease: comparison of dynamic gadolinium-enhanced subtraction MRI with bone scintigraphy. *Pediatr Radiol.* 2002;32(8):580–585.

22. Hochbergs P, Eckerwall G, Egund N, Jonsson K, Wingstrand H. Synovitis in Legg-Calvé-Perthes disease. Evaluation with MR imaging in 84 hips. *Acta Radiol.* 1998;39:532–537.

23. Buchmann RF, Jaramillo D. Imaging of articular disorders in children. *Radiol Clin North Am.* 2004;42(1):151–168.

24. Gash A, Walker CR, Carty H. Case report: complete photopenia of the femoral head on radionuclide bone scanning in septic arthritis of the hip. *Br J Radiol.* 1994;67:816–818.

25. Oka M, Monu JU. Prevalence and patterns of occult hip fractures and mimics revealed by MRI. *AJR Am J Roentgenol.* 2004;182(2):283–288.

26. Hirata T, Konishiike T, Kawai A, Sato T, Inoue H. Dynamic magnetic resonance imaging of femoral head perfusion in femoral neck fracture. *Clin Orthop.* 2001;(393):294–301.

27. Scott SM, Manaster BJ, Alazraki N, Wooten WW, Murphy K. Technetium 99m imaging of bone trauma: reduced sensitivity caused by hydrocortisone in rabbits. *AJR Am J Roentgenol.* 1987;148:1175–1178.

28. Hetsroni I, Shabat S, Mann G. A false negative technetium 99m bone scan in a 53-year-old man with a fractured tibia and fractured clavicles conducted 88 h after the accident. *Injury.* 2004;35(2):199–202.

29. Tuite MJ, De Smet AA, Gaynon PS. Tibial stress fracture mimicking neuroblastoma metastasis in two young children. *Skeletal Radiol.* 1995;24:287–290.

30. Hayes CW, Conway WF, Sundaram M. Misleading aggressive MR imaging appearance of some benign musculoskeletal lesions. *Radiographics.* 1992;12:1119–1134.

31. Sankaran-Kutty M, Corea JR, Ali MS, Kutty MK. Squamous cell carcinoma in chronic osteomyelitis. Report of a case and review of the literature. *Clin Orthop Rel Res.* 1985;198:264–267.

32. McGrory JE, Pritchard DJ, Unni KK, Ilstrup D, Rowland CM. Malignant lesions arising in chronic osteomyelitis. *Clin Orthop.* 1999;(362):181–189.

33. Wuk K. Squamous cell carcinoma arising from chronic osteomyelitis of the ankle region. *J Foot Ankle Surg.* 1990;29:608–612.

34. Swash M, Brown MM, Thakkar C. CT muscle imaging and the clinical assessment of neuromuscular disease. *Muscle Nerve.* 1995;18:708–714.

35. Vliet AM, Thijssen HO, Joosten E, Merx JL. CT in neuromuscular disorders: a comparison of CT and histology. *Neuroradiology.* 1988;30:421–425.

36. Enneking WF, Kagan A. Skip metastases in osteosarcoma. *Cancer.* 1975;36:2192–2205.

37. Davies AM, Makwana NK, Grimer RJ, Carter SR. Skip metastases in Ewing's sarcoma: a report of three cases. *Skeletal Radiol.* 1997;26:379–384.

38. Saifuddin A. The accuracy of imaging in the local staging of appendicular osteosarcoma. *Skeletal Radiol.* 2002;31(4):191–201.

39. Daffner RH, Lupetin AR, Dash N, Deeb ZL, Sefczek RJ, Schapiro RL. MRI in the detection of malignant infiltration of bone marrow. *AJR Am J Roentgenol.* 1986;146:353–358.

40. Uetani M, Hashmi R, Hayashi K. Malignant and benign compression fractures: differentiation and diagnostic pitfalls on MRI. *Clin Radiol.* 2004;59(2):124–131.

41. Terpos E, Rahemtulla A. Bisphosphonate treatment for multiple myeloma. *Drugs Today (Barc).* 2004;40(1):29–40.

42. Bredella MA, Caputo GR, Steinbach LS. Value of FDG positron emission tomography in conjunction with MR imaging for evaluting therapy response in patients with musculoskeletal sarcomas. *AJR Am J Roentgenol.* 2002;179:1145–1150.

43. Bastiaannet E, Groen H, Jager PL, et al. The value of FDG-PET in the detection, grading and response to therapy of soft tissue and bone sarcomas: a systematic review and meta-analysis. *Cancer Treat Rev.* 2004;30:83–101.

44. Cohen EK, Kressel HY, Frank TS, et al. Hyaline cartilage origin of bone and soft tissue neoplasms: MR appearance and histologic correlation. *Radiology.* 1988;167:477–481.

45. Rahmouni A, Montazel JL, Divine M, et al. Bone marrow with diffuse tumor infiltration in patients with lymphoproliferative diseases: dynamic gadolinium-enhanced MR imaging. *Radiology.* 2003;229(3):710–717.

46. Roodman GD. Mechanisms of bone lesions in multiple myeloma and lymphoma. *Cancer.* 1997;80(suppl 8):1557–1563.

47. Hong SP, Hahn JS, Lee JD, Bae SW, Youn MJ. 18F-fluorodeoxyglucose-positron emission tomography in the staging of malignant lymphoma compared with CT and 67Ga scan. *Yonsei Med J.* 2003;44(5):779–786.

48. Levine E, De Smet AA, Huntrakoon M. Juxtacortical osteosarcoma: a radiologic and histologic spectrum. *Skeletal Radiol.* 1985;14:38–46.

49. Murphey MD, Robbin MR, McRae GA, Flemming DJ, Temple HT, Kransdorf MJ. The many faces of osteosarcoma. *Radiographics.* 1997;17:1205–1231.

50. States LJ. Imaging of metabolic bone disease and marrow disorders in children. *Radiol Clin North Am.* 2001;39(4):749–772.

51. Deely DM, Schweitzer ME. MR imaging of bone marrow disorders. *Radiol Clin North Am.* 1997;35:193–212.

52. Tardivon AA, Vanel D, Munck JN, Bosq J. Magnetic resonance imaging of the bone marrow in lymphomas and leukemias. *Leuk Lymphoma.* 1997;25:55–68.

53. Biesecker JL, Marcove RC, Huvos AG, Mike V. Aneurysmal bone cysts. A clinicopathologic study of 66 cases. *Cancer.* 1970;26:615–625.

54. Hudson TM. *Radiologic-Pathologic Correlation of Musculoskeletal Lesions.* Baltimore: Williams & Wilkins; 1987;261–285.

55. Kransdorf MJ, Sweet DE. Aneurysmal bone cyst: concept, controversy, clinical presentation, and imaging. *AJR Am J Roentgenol.* 1995;164:573–580.

56. Ragsdale BD. Polymorphic fibro-osseous lesions of bone: an almost site-specific diagnostic problem of the proximal femur. *Hum Pathol.* 1993;24:505–512.

57. Gilkey FW. Liposclerosing myxofibrous tumor of bone. *Hum Pathol.* 1993;24:1264.

58. Kransdorf MJ, Murphey MD, Sweet DE. Liposclerosing myxofibrous tumor: a radiologic-pathologic-distinct fibro-osseous lesion of bone with a marked predilection for the intertrochanteric region of the femur. *Radiology.* 1999;212(3):693–698.

59. O'Connell JX, Nanthakumar SS, Nielsen GP, Rosenberg AE. Osteoid osteoma: the uniquely innervated bone tumor. *Mod Pathol.* 1998;11:175–180.

60. Liu PT, Chivers FS, Roberts CC, Schultz CJ, Beauchamp CP. Imaging of osteoid osteoma with dynamic gadolinium-enhanced MR imaging. *Radiology.* 2003;227(3):691–700.

61. Rosenthal DI, Hornicek FJ, Torriani M, Gebhardt MC, Mankin HJ. Osteoid osteoma: percutaneous treatment with radiofrequency energy. *Radiology.* 2003;229(1):171–175.

62. Murphey MD, Gross TM, Rosenthal HG. Musculoskeletal malignant fibrous histiocytoma: radiologic-pathologic correlation. *Radiographics.* 1994;14:807–826.

63. Jelinek J, Kransdorf MJ. MR imaging of soft-tissue masses. Mass-like lesions that simulate neoplasms. *Magn Reson Imaging Clin N Am.* 1995;3:727–741.

64. Parikh J, Hyare H, Saifuddin A. The imaging features of post-traumatic myositis ossificans, with emphasis on MRI. *Clin Radiol.* 2002;57(12):1058–1066.

65. Varma DG, Moulopoulos A, Sara AS, et al. MR imaging of extracranial nerve sheath tumors. *J Comput Assist Tomogr.* 1992;16:448–453.

66. Kudawara I, Ueda T, Yoshikawa H. Granular cell tumor of the subcutis: CT and MRI findings. A report of three cases. *Skeletal Radiol.* 1999;28(2):96–99.

67. Jardines L, Cheung L, LiVols V, et al. Malignant granular cell tumors: a report of a case and review of the literature. *Surgery.* 1994;116:49–54.

68. Lack EE, Worsham GF, Callihan MD, et al. Granular cell tumor: a clinicopathologic study of 110 patients. *J Surg Oncol.* 1980;13:301–316.

69. Wold LE, Swee RG, Sim FH. Vascular lesions of bone. *Pathol Ann.* 1985;20:101–137.

70. Jones BC, Sundaram M, Kransdorf MJ. Synovial sarcoma: MR imaging findings in 34 patients. *AJR Am J Roentgenol.* 1993;161:827–830.

71. Kransdorf M, Murphey MD. *Imaging of Soft Tissue Tumors.* Philadelphia: WB Saunders; 1997:79–94.

72. Jelinek JS, Kransdorf MJ, Shmookler BM, Aboulafia AJ, Malewer MM. Liposarcoma of the extremities: MR and CT findings in the histologic subtypes. *Radiology.* 1993;186:455–459.

73. Peterson JJ, Kransdorf MJ, Bancroft LW, O'Connor MI. Malignant fatty tumors: classification, clinical course, imaging appearance and treatment. *Skeletal Radiol.* 2003;32(9):493–503.

74. Hernandez MV, Peris P, Guanabens N, et al. Biochemical markers of bone turnover in Camurati-Engelmann disease: a report on four cases in one family. *Calcif Tissue Int.* 1997;61:48–51.

75. Saraiva JM. Progressive diaphyseal dysplasia: a three-generation family with markedly variable expressivity. *Am J Med Genet.* 1997;71:348–352.

76. Veyssier-Belot C, Cacoub P, Caparros-Lefebvre D, et al. Erdheim-Chester disease. Clinical and radiologic characteristics of 59 cases. *Medicine (Baltimore).* 1996;75(3):157–169.

77. Evans S, Williams F. Case report: Erdheim-Chester disease: polyostotic sclerosing histiocytosis. *Clin Radiol.* 1986;37(1):93–96.

78. Brower AC, Worsham GF, Dudley AH. Erdheim-Chester disease: a distinct lipoidosis or part of the spectrum of histiocytosis? *Radiology.* 1984;151(1):35–38.

79. Dimopoulos MA, Alexanian R. Waldenstrom's macroglobulinemia. *Blood.* 1994;83(6):1452–1459.

80. Moulopoulos LA, Dimopoulos MA, Varma DG, et al. Waldenstrom macroglobulinemia: MR imaging of the spine and CT of the abdomen and pelvis. *Radiology.* 1993;188:669–673.

81. Hoekstra HJ, Ham SJ, van der Graaf WT, Kamps WA, Molenaar WM, Schraffordt Koops H. Malignant fibrous histiocytoma of bone: a clinicopathologic study of 81 patients. *Cancer.* 1998;82:993–994.

82. Picci P, Bacci G, Ferrari S, Mercuri M. Neoadjuvant chemotherapy in malignant fibrous histiocytoma of bone and in osteosarcoma located in the extremities: analogies and differences between the two tumors. *Ann Oncol.* 1997;8:1107–1115.

83. Galli SJ, Weintraub HP, Proppe KH. Malignant fibrous histiocytoma and pleomorphic sarcoma in association with medullary bone infarcts. *Cancer.* 1978;41:607–609.

84. Desai P, Perino G, Present D, Steiner GC. Sarcoma in association with bone infarcts. Report of five cases. *Arch Pathol Lab Med.* 1996;120:482–489.

85. Gaucher AA, Regent DM, Gillet PM, Pere PG, Aymard BM, Clement V. Case report 656: malignant fibrous histiocytoma in a previous bone infarct. *Skeletal Radiol.* 1991;20(2):137–140.

86. Pritchard RS, Shah HR, Nelson CL, FitzRandolph RL. MR and CT appearance of iliopsoas bursal distention secondary to diseased hips. *J Comput Assist Tomogr.* 1990;14(5):797–800.

87. Steinbach LS, Schneider R, Goldman AB, Kazam E, Ranawat CS, Ghelman B. Bursae and abscess cavities communicating with the hip. Diagnosis using arthrography and CT. *Radiology.* 1985;156(2):303–307.

88. Varma DG, Richli WR, Charnsangavej C, Samuels BI, Kim EE, Wallace S. MR appearance of the distended iliopsoas bursa. *Am J Roentgenol.* 1991;156(5):1025–1028.

89. Janus C, Hermann G. Enlargement of the iliopsoas bursa: unusual cause of cystic mass on pelvic sonogram. *J Clin Ultrasound.* 1982;10(3):133–135.

90. Bianchi S, Martinoli C, Keller A, Bianchi-Zamorani MP. Giant iliopsoas bursitis: sonographic findings with magnetic resonance correlations. *J Clin Ultrasound.* 2002;30(7):437–441.

CHAPTER SIX
KNEE

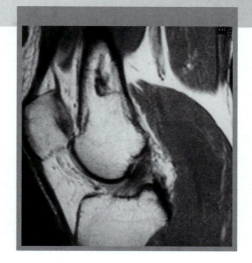

CASE 6-1

Clinical History: 3-year-old boy with swelling of the left knee.

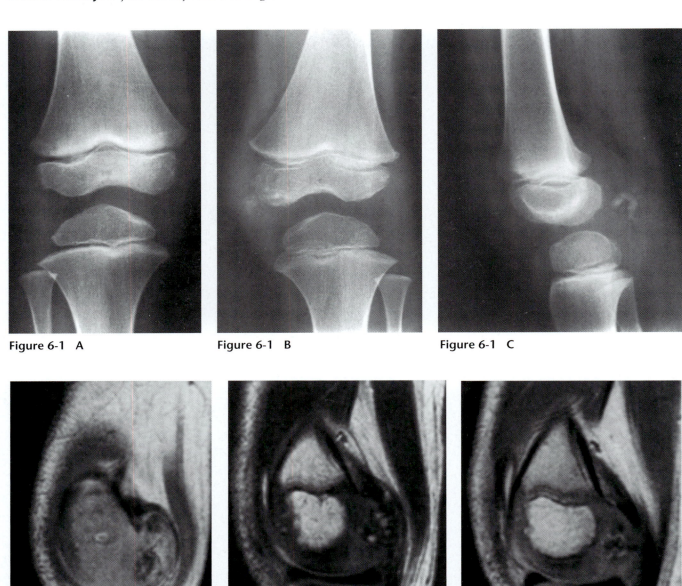

Figure 6-1   A

Figure 6-1   B

Figure 6-1   C

Figure 6-1   D

Figure 6-1   E

Figure 6-1   F

Findings: (A) Anteroposterior (AP) radiograph of the right knee is normal. (B, C) AP and lateral radiographs of the left knee demonstrate small, multifocal ossifications seen medial and posterior to the normal epiphysis. (D–F) Sagittal magnetic resonance imaging (MRI) through the medial femoral condyle using T1-weighting, proton density, and T1-weighting after intravenous gadolinium demonstrates cartilaginous overgrowth of the posterior aspect of the femoral epiphysis, with a secondary center of ossification. There is no mass lesion separate from this epiphyseal overgrowth.

Differential Diagnosis: Articular chondroma, loose body, osteochondritis dissecans.

Diagnosis: Articular chondroma (dysplasia epiphysealis hemimelica).

Discussion: Articular chondroma, also called dysplasia epiphysealis hemimelica or Trevor's disease [1], histologically consists of hyaline cartilage. It may be considered an epiphyseal form of osteochondroma. It is unilateral and typically affects only one-half of the epiphysis of a long bone (usually the medial portion), as seen here. The most common location is in the lower extremity, particularly about the ankle, which explains the alternate term of tarsal aclasis. It may or may not be associated with multiple exostoses. It is usually manifested in childhood. Complications include impaired growth and joint abnormalities, particularly deformities of alignment from the asymmetric growth. MRI is the most helpful imaging study in evaluating these lesions [2].

Clinical History: 22-year-old man with knee pain.

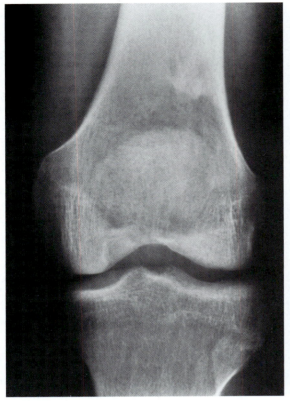

Figure 6-2   A

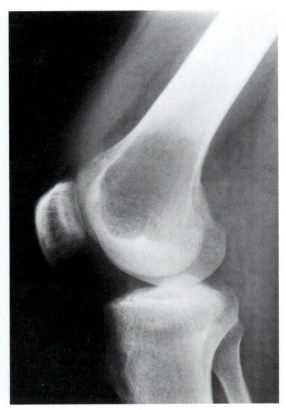

Figure 6-2   B

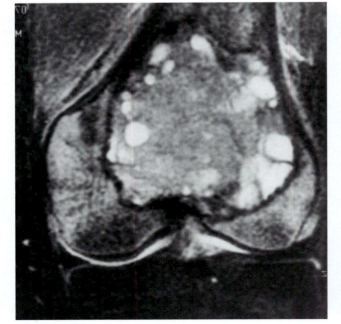

Figure 6-2   C

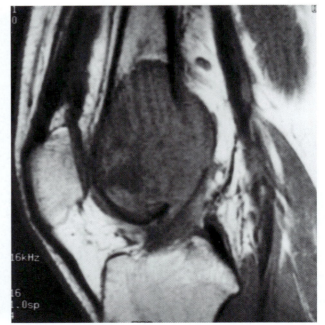

Figure 6-2   D

Findings: (A, B) AP and lateral radiographs of the knee. There is a lucent lesion in the lateral femoral condyle. There is very little reactive bone, if any. The posterior cortex may be violated on the lateral view. (C, D) Coronal T2-weighted and sagittal T1-weighted MRI demonstrates T1 hypointensity and T2 isointensity to muscle, with multiple round areas of T2 hyperintensity at the margins.

Differential Diagnosis: Giant cell tumor, chondroblastoma, clear cell chondrosarcoma.

Diagnosis: Giant cell tumor.

Discussion: The diagnostic possibilities for a large, solitary epiphyseal lesion in an adult include giant cell tumor, chondroblastoma, and clear cell chondrosarcoma. Chondroblastomas usually have sclerotic borders. Calcification is seen in 50% of patients and periosteal reaction is seen in 50% of patients. Clear cell chondrosarcoma typically occurs in the proximal femur or proximal humerus. Therefore, the most likely diagnosis is giant cell tumor.

Giant cell tumor of bone (osteoclastoma) is an uncommon lesion thought to arise from osteoclasts. The presence of giant cells is only one histologic component of the tumor, and other types of tumors may have giant cells. Giant cell tumors can occur at any age, but the typical patient is a young adult. The location is almost invariably in the epiphysis, with extension to the subchondral cortex and into the metaphysis. Less than 2% of these tumors occur adjacent to open growth plates. Giant cell tumors probably arise in the cutback zone of the metaphysis, where osteoclasts are plentiful and active. About 50% of tumors are found about the knee, but other long bones and the sacrum are also commonly involved.

The typical radiographic appearance is a geographic, lytic tumor near the end of a long bone, extending to or very close to the subarticular cortex. Lytic regions correspond to nonmineralized tumor tissue, destroying and replacing cancellous bone. A lobular pattern of growth may leave ridges or trabeculations in surrounding bone. Giant cell tumors are often expansile and may have cystic blood-filled regions similar to aneurysmal bone cysts. The zone of transition from tumor to normal bone is usually sharp and abrupt, but without a sclerotic margin (growth rate I-B). Some lesions erode from the epiphysis into the joint cavity and provoke synovitis. Approximately 10% of patients present with pathologic fracture. Computed tomography (CT) or MRI may be required to show the extent of tumor and the relationship to the adjacent joint. Giant cell tumors appear as areas of intense isotope uptake on bone scan and sometimes have a doughnut appearance, with greater activity at the margins.

The typical treatment of giant cell tumor is curettage, adjuvant treatment of the surgical bed with a high-speed burr, phenol or cryotherapy, and packing with methylmethacrylate. The reported overall rate of recurrence is about 25%. There are case reports of pulmonary and skin metastases from giant cell tumors [3,4]. Older literature suggests the existence of malignant giant cell tumors, but these may have represented primary malignant lesions such as osteosarcoma or malignant fibrous histiocytoma (MFH) that have prominent giant cells at histology. Spontaneous malignant transformation of a conventional giant cell tumor is rare [5].

Clinical History: 6-year-old boy with pain and swelling at the knee for several months.

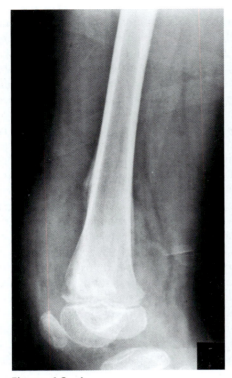

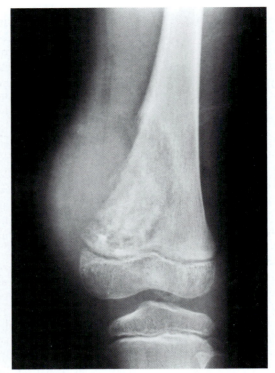

Figure 6-3   A   **Figure 6-3   B**

Findings: Lateral and AP radiographs of the knee. There is a large, destructive lesion involving the medial aspect of the distal femoral metaphysis, with cortical destruction and large soft tissue mass. The lesion extends to the growth plate but does not appear to cross into the epiphysis. Laminated, interrupted periosteal reaction is seen at the superior margin of the tumor. The margins of the lesion are poorly defined. Dense, amorphous regions of mineralization are present within the lesion.

Differential Diagnosis: Osteosarcoma, Ewing's sarcoma, lymphoma, metastasis.

Diagnosis: Osteosarcoma, high-grade intramedullary type.

Discussion: This destructive lesion should be unmistakable for a bone tumor. The lesion is moderately mineralized, and the mineralization has the dense, amorphous, cloud-like pattern characteristic of osteoid matrix. The location of the lesion and age of the patient is typical for the diagnosis. The age distribution of osteosarcoma has a sharp peak (46% of cases) between the ages of 10 and 20, but it has been described in very young children and in elderly adults. Osteosarcomas have been described in virtually every part of the skeleton, but the least common sites are probably the hands and feet.

In the Mayo Clinic series of bone tumors [6], the most common anatomic sites of osteosarcomas were distal femur (31%), proximal tibia (15%), proximal humerus (8%), pelvis (7%), proximal femur (5%), and femoral shaft (4%). Of osteosarcomas that occur in the long bones, only about 10% are found in the diaphysis alone, without extension to the metaphysis or epiphysis. The majority of osteosarcomas have no known cause, but in this series, more than 5% were found in irradiated bone, and more than 3% were found in regions of Paget's disease. Patients older than 60 are much more likely to have a preexisting condition (38%).

CASE 6-4

Clinical History: Young adult woman with headache, dizziness, prolonged bleeding time, and hypertension.

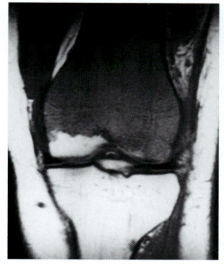

Figure 6-4 A

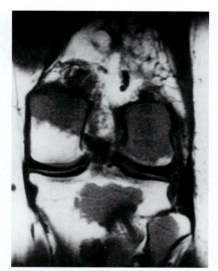

Figure 6-4 B

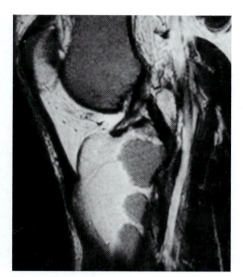

Figure 6-4 C

Findings: Select coronal and sagittal T1-weighted MRI demonstrate replacement of the normal fatty high-signal-intensity marrow with conglomerate deposits of low-signal-intensity material in both the femur and tibia. The visualized articular surfaces are normal.

Differential Diagnosis: Polycythemia vera, multiple myeloma, lymphoma, leukemia, hemoglobinopathies.

Diagnosis: Polycythemia vera.

Discussion: Polycythemia vera is an idiopathic mono-clonal marrow-proliferating process. Hyperplasia is most pronounced in the red blood cell constituents of the bone marrow. The main complications are thrombosis and bleed-ing diathesis. Multiple focal lytic lesions are characteristic.

On MRI, replacement of the normal fatty marrow is re-flected by decreased signal intensity on T1-weighted imag-ing, as seen here, showing an intermediate signal intensity on T2-weighted MRI between muscle and fat [19]. Later in the disease, marrow may be replaced by fibrosis and pro-duce a clinical and radiologic appearance of myelofibro-sis with extramedullary hematopoiesis. In this phase, there is decreased signal intensity in the bone marrow on both T1-weighted and T2-weighted MRI [20,21]. Secondary forms of polycythemia may occur and give rise to similar features. Gout, due to hyperuricemia, may complicate the ra-diographic findings. Definitive diagnosis is by bone marrow biopsy.

Clinical History: 20-year-old woman with knee pain and swelling for 3 months.

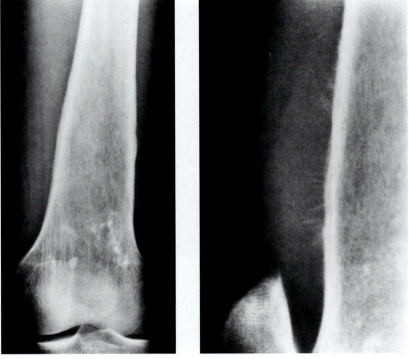

Figure 6-5   A   Figure 6-5   B

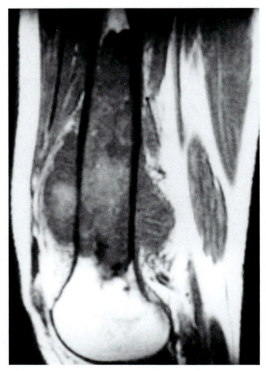

Figure 6-5   C

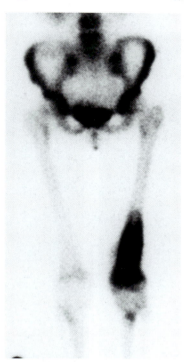

Figure 6-5   D

Findings: (**A**) AP radiograph of the distal femur. There is a mildly expansile lesion in the distal femur causing slight irregularity of the texture of the cortical bone, with a few localized areas of amorphous mineralization distally. There is subtle periosteal elevation medially and laterally at the distal shaft. The proximal and distal intramedullary extent of the lesion is imperceptible. (**B**) Lateral radiograph of the distal femur, photographic detail. There is permeation of tumor through the anterior femoral cortex into the soft tissues, with sunburst periosteal reaction and soft tissue mass. The destruction of the cortex is evident as unsharpness of its margins and vague lucency; the overall structure of the cortex remains intact. (**C**) Sagittal T1-weighted MRI shows an extensive intramedullary lesion with heterogeneous signal. The lesion penetrates the cortex anteriorly and posteriorly to form large soft tissue masses. Small regions of very low signal at the inferior extent of the tumor correspond to the mineralized matrix seen on the AP radiograph. (**D**) Radionuclide bone scan. Anterior whole-body scan (photographic detail) shows intense activity in the distal femur, corresponding to the tumor. There is also a modest regional increase in activity in the proximal femur and proximal tibia.

Differential Diagnosis: Osteosarcoma, Ewing's sarcoma, lymphoma, metastasis.

Diagnosis: Osteosarcoma, high-grade intramedullary type.

Discussion: This case illustrates a high-grade intramedullary osteosarcoma whose radiographic features are more subtle but nonetheless highly aggressive. The true extent of the lesion is shown dramatically by the MRI. The radionuclide bone scan shows a pattern of falsely extended uptake that corresponds to hyperemia and osteoporosis in the otherwise normal adjacent bone [7]. In contrast to the preceding cases, the lesion in this case is only slightly ossified.

Clinical History: 24-year-old woman with mass behind her left knee.

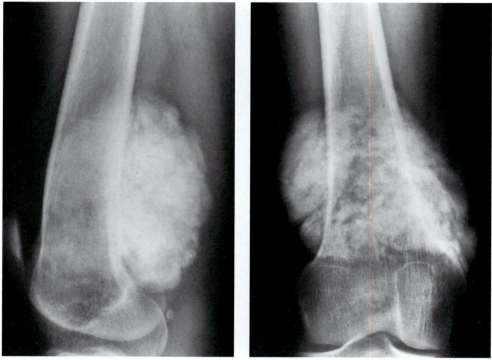

Figure 6-6   A

Figure 6-6   B

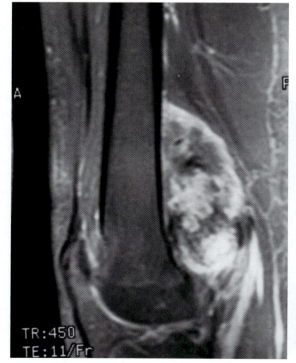

Figure 6-6   C

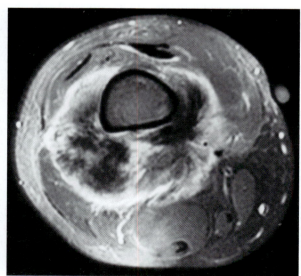

Figure 6-6   D

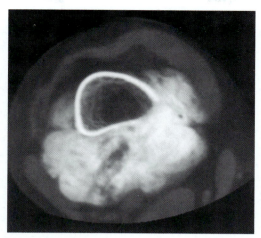

Figure 6-6 E

Findings: (**A**, **B**) Lateral and AP radiographs of the knee reveal a densely ossified mass arising from the posterior cortex of the distal femur, above the level of the condyles. (**C**, **D**) Sagittal and axial T1-weighted MRI with fat saturation after intravenous gadolinium injection shows the large cortically based mass wrapping around the femoral shaft. The lesion shows regions of dense mineralization (low signal) as well as enhancement. (**E**) Axial CT (bone windows) shows a dense lesion arising from the posterior cortex of the left knee. The lesion has destroyed the cortex at the posterior medial margin of the femoral shaft, but there is little, if any, tumor extending into the medullary space. The bulk of the tumor appears to be densely mineralized.

Differential Diagnosis: Parosteal osteosarcoma, osteochondroma, periosteal osteosarcoma, myositis ossificans, tumoral calcinosis.

Diagnosis: Parosteal osteosarcoma (juxtacortical osteosarcoma).

Discussion: Parosteal osteosarcomas represent approximately 5% of osteosarcomas. They differ from the conventional high-grade intramedullary osteosarcoma in several significant ways. Parosteal osteosarcoma arises on the cortical surface rather than within the medullary space, and virtually all are found in the metaphysis of a long bone, especially the posterior surface of the distal femoral metaphysis (66% of cases). The peak age at diagnosis is in the third decade, with more than 80% of patients older than 20. The presentation is nonspecific—often dull aching pain or mechanical difficulties caused by the mass itself. The lesions are commonly diagnosed and treated incorrectly for years as atypical osteochondromas that somehow recur locally. Even with late diagnosis, the prognosis is often better than for conventional osteosarcoma because they are, by definition, of low histologic grade (a higher-grade osteosarcoma arising on the surface of bone would be classified by the pathologist as either a periosteal osteosarcoma or a high-grade surface osteosarcoma).

The radiographic appearance is a lobulated, juxtacortical mass with densely ossified tumor tissue attached to the cortex, often by a stalk. Variable amounts of lucent, nonossified tissue are usually present, making the lesion larger than apparent on plain radiographs. The peripheral portions of the lesion tend to have the least ossification. A cleavage plane between tumor and underlying bone may be visible at the edge of the stalk in approximately two-thirds of cases, and it is characteristic of the slow, lobular growth of the tumor as it becomes larger than its attachment to the bone. Tumor invasion of the medullary cavity may occur by direct extension through the stalk. Such invasion is found in the minority of cases and can often be documented by CT or MRI. Localized regions of histopathologic dedifferentiation to high-grade spindle cell sarcoma is not uncommon (28%), either at presentation or at local recurrence [8]. The presence of a poorly defined soft tissue component distinct from the mineralized matrix is suggestive of a high-grade focus [9] (14).

Parosteal osteosarcoma is the only malignant primary bone tumor that is more common in females than males (by a ratio of nearly 2:1 in the Mayo Clinic series. Adamantinoma has an equal sex predilection, and all other malignant primary bone tumors are more common in males. Benign bone lesions that are more common in females include giant cell tumor, aneurysmal bone cyst, and hemangioma. The treatment of parosteal osteosarcoma is surgical. Recurrences with simple curettage are common, but wide excision with clear surgical margins may be curative. Long-term survival rates of 80% to 90% may be expected for patients without regions of dedifferentiation.

Clinical History: 35-year-old man with chronic, aching knee pain.

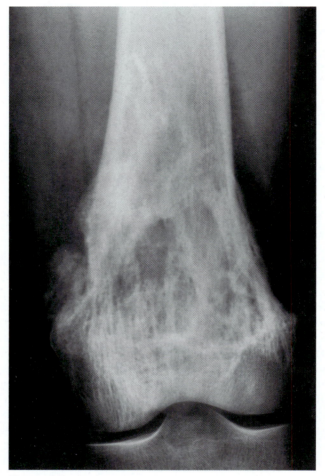

Figure 6-7   A

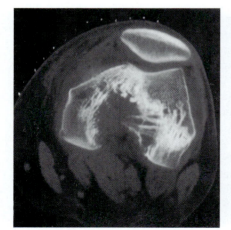

Figure 6-7   B

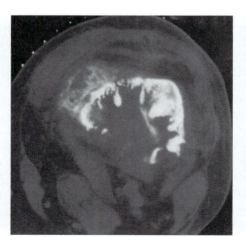

Figure 6-7   C

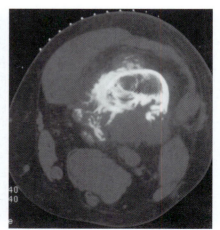

Figure 6-7   D

Findings: (A) AP radiograph of the knee. Bone loss is present at the intercondylar portion of the distal femur, probably extending to the medial cortex, with prominent reinforcement of the remaining trabeculae. Amorphous sclerosis is seen at the medial edge of the femur and along the more superior portion of the cortex adjacent to the intercondylar bone defect. (B) Axial noncontrast CT at the level of the femoral condyles shows a central destructive lesion with surrounding, sclerotic, reinforced trabecular bone. At the anteromedial cortex is a small, faintly mineralized soft tissue mass. (C) CT at the distal shaft shows extensive cortical bone destruction with prominent reinforced trabecular bone. Dense amorphous mineralization is seen on the endosteal surface of the anterior cortex. A mineralized soft tissue mass is present. (D) CT more proximally along the femoral shaft shows a large, partially mineralized soft tissue mass.

Differential Diagnosis: Osteosarcoma, chondrosarcoma, lymphoma, metastasis, desmoplastic fibroma.

Diagnosis: Osteosarcoma, low-grade intramedullary type.

Discussion: This case has features of an aggressive lesion as well as an indolent lesion. The presence of cortical destruction, cortical penetration, and formation of soft tissue mass suggests an aggressive process. The presence of reinforced trabeculae compensating structurally for the regions of cortical destruction suggests a lesion that has been present for some time. The mineralization of the soft tissue portion of the lesion suggests a bone-forming tumor.

Low-grade osteosarcomas are well-differentiated bone-forming malignancies whose radiologic and histopathologic appearances are challenging to the diagnostician [10]. Rare lesions, they occur in adults and are typically found around the knee. The prognosis for long-term survival is excellent, but local recurrences may be accompanied by dedifferentiation to high-grade tumor and metastatic spread.

CASE 6-8

Clinical History: 47-year-old man with knee pain.

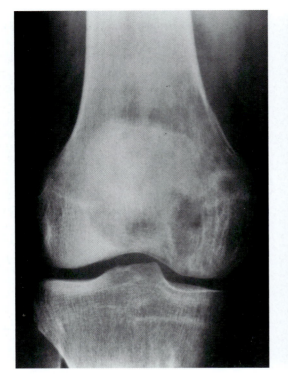

Figure 6-8   A

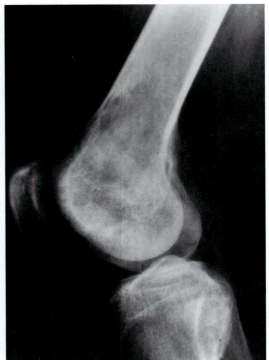

Figure 6-8   B

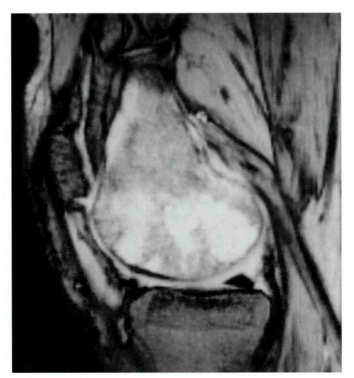

Figure 6-8   C

Findings: (A, B) AP and lateral radiographs show a lytic lesion in the medial femoral condyle with ill-defined borders, but extending to the articular surface. An associated soft tissue mass is not noted, and there is no associated periostitis. (C) Sagittal T2-weighted MRI demonstrates high signal intensity in this lesion, without definite cortical violation.

Differential Diagnosis: Malignant fibrous histiocytoma (MFH) of bone, metastasis, osteosarcoma, fibrosarcoma, chondrosarcoma, lymphoma.

Diagnosis: Malignant fibrous histiocytoma of bone.

Discussion: MFH is a lesion that may occur in soft tissue or bone. MFH is considered to be of histiocytic origin. Histologically, the lesions show fibrogenic differentiation, and multinucleated malignant giant cells may be a prominent feature. MFH arising in bone is relatively rare, comprising only 1% of primary malignant bone tumors [11]. MFH more frequently arises in the soft tissues. The age range of patients is wide, but most patients are adults. Although most lesions occur around the knee, lesions have been reported in the extremities, spine, and skull. In long bones, the lesions are usually metaphyseal. As with other types of bone tumors, the typical clinical presentation is pain and swelling. Approximately 25% of MFH in bone is secondary to a preexisting pathologic process, most commonly previous radiation therapy, Paget's disease, or bone infarction. Joint implants or their alloys have also been named as an inciting factor for MFH of bone [12].

The radiographic appearance is usually one of aggressive bone destruction with a moth-eaten or permeative pattern, as seen here. Reactive bone tends to be scant, and there will be no mineralized tumor matrix. The differential diagnosis includes metastasis, osteosarcoma, fibrosarcoma, chondrosarcoma, and lymphoma. The pathologic distinction between MFH and other bone sarcomas may be difficult. The presence of even microscopic foci of neoplastic osteoid or chondroid would cause the lesion to be classified as an osteosarcoma or chondrosarcoma, respectively. The distinction between MFH and fibrosarcoma is considered by some to be arbitrary, and they are radiologically indistinguishable.

Clinical History: 67-year-old woman with knee pain for several weeks, without a precipitating episode of trauma.

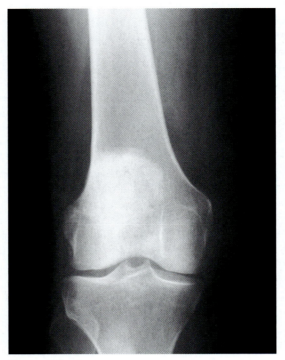

Figure 6-9   A

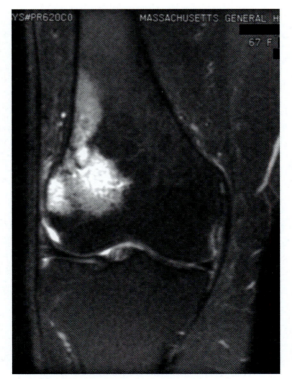

Figure 6-9   B

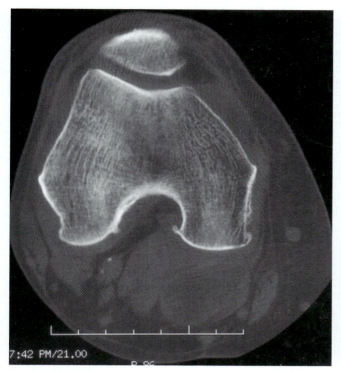

Figure 6-9   C

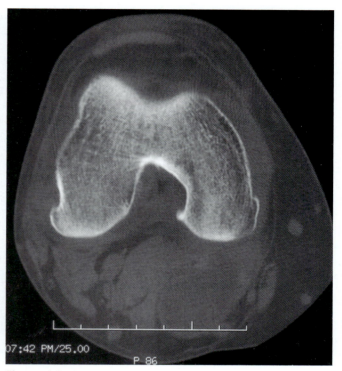

Figure 6-9   D

Findings: (**A**) AP radiograph of the knee shows very subtle periosteal elevation along the lateral cortex of the femoral metaphysis. (**B**) Coronal short-tau inversion-recovery MRI shows a large, bright region in the lateral metaphysis extending into the lateral femoral condyle. (**C**) Axial CT shows a minimal increase in sclerosis involving the lateral femoral condyle, corresponding to the abnormality on MRI. (**D**) A small portion of the lateral cortex is irregular and decreased in density, reflecting permeated destruction.

Differential Diagnosis: Lymphoma, metastases, osteosarcoma, infection.

Diagnosis: Primary lymphoma of bone.

Discussion: Primary lymphoma of bone can have a near normal appearance on radiographs [13]. MRI, as seen here, can show a large abnormality. In this case, the diagnosis was made by CT-guided needle biopsy. Sclerotic lymphoma of bone is one circumstance in which the percutaneously guided needle biopsy can be falsely negative. The infiltrative nature of the disease and the fragility of the cells may result in such severe crush artifacts that evidence of malignancy may be destroyed during the process of obtaining the specimen.

Patients with lymphoma involving bone may present with symptoms related to a bone lesion, or bone lesions may be discovered during staging after the diagnosis has been made from an extraskeletal site. Patients presenting with a bone lesion in whom there is no evidence of disease found elsewhere are considered to have primary lymphoma of bone, and they comprised only 3% of lymphomas of bone in the Mayo Clinic series [14]. There is a broad age range at time of diagnosis, and most lymphomas involve the portion of the skeleton containing red marrow. Bone destruction is the primary radiographic feature of primary lymphoma, and generally results in a permeated destruction of cortical and trabecular bone. A mottled and patchy appearance is typical. Approximately 50% of cases may have evidence of reactive bone or thickening of the cortex, but this reactive bone is typically sparse, and periosteal bone formation as might be seen in Ewing's sarcoma is notably unusual. Soft tissue extension may be obvious, large, and asymmetric. Pathologic fracture is common. In a minority of cases, irregular sclerosis is present at the affected site, rather than a mixture of lysis and sclerosis.

Clinical History: Female college varsity soccer player with persistent pain after injury. The team doctor ordered an MRI.

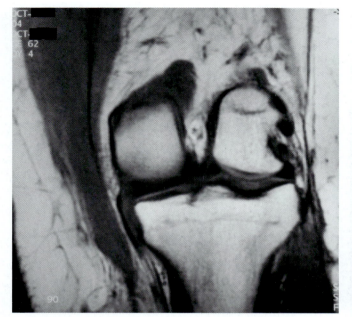

Figure 6-10   A

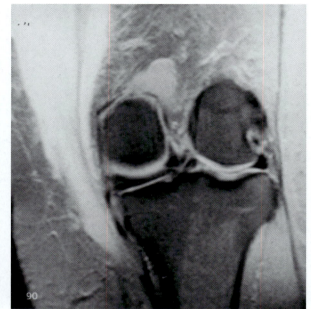

Figure 6-10   B

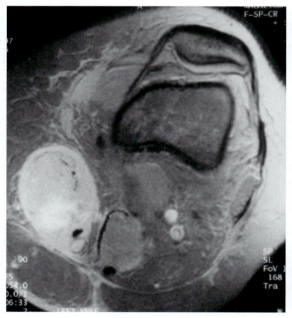

Figure 6-10   C

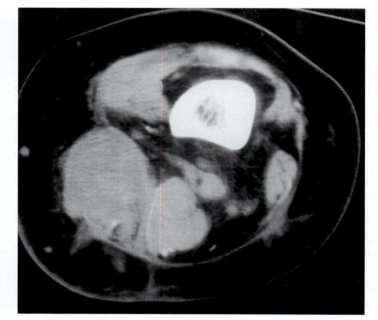

Figure 6-10   D

Findings: (A) Coronal T1-weighted MRI shows enlargement of the sartorius muscle. The margins of the muscle are slightly irregular, and subcutaneous edema is present. (B) Coronal T2-weighted MRI shows high signal intensity in the sartorius muscle. (C) Axial T2-weighted MRI shows the enlargement of the sartorius, with high signal intensity and surrounding edema. (D) Axial CT at the time of needle biopsy shows enlargement of the sartorius.

Differential Diagnosis: Non-Hodgkin's lymphoma, intramuscular metastasis, soft tissue sarcoma, inflammatory disease, intramuscular tear and/or hemorrhage.

Diagnosis: Non-Hodgkin's lymphoma of sartorius muscle.

Discussion: Factors that favor malignancy in a soft tissue mass are large size, deep location (e.g., intramuscular), and surrounding edema. The abnormality of the sartorius in this case has an aggressive appearance because of the diffuse nature of the enlargement and the markedly irregular margins around the muscle belly. The differential diagnosis includes inflammatory disease, intramuscular tear and/or hemorrhage, intramuscular metastasis, and soft tissue sarcoma. Lymphoma, presenting as an intramuscular mass without evidence of disease elsewhere, is a distinctly rare entity. Primary intramuscular non-Hodgkin's lymphoma has a good prognosis, and because the treatment is not surgical, percutaneous needle biopsy is the key diagnostic procedure in this circumstance [15].

Clinical History: 9-year-old boy with swollen and painful knee.

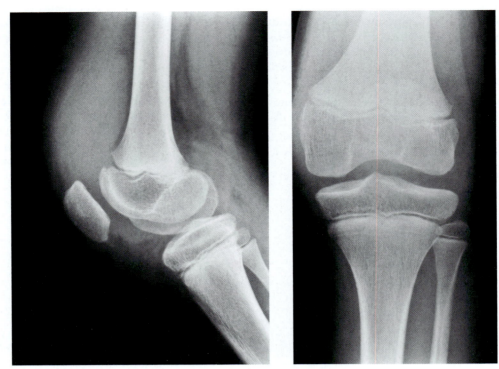

Figure 6-11   A

Figure 6-11   B

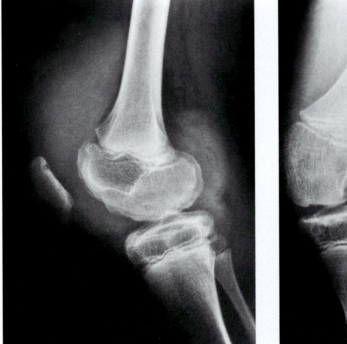

Figure 6-11   C

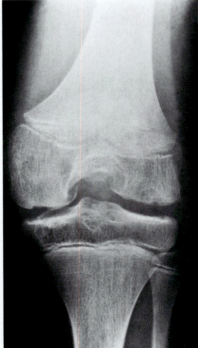

Figure 6-11   D

Findings: (A) Lateral radiograph of the knee shows marked synovial hypertrophy and effusion, with epiphyseal overgrowth. (B) AP radiograph shows squaring of the condyles and degenerative changes. (C, D) One year later. Lateral and AP radiographs demonstrate the progression of the findings, with the additional feature of erosions of the articular surface.

Differential Diagnosis: Hemophilia, juvenile idiopathic arthritis, postinfectious arthropathy.

Diagnosis: Hemophiliac knee.

Discussion: The early findings in this case may be attributable to juvenile idiopathic arthritis or hemophilia. Juvenile idiopathic arthritis is more common in females and generally shows osteoporosis as an early finding. Erosive changes are frequent in juvenile idiopathic arthritis and are not noted in the initial film, although joint destruction is already evident.

Hemophilia A is a clotting disorder related to factor VIII deficiency. It is transmitted as an X-linked disorder and therefore occurs almost exclusively in males. Although other varieties of hemophilia exist, this is the most common type. The primary radiographic feature of this disorder is hemarthrosis, as seen on the lateral views in this instance, with joint destruction after repeated episodes [16]. Some cardinal features include squaring of the inferior pole of the patella and widening of the intercondylar notch. These findings, however, can also be observed in juvenile idiopathic arthritis [17]. Differentiating features include subperiosteal hemorrhage and intraosseous cystic lesions that are not subarticular. The latter finding is related to intraosseous hemorrhage and, when substantial in size, is referred to as a pseudotumor. These are seen most often in the ilium and calcaneus. Extremity overgrowth or undergrowth may occur, depending on whether hyperemia or early fusion of the growth plate is the predominant effect of the disorder. Avascular necrosis of the epiphysis can occur secondary to elevated intraarticular pressures from hemarthrosis [18]. Avascular necrosis may occur in juvenile idiopathic arthritis as a result of steroid treatment.

Clinical History: 7-year-old girl with joint swelling.

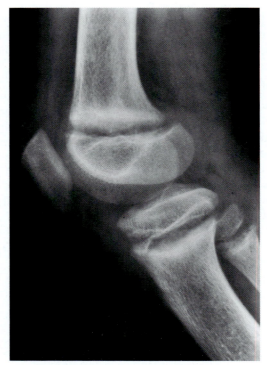

Figure 6-12   A

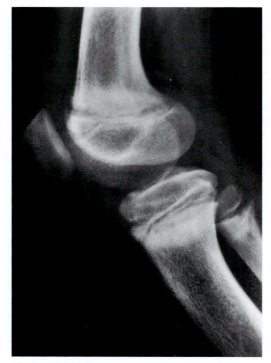

Figure 6-12   B

Findings: (A) Lateral knee radiograph taken at presentation. There is widening and fraying of the distal femur, proximal fibula, and tibia physes. (B) Lateral knee radiograph taken 7 months later. There is interval sclerosis and filling in of the physeal widening.

Differential Diagnosis: Rickets, metaphyseal dysplasia.

Diagnosis: Rickets.

Discussion: Rickets and osteomalacia are childhood and adult manifestations, respectively, of a systemic disease in which the calcification of osteoid is deficient. The common final pathway in both conditions is the lack of available calcium or phosphorus (or both) for mineralization of osteoid. In rickets, the predominant effect is on the growth plates; in osteomalacia, the predominant effect is on remodeling of mature bone. When rickets or osteomalacia occurs in conjunction with chronic renal failure, the condition is called renal osteodystrophy.

Dietary deficiency of vitamin D, usually coupled with inadequate exposure to sunlight so that photochemical synthesis of vitamin D in the skin does not occur, results in reduced gastrointestinal calcium absorption, hypocalcemia, and secondary hyperparathyroidism to mobilize calcium from the skeleton. Pure vitamin D deficiency-induced rickets and osteomalacia is relatively rare in the United States, except among immigrants, food faddists, the institutionalized elderly, and patients on total parenteral nutrition. Other causes include failure of enzymatic conversion of 25-hydroxyvitamin D to its physiologically more active metabolite 1,25-dihydroxyvitamin D, end-organ insensitivity to 1,25-dihydroxyvitamin D, genetic and acquired renal tubular reabsorption defects, and gastrointestinal malabsorption of dietary calcium or phosphorus. In the United States, gastrointestinal malabsorption from a variety of etiologies is the most common cause of rickets and osteomalacia. Rickets and osteomalacia may occur in association with polyostotic fibrous dysplasia and neurofibromatosis, and may be caused by chronic use of anticonvulsant medications or aluminum-containing antacids.

In rickets, there is widening of the growth plate because of continued cartilage growth in the absence of normal mineralization and ossification. Radiographic findings are most apparent in the most active regions of growth, and the uncalcified cartilage may become quite bulky. Frequent sites of radiographic abnormalities include the costochondral junctions of ribs, the distal femur, both ends of the tibia, the proximal humerus, the distal radius, and the ulna. Irregular, disorganized mineralization of the zone of provisional calcification creates a frayed appearance. Mechanical stress on the thickened growth plate may lead to widening, cupping, and bowing deformities. Bone texture (trabecular pattern) appears coarsened, and there is a delayed appearance of ossification centers. Rachitic bone is less resistant to bending and shearing loads, and stress fractures and bowing deformities are common. Transverse zones of lucency on the concave side of long bones, called Milkman's pseudofractures or Looser's zones, are focal collections of nonmineralized osteoid; they probably do not represent insufficiency injuries. After the initiation of successful treatment of rickets, the uncalcified osteoid calcifies, so that the zone of provisional calcification appears as a wide band that narrows the growth plate to its normal thickness. Ossification of nonmineralized subperiosteal osteoid is apparent as new periosteal bone.

Metaphyseal dysplasia is a rare disorder caused by an inborn error in enchondral ossification that results in widened, irregular-appearing growth plates. Laboratory values are normal, however.

Clinical History: 3-year-old boy with anemia and a companion case.

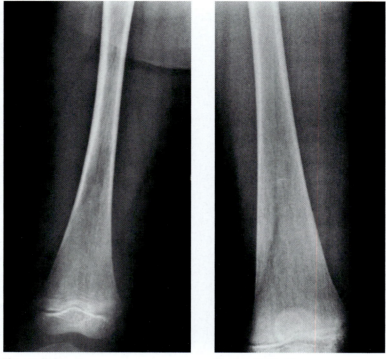

Figure 6-13   A   Figure 6-13   B

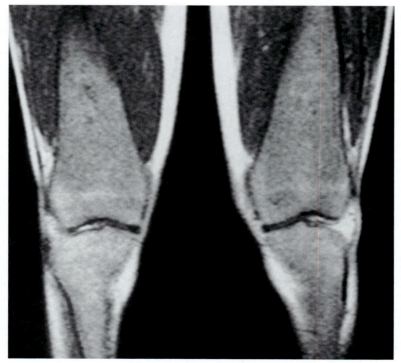

Figure 6-13 ` C

Findings: (A) AP radiograph of a knee taken at age 3 shows Erlenmeyer flask deformities of the femur and tibia. (B) AP radiograph of the knee taken at age 12 shows a progressive Erlenmeyer flask deformity. (C) Companion case. Coronal T1-weighted MRI of a young adult shows diffuse replacement of the fatty marrow, with intermediate signal and Erlenmeyer flask deformities.

Differential Diagnosis: Gaucher's disease, chronic anemias, Pyle's disease, Niemann-Pick disease.

Diagnosis: Gaucher's disease.

Discussion: Anemias, Pyle's disease, Niemann-Pick disease, and Gaucher's disease can produce Erlenmeyer flask deformities. The bone marrow is one of the largest organs of the body. Confined to the intramedullary space of bone, it consists of a meshwork of trabecular bone with fat cells, myeloid cells, reticulum cells, and supporting structures. At birth, the marrow cavities of the tubular bones, the flat bones, and the vertebrae have a predominance of hematopoietic cells. With advancing age, the hematopoietic marrow regresses and is replaced by fatty marrow, beginning distally in the extremities and progressing to incompletely encompass the pelvis, spine, and cranium. The process may reverse (called marrow reconversion) when there is an increased demand for hematopoiesis, as might occur in anemia or replacement of normal hematopoietic marrow by a pathologic process. Radiographic findings of marrow disorders are indirect and nonspecific.

When chronic marrow space expansion occurs in the growing skeleton, adaptive bone changes may occur during the development of the bone. Actual enlargement of the marrow space will alter the normal bony contours; such changes do not occur acutely nor do they occur in the adult. MRI is the best method for direct imaging of the bone marrow. Because marrow is a conglomeration of different tissues, the appearance on MRI may vary, both with the composition of the marrow as well as the particular technical parameters. In general, fatty marrow has the predominant signal characteristics of fat, and hematopoietic marrow has signal characteristics more similar to muscle. Nuclear scans with technetium Tc 99m sulfur colloid or technetium Tc 99mTc methylene diphosphonate can provide physiologic assessments of the reticuloendothelial marrow elements and the surrounding bone, respectively.

The prototype for the lipid storage diseases is Gaucher's disease (glucocerebroside lipidosis). In this autosomal recessive condition, deficiency of glucocerebrosidase results in the progressive accumulation of histiocytes laden with glucocerebroside lipids in the bone marrow and other organs and tissues. Secondary changes in bone are observed [22]. The classic radiographic finding is the Erlenmeyer flask deformity, which is undermodeling of the metaphysis due to marrow space packing. Cortical thinning by endosteal erosion and osteopenia are additional radiographic abnormalities that may be evident. Osteonecrosis of the femoral head is a common association, and is usually bilateral. After prolonged enzyme replacement therapy with macrophage-targeted glucocerebrosidase (glucosylceramidase), marrow composition, bone mass, and bone morphology revert toward normal.

Clinical History: 65-year-old woman with chronic knee pain.

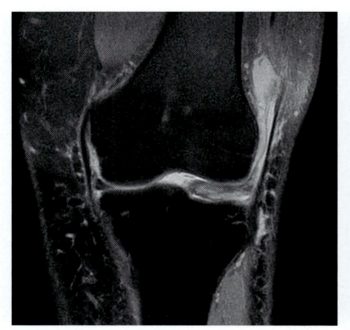

Figure 6-14   A

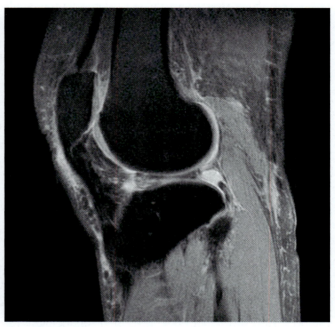

Figure 6-14   B

Findings: (A, B) Coronal and sagittal proton-density, fat-suppressed MRI demonstrates a large lateral meniscus with diffusely abnormal signal.

Differential Diagnosis: Discoid meniscus, complex meniscal tear.

Diagnosis: Discoid meniscus with complex tear.

Discussion: A discoid meniscus is a developmental anomaly that predisposes the patient to meniscal tears. Instead of the meniscus being C-shaped, it is shaped like a disc. With meniscal tissue now present in the joint space, it is more likely to degenerate and tear. The majority of adolescent patients with a meniscal tear have this anomaly. A discoid meniscus appears abnormally large on MRI. It will measure at least 12 mm wide on coronal images and have three or more sagittal images (4 mm thickness each) with a bowtie appearance. The discoid meniscus is typically lateral in location and does not predispose the patient to tears of the non-discoid medial meniscus [23]. Treatment of symptomatic patients includes repair of a tear, if present, and saucerization of the excess meniscal tissue [24].

Clinical History: 8-year-old boy with knee pain, radiographs are five months a part.

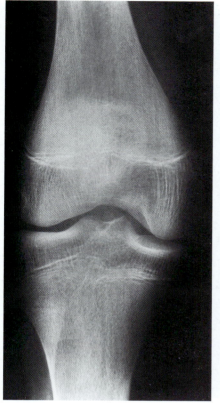

Figure 6-15   A

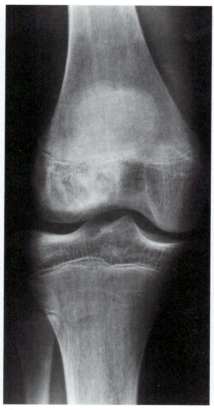

Figure 6-15   B

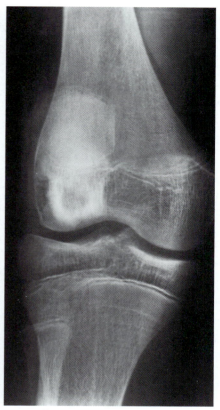

Figure 6-15   C

Findings: (A) AP film of the right knee demonstrates normal articular surfaces, but medial femoral condyle overgrowth. (B) AP radiograph of the right knee taken 5 months later demonstrates increased density to the lateral femoral condyle, with a smooth subarticular band. (C) AP radiograph of the right knee taken 10 months later demonstrates a more defined, solid band of sclerosis within the femoral condyle.

Differential Diagnosis: Bone infarct due to hemoglobinopathy, Gaucher's disease, steroid medication, trauma, pancreatitis.

Diagnosis: Sickle cell anemia.

Discussion: Sickle cell anemia occurs when valine is substituted for glutamate in the beta-chain of hemoglobin. The result is an abnormal form of hemoglobin that is less effective at carrying oxygen and predisposed to causing thromboses. The skeletal manifestations of this process include widening of the marrow space, bone infarcts, and an overall dense appearance of the bones. H-shaped vertebra and a snow-capped appearance of the humeral heads is classic. Osteomyelitis is not uncommon, and the diaphysis represents a common site for its occurrence in this condition. Salmonella is a more frequent pathogen in these cases. The main complication is infarctions due to the abnormal configuration of the hemoglobin, as seen here.

Clinical History: 38-year-old woman treated with corticosteroids for inflammatory arthritis.

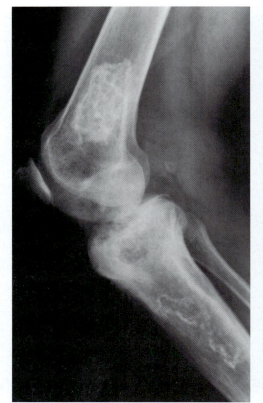

Figure 6-16   A

Figure 6-16   B

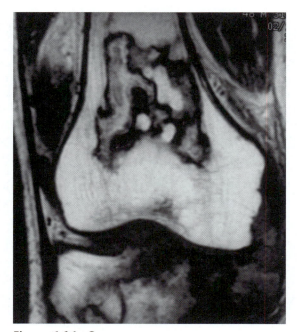

Figure 6-16   C

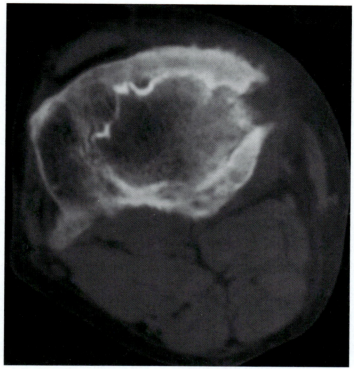

Figure 6-16   D

Findings: (**A, B**) Lateral and AP radiographs of knee. There are extensive regions of irregular calcification in the distal femur and proximal tibia. There is no mass effect or bone destruction. (**C**) Coronal T1-weighted MRI shows the lesions with low-signal-intensity borders and fatty centers. (**D**) Axial CT through the tibial epiphysis shows a calcified central lesion with well-defined, serpentine, sclerotic borders and more irregular sclerosis in the surrounding bone.

Differential Diagnosis: None.

Diagnosis: Calcified medullary infarcts with subchondral collapse of the tibial articular surface.

Discussion: Ossification around the margins of medullary infarcts occurs after revascularization and repair. Bone repair occurs as a process of creeping substitution, and the sclerotic margin represents the portion being repaired. New bone is layered on the infarcted trabeculae, which are then removed very slowly and replaced by living bone. This process is generally too slow to observe progression on serial radiographs. Complications related to bone infarction include subchondral collapse, secondary osteoarthrosis and related sequelae, and the rare development of sarcomas such as osteosarcoma or MFH [25].

Clinical History: 30-year-old woman with history of lymphoma.

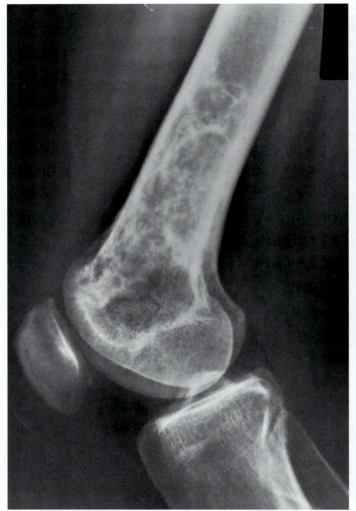

Figure 6-17   A

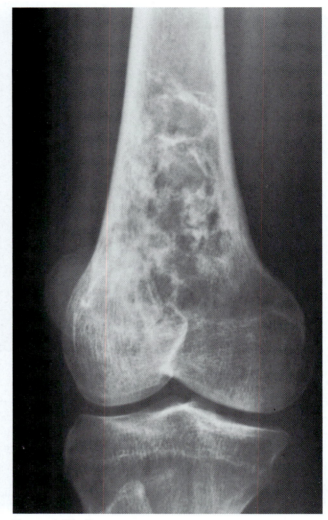

Figure 6-17   B

Findings: Lateral and AP radiographs of the knee. There are sclerotic and cystic-appearing changes in distal femoral metaphysis. The trabecular pattern appears coarsened. There is no cortical destruction, periosteal reactive bone, or soft tissue involvement.

Differential Diagnosis: Radiation changes, marrow infarcts, Paget's disease, metastases, osteosarcoma, lymphoma, infection.

Diagnosis: Radiation changes.

Discussion: A mixed lytic and sclerotic pattern may be seen in Paget's disease, metastases, certain primary bone tumors, infection, and radiation. There is no cortical thickening, however, making Paget's disease less likely. There is no cortical destruction to suggest tumor or infection.

Therapeutic irradiation is a common treatment for osseous metastases. Sites of bone pain confirmed as abnormal by radiographs or bone scan in patients with known metastases are often radiated as palliative treatment. Irradiated osseous lesions heal by sclerosis and filling in of lytic areas. Radiation effects are independent of the source of the radiation. In the immature skeleton, radiation in total doses of 2,000 cGy or more impairs bone growth. The epiphysis is particularly sensitive, since radiation causes direct cellular injury to chondrocytes, and possibly vascular damage to fine physeal blood vessels. The greater the growth potential at the time of irradiation, the more profound the effect. If an entire growing bone is irradiated, loss of bone growth in the whole bone results in a small bone. Focal doses affect the irradiated portion; for example, angular deformities could result from an asymmetrically irradiated growth plate. Radiotherapy also increases the risk for epiphyseal plate trauma, including the occurrence of slipped capital femoral epiphysis and avascular necrosis. Scoliosis may follow irradiation of the spine.

In the mature skeleton, the primary complication is radiation osteonecrosis. This is a dose-related effect and occurs due to effects on osteoblasts. The mandible is a common site in the jaw, and occurs more frequently after treatment for oral cancers as opposed to other head and neck tumors [26]. Treatment of radiation-induced osteonecrosis with hyperbaric oxygen may be of benefit [27]. Radiographs and CT will show irregular sclerosis in the irradiated bone. Radiation osteitis shows predominantly sclerosis and periostitis, and predisposes the patient to ischemic necrosis, infection, and fracture.

On bone scan, irradiated bone may initially show increased radionuclide accumulation from hyperemia and new bone formation. After several weeks or months, the bone scan will show decreased radionuclide accumulation due to decreased bone formation and decreased vascularity. On MRI, irradiated bone has the signal characteristics of fatty marrow. The anatomic location and extent of these changes conforms to the size and shape of the radiation portal.

Clinical History: Adult woman with grating sensation in knee.

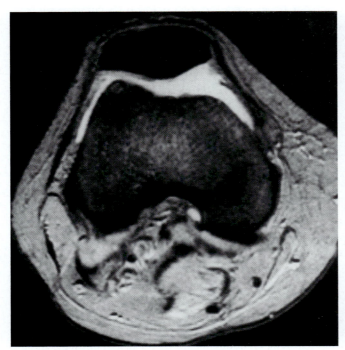

Figure 6-18   A

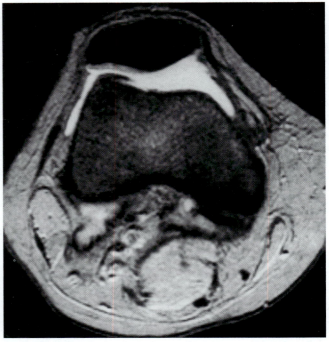

Figure 6-18   B

Findings: (A, B) Axial T2-weighted MRI demonstrates a deficiency of the articular cartilage along the medial patellar facet.

Differential Diagnosis: None.

Diagnosis: Chondromalacia patellae.

Discussion: Chondromalacia patellae refers to patellar cartilage damage causing pain. Many different staging methods have been proposed. A method described by Outerbridge [28] is commonly used.

• Stage 1: Softening or swelling of the cartilage, seen as signal intensity changes on MRI.

• Stage 2: Fragmentation or fissuring of the cartilage measuring half an inch or less.
• Stage 3: Fragmentation or fissuring of the cartilage measuring greater than half an inch.
• Stage 4: Full thickness cartilage loss.

Changes in the subchondral bone may be seen. MRI and arthroscopy correlation is better with higher stages [29]. The medial facet, as seen this case, is a common location [30]. Causes include patellar tracking disorders and trauma.

CASE 6-19

Clinical History: 55-year-old woman with knee pain.

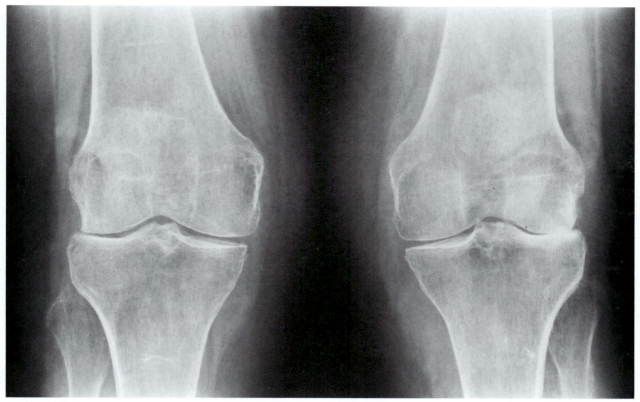

Figure 6-19

Findings: AP standing radiograph of both knees. The bones are osteoporotic. Uniform joint space loss is present with minimal proliferative bone changes. Some secondary osteoarthritic changes are present in the lateral compartment of the left knee, but these are rather modest compared to the amount of joint space loss.

Differential Diagnosis: Rheumatoid arthritis, osteoarthritis, pyrophosphate arthropathy.

Diagnosis: Rheumatoid arthritis.

Discussion: This case shows features of systemic inflammatory arthritis, with uniform cartilage space loss and osteoporosis. The presence of subchondral sclerosis and modest osteophyte formation is indicative of secondary degenerative changes, a common feature in rheumatoid arthritis that involves the hips and knees.

Rheumatoid arthritis is a systemic autoimmune disease manifested in the musculoskeletal system by inflammatory polyarthritis of the small synovial joints. The pathogenesis is not understood and no causative agent has been proven. Genetic factors affect the susceptibility to, and expression of, the disease. Rheumatoid arthritis is generally distinguished from other arthritides by the presence of rheumatoid factor

(RF) in the serum. Rheumatoid arthritis has a prevalence of 1% in the general population, with women affected more often than men by a ratio of 3:1. High RF titers often correlate with more severe disease.

The typical age of presentation is 25 to 55 years old. In 70% of cases the onset is insidious and occurs over weeks to months, in 20% of cases the onset occurs over days to weeks, and in 10% of cases the onset is acute and occurs over hours to days. The acute onset mimics the onset of septic arthritis. The clinical course of rheumatoid arthritis is progressive in 70% of cases, leading to disabling, destructive disease. The clinical progression may be rapid or slow. In 20% of cases the disease is intermittent, with remissions generally lasting longer than exacerbations, but in 10% of cases the remissions last several years. The clinical diagnosis is based on criteria that include morning stiffness; symmetric swelling of the proximal interphalangeal, metacarpophalangeal, or wrist joints; rheumatoid nodules; serum RF; and specific radiographic findings. In the knee, the typical inflammatory changes are commonly superimposed on secondary degenerative changes, but the proliferative bone response tends to be disproportionately modest in comparison to the loss of joint space.

CASE 6-20

Clinical History: 37-year-old man with chronically swollen knee.

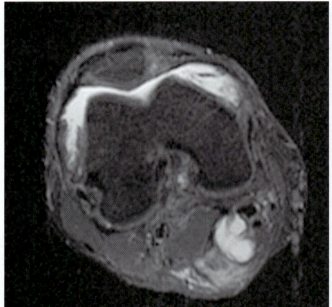

Figure 6-20   A

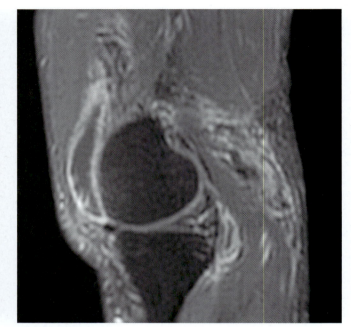

Figure 6-20   B

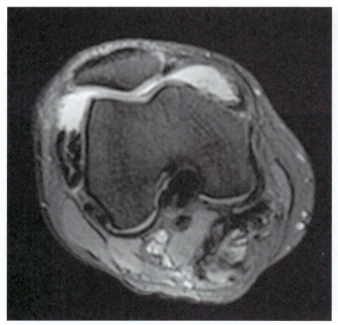

Figure 6-20   C

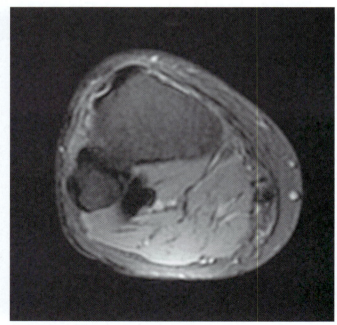

Figure 6-20   D

Findings: (**A**) Axial T2-weighted MRI shows a large effusion and a Baker's cyst. The synovium is thickened, particularly in the lateral aspect. (**B**) Sagittal T1-weighted, fat-saturated, post-gadolinium MRI shows synovial enhancement. (**C**) Axial T2*-weighted gradient-recalled echo (GRE) MRI shows low signal blooming of portions of the synovium, corresponding to the regions of synovial thickening seen on the T2-weighted MRI. (**D**) Axial T2*-weighted GRE MRI shows the abnormality extending into the proximal tibial-fibular joint.

Differential Diagnosis: Pigmented villonodular synovitis (PVNS), hemophilia, synovial hemangiomatosis.

Diagnosis: Pigmented villonodular synovitis, diffuse form.

Discussion: The knee is the most common location for PVNS. It may present in diffuse or localized (nodular) forms. The differential diagnosis includes other causes of synovial hemosiderin deposition, but these can be easily dismissed in this case. Hemophilia causes a degenerative arthropathy that should be advanced by adulthood, which is not seen here. The slow-flowing, blood-filled venous spaces of synovial hemangiomatosis should be evident, but are absent here as well [31]. A degenerative arthropathy that resembles hemophilia has also been described in synovial hemangiomatosis [32]. PVNS does not generally cause bony erosions in the knee because it has a loose joint capsule, unlike most other joints where erosions are common. Hemosiderin depositions are particularly evident on T2*-weighted GRE MRI.

Clinical History: 8-year-old boy with swollen knee (his other joints feel fine), and a companion case.

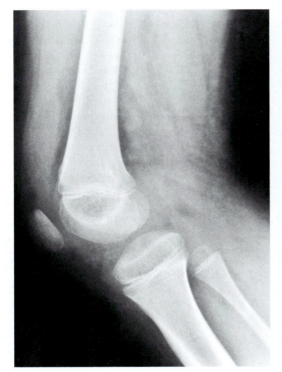

Figure 6-21   A

Figure 6-21   B

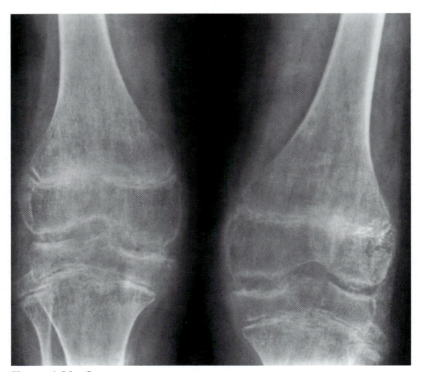

Figure 6-21   C

Findings: (A, B) Lateral and AP radiographs of the knee show effusion only. (C) Companion case: boy with the same disease for 2 years. AP radiograph of both knees shows profound osteopenia. The epiphyses are symmetrically overgrown, and irregularity of the subchondral bone is present.

Differential Diagnosis: Juvenile idiopathic arthritis, hemophilia, trauma, infection.

Diagnosis: Juvenile idiopathic arthritis.

Discussion: The findings in this case, a monoarticular arthritis of a large joint in a child manifested by effusion, represent the initial presentation of juvenile idiopathic arthritis and are entirely nonspecific. The differential diagnosis would include trauma and infection, as well as systemic disease such as juvenile idiopathic arthritis and hemophilia. The companion case shows the same disease process at a more advanced stage, where the systemic nature of the condition is evident in the bilateral symmetric involvement of both knees. Also evident is the superimposition of inflammatory arthritis on growing joints.

Juvenile idiopathic arthritis has formerly been referred to as juvenile chronic arthritis and juvenile rheumatoid arthritis [33,34]. Unlike adult rheumatoid arthritis, juvenile idiopathic arthritis has a predilection for large joints. Because the disease has its onset in the skeletally immature child, growth disturbances are typically present, as either overgrowth or undergrowth. If hyperemia is the predominant effect, as is typically the case in the knees, overgrowth of the femoral condyles and proximal tibia occurs and is recognized radiographically by disproportionate enlargement of the ends of the bones at the knee as compared with the widths of the femoral and tibial shafts. If erosion of cartilage by inflammatory pannus and consequent epiphyseal destruction is the predominant effect, undergrowth occurs. A common location for undergrowth is the distal ulna, resulting in ulnar minus variance.

Clinical History: 18-year-old man with chronic disease and short stature, and a companion case.

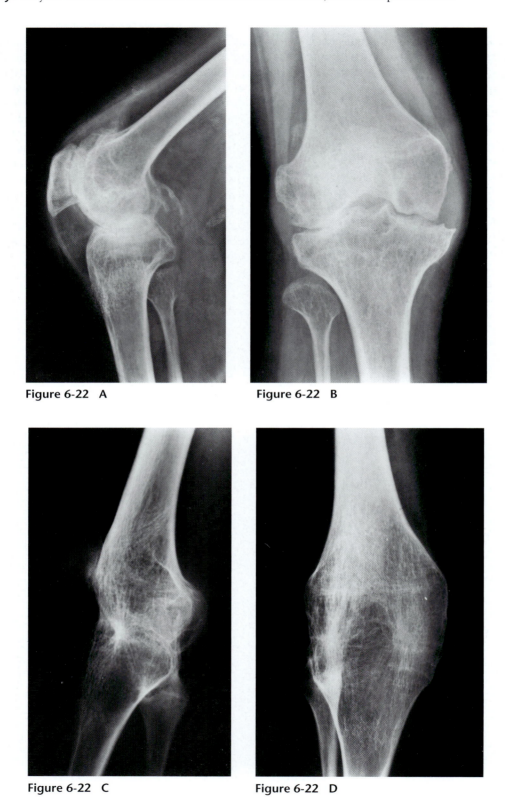

Figure 6-22   A

Figure 6-22   B

Figure 6-22   C

Figure 6-22   D

Findings: (A, B) Lateral and AP radiographs of the knee. There is marked overgrowth of the femoral epiphysis, tibial epiphysis, fibular epiphysis, and patella. There is osteoporosis. The cartilage spaces are narrowed diffusely, and there is subchondral sclerosis and irregularity of all the articular surfaces. The musculature is atrophic, and there is a small effusion. (C, D) Companion case. Lateral and AP radiographs of the knee. There is ankylosis of the joint, with remodeled trabecular bone flowing continuously across the site of the joint. Diffuse osteoporosis is present.

Differential Diagnosis: Juvenile idiopathic arthritis, hemophilia, septic arthritis.

Diagnosis: Juvenile idiopathic arthritis.

Discussion: In this case, the stigmata of inflammatory joint disease in the growing skeleton—marked overgrowth from prolonged hyperemia—are present. Diffuse cartilage loss is a result of the inflammatory joint disease itself, and early secondary degenerative change follows. Osteoporosis and muscular atrophy may result from hyperemia, chronic disease, and disuse, but they may also result from the systemic corticosteroids used to treat the disease. Other skeletal complications of treatment include osteonecrosis and insufficiency fractures.

The companion case shows one of the end-stage sequela of juvenile idiopathic arthritis: bony ankylosis. Bony ankylosis is a common characteristic of end-stage juvenile idiopathic arthritis, but it is very unusual in adult-onset rheumatoid arthritis. Other findings, similar to conventional adult-onset rheumatoid arthritis, are not uncommon, including bursal cyst formation, subchondral cysts, muscle and ligamentous atrophy, cortical erosions at capsular attachment sites, protrusio acetabuli, and soft tissue swelling.

Clinical History: 81-year-old woman with swollen, painful knees.

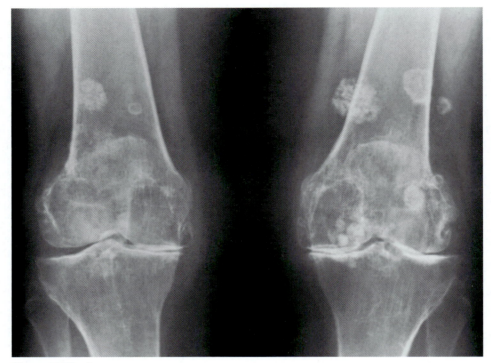

Figure 6-23   A

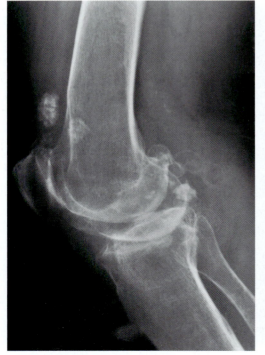

Figure 6-23   B

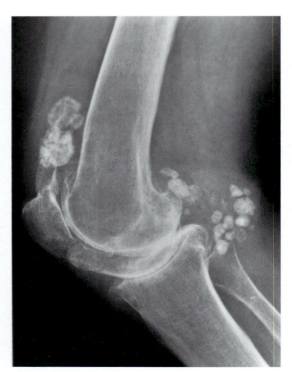

Figure 6-23   C

Findings: (A) AP and (B–C) lateral radiographs of both knees. There are multiple round, dense, loose bodies within the joint, with a lamellated appearance. Both knees show degenerative changes, with asymmetric joint space narrowing, subchondral sclerosis, and osteophyte formation.

Differential Diagnosis: Primary or secondary synovial osteochondromatosis, trauma.

Diagnosis: Secondary synovial osteochondromatosis.

Discussion: The presence of bilateral calcified loose bodies in the setting of osteoarthritis suggests secondary synovial osteochondromatosis. In this circumstance, fragments of bone and cartilage from the margins of the articular surfaces where osteophyte formation occurs become detached. Loose in the joint capsule, the cartilaginous portions may continue to grow. Other preexisting articular derangements that may be associated with secondary osteochondromatosis include avascular necrosis, osteochondritis dissecans, neuropathic arthropathy, trauma, and rheumatoid arthritis [35]. Bursal synovial osteochondromatosis has been reported to develop secondary to underlying osteochondromas [36]. In the secondary form, loose bodies tend to be highly variable in size and relatively few in number, as in this case.

Primary synovial osteochondromatosis occurs by synovial metaplasia that gives rise to cartilaginous bodies that frequently calcify. The loose bodies tend to be more or less uniform in size and are typically present in large numbers. The process evolves in stages, from synovial metaplasia to synovial metaplasia with intraarticular bodies. In the inactive stage, bodies are present without synovial metaplasia [37]. The knees and hips are sites of predilection, and typically only one joint is involved. Although principally an intraarticular process, bursal and tenosynovial forms have been documented [38,39].

Plain films fail to show calcification in 5% to 30% of cases [40]. Adjacent bone erosions may occur, and CT may demonstrate these latter findings to better advantage. Early on, the joint space may be enlarged. Later, secondary degenerative changes may predominate, causing joint space narrowing. Clinical symptoms include limitation of motion and pain. After resection, recurrences may occur, and rare instances of malignant transformation to chondrosarcoma have been described [41]. With the intraarticular form, men are affected twice as often as women, whereas the extraarticular variety displays no sex predilection.

Clinical History: 56-year-old man with recurrent episodes of knee pain, and a companion case.

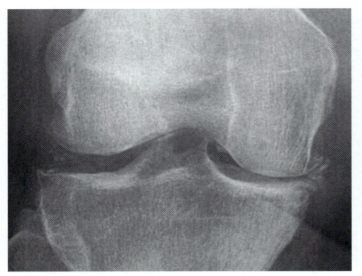

Figure 6-24   A

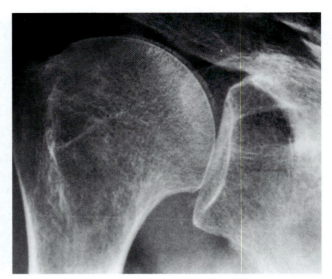

Figure 6-24   B

Findings: (A) Knee radiograph shows chondrocalcinosis of the medial and lateral menisci. Chondrocalcinosis of the articular cartilage is also evident, particularly in the femur. Medial joint space narrowing and osteophyte formation are present. (B) Companion case. AP radiograph of the shoulder shows chondrocalcinosis of the articular cartilage of the humerus.

Differential Diagnosis: None.

Diagnosis: Calcium pyrophosphate dihydrate (CPPD) crystal deposition disease.

Discussion: CPPD crystal deposition disease is a polyarticular arthritis with deposition of CPPD crystals in articular tissues. Its initial presentation may be monoarticular. The definitive clinical diagnosis requires the identification of CPPD crystals from joint fluid, but the radiologic findings can be diagnostic. CPPD deposition disease has been associated with hyperparathyroidism, hemochromatosis, aging, and osteoarthritis. It has been weakly associated with hypothyroidism, ochronosis, Paget's disease, Wilson's disease, acromegaly, diabetes, and gout. CPPD crystal deposition disease has three manifestations: chondrocalcinosis, crystal-induced synovitis, and pyrophosphate arthropathy.

CPPD crystals are generated locally in the articular tissues, where asymptomatic deposits may accumulate in cartilage, joint capsules, intervertebral discs, tendons, and ligaments. In cartilage, these deposits may be evident radiographically as chondrocalcinosis. Chondrocalcinosis is most common in the knees, wrists, elbows, and hips. It is found in both fibrocartilage and hyaline cartilage.

Shedding of crystals into the joint space after rupture of a deposit causes an acute, self-limited, crystal-induced synovitis. This acute synovitis is clinically similar to acute gouty arthritis and has been known as pseudogout. As with gouty arthritis, acute episodes of inflammatory synovitis may recur intermittently. During an acute episode, CPPD crystals can be recovered by joint aspiration and identified by polarized light microscopy or more definitive physical means. Uncommonly, these episodes can run together into a subacute or chronic crystal synovitis that resembles rheumatoid arthritis, except the large joints of the limbs tend to be involved, rather than the small joints of the hands and feet.

CASE 6-25

Clinical History: 43-year-old woman with recurrent episodes of knee pain.

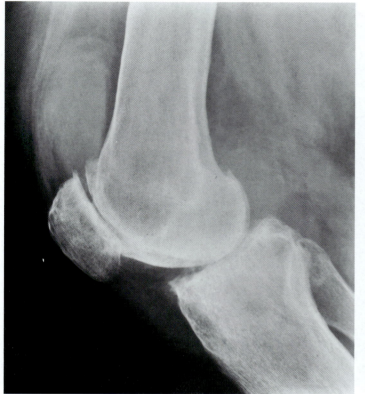

Figure 6-25   A

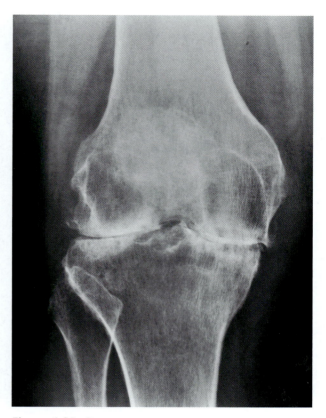

Figure 6-25   B

Findings: Lateral and AP radiographs of the knee show a large joint effusion. There is uniform loss of the cartilage space in both medial and lateral compartments, subchondral sclerosis, osteophyte formation, and subchondral cyst formation. The overall mineralization of the bones is normal. Involvement of the medial, lateral, and patellofemoral compartments is more or less symmetric.

Differential Diagnosis: Primary or secondary osteoarthritis, pyrophosphate arthropathy, rheumatoid arthritis.

Diagnosis: Pyrophosphate arthropathy.

Discussion: Pyrophosphate arthropathy refers to the pattern of degenerative joint disease resulting from CPPD crystal deposition disease [42]. Deposition of CPPD crystals in the cartilage (chondrocalcinosis) and recurrent episodes of crystal-induced inflammatory arthritis leads to degenerative joint disease. Unlike primary osteoarthritis, pyrophosphate arthropathy of the knee typically involves medial, lateral, and patellofemoral joint compartments uniformly. Hypertrophic bone changes tend to be florid, with extensive subchondral sclerosis, prominent osteophyte formation, and subchondral cyst formation. Fragmentation resembling neuropathic arthropathy may occur. Involvement is often not bilaterally symmetric. Because chondrocalcinosis will not be present in advanced pyrophosphate arthropathy (cartilage will have been destroyed), the radiographic differential diagnosis of three-compartment degenerative change at the knee is primary osteoarthritis, or secondary osteoarthritis after inflammatory arthritis such as infection.

Clinical History: 44-year-old man who is wheelchair-bound.

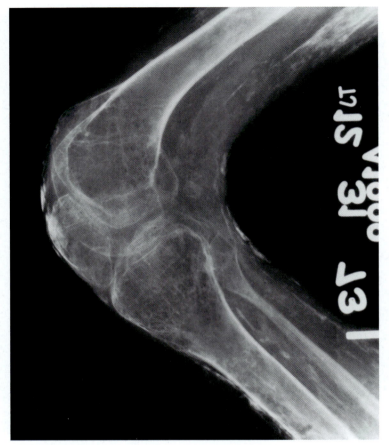

Figure 6-26

Findings: Lateral radiograph of the knee shows soft tissue calcification, soft tissue atrophy, and osteoporosis. A flexion contracture is present.

Differential Diagnosis: Dermatomyositis, polymyositis, scleroderma, burns.

Diagnosis: Dermatomyositis.

Discussion: Dermatomyositis and polymyositis are diseases of unknown etiology, thought to occur on an autoimmune basis, affecting striated muscle by diffuse, nonsuppurative inflammation and degeneration. The pathogenesis involves an autoimmune mechanism. There may be some overlap with other collagen vascular disorders, which is considered as a specific subtype of polymyositis and is most notable in Sjögren's syndrome. In dermatomyositis, the skin is also involved. Multiple clinical classifications are based on various features, particularly progressive muscle weakness and rash. There is an associated risk of malignancy in patients with dermatomyositis who are older than 40, particularly men. The diagnosis is made by serum enzyme studies, electromyogra-phy, and muscle biopsy. MRI may be more sensitive, although less specific, than biopsy [43,44].

Early on, manifestations include deep and superficial soft tissue edema. The process may be halted with treatment or may progress to further changes. This will show increased signal intensity on T2-weighted images, and short-tau inversion recovery pulse sequences with MRI. Later stages are characterized by muscle atrophy and fibrosis. Although not common, articular abnormalities may also be seen. The characteristic radiographic abnormality is widespread soft tissue calcification, particularly of intermuscular fascial planes between large proximal limb muscles. There may be subcutaneous calcifications similar to those in scleroderma. Bone scanning may detect uptake of radionuclide.

Location and distribution may help differentiate this entity from other forms of autoimmune myopathies. Changes in dermatomyositis are typically symmetric in a proximal distribution, with particular predilection for the vasti, glutei, adductors, and hamstrings [45,46].

Clinical History: 6-year-old boy with leg-length discrepancy.

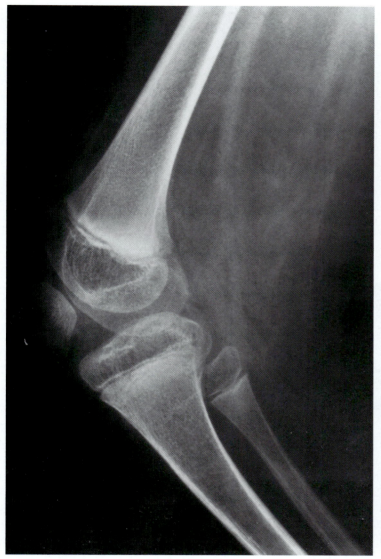

Figure 6-27   A

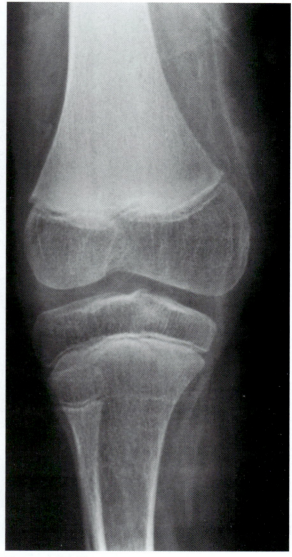

Figure 6-27   B

Findings: Lateral and AP radiographs of the right knee demonstrate osteopenia with atrophy of the soft tissues. The diaphyses are gracile. No articular erosions or joint space narrowing is identified.

Differential Diagnosis: Poliomyelitis, paralysis (from any cause), osteogenesis imperfecta.

Diagnosis: Poliomyelitis.

Discussion: Poliomyelitis is a viral infection that causes acute flaccid paralysis. Once a common childhood epidemic disease of worldwide proportions, endemic polio has been eliminated from the Western Hemisphere since 1991. Global eradication is considered feasible, but the disease remains endemic in Afghanistan and Pakistan [47]. Many patients who have recovered from poliomyelitis will continue to present with musculoskeletal sequela. Poliomyelitis classically demonstrates unilateral hypoplasia of the lower extremity. There is atrophy of the surrounding muscles with fatty infiltration. Other skeletal manifestations are clubfoot, hip dislocations, and scoliosis. Postpoliomyelitis syndrome is a weakness described in patients who have been recovered from their initial paralysis for 10 to 15 years; the knee is a particularly symptomatic joint in this condition [48].

Clinical History: 89-year-old man with knee pain.

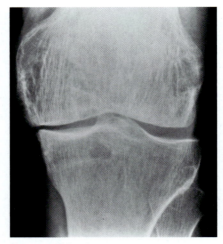

Figure 6-28 A

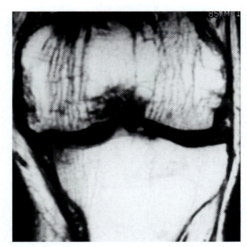

Figure 6-28 B

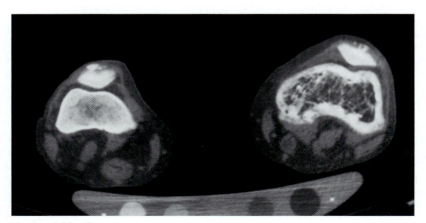

Figure 6-28 C

Findings: (A) AP radiograph of the knee demonstrates coarsening of the vertical trabecular pattern, with obliteration of the intercondylar notch. (B) Coronal T1-weighted MRI of the knee shows enlargement of the entire distal femur. The trabecular bone pattern is prominent and outlined by the bright signal of the fatty marrow. Degenerative changes are present in the medial compartment of the knee. (C) Axial CT shows enlargement of the involved distal femur compared to the opposite side. The cortical thickening is quite striking.

Differential Diagnosis: None.

Diagnosis: Paget's disease of the femur, with secondary osteoarthritis.

Discussion: Paget's disease (osteitis deformans) is a bone disease seen in middle-aged and elderly individuals. It is characterized by excessive and abnormal remodeling of bone. Usually asymptomatic, Paget's disease has a prevalence of 3% in the adult population older than 40. In most cases, involvement is polyostotic. Although any bone may be involved, the majority of cases involve the pelvis, spine, skull, femur, or tibia.

Current evidence suggests that Paget's disease is a slowly developing viral infection of osteoclasts. The disease has active and quiescent (inactive) phases. The active phase begins with a focus of excessive osteoclastic activity, resulting in a localized area of osteolysis where bone is replaced by nonossified fibrovascular tissue. The demarcation between normal uninvolved bone and the area of osteolysis is typically quite sharp. Subsequently, the areas of osteolysis are filled in with pagetoid bone, even as the osteoclastic activity continues. Pagetoid bone consists of layers of disorganized woven bone separated by resorption cavities and nonossified fibrovascular tissue. Bone is formed both endosteally and periosteally. The combination of osteoclastic and osteoblastic activity results in rapid remodeling and turnover of bone. Eventually, for unknown reasons, the osteoclastic activity moderates and, after the osteolytic areas have filled with bone, the rate of bone turnover decreases. With the decrease in turnover, the bone enters the quiescent phase of Paget's disease. Focal areas of pagetoid bone may be replaced by islands of lamellar bone, but haversian systems and remodeling along lines of stress does not occur. Slow endosteal and periosteal apposition of bone may continue to thicken the cortex and enlarge the bone, sometimes obliterating the marrow space.

Paget's disease involving subchondral bone is thought to result in accelerated osteoarthritis in the adjacent joint [49], although the magnitude of the association is uncertain [50]. Biomechanical modification of the articular surface is thought to be the pathogenesis of the early joint degeneration. Insufficiency microfractures of the subchondral bone may also contribute, as pagetoid bone does not remodel along lines of stress and is weaker than normal bone.

Clinical History: 40-year-old man twisted knee and fell.

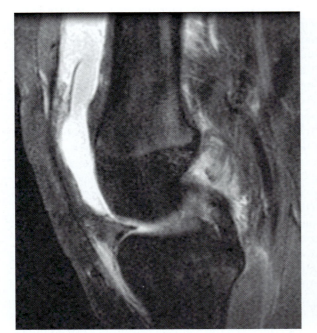

Figure 6-29 A

Figure 6-29   B

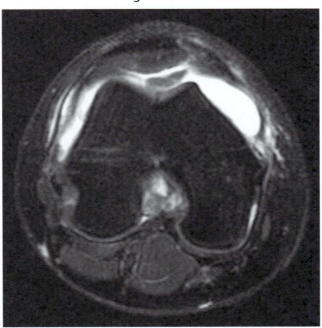

Figure 6-29   C

Findings: Sagittal proton-density (**A**), coronal T1-weighted (**B**), and axial T2-weighted fat-suppressed (**C**) MRI of the knee shows intermediate intensity material within the intercondylar notch. The sagittal image shows no normal anterior cruciate ligament (ACL) fibers. Coronal images also demonstrate no definitive ACL fibers within the intercondylar notch adjacent to the posterior cruciate ligament. This is known as the empty notch sign. Axial images show a normal posterior cruciate ligament with no normal ACL fibers visualized.

Differential Diagnosis: None.

Diagnosis: Full thickness anterior cruciate ligament tear.

Discussion: The ACL is a straight, predominantly low-signal ligament which fans distally as it attaches to the anterior tibial plateau. Usually when there is a complete tear of the ACL, it is simply not visualized. ACL tears are mechanically caused from a valgus force with a rotatory motion resulting in anteromedial rotary instability. Most commonly, ACL tears occur at its proximal femoral attachment; however, they may also occur at its midportion, and rarely at its distal tibial attachment. Characteristic bone bruise pattern includes marrow edema at the posterolateral tibial plateau and the mid-portion of the lateral femoral condyle [51]. An important associated condition is the Segond fracture [52]. This fracture is an avulsion fracture of the lateral tibial plateau at the insertion of the meniscotibial portion of the lateral capsular ligament.

Clinical History: 15-year-old adolescent boy injured playing sports.

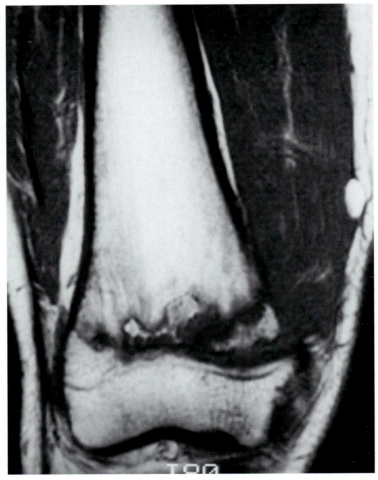

Figure 6-30

Findings: Coronal T1-weighted MRI demonstrates widening of the medial growth plate of the distal femur with low-density material, and continuation with linear extension into the medial femoral metaphysis.

Differential Diagnosis: None.

Diagnosis: Salter type II fracture.

Discussion: Growth plate injuries have been categorized into five basic types in the Salter-Harris system.

- Type I Salter injuries are noted radiographically by widening of the growth plate and soft tissue swelling. The injury is usually by a shearing mechanism through the zone of hypertrophy. These typically occur in children less than 5 years old.
- Type II Salter injuries are the most common type, typically occurring at the end of long bones. Avulsion of the

growth plate occurs with the line of fracture then extending through the metaphysis, as seen here. The prognosis for these injuries is good.

- Type III Salter injuries involve a vertical component through the epiphysis and growth plate, and separation of the growth plate with sparing of the adjacent metaphysis.
- Type IV Salter injuries are similar to type III, but also disrupt the underlying metaphysis.
- Type V Salter injuries constitute isolated compression of the growth plate. As a result of these injuries to the growth plate, physeal bars may form and interfere with subsequent growth in that location. This complication is generally more common with higher level Salter injuries.

MRI may demonstrate a different Salter-Harris class of injury than radiography in up to 50% of cases of physeal trauma [53].

CASE 6-31

Clinical History: 78-year-old woman with knee pain.

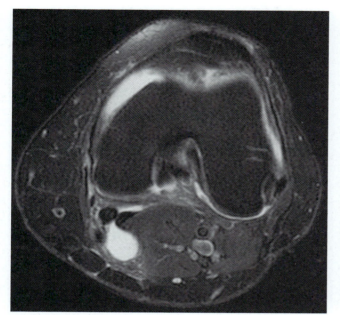

Figure 6-31   A

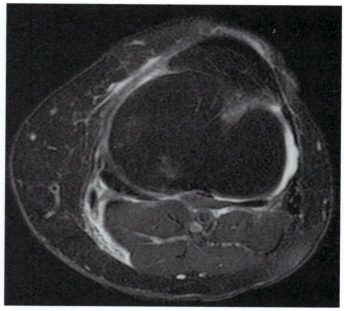

Figure 6-31   B

Findings: Axial T2-weighted MRI demonstrates a small joint effusion, with fluid tracking between the semimembranosus and medial head of the gastrocnemius. The second image demonstrates fluid tracking in the medial fascial plane, distal to this collection.

Differential Diagnosis: Ruptured Baker's cyst, thrombophlebitis, cellulitis, fasciitis, myositis.

Diagnosis: Ruptured Baker's cyst.

Discussion: An outpouching of synovial lining into a bursa causes a Baker's cyst. The most common location for its occurrence is in the semimembranosus-gastrocnemius bursa. It is classically situated, as seen here, between the semimembranosus tendon and the medial head of the gastrocnemius muscle group. The neck of the cyst can frequently be seen on MRI, confirming communication with the joint space. Popliteal cysts can be readily detected with ultrasound or MRI, showing a smooth, thin-walled collection of fluid that may contain septations, synovial tissues, or loose bodies. The point of communication may become constricted or oblit-

erated, and a clear communication with the joint may not be demonstrated. Inflammatory conditions such as rheumatoid arthritis and osteoarthritis are common predisposing factors. Ligamentous and meniscal tears, chronic effusions, and increased age are other associations.

Sometimes, as in this case, the cyst may rupture and a well-defined collection may not be appreciated. Fluid in these cases may be detected in the bursa and adjacent interstitial tissues. Fluid can track extensively along the fascial planes, usually coursing inferiorly due to the effects of gravity. The primary differential diagnosis for an unruptured popliteal cyst is ganglion cyst. These are usually related to the cruciate ligaments, more often the PCL than the ACL [61]. The main distinguishing feature for a popliteal cyst is its predilection for the semimembranosus-gastrocnemius bursa. A ruptured cyst shows edema in the medial soft tissues, which can be seen with trauma; however, the preponderance of fluid coupled with the absence of bone bruises or muscle/ligamentous injury suggests that this process originated in the bursa and favors the diagnosis of Baker's cyst.

Clinical History: 28-year-old woman with severe knee pain and swelling after a fall.

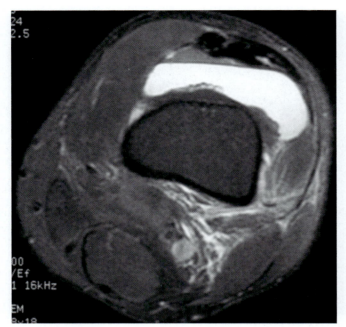

Figure 6-32   A

Figure 6-32   B

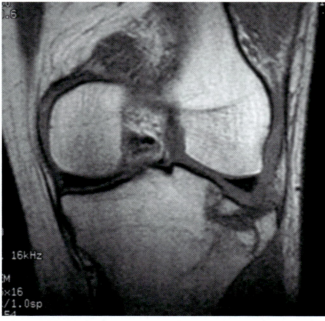

Figure 6-32   C

Findings: (A) Axial T2-weighted MRI of the knee at the level of the suprapatellar recess shows a large effusion distending the suprapatellar recess. Fluid-fluid levels are present extending horizontally across the recess, with fluid of suppressed signal intensity layered on fluid of very high signal intensity. (B) Axial T2-weighted MRI of the knee at the level of the patella shows a large effusion with a horizontal serum-sediment level. (C) Coronal T1-weighted MRI shows a depressed lateral tibial plateau fracture.

Differential Diagnosis: None.

Diagnosis: Depressed lateral tibial plateau fracture with lipohemarthrosis.

Discussion: Tibial plateau fractures are the result of compressive loading of the tibia. Approximately 76% of cases involve the lateral tibial plateau alone, 11% involve the medial condyle alone, 10% involve both condyles, and 3% of cases involve the posterior margin. Lipohemarthrosis is a manifestation of an intraarticular fracture and, at the knee, most commonly occurs with fractures of the tibial plateau.

Traumatic disruption of the cortex allows liquid marrow to extrude into the joint, where it layers on top of blood because of its lesser density. A second fluid-fluid level may be seen as the cellular elements of blood sediment dependently and separate from the serum, but this is not evident in this case.

A linear demarcation between fat and blood may be seen on the radiograph if the exposure was made with a horizontal beam. Because the suprapatellar recess is the most anterior part of a distended knee joint capsule when the knee is extended, the fat will collect in that specific location. On MRI, a similar demarcation is seen as a fluid-fluid level, with the fatty component occupying the nondependent portion of the joint capsule. The fatty layer should follow the signal characteristics of marrow fat or subcutaneous fat on various imaging parameters. Chemical shift artifact, seen here as a dark line between the fat and the blood, may enhance the separation. The distinction is made most easily on sagittal or axial images. Only one-third of intraarticular fractures of the knee will be associated with a lipohemarthrosis.

Clinical History: 25-year-old man with knee injury.

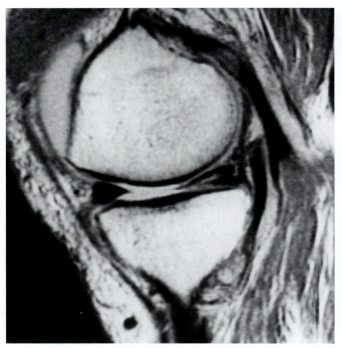

Figure 6-33 A

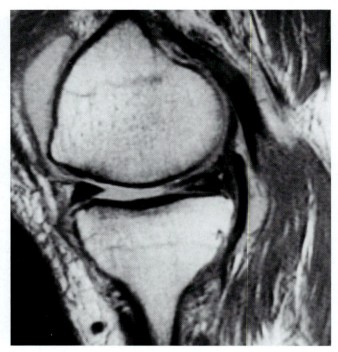

Figure 6-33 B

Findings: Sagittal proton-density MRI of the knee through the medial compartment. The posterior horn of the medial meniscus has a band of high signal extending horizontally and obliquely to the inferior articular surface. The anterior horn is normal. There is a large effusion.

Differential Diagnosis: Meniscal tear, meniscal degeneration.

Diagnosis: Medial meniscal tear, posterior horn.

Discussion: On MRI, the normal menisci and ligaments are visualized as low-signal structures. Meniscal tears are evident as high-signal regions on T1-weighted or proton-density MRI that involves an articular margin. Gross distortions of meniscal shape or intrameniscal fluid collections indicate meniscal tears with displaced fragments. Torn meniscal fragments can interfere with motion, causing locking, and may erode the articular cartilage, leading to early degenerative arthritis. Acute traumatic meniscal tears generally occur in young people when the meniscus is compressed between the femoral condyle and tibial plateau during crush and twisting injuries. In older individuals, degen-erative meniscal tears are thought to result from multiple subacute traumatic episodes that lead to chondrocyte death, increased mucinous ground substance (myxoid degeneration), and loss of mechanical integrity.

The appearance of increased intrameniscal signal intensity on MRI has been divided into three grades, with histologic correlation [54]. The normal meniscus has uniformly low signal intensity.

- In MRI grade 1, globular increased-signal-intensity region is present within the meniscus and corresponds histologically to early mucinous degeneration.
- In MRI grade 2, a horizontal, linear increased-signal-intensity region is present, without involvement of an articular surface, and corresponds to more advanced meniscal degeneration.
- In MRI grade 3, the increased-signal-intensity region communicates with at least one articular surface and corresponds to a tear; in 5% to 6% of these, the tears are considered intrasubstance cleavage tears and may not be visible on arthroscopy.

Clinical History: 35-year-old man with knee trauma, locking, and effusion.

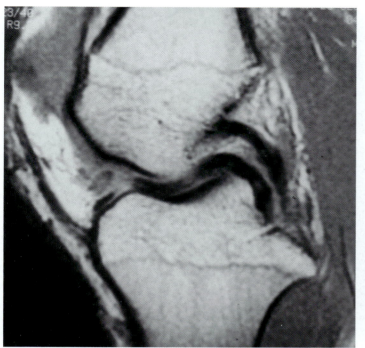

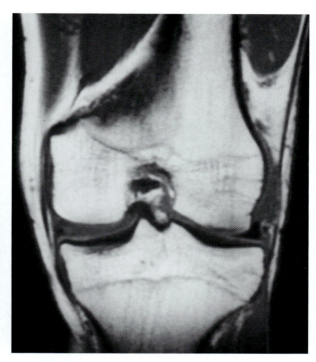

Figure 6-34   A

Figure 6-34   B

Findings: (A) Sagittal T1-weighted MRI demonstrates double posterior cruciate ligament (PCL) sign. (B) Coronal T1-weighted MRI demonstrates an extra density inferior to the ACL origin.

Differential Diagnosis: Tear of the ACL, bucket-handle tear of the meniscus.

Diagnosis: Bucket-handle tear.

Discussion: The differential diagnosis for the double PCL sign includes tear of the ACL and bucket-handle tear of the meniscus. The ACL in this case is intact.

Bucket-handle tears consist of vertical tears of the meniscus with translocation of the medial fragment. This is an unstable injury. The meniscal fragment generally demonstrates low signal intensity on all pulse sequences. When the medial fragment lies in the intercondylar region, it may parallel the course of the PCL, as seen here. Additional signs of a bucket-handle tear include an anteriorly flipped meniscal fragment, a fragment flipped into the intercondylar notch, and an absent bowtie on sagittal images [55].

Traumatic acute meniscal tears occur in younger patients, basically by a compressive mechanism at the femorotibial articulation. Acute traumatic meniscal tears generally occur in young people when the meniscus is compressed between the femoral condyles and tibial plateaus during crush and twisting injuries. In older individuals, degenerative meniscal tears are thought to result from multiple subacute traumatic episodes that lead to chondrocyte death, increased mucinous ground substance, and loss of mechanical integrity. MRI and arthroscopy dominate the workup for internal derangement of the knee. On MRI, the normal menisci and ligaments are visualized as low-signal structures. Meniscal tears are evident as high-signal regions on T1 or proton-density sequences that involve an articular margin. Gross distortions of meniscal shape or intrameniscal fluid collections indicate meniscal tears with displaced fragments.

Clinical History: 21-year-old woman with knee injury, and a companion case.

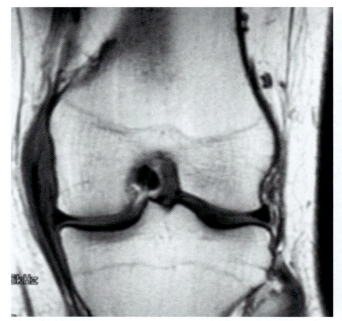

Figure 6-35   A

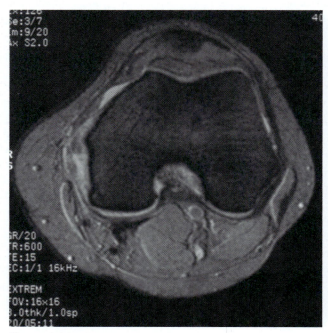

Figure 6-35   C

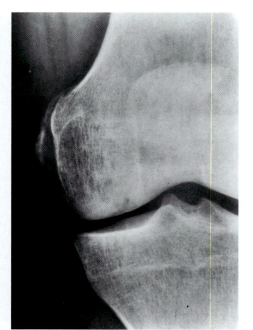

Figure 6-35   B

Figure 6-35   D

Findings: (**A, B**) Coronal T1-weighted and T2-weighted MRI shows hemorrhage in the medial collateral ligament (MCL), with tear through the proximal origin. Abnormal signal is present at the expected location of the ACL. (**C**) Axial T2-weighted MRI shows edema and hemorrhage at the medial aspect of the distal femur where the MCL should originate. (**D**) Companion case. Detail of AP radiograph of the knee demonstrates calcification of the proximal portion of the MCL.

Differential Diagnosis: None.

Diagnosis: Acute medial collateral ligament sprain. An ACL sprain is present. Not shown but also present was a tear of the posterior horn of the medial meniscus. The companion case is an old MCL sprain with heterotopic ossification (Pellegrini-Stieda disease).

Discussion: Injury of the collateral ligaments may be imaged directly with MRI, which has been demonstrated to have 87% accuracy in identifying these injuries [56]. Partial tears are thickened and edematous, and they may contain hemorrhage, whereas complete tears are discontinuous. The MCL is comprised of superficial and deep fibers, with the latter tenaciously fixed to the capsule and medial meniscus. This imparts a degree of rigidity to this structure, which renders it more susceptible to tears with associated injuries than its lateral counterpart. Valgus stress in flexion is a common mechanism for precipitating injury to the MCL. O'Donoghue's unhappy triad, present in this particular case, is a common set of associated injuries that consists of medial meniscal tear, ACL tear, and MCL disruption [57].

Conservative treatment is advocated for isolated tear of the MCL, whereas surgical treatment is recommended when associated injuries are present. The MCL may calcify as a sequela of trauma, which is radiographically detectable as a curvilinear density. Maturation with trabecular bone formation and frank ossification may occur, resulting in an appearance called Pellegrini-Stieda disease. Bone spurs at tendinous and ligamentous insertion sites, or enthesopathies, should be distinguished from this entity. Enthesophytes typically do not run the entire course of the ligament, and frequently occur at symmetric multiple sites in conjunction with an underlying condition such as spondyloarthropathy or diffuse idiopathic skeletal hyperostosis.

Clinical History: 58-year-old woman twisted knee while playing tennis.

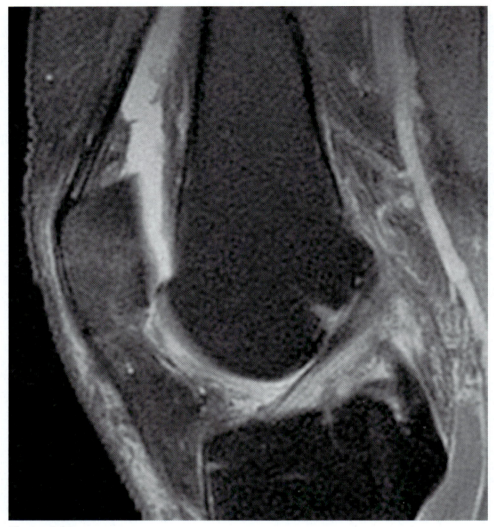

Figure 6-36

Findings: Sagittal proton-density fat-saturated MRI shows abnormal increased signal in the ACL. There is a moderate knee effusion.

Differential Diagnosis: None.

Diagnosis: Sprain (partial thickness tear) of the anterior cruciate ligament

Discussion: Because the ACL is active throughout the knee's range of motion, it can be injured by a variety of non-contact, deceleration, hyperextension, twisting, and pivoting mechanisms. The ACL is the most frequently injured knee ligament, and is commonly associated with medial meniscal tears, capsular tears, and transchondral impaction fractures. O'Donoghue's triad, a frequent association of injuries, consists of ACL tear, MCL tear, and medial meniscal tear [58,59]. Occasionally, loading of the ACL will result in an avulsion fracture of its insertion at the medial tibial spine. An avulsion fracture at the margin of the lateral tibial plateau where the knee capsule attaches (Segond fracture) is indicative of severe internal derangement, including ACL tear. PCL sprains are less common than ACL sprains by at least one-tenth. Trabecular microfractures (also called bone bruises) are seen on MRI as regions of localized edema, with intact overlying articular cartilage and subcortical bone. They occur from impaction trauma and are commonly associated with meniscal tears and ACL sprains.

Clinical History: 38-year-old woman with positive posterior drawer test after knee hitting dashboard in a recent motor vehicle accident.

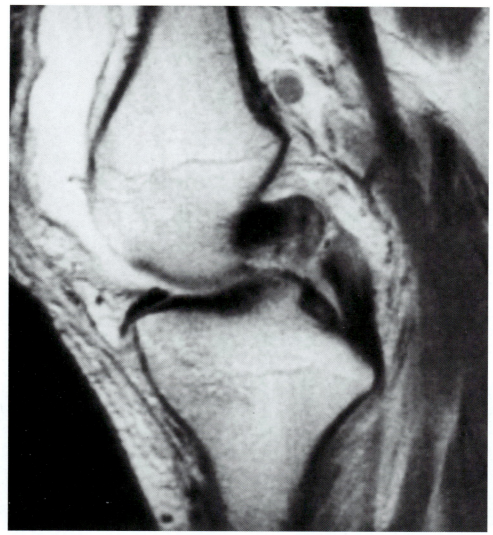

Figure 6-37

Findings: Sagittal T2-weighted MRI demonstrates focal discontinuity of the midportion of the PCL. A moderate joint effusion is present.

Differential Diagnosis: None.

Diagnosis: Posterior cruciate ligament tear.

Discussion: Acute PCL tear is characterized by increased signal intensity and disruption of the fibers of the PCL. The PCL is disrupted in its midsubstance in this instance, the most common location for its occurrence [60]. These tears are generally precipitated by hyperextension or a posterior impact during flexion. The posterior drawer sign in PCL tears refers to the posterior translation of the tibia relative to the femur seen with PCL disruption. The PCL is a much sturdier and thicker ligament than the ACL; therefore, PCL tears are often accompanied by other ligamentous and meniscal injuries, including ACL tears. As many as 50% of PCL sprains are isolated and are sustained in a dashboard injury or a fall directly on to a flexed knee. The remaining PCL sprains have complex mechanisms of injury and are associated with injuries of the ACL, MCL, medial meniscus, or other structures.

Clinical History: 77-year-old man with chronic knee pain.

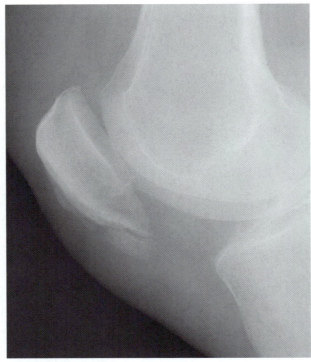

Figure 6-38   A

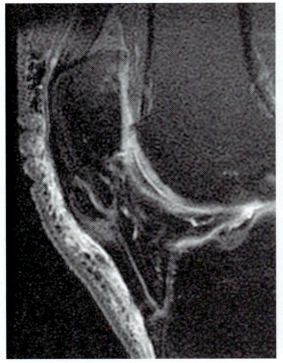

Figure 6-38   B

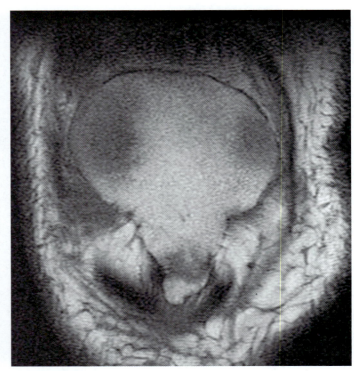

Figure 6-38   C

Findings: (A) Lateral radiograph of the anterior knee shows elongation and fragmentation of the patellar distal pole. (B) Sagittal proton-density, fat-suppressed MRI demonstrates the low-signal deformity of the patella. Increased signal in the proximal patellar tendon is likely due to magic angle artifact. (C) Coronal T1-weighted MRI shows the elongated distal patellar pole.

Differential Diagnosis: Chronic Sinding-Larsen-Johansson (SLJ) disease, old patellar fracture.

Diagnosis: Sinding-Larsen-Johansson disease.

Discussion: SLJ disease is an osteochondrosis of the distal patellar pole. This occurs as a result of repetitive traction microtrauma from the patellar tendon. SLJ is sometimes referred to as jumper's knee. Osgood-Schlatter disease is a similar entity located at the tibial tubercle. SLJ disease appears radiographically as fragmentation of the ossification center, with subsequent formation of separate bony fragments and elongation of the distal patellar pole. On MRI and ultrasound, soft tissue swelling, patellar tendon edema, and bursitis can be seen, in addition to the fragmented ossification center [62]. This is a self-limited process that requires no treatment [63].

Clinical History: 17-year-old adolescent boy with chronic knee pain following injury, and a companion case.

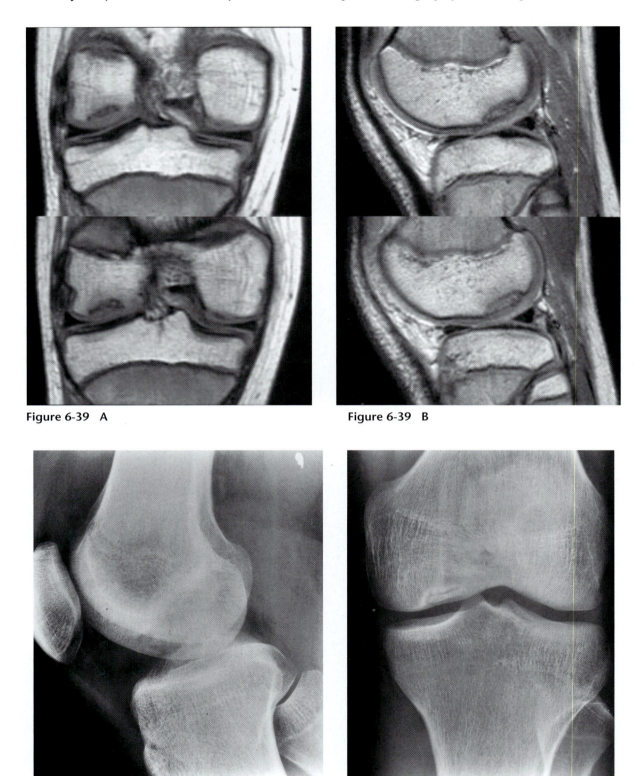

Figure 6-39 A

Figure 6-39 B

Figure 6-39 C

Figure 6-39 D

Findings: (A) Coronal T1-weighted MRI through the femoral condyles shows a low-signal osteochondral lesion in the central articular surface of the lateral femoral condyle. (B) Sagittal proton-density MRI through the lateral compartment shows the osteochondral lesion. (C, D) Companion case. Radiographs of the knee show a focal sclerotic lesion in the articular surface of the lateral aspect of the medial femoral condyle.

Differential Diagnosis: None.

Diagnosis: Osteochondral fracture (osteochondritis dissecans).

Discussion: The lateral aspect of the medial femoral condyle is a prime location for osteochondritis dissecans. The irregularity of the articular surface in this location is classic for this entity. Although spontaneous osteonecrosis of the knee may produce similar findings, it tends to involve the weight-bearing portion of the medial femoral condyle and occurs in an older population.

Osteochondritis dissecans is subsumed under the more general category of osteochondral injuries. The primary etiology for its occurrence is trauma. It is observed more frequently in males, has a peak incidence in the second decade, and can be bilateral in 25% of cases. The histologic appearance may be confusing; therefore, radiologic findings may be more reliable. Irregularity and fragmentation of the articular surface of the medial femoral condyle on its lateral aspect is classic [64]. The lateral femoral condyle and patella are other favored locations. On occasion, a curvilinear subchondral lucency or fracture may be detected. When the injury is strictly chondral, radiographs will appear normal. Conversely, a subchondral injury may occur without damage to the overlying cartilage.

The fragment may be in situ or detached. Secondary signs include soft tissue swelling and effusion. On MRI, when fluid is seen surrounding an in situ fragment, it is felt to be unstable. Detached fragments may become resorbed or may persist as intraarticular bodies. In the latter instance, the fragment may grow by apposition of cartilage and bone. Treatment is determined by manifested symptoms. Pain and instability may warrant surgery. The size of the lesion may predict instability—lesions larger than 8 × 8 mm are associated with instability [65]. Long-term complications include osteoarthritis [66].

Clinical History: 16-year-old male with knee trauma.

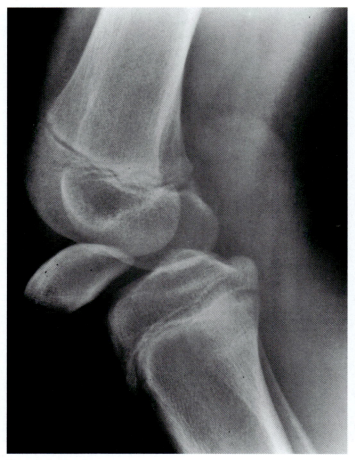

Figure 6-40   A

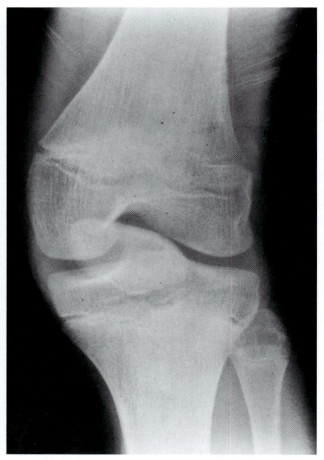

Figure 6-40   B

Findings: Lateral and AP radiographs of the knee show that the patella has assumed a horizontal orientation within the joint. No fracture is identified.

Differential Diagnosis: None.

Diagnosis: Horizontal intercondylar dislocation of the patella.

Discussion: Patellar dislocations are usually the result of a direct blow to the patella. The common patellar dislocation is to the lateral side, with the patella retaining its normal orientation relative to the knee. Unusual forms of patellar dislocation exist, including horizontal dislocation [67], vertical axis rotation, and superior dislocation. Horizontal intercondylar dislocation of the patella occurs when the patella is rotated 90 degrees along its horizontal axis, so that the articular surface faces inferiorly (as in most reported cases) or superiorly (extremely rare).

The mechanism of injury is thought to be direct blow to the superior pole of the patella in the flexed knee, of sufficient force to displace the upper bony margin of the patella

into the intercondylar notch of the femur. When the knee is subsequently extended, the femur acts like a bottle opener to avulse the patella from its attachment to the quadriceps mechanism. The detached patella is thereby dislocated between the femur and the tibia into the intercondylar notch, with the articular surface facing inferiorly and the superior pole pointing posteriorly. The patella is generally detached incompletely from the quadriceps mechanism, forcing it to retain its abnormal orientation. Male adolescents are the most prone to this type of injury.

In vertical axis dislocation, a direct blow to the patella while the knee is extended rotates the patella along its long (vertical) axis, so that the medial edge becomes lodged in the patellofemoral groove [68–70]. In vertical patellar dislocation, a direct blow to the inferior pole of the patella while the knee is extended may displace the patella superior to the patellofemoral groove. If degenerative change is preexisting, interlocking osteophytes may prevent the patella from returning to the normal position [71].

CASE 6-41

Clinical History: 24-year-old man with large knee effusion and pain.

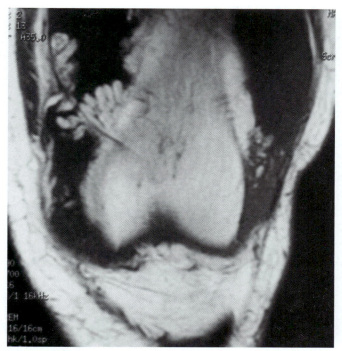

Figure 6-41 A

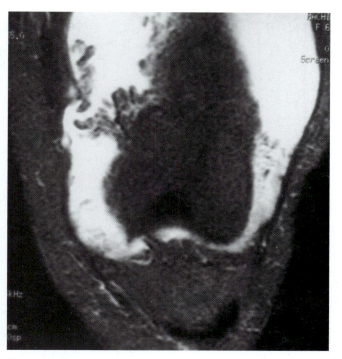

Figure 6-41 B

Findings: (A) Coronal T1-weighted MRI through the patellofemoral groove of the distal femur shows arborizing, villous, fatty proliferation of the synovium. A large effusion is present. (B) Coronal T2-weighted MRI with fat suppression shows the effusion outlining the fatty synovial proliferation. The signal within the proliferation has been suppressed similar to the subcutaneous fat.

Differential Diagnosis: Lipoma arborescens, pigmented villonodular synovitis, synovial chondromatosis, rheumatoid arthritis, synovial hemangiomatosis, amyloid arthropathy.

Diagnosis: Lipoma arborescens.

Discussion: Although the differential diagnosis for synovial masses includes several possibilities, the fatty composition of the lesion provides the correct diagnosis. Lipoma arborescens (lipomatosis of the synovium) is characterized by multiple, swollen, synovial villous projections of fatty tissue, with a tree-like branching pattern that gives it its name. Diffuse replacement of subsynovial tissue by mature fat cells produces a villous transformation of the synovium. It may begin de novo, but has also been associated with degenerative joint disease, rheumatoid arthritis, and posttraumatic conditions [83]. Although the etiology is unknown, it is thought to be a nonneoplastic reactive process. The condition is typically monoarticular and involves the knee, but involvement of multiple joints and involvement of the wrist, shoulder, and hip have been described.

Patients present with long-standing, slowly progressive joint swelling and pain. Radiographs typically show effusion and any associated articular disease. MRI always shows effusions and lipomatous proliferation with a villous morphology; the signal intensity is similar to that of fat on T1-weighted and T2-weighted images [84–87]. The proliferation may have broad-based polypoid morphology or a thin papillary one. Mass-like subsynovial fat deposition, erosive bone changes at articular margins, synovial cysts, and degenerative changes may be found in a minority of cases. The treatment is local excision of the lesion.

Clinical History: 6-month-old girl with failure to thrive.

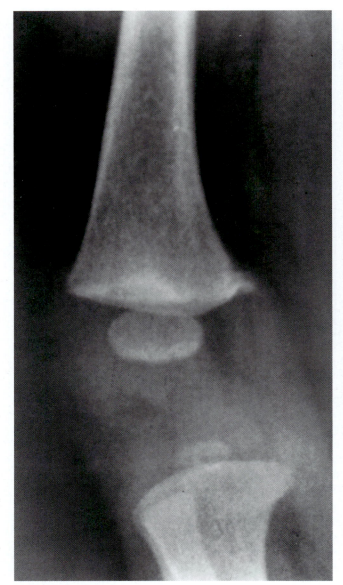

Figure 6-42   A

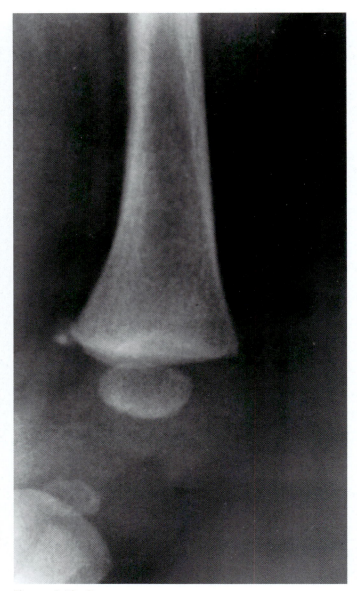

Figure 6-42   B

Findings: (A) AP radiograph of the right knee. There is a small bony excrescence extending medially from the distal femoral metaphysis. (B) AP radiograph of the left knee. There is a triangular fragment of bone adjacent to the medial aspect of the distal metaphysis of the femur. The fragment is slightly displaced and has unsharp margins.

Differential Diagnosis: None.

Diagnosis: Battered child with corner fractures of different ages.

Discussion: Corner fractures in a very young child are virtually pathognomonic for child abuse. However, the most common fractures seen in child abuse [72] are spiral fractures of the long bones of the lower limb in toddlers, fractures of the clavicle, and simple linear fractures of the skull outside the occiput. These fractures are not specific to child abuse and may occur with accidental trauma. Child abuse is likely when injuries are discovered that are more extensive or more severe than the history given for the trauma; when the injuries are of different ages, indicating prior episodes of trauma; or when there is fracture without adequate explanation.

Corner fractures are caused by indirect torsional, acceleration, and deceleration forces generated when an infant is shaken violently. Massive forces develop as the head and extremities flail about. In the long bones of the extremities, radiologic-pathologic studies have shown the fundamental lesion to be a series of microfractures occurring in a plane through the immature metaphyseal primary spongiosa, which is the zone of growing bone where delicate trabeculae are first apposed to central calcified cores. The fracture fragment consists of a thin plate of bone, calcified cartilage, the growth plate, and the attached epiphysis. This fracture is recognized as a transverse subepiphyseal lucency with an adjacent linear density abutting the growth plate. If the fragment is tipped or viewed obliquely, it will have a bucket-handle appearance. If the periphery is thicker than the central portion, it will have a corner fracture appearance. These metaphyseal lesions are injuries highly specific for intentional injury and differ from the usual Salter types of growth plate fractures, in which the fracture plane is between the calcified and uncalcified zones of cartilage. Shaking may separate a long bone from its periosteal envelope, leading to subperiosteal hemorrhage and periosteal elevation. Once the periosteum begins to make new reactive bone, its displaced position will become evident.

It may become critical to establish the age of a fracture by radiologic appearance in relation to the historical timing of the trauma. Dating fractures by roentgenography is imprecise. In general, a fracture with definite but slight periosteal new bone may be as recent as 4 to 7 days old; unless immobilized or internally fixed, a fracture 20 days old will almost always have well-defined periosteal new bone and soft callus. A fracture with a large amount of periosteal new bone or callus is more than 14 days old. Long bone fractures in infants heal with widespread periosteal new bone formation.

CASE 6-43

Clinical History: 67-year-old woman with total knee replacement.

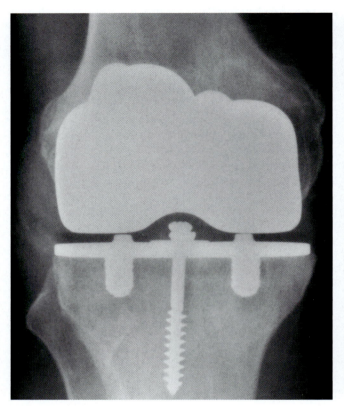

Figure 6-43   A

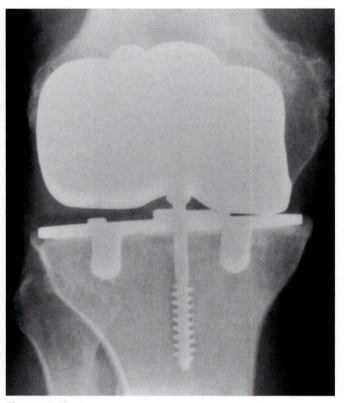

Figure 6-43   B

Findings: (A) AP radiograph of weight-bearing knee shortly after initial surgery for total knee replacement shows normal position and alignment of the components. (B) AP radiograph of weight-bearing knee 2 years later shows marked narrowing of the medial joint space, with metal articulating with metal. A varus deformity results.

Differential Diagnosis: None.

Diagnosis: Total knee replacement with failure of tibial polyethylene.

Discussion: The radiographic joint space in a total knee replacement is the space between the metal components that is normally occupied by a polyethylene liner. Polyethylene, like other plastics, is radiolucent on radiographs and can generally be distinguished from joint fluid. Narrowing of the joint space in a total knee replacement is indicative of failure of the polyethylene, due to excessive wear from the surface, fragmentation, or even dislocation. Loss of polyethylene from the patellar component may be difficult to demonstrate on radiographs. Other complications involving total knee replacement include infection, osteolysis and component loosening, instability, and metallosis.

CASE 6-44

Clinical History: 74-year-old woman with acute knee pain.

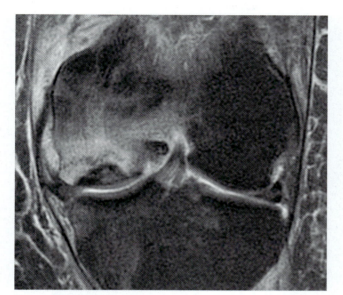

Figure 6-44   A

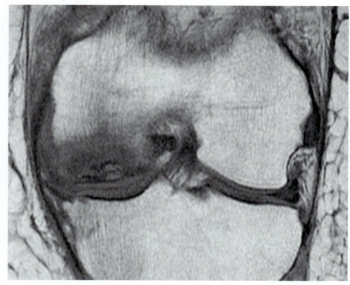

Figure 6-44   B

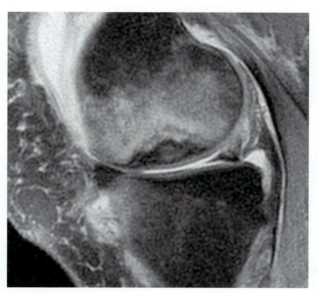

Figure 6-44   C

Findings: Coronal fat-suppressed, proton-density (A), coronal T1-weighted (B), and sagittal fat-suppressed proton-density (C) MRI shows abnormal signal in the weight-bearing surface of the medial femoral condyle. A serpiginous low-signal region is surrounded by edema. There is no collapse of the articular surface.

Differential Diagnosis: Subchondral fracture, osteonecrosis, osteochondritis dissecans, osteoarthritis, contusion, transient bone marrow edema.

Diagnosis: Spontaneous osteonecrosis of the knee (SONK).

Discussion: SONK is typically seen in elderly women with acute knee pain. The etiology is controversial. The leading theory is that SONK is an insufficiency fracture [73,74], such as those seen in the pelvis, although others believe it is due to venous thrombosis. SONK can be seen along the weight-bearing surface of either femoral condyle. Osteochondritis dissecans would typically be in a younger patient, with a similar-appearing lesion along the lateral aspect of the medial femoral condyle. Collapse of the subchondral bone can lead to accelerated osteoarthritis. Approximately 20% of cases resolve spontaneously [75].

Clinical History: 73-year-old woman 10 years after total knee replacement.

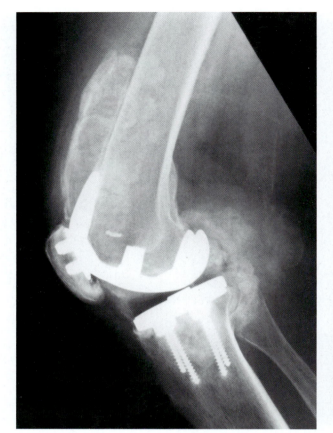

Figure 6-45   A

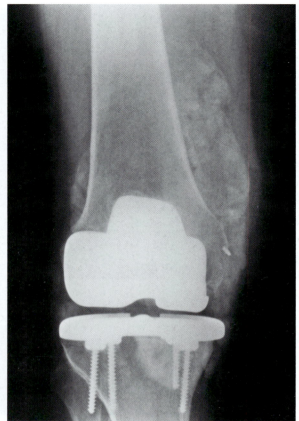

Figure 6-45   B

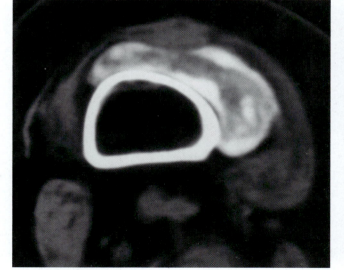

Figure 6-45   C

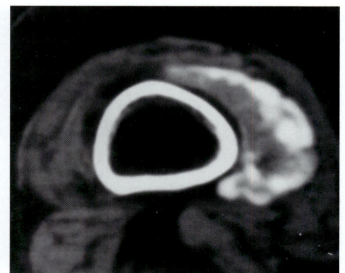

Figure 6-45   D

Findings: (A, B) Lateral and AP radiographs show a total knee prosthesis. Radiodense material outlines a distended joint capsule. (C, D) Axial CT without the use of contrast material demonstrates that the radiodense material seen on the radiographs is metallic.

Differential Diagnosis: None.

Diagnosis: Metallosis.

Discussion: The initial thought on encountering metallic density in a joint capsule is that radiographic contrast has been injected or secreted into the joint. Once it has been established that this is not the case, the obvious source of the metallic density is the metal that is already present within the joint, namely, the components of the knee prosthesis.

Metallosis is a complication of total joint replacements caused by abrasion of metal components, typically after failure of interposed polyethylene-bearing surfaces. In one series, metallosis was present in 7 of 30 patients with total knee replacements using metal-backed patellar components [76].

Microscopic particles abraded from polyethylene surfaces are known to provoke a giant cell foreign body reaction that results in osteolysis and implant loosening, but a major role for metal debris-containing histiocytes in this process has also been suggested [77]. Metal and polyethylene particles may be carried away from joint replacements by lymphatics [78], but with uncertain systemic effects.

The characteristic radiographic finding of metallosis after total knee replacement is a radiodensity outlining the suprapatellar recess of the joint capsule caused by the presence of embedded metal particles [79]. Arthrocentesis produces a thick, dark gray or black fluid. At surgery, the joint capsule is typically filled with dark fluid and metallic debris, with a grossly blackened and hypertrophic synovium. Metallosis is treated by synovectomy and revision of the prosthesis. Although the metal-backed patellar component is no longer in use, patients with this implant are still common, and metallosis may follow failure of tibial polyethylene components.

Clinical History: 34-year-old woman with left knee pain resembling intermittent claudication.

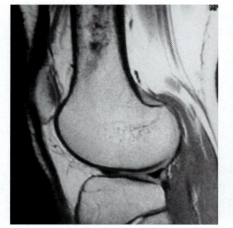

Figure 6-46   A

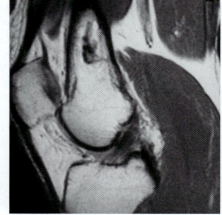

Figure 6-46   B

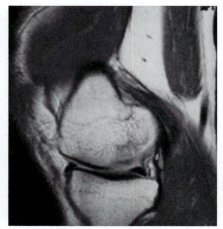

Figure 6-46   C

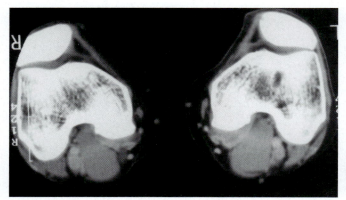

Figure 6-46   D

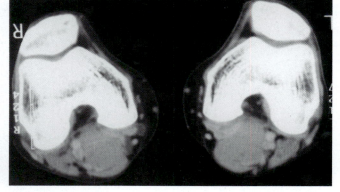

Figure 6-46   E

Findings: (A–C) Sagittal proton-density MRI of the left knee through the lateral femoral condyle, intercondylar notch, and medial condyle shows diminutive heads of the lateral and medial gastrocnemius muscle, with a large, anomalous muscle arising from the posterior aspect of the distal femoral shaft. An incidental enchondroma is present in the more proximal femoral shaft. (D, E) Axial CT, after intravenous contrast medium injection of both knees at the level of the popliteal fossa, shows on each side an anomalous muscle occupying the popliteal fossa, displacing the popliteal vessels laterally.

Differential Diagnosis: None.

Diagnosis: Popliteal entrapment syndrome.

Discussion: Various anomalies of the origin of the medial of the gastrocnemius may result in aberrant location of the muscle belly [80,81,82]. In some circumstances, this aberrant location may result in compression of the popliteal vessels between the aberrant medial and lateral heads of the gastrocnemius muscle. Functional segmental occlusion of the popliteal artery with flexion may cause ischemic symptoms in the lower extremities. In the most common anomaly, a portion of the medial head of the gastrocnemius originates along the posterior aspect of the distal femoral shaft, proximal and lateral to its normal origin on the posterior face of the medial femoral condyle. This muscle then courses inferiorly in the popliteal fossa to join the remaining fibers of the gastrocnemius in the calf. The medial and lateral heads may be smaller than normal, so that the overall bulk of the muscle is normal. The symptoms of claudication may be atypical, with symptoms related more to the degree of knee flexion than actual exertion.

Thrombotic and embolic complications may occur in the distal arteries. Popliteal artery entrapment may result when the artery has an atypical course, either with or without an aberrant gastrocnemius origin. Patients are typically adults, men more commonly than women, who are physically active. Symptoms usually begin when the patients are in their early 30s, with the diagnosis not made until their late 30s. Radiographs are normal, but cross-sectional imaging will show the anomaly. Angiograms may be normal if they are done with the patient at rest with the knee in extension. The treatment is surgical.

Clinical History: 45-year-old man with knee pain.

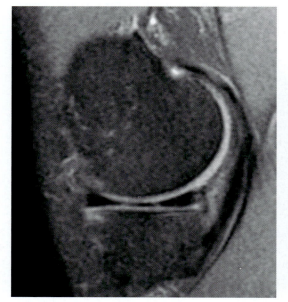

Figure 6-47   A

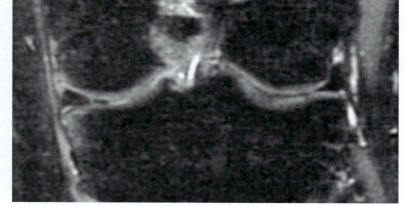

Figure 6-47   B

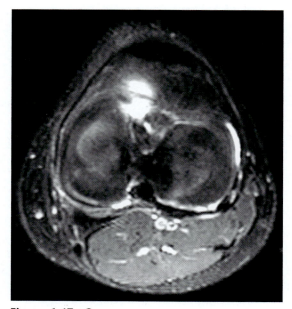

Figure 6-47   C

Findings: Sagittal (**A**), coronal (**B**), and axial (**C**) T2-weighted fat-saturated images of the knee show small vertical areas of high signal within the body of the medial meniscus. The middle third of the medial meniscus is irregular in shape and does not resemble a normal bowtie configuration. The axial image demonstrates an oblique irregular area of high signal extending perpendicular to the horizontal axis of the meniscus.

Differential Diagnosis: None.

Diagnosis: Radial/flap tear of the medial meniscus.

Discussion: A radial tear is defined as a tear perpendicular to the free edge of the meniscus. When a tear has both a radial and a longitudinal component, it is referred to as a flap tear. On sagittal sequences, a radial tear may be manifested by a few vertical striations of high signal on peripheral sections. When a radial tear occurs in the medial meniscus, the posterior horn is usually involved. This usually presents in older patients. However, the most common location of a radial/flap tear is the middle third of the meniscus, most likely due to the large curvature in this region. Radial tears are more common in patients who have undergone a prior partial meniscectomy [88]. ACL tears may be associated with radial tears occurring at the posterior horn of the lateral meniscus.

Clinical History: 55-year-old man injured knee 6 months earlier.

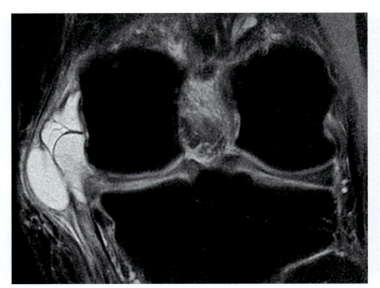

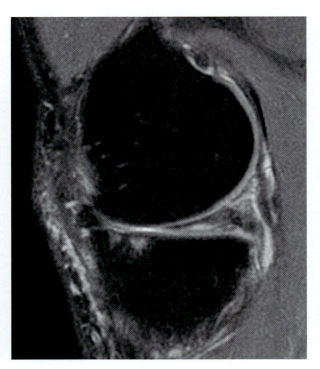

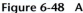

Figure 6-48 A

Figure 6-48 B

Findings: Coronal and sagittal (**A, B**) proton-density, fat-suppressed images of the knee show a multilobulated cystic structure adjacent to the medial meniscus. This structure displaces the MCL. There is high signal in the posterior horn of the medial meniscus.

Differential Diagnosis: None.

Diagnosis: Peripheral medial meniscal tear with associated meniscal cyst.

Discussion: The normal meniscus remains low signal on all pulse sequences. High signal on T2-weighted images within the meniscus must reach an articular surface to fulfill the criteria for a meniscal tear. Areas of high signal on T2-weighted imaging within the substance of the meniscus that does not reach an articular surface are usually classified as mucoid degeneration.

A complication of a meniscal tear is a meniscal cyst. The communication between the cyst and the tear allows joint fluid to enter using a ball-valve mechanism; therefore, the cyst continues to grow and may become symptomatic. The posterior horn of the medial meniscus and anterior horn of the lateral meniscus are common locations for the development of a meniscal cyst. Meniscal cysts that are medially located tend to be more symptomatic due to the close proximity to the MCL. Medial meniscal cysts are twice as common as lateral meniscal cysts [89]. Meniscal cysts may be asymptomatic [90].

SOURCES AND READINGS

1. Trevor D. Tarso-epiphyseal aclasis: a congenital error of epiphyseal development. *J Bone Joint Surg Br.* 1950;32-B:204–213.

2. Schoenberg NY, Lehman WB. Magnetic resonance imaging of pediatric disorders of the ankle and foot. *Magn Reson Imaging Clin N Am.* 1994;2:109–122.

3. Tyler W, Barrett T, Frassica F, McCarthy E. Skin metastasis from conventional giant cell tumor of bone: conceptual significance. *Skeletal Radiol.* 2002;31:166–170.

4. Kitano K, Shiraishi T, Okabayashi K, Iwasaki A, Kawahara K, Shirakusa T. A lung metastasis from giant cell tumor of bone at eight years after primary resection. *Jpn J Thorac Cardiovasc Surg.* 1999;47:617–620.

5. Grote HJ, Braun M, Kalinski T, et al. Spontaneous malignant transformation of conventional giant cell tumor. *Skeletal Radiol.* 2004;33:169–175.

6. Unni KK. *Dahlin's Bone Tumors: General Aspects and Data on 11,087 Cases.* 5th ed. Philadelphia: Lippincott-Raven Publishers; 1996:143–181.

7. Chew FS, Hudson TM. Radionuclide bone scanning of osteosarcoma: falsely extended uptake patterns. *AJR Am J Roentgenol.* 1982;139:49–54.

8. Unni KK. *Dahlin's Bone Tumors: General Aspects and Data on 11,087 Cases.* 5th ed. Philadelphia: Lippincott-Raven Publishers; 1996:185–196.

9. Jelinek JS, Murphey MD, Kransdorf MJ, Shmookler BM, Malawer MM, Hur RC. Parosteal osteosarcoma: value of MR imaging and CT in the prediction of histologic grade. *Radiology.* 1996;201:837–842.

10. Murphey MD, Robbin MR, McRae GA, Flemming DJ, Temple HT, Kransdorf MJ. The many faces of osteosarcoma. *Radiographics.* 1997;17:1205–1231.

11. Unni KK. *Dahlin's Bone Tumors: General Aspects and Data on 11,087 Cases.* 5th ed. Philadelphia: Lippincott-Raven Publishers; 1996:217–224.

12. Schuh A, Zeiler G, Holzwarth U, Aigner T. Malignant fibrous histiocytoma at the site of a total hip arthroplasty. *Clin Orthop.* 2004;425:218–222.

13. Krishnan A, Shirkhoda A, Tehranzadeh J, Armin AR, Irwin R, Les K. Primary bone lymphoma: radiographic-MR imaging correlation. *Radiographics.* 2003;23:1371–1383.

14. Unni KK. *Dahlin's Bone Tumors: General Aspects and Data on 11,087 Cases.* 5th ed. Philadelphia: Lippincott-Raven Publishers; 1996:237–248.

15. Hill S, Dunn A, Thomas JM. Lymphoma presenting as an intramuscular mass. *Br J Surg.* 1997;84:1741–1743.

16. Kerr R. Imaging of musculoskeletal complications of hemophilia. *Semin Musculoskelet Radiol.* 2003;7:127–136.

17. Boldero JL, Kemp HS. The early bone and joint changes in hemophilia and similar blood dyscrasias. *Br J Radiol.* 1966;39:172–180.

18. Paton RW, Evans DK. Silent AVN of the femoral head in hemophilia. *J Bone Joint Surg.* 1988;70B:737–739.

19. Kaplan PA, Asleson RJ, Klassen CW, Duggan MJ. Bone marrow patterns in aplastic anemia: observations with 1.5 T MRI. *Radiology.* 1987;164:441–444.

20. Steiner RM, Mitchell DG, Reno VM, et al. MRI of bone marrow: diagnostic value in diffuse hematologic disorders. *Mag Res Q.* 1990;6:17–34.

21. Jensen KE, Nielssen A, Thomsen C. In vivo measurements of T1 relaxation processes in the bone marrow in patients with myelodysplastic syndrome. *Acta Radiol.* 1989;30:365–368.

22. McHugh K, Olsen ØE, Vellodi A. Gaucher disease in children: radiology of non-central nervous system manifestations. *Clin Radiol.* 2004;59:117–123.

23. Rohren EM, Kosarek FJ, Helms CA. Discoid lateral meniscus and the frequency of meniscal tears. *Skeletal Radiol.* 2001;30:316–320.

24. Youm T, Chen AL. Discoid lateral meniscus: evaluation and treatment. *Am J Orthop.* 2004;33:234–238.

25. Duong S, Sallis JG, Zee SY. Malignant fibrous histiocytoma arising within a bone infarct in a patient with sickle cell trait. *Int J Surg Pathol.* 2004;12:67–73.

26. Curi MM, Dib LL. Osteoradionecrosis of the jaws: a retrospective study of the background factors and treatment in 104 cases. *Maxillofac Surg.* 1997;55:540–546.

27. Wood GA, Liggins SJ. Does hyperbaric oxygen have a role in the management of osteoradionecrosis? *Br J Oral Maxillofac Surg.* 1996;34:424–427.

28. Outerbridge R. The aetiology of chondromalacia patellae. *J Bone Joint Surg Br.* 1961;43:752–757.

29. van Leersum M, Schweitzer ME, Gannon F, Finkel G, Vinitski S, Mitchell DG. Chondromalacia patellae: an in vitro study. Comparison of MR criteria with histologic and macroscopic findings. *Skeletal Radiol.* 1996;25:727–732.

30. Elias DA, White LM. Imaging of patellofemoral disorders. *Clin Radiol.* 2004;59:543–557.

31. Greenspan A, Azouz EM, Matthews J II, Decarie JC. Synovial hemangioma: imaging features in eight histologically proven cases, review of the literature, and differential diagnosis. *Skeletal Radiol.* 1995;24:583–590.

32. Price NJ, Cundy PJ. Synovial hemangioma of the knee. *J Pediatr Orthop.* 1997;17:74–77.

33. Olson JC. Juvenile idiopathic arthritis: an update. *WMJ.* 2003;102:45–50.

34. Johnson K, Gardner-Medwin J. Childhood arthritis: classification and radiology. *Clin Radiol.* 2002;57:47–58.

35. Murphy FP, Dahlin DC, Sullivan CR. Articular synovial chondromatosis. *J Bone Joint Surg Am.* 1962;44:77–86.

36. Peh WC, Shek TW, Davies AM, Wong JW, Chien EP. Osteochondroma and secondary synovial osteochondromatosis. *Skeletal Radiol.* 1999;28:169–174.

37. Milgram JW, Dunn EJ. Periarticular chondromas and osteochondromas: a report of three cases. *Clin Orthop.* 1989;148:147–151.

38. DeBenedetti MJ, Schwinn CP. Tenosynovial chondromatosis in the hand. *J Bone Joint Surg Am.* 1979;61:898–903.

39. Lynn MD, Lee J. Periarticular tenosynovial chondrometaplasia: report of a case at the wrist. *J Bone Joint Surg Am.* 1972;54:450–452.

40. Manco LG, DeLuke DM. CT diagnosis of synovial chondromatosis of the TMJ. *AJR Am J Roentgenol.* 1987;148:574–576.

41. Kenan S, Abdelwahab IF, Klein MJ, Lewis MM. Case report 817: Synovial chondrosarcoma secondary to synovial chondromatosis. *Skeletal Radiol.* 1993;22:623–626.

42. Bencardino JT, Hassankhani A. Calcium pyrophosphate dihydrate crystal deposition disease. *Semin Musculoskelet Radiol.* 2003;7:175–185.

43. Adams EM, Chow CK, Premkumar A, Plotz PH. The idiopathic inflammatory myopathies: spectrum of MR imaging findings. *Radiographics.* 1995;15:563–574.

44. Fraser DD, Frank JA, Dalakas M, et al. MRI in the inflammatory myopathies. *J Rheumatol.* 1991;18:1693–1700.

45. Hernandez RJ, Keim DR, Sullivan DB, et al. MRI appearance of the muscles in childhood dermatomyositis. *J Pediatr.* 1990;117:546–550.

46. Christopher-Stine L, Plotz PH. Adult inflammatory myopathies. *Best Pract Res Clin Rheumatol.* 2004;18:331–344.

47. Centers for Disease Control and Prevention (CDC). Progress toward poliomyelitis eradication—Afghanistan and Pakistan, January 2003–May 2004. *MMWR Morb Mortal Wkly Rep.* 2004;53:634–637.

48. Grant AD, Atar D, Lehman WB. Postpoliomyelitis syndrome problems of knee function: a review. *Bull Hosp Joint Dis.* 1993;53:27–29.

49. Altman RD. Articular complications of Paget's disease of bone. *Semin Arthritis Rheum.* 1994;23:248–249.

50. Helliwell PS. Osteoarthritis and Paget's disease. *Br J Rheumatol.* 1995;34:1061–1063.

51. Zeiss J, Paley K, Murray K, Saddemi SR. Comparison of bone contusion seen by MRI in partial and complete tears of the anterior cruciate ligament. *J Comput Assist Tomogr.* 1995;19:773–776.

52. Goldman AB, Pavlov H, Rubenstein D. The Segond fracture of the proximal tibia: a small avulsion that reflects major ligamentous damage. *AJR Am J Roentgenol.* 1988;151:1163–1167.

53. Jaramillo D, Hoffer FA, Shapiro F, Rand F. MRI of fractures of the growth plate. *AJR Am J Roentgenol.* 1990;155:1261–1265.

54. Stoller DW, Cannon WD Jr, Anderson LJ. The knee. In: Stoller DW, ed. *Magnetic Resonance Imaging in Orthopaedics and Sports Medicine.* Philadelphia: Lippincott-Raven Publishers; 1993:177–178.

55. Dorsay TA, Helms CA. Bucket-handle meniscal tears of the knee: sensitivity and specificity of MRI signs. *Skeletal Radiol.* 2003;32:266–272.

56. Yao L, Dungan D, Seegar LL. MRI of tibial collateral ligament injury: comparison with clinical examination. *Skeletal Radiol.* 1994;23:521–524.

57. Staron RB, Haramati N, Feldman F, et al. O'Donoghue's triad: MRI evidence. *Skeletal Radiol.* 1994;23:633–636.

58. O'Donoghue DH. Surgical treatment of fresh injuries to the major ligaments of the knee. *J Bone Joint Surg Am.* 1950;32:721–731.

59. Kaplan PA, Dussault RG. MRI of the knee: menisci, ligaments, tendons. *Topics Magn Reson Imaging.* 1993;5:228–248.

60. Sonin AH, Fitzgerald SW, Friedman H, et al. PCL injuryMRI diagnosis and patterns of injury. *Radiology.* 1994;190:455–458.

61. Recht MP, Applegate G, Kaplan P, et al. The MR appearance of cruciate ganglion cysts: a report of 16 cases. *Skeletal Radiol.* 1994;23:597–600.

62. De Flaviis L, Nessi R, Scaglione P, et al. Ultrasonic diagnosis of Osgood-Schlatter and Sinding-Larsen-Johansson diseases of the knee. *Skeletal Radiol.* 1989;18:193–197.

63. Medlar RC, Lyne ED. Sinding-Larsen-Johansson disease. Its etiology and natural history. *J Bone Joint Surg Am.* 1978;60:1113–1116.

64. Aichroth P. Osteochondritis dissecans of the knee: a clinical study. *J Bone Joint Surg Br.* 1971;53:440–447.

65. Mesgarzadeh M, Schneck CD, Bonakdarpour A. MRI of the knee and correlation with normal anatomy. *Radiographics.* 1988;8:707–733.

66. Linden B. Osteochondritis dissecans of the femoral condyles. A long-term follow up study. *J Bone Joint Surg Am.* 1977;59:769–776.

67. Brady TA, Russell D. Interarticular horizontal dislocation of the patella. *J Bone Joint Surg Am.* 1965;47:1393–1396.

68. Corso SJ, Thal R, Forman D. Locked patellar dislocation with vertical axis rotation. A case report. *Clin Orthop.* 1992;279:190–193.

69. Rao R, Bains RS, Lum G. Acute traumatic vertical axis rotational dislocation of the patella. *Orthopedics.* 1997;20:713–715.

70. Corfield AR, Stevenson J. Vertical patellar dislocation: a case report. *Eur J Emerg Med.* 2004;11:170–171.

71. Hanspal RS. Superior dislocation of the patella. *Injury.* 1985;16:487–488.

72. Kleinman PK. *Diagnostic Imaging of Child Abuse.* Baltimore: Williams & Wilkins; 1987:5–28.

73. Yamamoto T, Bullough PG. Spontaneous osteonecrosis of the knee: the result of subchondral insufficiency fracture. *J Bone Joint Surg Am.* 2000;82:858–866.

74. Sokoloff RM, Farooki S, Resnick D. Spontaneous osteonecrosis of the knee associated with ipsilateral tibial plateau stress fracture: report of two patients and review of the literature. *Skeletal Radiol.* 2001;30:53–56.

75. Soucacos PN, Johnson EO, Soultanis K, Vekris MD, Theodorou SJ, Beris AE. Diagnosis and management of the osteonecrotic triad of the knee. *Orthop Clin North Am.* 2004;35:371–381.

76. Rader CP, Lohr H, Whittmann R, Eulert J. Results of total knee arthroplasty with a metal-backed patellar component: a 6-year follow-up study. *J Arthroplasty.* 1996;11:923–930.

77. Al Saffar N, Revel PA. Interleukin-1 production by activated macrophages surrounding loosened orthopaedic implants: a potential role in osteolysis. *Br J Rheumatol.* 1994;33:309–316.

78. Shinto Y, Uchida A, Yoshikawa H, et al. Inguinal lymphadenopathy due to metal release from a prosthesis: a case report. *J Bone Joint Surg Br.* 1993;75-B:266–269.

79. Weissman BN, Scott RD, Brick GW, Corson JM. Radiographic detection of metal-induced synovitis as a complication of arthroplasty of the knee. *J Bone Joint Surg Am.* 1991;73-A:1002–1007.

80. Atilla S, Akpek ET, Yucel C, Tali EK, Isik S. MR imaging and MR angiography in popliteal artery entrapment syndrome. *Eur Radiol.* 1998;8:1025–1029.

81. Hoelting T, Schuermann G, Allenberg JR. Entrapment of the popliteal artery and its surgical management in a 20-year period. *Br J Surg.* 1997;84:338–341.

82. Murray A, Halliday M, Croft RJ. Popliteal artery entrapment syndrome. *Br J Surg.* 1991;78:1414–1419.

83. Resnik D. Tumors and tumor-like lesions in or about joints. In: Resnick D, ed. *Diagnosis of Bone and Joint Disorders.* 4th ed. Philadelphia: WB Saunders; 2002:4160–4161.

84. Martin S, Hernandez L, Romero J, et al. Diagnostic imaging of lipoma arborescens. *Skeletal Radiol.* 1998;27:325–329.

85. Soler T, Rodriguez E, Bargiela A, Da Riba M. Lipoma arborescens of the knee: MR characteristics in 13 joints. *J Comput Assist Tomogr.* 1998;22:605–609.

86. Kloen P, Keel SB, Chandler HP, Geiger RH, Zarins B, Rosenberg AE. Lipoma arborescens of the knee. *J Bone Joint Surg Br.* 1998;80:298–301.

87. Vilanova JC, Barcelo J, Villalon M, Aldoma J, Delgado E, Zapater I. MR imaging of lipoma arborescens and the associated lesions. *Skeletal Radiol.* 2003;32:504–509.

88. Magee T, Shapiro M, Williams D. Prevalence of meniscal radial tears of the knee revealed by MRI after surgery. *AJR Am J Roentgenol.* 2004;182:931–936.

89. Campbell SE, Sanders TG, Morrison WB. MR imaging of meniscal cysts: incidence, location, and clinical significance. *AJR Am J Roentgenol.* 2001;177:409–413.

90. Tschirch FT, Schmid MR, Pfirrmann CW, Romero J, Hodler J, Zanetti M. Prevalence and size of meniscal cysts, ganglionic cysts, synovial cysts of the popliteal space, fluid-filled bursae, and other fluid collections in asymptomatic knees on MR imaging. *AJR Am J Roentgenol.* 2003;180:1431–1436.

CHAPTER SEVEN
LOWER LEG

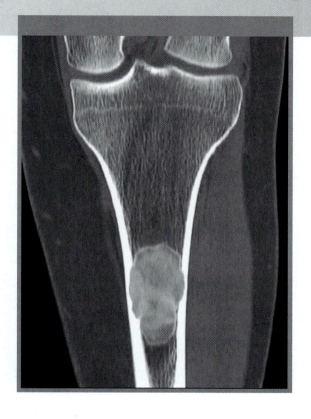

Clinical History: 3-year-old boy with progressive bowing deformity.

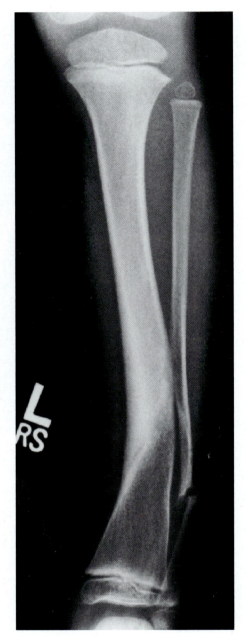

Figure 7-1

Findings: Anteroposterior (AP) radiograph of the lower extremity. There is an angular deformity of the tibia, with increased sclerosis at the site of the deformity. A fracture of the fibula is noted distal to the angular deformity.

Differential Diagnosis: Neurofibromatosis, osteogenesis imperfecta, fibrous dysplasia.

Diagnosis: Pseudoarthrosis of neurofibromatosis.

Discussion: Neurofibromatosis is one of the many conditions known in the group of phakomatoses. Neurofibromatosis is an autosomal dominant disorder with many different subtypes. Type I is associated with bone deformities and cafe-au-lait spots. Anterolateral bowing of the tibia is a characteristic feature and is due to an underlying mesodermal dysplasia. These abnormal bones are prone to fractures and development of a pseudoarthrosis, although the precise cause for the development of the pseudoarthrosis is not clear.

Clinical History: 4-year-old girl with multiple orthopedic problems.

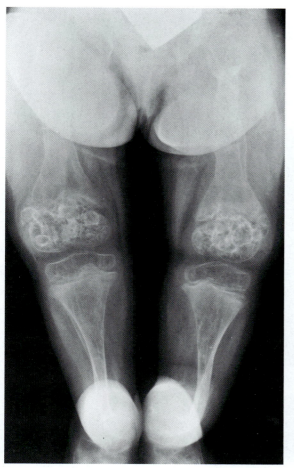

Figure 7-2   A

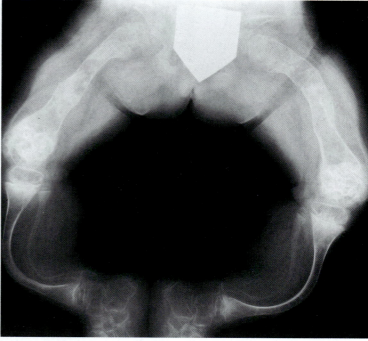

Figure 7-2   B

Findings: (**A**) AP radiograph of the legs. The bones are osteoporotic. There are multiple healed femoral shaft fractures, and severe posterior bowing deformities of the lower legs. The epiphyses at the knees are enlarged and have a popcorn appearance. (**B**) Frog lateral radiograph of both lower extremities shows osteoporosis, bowing deformities of the femurs, tibias, and fibulas, and multiple healed fractures.

Differential Diagnosis: Osteogenesis imperfecta, fibrous dysplasia.

Diagnosis: Osteogenesis imperfecta.

Discussion: Osteogenesis imperfecta is a group of inborn connective tissue disorders characterized by radiographically decreased bone density. The underlying problem is one of abnormal collagen synthesis, in which a variety of different molecular defects in collagen produce a continuous spectrum of phenotypes. In the skeleton, the bone matrix is deficient, resulting in thin, osteoporotic, and fragile bones that are subject to repeated insufficiency fractures and consequent deformity. The condition is heritable, but cases are often sporadic. In general, there are autosomal recessive severe forms that present at birth, and autosomal dominant forms that present later and have a mild course. The condition ranges from severe, congenital involvement with multiple fractures in utero and perinatal death, to mild, late manifestations in adulthood. The severe forms account for 10% of cases, and the less severe forms account for 90% of cases. The incidence of osteogenesis imperfecta is 1 per 20,000 to 60,000 live births. Associated clinical features, with variable expression, include blue sclerae (90%); thin, translucent skin; hypermobile, lax peripheral joints; abnormal teeth (dentinogenesis imperfecta); and deafness (fragile otic bones). Bisphosphonate treatment has been helpful for patients with moderate to severe disease [1].

Clinical History: 18-year-old man with short stature.

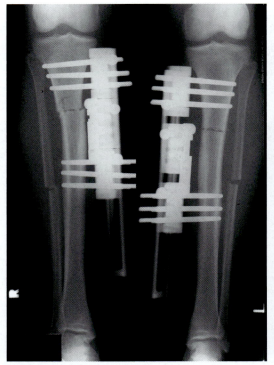

Figure 7-3   A

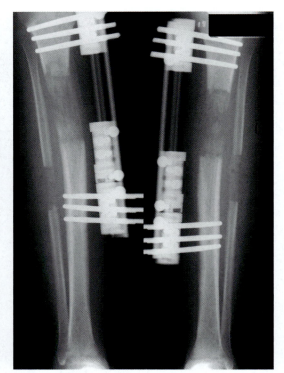

Figure 7-3   B

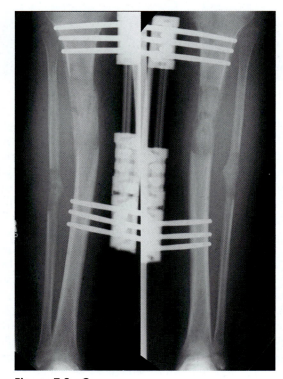

Figure 7-3   C

Findings: AP radiographs of the lower legs. (**A**) Pin-rod external fixators are present bilaterally, and osteotomies have just been performed through the proximal tibial and fibular shafts. (**B**) After 5 months of treatment, there has been a 6-cm gain in length. (**C**) After 7 months of treatment, the distracted fragments are bridged by remodeling bone.

Differential Diagnosis: Limb lengthening for short stature (from any cause).

Diagnosis: Congenital adrenocortical hyperplasia with limb lengthening.

Discussion: Congenital adrenal hyperplasia is an autosomal recessive defect, involving the enzyme 21-hydroxylase, that results in failure to synthesize cortisol. There is a secondary overproduction of androgenic hormones that cause precocious puberty. The effect on the growing skeleton is rapid growth but premature closure of the epiphyses, so that a tall child becomes a short adult. The incidence of congenital adrenal hyperplasia is approximately 1 in 16,000, with a salt-wasting form from adrenal insufficiency and a simply virilizing form from excess androgens [2]. Conventional treatment is steroid replacement with exogenous corticosteroids. Surgical limb lengthening using the callus distraction (callotasis) has been applied to patients with developmentally short stature, such as those with achondroplasia [3,4,5]. In this technique, the cortex of the bone is partially cut, leaving the medullary contents intact. After 2 weeks, as soft callus forms, the two bone segments are slowly distracted by means of an external fixator, stretching out the callus as the gap between the fragments is increased 1 mm or so per day to lengthen the bone. Several centimeters of length can be gained and the complication rate is relatively low. Once the desired length has been attained, healing and remodeling ultimately results in cortical bone formation. In this case, pin-rod external fixators have been used and both tibias have been lengthened symmetrically.

Clinical History: Young child with multiple orthopedic problems.

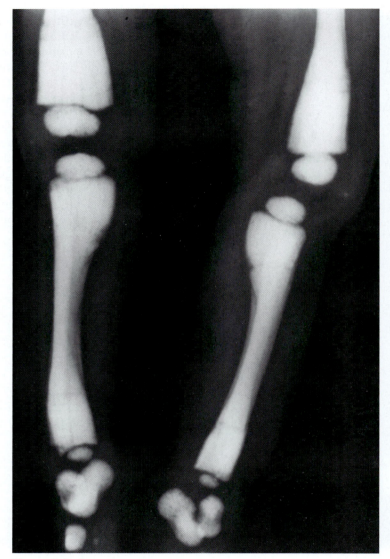

Figure 7-4 A

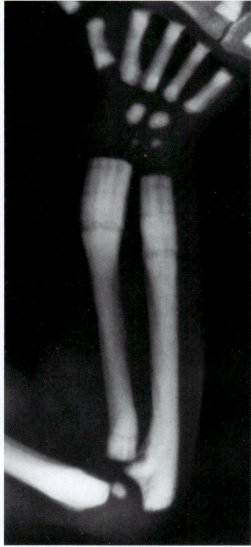

Figure 7-4 B

Findings: (**A**) AP radiograph of the lower extremities shows diffusely sclerotic bones without development of the medullary space. The metaphyses are undertubulated and club-shaped. (**B**) Radiograph of an upper extremity of the same patient shows similar findings.

Differential Diagnosis: Osteopetrosis, pyknodysostosis.

Diagnosis: Osteopetrosis, precocious form.

Discussion: All of the bones in this very young child show a generalized chalk-white density. The medullary cavity seems obliterated by the uniform density. The bone has a shape similar to a juggling club, with a narrow middle portion and a wider distal portion of uniform diameter. This shape is the result of longitudinal growth at the physis without bone resorption and remodeling in the cutback zone of the metaphysis, leaving the new bone the same diameter as the physis.

Osteopetrosis is a disorder due to abnormal function of the osteoclasts. There are autosomal recessive and dominant types. The autosomal dominant, or delayed form, is the most common. The precocious form (shown in this case) is inherited as an autosomal recessive trait and is usually lethal due to obliteration of the marrow. The osteoclasts fail to normally remodel bone. The unopposed osteoblastic activity leads to the generalized increase in bone density. The autosomal dominant form, of which there are two distinct genetic entities, was formerly known as marble bone disease or Albers-Schoenberg's disease [6].

Clinical History: Progressive bowing of lower extremities.

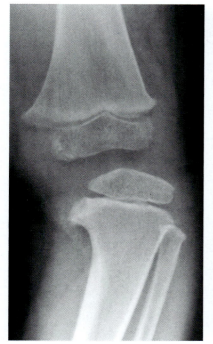

Figure 7-5   A

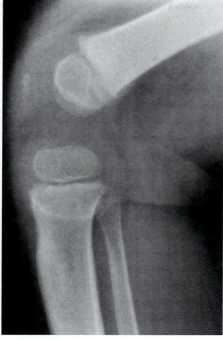

Figure 7-5   B

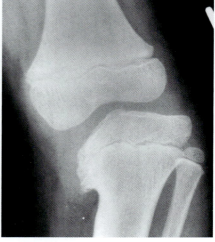

Figure 7-5   C

Findings: (A, B) AP and lateral radiographs of the left knee at age 3 years demonstrate a varus deformity of the tibia with a prominent medial metaphyseal beak. (C) AP radiograph of the knee at age 7 years shows progression of the varus deformity, slanting of the medial tibial plateau, with persistent metaphyseal beak.

Differential Diagnosis: Blount's disease, posttraumatic deformity, rickets, physiologic bowing.

Diagnosis: Blount's disease.

Discussion: The diagnosis in this case is made by recognizing the abnormally small, beaked appearance of the medial portion of the tibial metaphysis, with genu varus. These findings, in conjunction with a normal appearance of the lateral portion of the tibial metaphysis and normal femoral metaphysis, lead to the correct diagnosis.

Blount's disease of the tibia is an entity subsumed within the larger group of disorders known as osteochondroses, recognized individually by the specific site of involvement within the skeleton. Other examples of osteochondroses include such entities as Legg-Calvé-Perthes disease of the capital femoral epiphysis and Kienböck's disease of the lunate. Blount's disease specifically affects the medial portion of the proximal tibial metaphysis. The etiology of the abnormal development of the medial portion of the metaphysis is unknown. Abnormal development of the medial metaphysis results in the characteristic metaphyseal beak and genu varus deformity. Magnetic resonance imaging (MRI) is helpful to evaluate the growth plate in patients who are already affected and in patients who are at risk, such as toddlers with delayed resolution of physiologic tibial bowing [7,8].

Clinical History: Bowed legs in an infant.

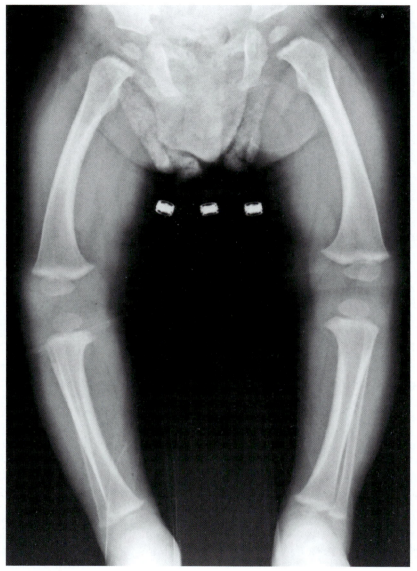

Figure 7-6

Findings: AP radiograph of both lower extremities demonstrates a mild tibia vara without beaking of the proximal medial metaphyses or widening of the physes.

Differential Diagnosis: Physiologic bowing, Blount's disease, rickets.

Diagnosis: Physiologic bowing.

Discussion: The diagnosis in this case is made by recognizing that this is a young child with slight bowing of femurs and tibias centered at the knee, without any intrinsic abnor-mality. In particular, there is no medial tibial metaphyseal fragmentation. Mild enlargement of the medial tibial metaphyses can be present [9].

Physiologic bowing is thought to be related to the fetal position within the close confines of the uterus. It is self-limited. Parents usually bring these children in for evaluation between 1 and 2 years of age because of their bowed legs. Once the toddler begins to stand and walk, normal weight-bearing stresses correct the slight bowing.

Clinical History: 4-year-old girl with short stature.

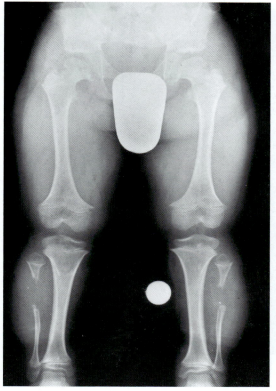

Figure 7-7   A

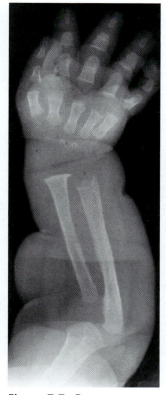

Figure 7-7   B

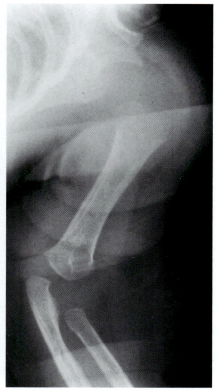

Figure 7-7   C

Findings: (A) Standing AP radiograph of the lower limbs. The long bones are short and thick with flared metaphyses. (B) Posteroanterior radiograph of the forearm and hand shows short but thick bones in the hand and forearm. The fingers have a stubby appearance. (C) AP radiograph of the upper arm shows a disproportionately short humerus. Note that with all the bones, there is a normal cortical and trabecular structure, and the bones have normal density.

Differential Diagnosis: None.

Diagnosis: Achondroplasia.

Discussion: Achondroplasia is a genetic disorder of abnormal enchondral ossification [10]. The long bones are abnormally short with metaphyseal flaring. Bone shortening is most prominent in the proximal aspect of the extremity (rhizomelic micromelia). The hand bones are short and broad, producing what is sometimes called a trident appearance. The acetabulae are flat and the iliac bones are squared. Additional findings in achondroplasia (not shown) include a large cranium compared with the face, a small foramen magnum, a narrowed interpediculate distance in the lower lumbar spine, and concavity of the posterior vertebral bodies. The limb shortness in achondroplasia is being treated with increasing frequency by surgical limb lengthening (callotasis).

Clinical History: 36-year-old woman with leg pain.

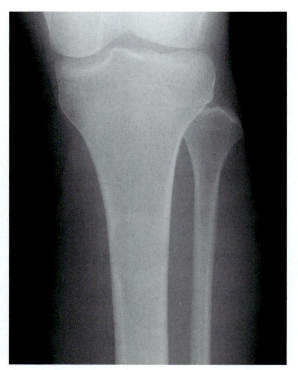

Figure 7-8   A

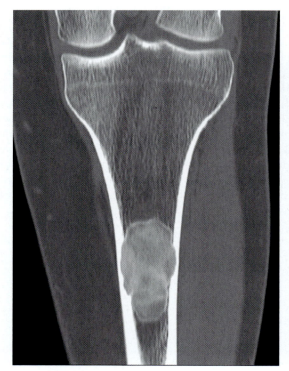

Figure 7-8   B

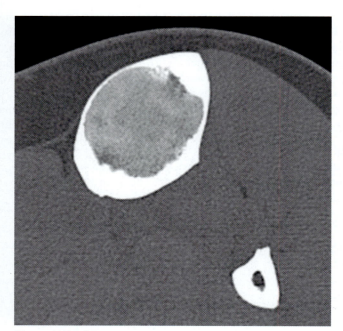

Figure 7-8   C

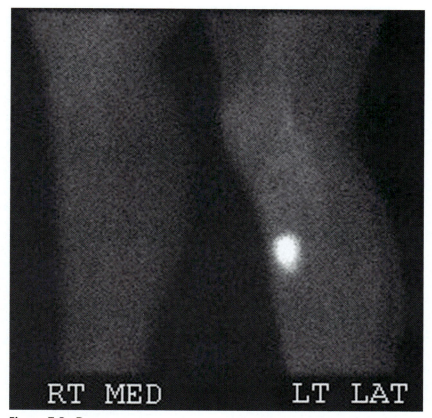

RT MED   LT LAT

Figure 7-8 D

Findings: An AP radiograph (**A**), coronal reconstructed computed tomography (CT) (**B**), and axial CT (**C**) of the proximal tibial diaphysis shows a focal lesion with ground-glass mineralization. The lesion has a faint sclerotic margin and is oriented along the long axis of the bone. Mild endosteal scalloping is present. Increased radiotracer uptake is seen in the lesion on bone scan (**D**).

Differential Diagnosis: None.

Diagnosis: Fibrous dysplasia.

Discussion: Fibrous dysplasia is a benign fibroosseous lesion that is neither familial nor hereditary. Fibrous dysplasia appears to be a developmental abnormality involving the proliferation and maturation of fibroblasts, in which benign fibrous tissue, with abnormally arranged, dysplastic trabeculae of immature woven bone, replaces normal bone. The dysplastic trabeculae are no thicker than 0.1 mm, so they are not individually visible on clinical radiographs. If present in

sufficient preponderance, however, they give the lesions a ground-glass density; if not, the lesions are radiolucent.

The lesions are medullary, but may replace both cancellous and cortical bone. The abnormal area may be sharply circumscribed and marginated by a thick layer of reactive bone, or it may blend gradually with the adjacent normal bone. The cortex may be either thickened or thinned, but frequently the outer size and shape of the affected bone is unchanged.

Bowing deformities result from biomechanically insufficient bone and from malunion of pathologic fractures. Lesions in the long bones are often discovered because of fracture or deformity. Therapy is restricted to orthopedic management of complications. The monostotic form is not associated with other abnormalities or disease. In this case, the patient underwent lesion curettage and bone grafting due to the risk of pathologic fracture.

Clinical History: 12-year-old boy with ankle swelling and tenderness.

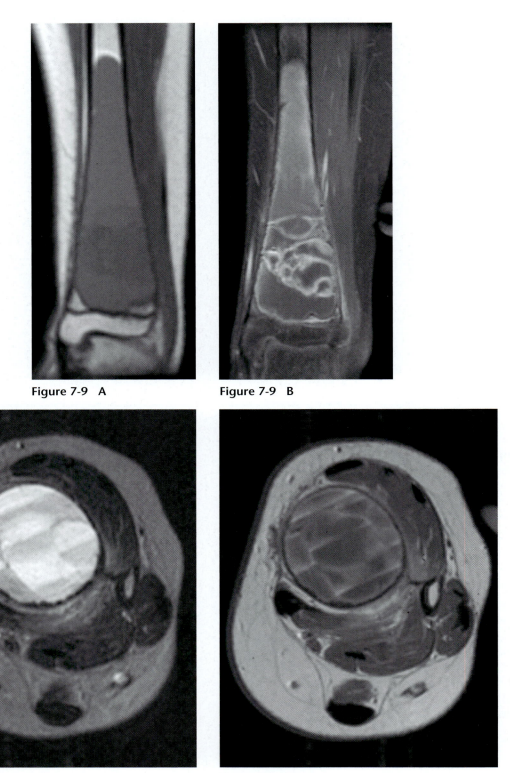

Figure 7-9   A

Figure 7-9   B

Figure 7-9   C

Figure 7-9   D

Findings: (A) Coronal T1-weighted MRI shows a long lesion in the distal tibia with mild expansion and heterogeneous internal signal. (B) Coronal T1-weighted, fat-suppressed, post-gadolinium MRI shows enhancement of the periphery of the lesion as well as complex curvilinear enhancement within its central portion. (C) Axial T2-weighted MRI shows multiple fluid-fluid levels within the lesion, corresponding to separate compartments. (D) Axial T1-weighted, fat-suppressed, post-gadolinium MRI shows enhancement of the septations between compartments.

Differential Diagnosis: Aneurysmal bone cyst, simple bone cyst.

Diagnosis: Aneurysmal bone cyst.

Discussion: Aneurysmal bone cysts are expansile, cystic lesions of bone. They probably result from a vascular disturbance caused by trauma [11] or underlying tumor. In one-third or more of cases, the pathologist can recognize an adjacent primary benign or malignant bone lesion. In this case, trauma as the antecedent event is well documented. Most cysts occur in patients between 10 to 20 years old, and patients typically present with pain and/or swelling of less than 6-months' duration. More than 50% of aneurysmal bone cysts are found in long bones, usually metaphyseal. Twelve to 30% are found in the spine, often the posterior elements, and the remainder are found in the pelvis or other flat bones.

Aneurysmal bone cysts are eccentric, lucent lesions that expand the host bone and give it a blown-out or ballooned appearance (hence the term aneurysmal). Sometimes the expanded cortical shell is interrupted when periosteal bone growth is outpaced by expansion of the lesion, but the periosteum remains intact, although radiographically invisible. The walls may have trabeculations, but true bony septations are rare. Aneurysmal bone cysts may also be located centrally within a long bone, as in this case. The lesion consists of sponge-like, fibrovascular tissue, with cystic spaces or cavities filled with blood or serosanguineous fluid. The growth plate may be invaded. CT or MRI may demonstrate fluid-fluid levels, often in multiple compartments, and the periphery of the lesion and septations will enhance following contrast injection. Aneurysmal bone cysts are treated in a manner similar to giant cell tumors, unless an underlying lesion is found that should be treated more aggressively. The clinical course may vary from indolent and self-healing to rapid, relentless growth. Aneurysmal bone cysts have no metastatic potential.

Clinical History: 24-year-old woman with a painless soft tissue mass in the calf.

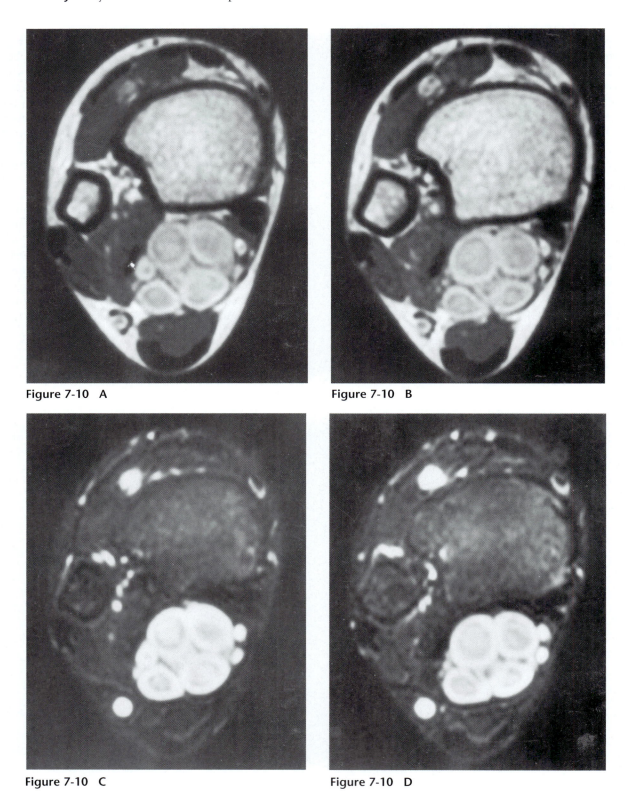

Figure 7-10   A

Figure 7-10   B

Figure 7-10   C

Figure 7-10   D

Findings: Axial T1-weighted (**A**, **B**) and T2-weighted (**C**, **D**) MRI shows a cluster of well-defined structures, demonstrating central relative hypointensity on T1 and T2 with rings of hyperintensity. Serial images establish the cylindrical nature of these structures.

Differential Diagnosis: Neurofibroma or schwannoma.

Diagnosis: Neurofibroma.

Discussion: The ring-like morphology and central foci of hypointensity seen in this case is typical of peripheral nerve sheath tumors. In conjunction with the cylindrical nature of the lesion on long axis images, the diagnosis is likely to be neurofibroma. Most neurofibromas (90%) are solitary, slow-growing lesions found in young adults. The lesions may be superficial or deep, and are usually painless. Because they are intimately associated with the underlying nerve, the patient may have dysesthesias. Because the lesion cannot be separated from the nerve, the nerve must be sacrificed at the time of surgical removal. MRI findings are often characteristic. The target appearance with a hyperintense rim and inner area of low signal intensity on T2 is typical of benign peripheral nerve tumors. It may be seen with either neurofibroma or schwannoma. Small foci of brighter signal intensity within the target area are said to represent thickened nerve bundles. This speckled appearance within a target lesion is characteristic of a peripheral nerve sheath tumor.

Clinical History: 16-year-old girl with leg swelling.

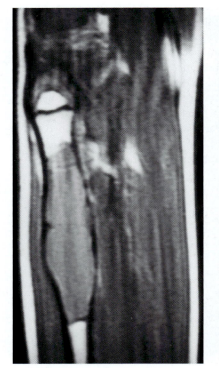

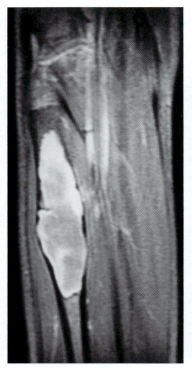

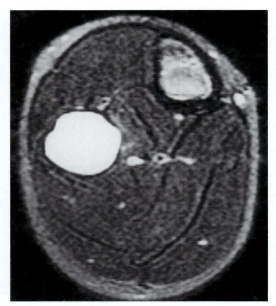

Figure 7-11 A   Figure 7-11 B   Figure 7-11 C

Findings: (A, B) Coronal T1-weighted MRI without and with gadolinium demonstrates T1 hypointensity and rim enhancement in a geographic, mildly expansile process of the proximal fibula diaphysis. (C) The T2 hyperintensity is homogeneous on the axial image. The lesion is central in transverse location.

Differential Diagnosis: Simple bone cyst, aneurysmal bone cyst, fibrous dysplasia.

Diagnosis: Simple bone cyst.

Discussion: The diagnosis is made in conjunction with a plain radiograph (not shown). The expansile lesion in the metaphysis or diametaphysis is homogenous, with fluid signal characteristics and no aggressive features. There is no solid component and no septations within the lesion. The lesion has no mineralization within.

Clinical History: 37-year-old woman with swelling, and a companion case.

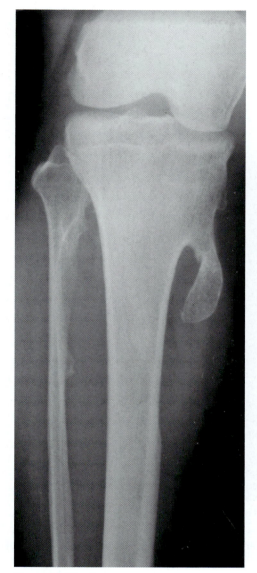

Figure 7-12   A

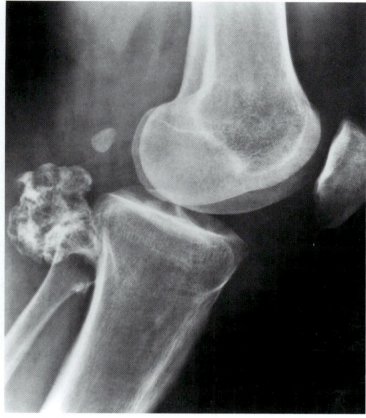

Figure 7-12   B

Findings: (A) AP radiograph of the lower leg. There is an exostotic bony lesion arising from the medial tibial metaphysis. The cortex and marrow space of the lesion is contiguous with that of the underlying bone. Broadening of the proximal fibula represents another en plaque lesion. (B) Companion case. Lateral radiograph of the knee shows a pedunculated lesion arising from the posterior aspect of the proximal tibial cortex. The cortex and medullary space of the stalk are contiguous with the cortex and medullary space of the tibia.

Differential Diagnosis: None.

Diagnosis: Osteochondroma.

Discussion: The diagnosis in this case is made by recognizing that the lesion is composed of mature bone, with cortex and medullary space that is contiguous with the underlying bone. This osteochondroma has a coat-hook morphology, whereas the companion case has a more pedunculated cauliflower morphology. Osteochondromas (also called benign exostoses) are outgrowths of histologically normal bone that arise in the vicinity of a growth plate.

Clinical History: 5-year-old boy with anterior leg mass.

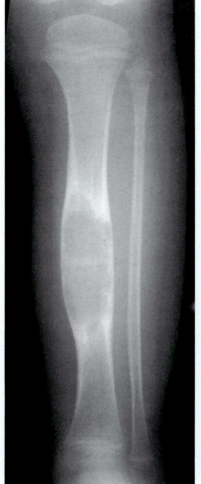 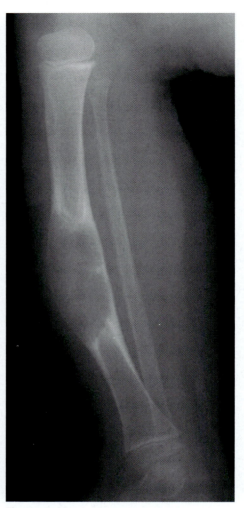

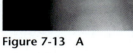

Figure 7-13   A   Figure 7-13   B

Findings: AP and lateral radiographs of the lower leg. There is an expansile lesion involving a long segment of the tibial diaphysis. The lesion has a hazy appearance and well-formed surrounding sclerosis. The lesion is somewhat asymmetric. There is no cortical penetration, periosteal reaction, or soft tissue mass.

Differential Diagnosis: Fibrous dysplasia, osteoblastoma, adamantinoma, osteofibrous dysplasia.

Diagnosis: Osteoblastoma.

Discussion: A specific diagnosis is not possible in this case, but an expansile lesion with hazy mineralization in the tibial midshaft of a child brings up the differential of fibrous dysplasia and osteoblastoma. Other midshaft tibial lesions in children include adamantinoma and osteofibrous dysplasia (ossifying fibroma), both of which should have a more bubbly or multilocular appearance, and are typically found in the cortex rather than the medullary space. Although osteoblastomas have a distinct predilection for the spine, of the approximately 30% that involve the long bones, the vast majority of these involve the lower extremities and are centered in the diaphysis. Most osteoblastomas are radiographically lucent, but mottled, stippled, or hazy ground-glass mineralization may be present. Osteoblastoma is unusual in children less than 5 years old, and there is a male predilection.

Clinical History: 26-year-old intoxicated woman who fell down the stairs.

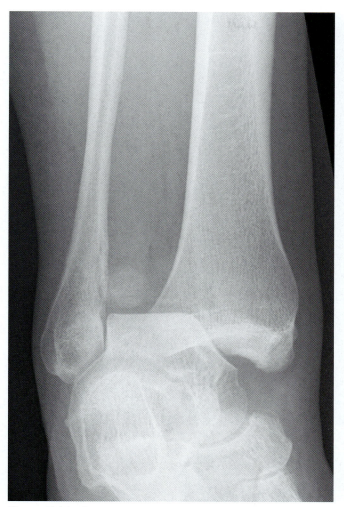

Figure 7-14 A

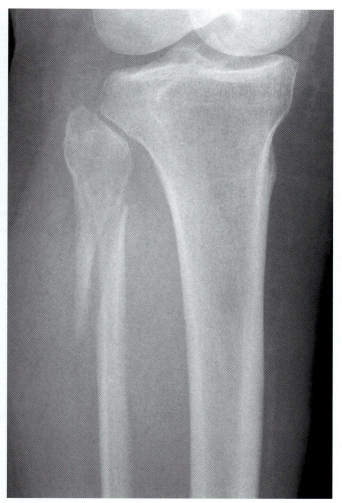

Figure 7-14 B

Findings: (A) Oblique radiograph of the ankle shows lateral dislocation of the talus and foot with disruption of the tibio-fibular syndesmosis, and gross separation of the distal fibula from the tibia. A bone fragment representing the posterior malleolus is seen en face between the tibia and the fibula. The relationship of the talus to the lateral malleolus has been maintained. The displacement of the talus indicates that the deltoid ligament must be disrupted. (B) Oblique radiograph of the proximal leg shows a fracture of the proximal fibular shaft.

Differential Diagnosis: None.

Diagnosis: Maisonneuve fracture.

Discussion: A Maisonneuve fracture occurs with abduction loading of the foot. The syndesmosis ruptures as the fibula is displaced laterally, but the strong posterior tibio-fibular ligaments remain intact and avulse the posterior malleolus. Loading forces extend proximally, tearing the interosseous membrane, and finally exiting with a proximal fibular fracture. The deltoid ligament is disrupted as the talus moves laterally out of the mortise. In this case, the talus became impacted against the lateral aspect of the tibia, but in the typical case, the talus relocates into the mortise on the rebound, reducing the posterior malleolar fragment.

Clinical History: 18-year-old woman with knee pain.

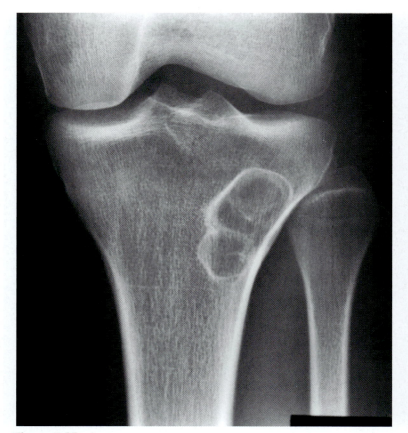

Figure 7-15   A

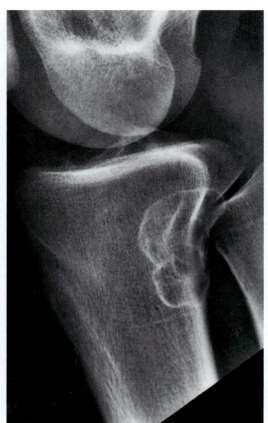

Figure 7-15   C

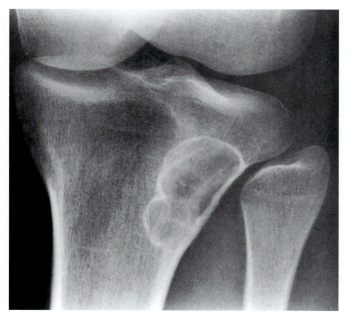

Figure 7-15   B

Findings: AP, lateral, and oblique radiographs of the knee show a well-defined, multiloculated, lucent lesion with sclerotic borders in the metadiaphysis. It is cortically based and eccentric, with extension into the medullary space. There is minimal expansion of the cortical surface.

Differential Diagnosis: None.

Diagnosis: Nonossifying fibroma (fibrous cortical defect).

Discussion: Nonossifying fibromas are histologically identical to fibrous cortical defects. Both are nonneoplastic proliferations of fibrous tissue and histiocytes that are self-limited and have no potential for growth or spread. Common radiologic usage of these terms refers to small, shallow, cortical lesions as fibrous cortical defects, and larger, multiloculated lesions as nonossifying fibromas. These lesions regress spontaneously, filling in with bone from the periphery and disappearing. The lesions are present at some time in perhaps one-third of all children. Fibrous cortical defects are seen mostly in children between 4 to 8 years old. Located on the cortical surface of the metaphysis at the attachment of a tendon or ligament, mostly around the knee, they produce a 1 cm to 4 cm scalloped defect in the underlying bone. They are round or oval, lucent, and sharply marginated by a sclerotic rim. Some have a bubbly appearance. Pathologic fractures may occur, but fibrous cortical defects are usually clinically silent. The distal femur, distal tibia, proximal tibia, and fibula are the reported locations for 90% of these lesions.

The lesion in this case has very indolent characteristics. The best way to estimate the rate of growth of a focal bone lesion is to evaluate the interface between the lesion and the host bone. The presence of a well-defined, thin, sclerotic rim of bone completely surrounding a lesion is indicative of a lesion whose rate of growth is slow enough to allow reactive osteoblastic activity. This rim of bone distributes biomechanical stress around the lesion and is typically better developed in weight-bearing bones. Lesions located in the diaphysis often do not have sclerotic margins, regardless of the growth rate.

Clinical History: 10-year-old boy with pain, restricted motion, and swelling.

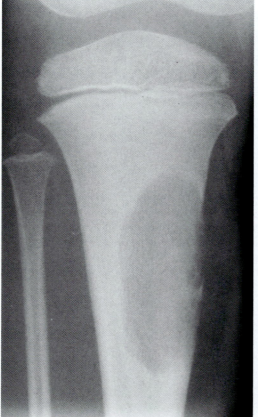

Figure 7-16   A

Figure 7-16   B

Findings: AP and lateral radiographs of the knee demonstrate a geographic, eccentric lesion in the proximal tibial metadiaphysis. There is mild expansion, trabeculation, and thinning of cortex. Small areas of cortical perforation are demonstrated laterally.

Differential Diagnosis: Nonossifying fibroma, enchondroma, chondroblastoma, fibrous dysplasia, chondromyxoid fibroma.

Diagnosis: Chondromyxoid fibroma.

Discussion: The diagnosis in this case is not easily made. Chondromyxoid fibroma is the rarest of all the cartilage tumors, and the imaging findings are nonspecific, so one should always expect to be wrong when proposing the diagnosis. However, the most common location for chondromyxoid fibroma is the proximal metaphysis of the tibia. The lesions are eccentric and often have a lobulated, well-defined margin. Cartilaginous matrix mineralization is not usually seen. Periosteal reaction is not a prominent feature. The first diagnostic consideration is usually nonossifying fibroma.

As the name indicates, histologically chondromyxoid fibroma is composed of a mixture of cartilaginous, myxoid, and fibrous elements. The lesion most commonly affects long bones, especially the tibia. In the Mayo Clinic series, [14] chondromyxoid fibroma was the least common of the benign cartilage tumors, comprising only 3%, compared with 9% for chondroblastoma, 24% for chondroma (including enchondroma and periosteal chondroma), and 64% for osteochondroma.

Clinical History: 8-year-old girl with anterior leg mass.

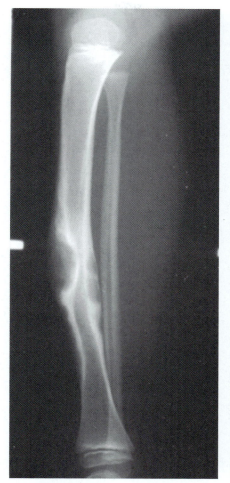

Figure 7-17   A

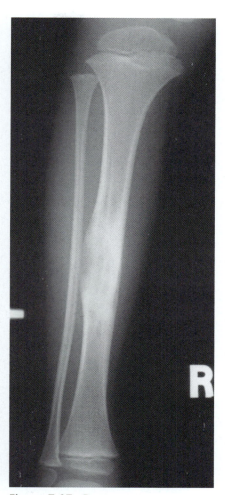

Figure 7-17   B

Findings: Lateral and AP radiographs of tibia show a bowing deformity, with the apex directed anteriorly. There is an anterior cortex lesion with multiple lucent regions and surrounding sclerosis.

Differential Diagnosis: Adamantinoma, ossifying fibroma, neurofibromatosis, fibrous dysplasia.

Diagnosis: Adamantinoma.

Discussion: The radiologic diagnosis may be suggested by the particular location of the lesion in the anterior cortex of the tibia at the mid diaphysis. Adamantinomas are malignant tumors thought to be of angioblastic or epithelioid origin. Most patients are adolescents or young adults. Ninety percent of these lesions are found in the tibia. The clinical course tends to be long, and most patients present with pain or swelling. The most common radiographic appearance is multiple, sharply circumscribed, lucent lesions of different sizes with surrounding sclerosis. Involvement of the bone is typically asymmetric, with the anterior tibial cortex virtually always the epicenter of the lesion. A relationship with ossifying fibroma has been postulated, because some regions of the tumors may have a histologic and radiologic resemblance. Whether ossifying fibroma represents a precursor to adamantinoma or whether it represents a reparative response is unknown; both possibilities have been suggested. The treatment of adamantinoma is surgical, but local recurrence, lymphatic metastases, and hematogenous metastases may occur.

Clinical History: 35-year-old man with intermittent swelling of the posterior calf.

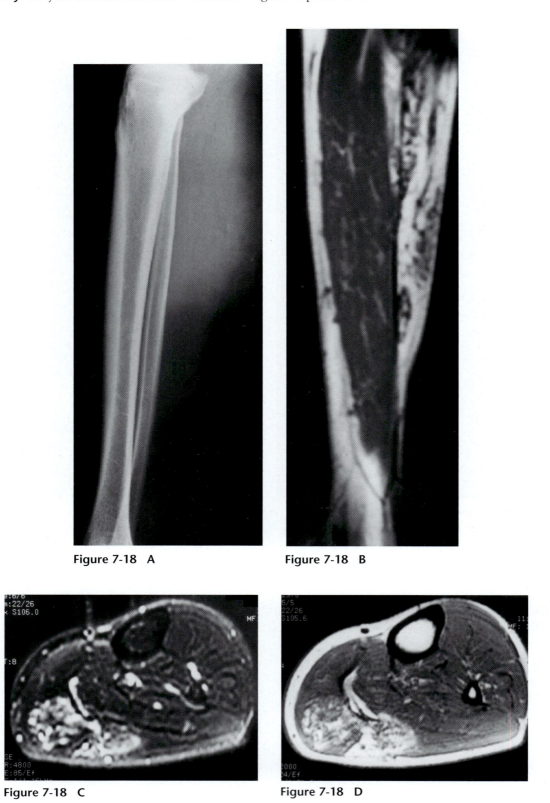

Figure 7-18   A   Figure 7-18   B

Figure 7-18   C   Figure 7-18   D

Findings: (**A**) Lateral radiograph demonstrates soft tissue swelling with a few phleboliths. The region of abnormality shows mottled densities within fat and loss of the normal sharp demarcation between the subcutaneous fat and the superficial fascia. (**B**) Sagittal T1-weighted MRI demonstrates tubular structures with low signal intensity in a base of high signal intensity (fat). (**C**) Axial T2-weighted MRI shows tubular structures of high-intensity signal posteriorly. (**D**) Axial T1-weighted MRI after intravenous gadolinium injection shows enhancement of the lesion.

Differential Diagnosis: Hemangioma, cellulitis.

Diagnosis: Hemangioma, soft tissue.

Discussion: Phleboliths within the soft tissue mass in the calf are suggestive of a vascular malformation. The MRI findings confirm the diagnosis. On T1-weighted MRI, hemangiomas characteristically have heterogenous signal intensity with some areas of fat-signal intensity. Low-intensity tubular structures of various sizes are usually evident. T2-weighted MRI shows fluid signal within the tubular structures, corresponding to sluggish blood flow. Hemangiomas may be classified histologically based on the predominant type of vascular channel [15]. The three main types are capillary, cavernous, and arteriovenous. The capillary type is most often found in the dermis or subcutaneous tissues, and typically does not undergo diagnostic imaging. The arteriovenous or venous types are rare. It is the cavernous type that often presents as a soft tissue mass requiring diagnostic imaging. Together, the classic radiographs and MRI findings are virtually diagnostic of cavernous hemangioma.

Clinical History: 15-year-old cross-country runner with lower leg pain.

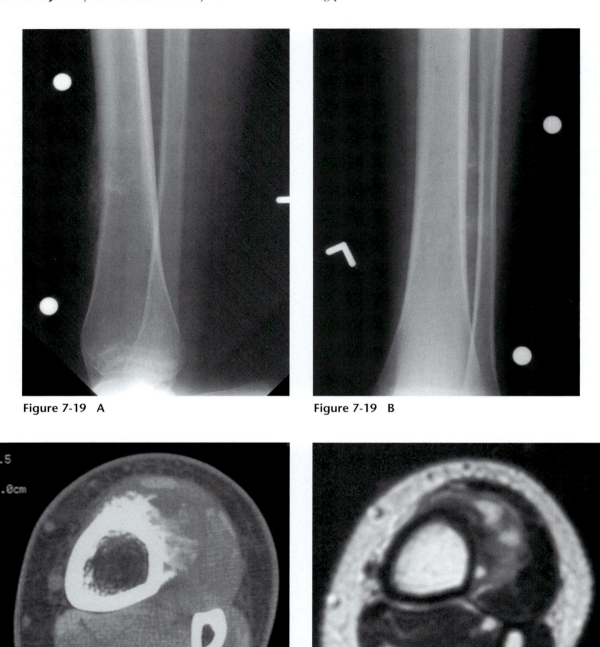

Figure 7-19   A

Figure 7-19   B

Figure 7-19   C

Figure 7-19   D

Findings: (**A, B**) Lateral and AP detail views of the lower tibia demonstrate a mass on the cortical surface of the distal tibia. There are lucent and sclerotic regions, with spicules of bone projecting away from the cortex into the soft tissues. (**C**) Axial CT with contrast enhancement shows the tumor mass extending from the cortical surface. (**D**) Axial T1-weighted MRI after gadolinium injection shows an enhancing mass apposed to an intact cortex, with low-signal regions within.

Differential Diagnosis: Parosteal osteosarcoma, periosteal osteosarcoma, high-grade surface osteosarcoma, lymphoma, juxtacortical chondroma.

Diagnosis: Periosteal osteosarcoma.

Discussion: Osteosarcoma is an uncommon, malignant, bone-forming tumor with three commonly recognized but rare variants that arise on the cortical surface: parosteal osteosarcoma, periosteal osteosarcoma, and high-grade surface osteosarcoma [16]. Periosteal osteosarcomas comprise about 1.5% of all osteosarcomas. Usually found in the diaphysis of the femur or tibia, the peak age of discovery is about 20 years old, and most patients present after a few weeks or months of pain, swelling, tenderness, or mass [17]. Periosteal osteosarcomas are moderately differentiated and chondroblastic, unlike the more common parosteal os-teosarcomas, which are well-differentiated and fibroblastic. The presence of any high-grade histologic features would cause the lesion to be classified as a high-grade surface osteosarcoma [18].

It is uncertain whether these surface osteosarcomas arise in the periosteum or in the outer layers of the cortex. On imaging, periosteal osteosarcomas appear as elongated, partially mineralized masses on the cortical surface of a long bone in the diaphyseal region, with thickened underlying cortex and solid periosteal reaction at the margins. Lucent regions within the tumor correspond to nonmineralized tumor cartilage, and brush-like spicules of bone extending from the underlying cortex into the tumor correspond mostly to trabeculae of reactive bone. Blotchy, punctate, and circular densities in the tumor represent mineralization of chondroid tumor matrix and reactive bone. The periphery of the lesion will have less mineralization. Periosteal osteosarcomas are much less dense radiographically than parosteal osteosarcomas, reflecting the difference in their histologic differentiation. Minimal involvement of the marrow space can be seen on CT or MRI [19]. Periosteal osteosarcomas are treated with wide excision. Their prognosis is better than that of high-grade intramedullary or high-grade surface osteosarcomas, but worse than parosteal osteosarcomas.

Clinical History: 8-year-old boy with painless swelling of the lower leg.

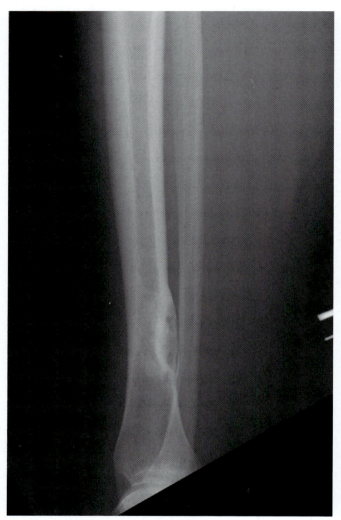

Figure 7-20   A

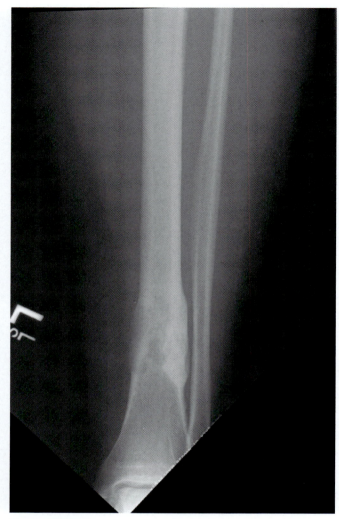

Figure 7-20   B

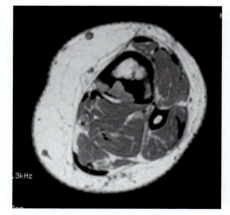

Figure 7-20   C

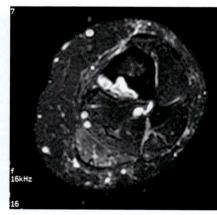

Figure 7-20   D

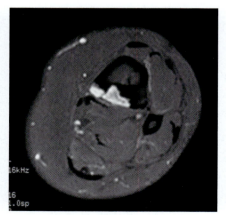

Figure 7-20   E

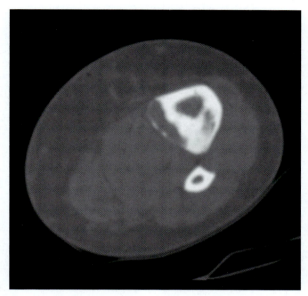

Figure 7-20   F

Findings: (**A, B**) Lateral and AP radiographs of the lower leg show an expansile cortical lesion of the distal tibial shaft. Mature periosteal bone is heaped up around the lesion. Axial proton density (**C**), T2-weighted (**D**), and T1-weighted gadolinium-enhanced (**E**) MRI of the lower leg shows a heterogeneous cortical lesion with solid surrounding periosteal reaction and intense enhancement. There are no extraosseous or intramedullary components. (**F**) Axial CT shows a thin rim of intact bone surrounding the superficial aspect of the lesion. The lateral portion of the lesion shows ground-glass mineralization.

Differential Diagnosis: Adamantinoma, ossifying fibroma, neurofibromatosis, fibrous dysplasia.

Diagnosis: Ossifying fibroma (osteofibrous dysplasia).

Discussion: Ossifying fibroma is considered a benign fibroosseous disorder that resembles fibrous dysplasia pathologically and radiologically except for its intracortical location. Campanacci rendered the first comprehensive description of this entity [20]. The lesions are slightly more common in males and generally occur when the patient is less than 10 years old. Involvement is virtually isolated to the tibia, usually in the mid diaphysis, although rarely fibular involvement may be seen. The lesions may resolve spontaneously or show some degree of progression. Although it appears to be a distinct entity, a relationship to adamantinoma and

fibrous dysplasia has been suggested. Osteofibrous dysplasia may be a precursor to malignant adamantinoma, and simultaneous occurrence of both lesions has been documented [21,22,23]. Bony resorption with subsequent fibrous repair may be responsible for these lesions, or they may represent a particular type of fibrous dysplasia.

Certain trisomies may be associated with osteofibrous dysplasia [24]. Pathologically, osteoblastic rimming and lamellar trabeculae are histologically distinguishing features from conventional fibrous dysplasia [25]. These lesions may have a radiographic appearance similar to that of adamantinoma; however, discriminating features include ground-glass texture of the bone, anterior bowing, and absence of destructive or periosteal changes. In addition, fibrous dysplasia generally occurs in a younger population. These features enabled proper identification of fibrous or osteofibrous dysplasia in 87% of cases and adamantinoma in 95% of cases in one study [26]. MRI is nonspecific and not particularly useful in the evaluation of these lesions [27], except perhaps for anatomic extent. Conservative treatment is advocated, since there is a high postsurgical recurrence rate [28]. Prevalent complications include pathologic fracture and pseudoarthrosis. In a series of 11 patients, four had pathologic fracture, complicated by pseudoarthrosis in two of these instances.

Clinical History: 80-year-old woman, profoundly ill.

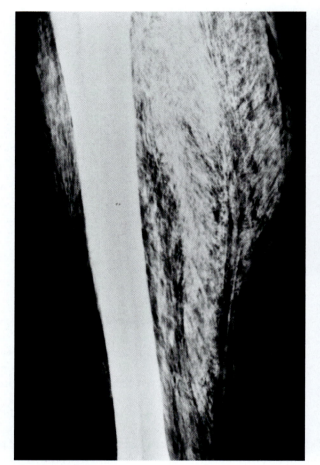

Figure 7-21   A

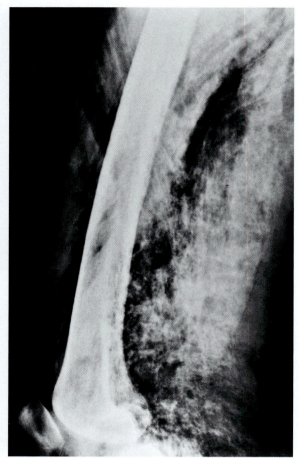

Figure 7-21   B

Findings: Lateral radiographs of the leg and thigh on the same side. Gas has dissected into the deep soft tissues outlining the muscle bundles and fascial planes.

Differential Diagnosis: Infection, penetrating trauma, ulceration.

Diagnosis: Clostridial myonecrosis (gas gangrene).

Discussion: Clostridial myonecrosis usually results from trauma. Clostridial contamination of traumatic wounds may produce extensive tissue damage and gas formation in devitalized tissues (gas gangrene). The most common causative agent, *Clostridium perfringens,* is widely distributed in nature. Clostridial myositis has a classic radiographic appearance of extensive linear collections of gas that are dispersed widely throughout the affected muscles.

Spontaneous, non-trauma-related clostridial myonecrosis has been associated with colorectal carcinoma, leukemia, diabetes mellitus, and drug-related immunosuppression [29,30]. The main underlying conditions in spontaneous clostridial myonecrosis consist of hematologic or gastrointestinal malignancy, and the most commonly implicated organisms are *C. perfringens* and *C. septicum* [31]. The mortality from spontaneous clostridial myonecrosis is higher than that occurring in the setting of trauma, with a survival rate of only 19% [32].

Symptoms consist of pain, edema, hemorrhagic bullae, and crepitus, frequently accompanied by shock. Gram-positive rods retrieved from the infected area help establish the diagnosis. *Clostridia* are gas-producing organisms, and the presence of gas, which may be suggested by crepitus in the infected area clinically and confirmed radiographically, should suggest the diagnosis.

Treatment is by debridement and antibiotic therapy. Hyperbaric oxygen therapy may be beneficial and has demonstrated a synergistic effect in decreasing morbidity and mortality in animal models. Retrospective human studies suggest this therapy may decrease mortality by a factor of two [33].

Clinical History: 10-year-old boy with leg pain and tenderness.

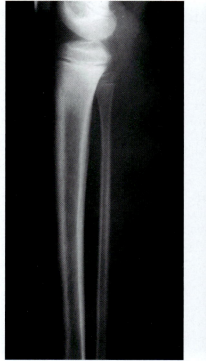

Figure 7-22   A

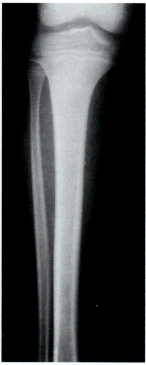

Figure 7-22   B

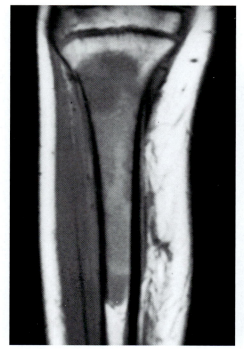

Figure 7-22   C

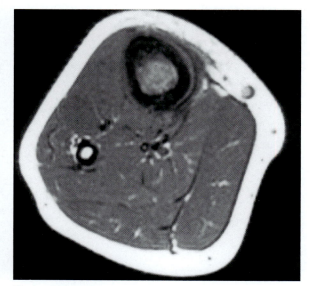

Figure 7-22   D

Findings: (A, B) Lateral and AP radiographs of the lower leg show a vague region of sclerosis in the proximal tibia and subtle periosteal reaction along the proximal shaft, seen posteriorly on the lateral radiograph and laterally on the AP radiograph. (C) Coronal T1-weighted MRI shows replacement of the fatty marrow in the proximal tibia. Periosteal reactive bone is present along both sides of the shaft, with a pathologic buckle fracture of the lateral cortex of the metaphysis. (D) Axial proton density MRI shows the intramedullary process permeating through the cortex into the surrounding soft tissues. Tiny focal regions of intermediate signal give the normally homogeneous low-signal cortical bone a mottled, blurred appearance. A layer of periosteal bone partially surrounds the tibia.

Differential Diagnosis: Osteosarcoma, Ewing's sarcoma, and lymphoma.

Diagnosis: Ewing's sarcoma.

Discussion: The radiographs are exceedingly subtle and could easily be passed as normal. The MRI shows an extensive intramedullary lesion with a permeative growth pattern, characteristic of a rapidly enlarging process. The differential diagnosis is that of an aggressive intramedullary lesion, and includes neoplasm as well as infection. The location is common for osteosarcoma, Ewing's sarcoma, and lymphoma, which are the most common bone tumors in the pediatric age group. Hematogenous osteomyelitis begins at the metaphyseal side of the growth plate and is unlikely for that reason. The lack of tumor ossification favors Ewing's sarcoma and lymphoma, but no CT was obtained, and small regions could easily be missed on radiographs or MRI. Clearly, the definitive diagnosis must be made by biopsy.

Clinical History: 55-year-old woman, and a companion case.

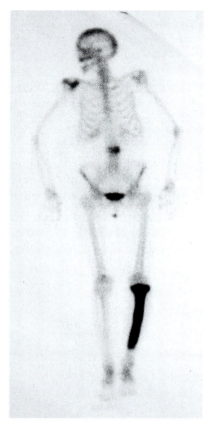

Figure 7-23   A

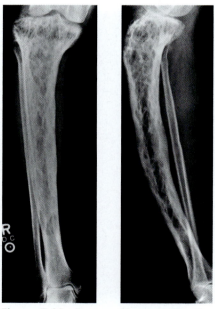

Figure 7-23   B   Figure 7-23   C

Findings: (A) Whole-body radionuclide bone scan shows intense activity in the tibia, extending from the knee almost to the ankle. There is a bowing deformity. Additional areas of abnormality are seen in the lumbar spine and right shoulder. (B, C) Companion case: 78-year-old woman. AP and lateral radiographs of the tibia show marked cortical and trabecular thickening, beginning at the proximal end of the tibia and extending to the distal metadiaphysis. At the distal interface between abnormal and normal bone is a flame-shaped region of osteolysis.

Differential Diagnosis: None.

Diagnosis: Paget's disease.

Discussion: The intense activity on bone scan involving a long bone from one end toward the other is diagnostic of Paget's disease. On the radiographs, the cortical thickening, coarse trabecular pattern, and the flame-shaped osteolysis are typical for Paget's disease.

Paget's disease commonly begins at the end of a long bone as a zone of osteolysis that is eventually replaced with cortical and trabecular thickening [34,35]. The new bone is weak bone—a highly vascular mosaic of woven and lamellar bone—and a characteristic lateral bowing of the femur or anterior bowing of the tibia ensues. At sites of tuberosities, primary involvement can begin in the diaphysis, as in this case. This is classically described in the tibial tuberosity, but is also present at the femoral trochanters or humeral tuberosities. This form of Paget's disease is most common in younger patients with monostotic disease who tend to have a normal alkaline phosphatase.

Differential considerations for unilateral anterior tibial bowing include the saber shin abnormality seen in syphilis, neurofibromatosis (in which case cortical thinning is more common), and amniotic band syndrome (obvious from birth). Treatment is usually supportive and directed at the complications of the disease; however, it is not clear who is at risk of complications or if the medication to decrease bone turnover is effective in decreasing the progression of the disease.

It is interesting to note that the initial site of Paget's disease is at the end of a long bone, an area with extensive vascularity but little hematopoietic marrow. Therefore, the primary inciting event seems to depend on vascularity, but propagation of the disease is dependent on the osteoclastic activity of the hematopoietic marrow.

Clinical History: 13-year-old girl with knee pain, and a companion case.

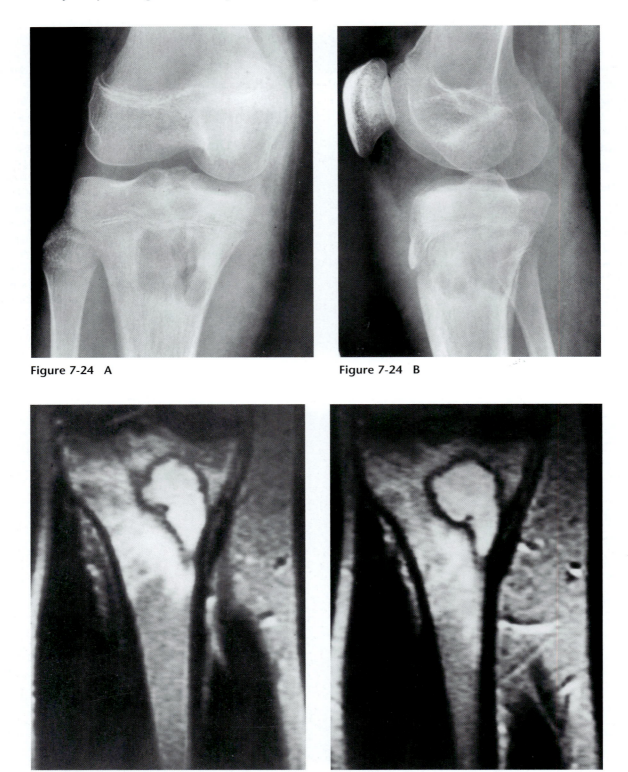

Figure 7-24   A

Figure 7-24   B

Figure 7-24   C

Figure 7-24   D

Findings: (A, B) AP and lateral radiographs of the knee. A lucent lesion in the proximal tibial metaphysis abutting the growth plate is present, with a somewhat lobular contour and surrounding sclerosis. The sclerosis merges imperceptibly with the surrounding bone. Soft tissue swelling is present, and a single layer of solid periosteal reactive bone is present posteriorly. There is no knee joint effusion. (C, D) Companion case: a young man with knee pain. T2 coronal MRI demonstrates a geographic area of high signal intensity, with a low-signal intensity rim in the metadiaphysis of the tibia and extension to the cortical surface. Extensive surrounding marrow edema is present.

Differential Diagnosis: Eosinophilic granuloma, infection, lymphoma, metastasis.

Diagnosis: Brodie's abscess.

Discussion: A Brodie's abscess is a local, subacute bone abscess that may present as a solitary bone lesion. Symptoms of recurrent pain and local tenderness with swelling and erythema may be present for months or years. Most cases occur in adolescents and young adults, but the reported age range is 6 to 61 years. Males are affected more often than females by a 2:1 ratio. The typical location is the metaphysis or diaphysis of the femur or tibia. A Brodie's abscess may begin de novo, it may develop in the same site as the preceding episode of acute osteomyelitis, or it may follow an acute episode of osteomyelitis at another site. Only 25% of patients have a history of antecedent infection or show systemic signs of infection. *Staphylococcus aureus* is the most common offending organism.

Radiographically, a Brodie's abscess appears as a well-defined lucent area in cancellous bone, with smooth, round, geographic margins and a thick sclerotic rind that may merge imperceptibly with the surrounding bone. The lesion may appear lobulated, with lucent serpentine tracts extending along the bone, sometimes leading to a draining sinus on the skin. CT is valuable for defining the reactive sclerosis, and it can permit identification of tracts in the bone. The corresponding pathology is an avascular cavity, typically 1 to 4 cm in size, lined with granulation tissue and filled with fluid but usually not frank pus. Thickening of trabeculae adjacent to the lesion by reactive endosteal bone formation may form a sclerotic rind about the cavity.

Although Brodie's abscesses have a characteristic appearance, they may be confused with other focal bone lesions, including tumors. The key radiologic feature of a Brodie's abscess is the extensive reactive bone formation that has a sharp interface with the lesion but merges gradually with surrounding normal bone.

Clinical History: 47-year-old man with knee pain for several weeks.

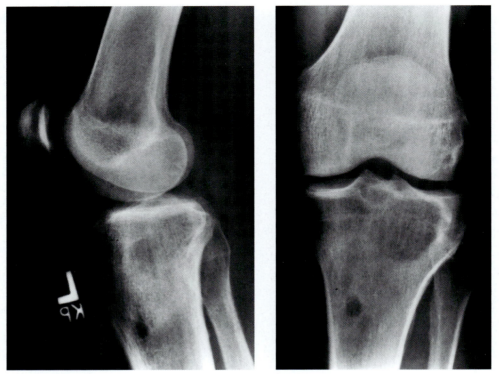

Figure 7-25   A

Figure 7-25   B

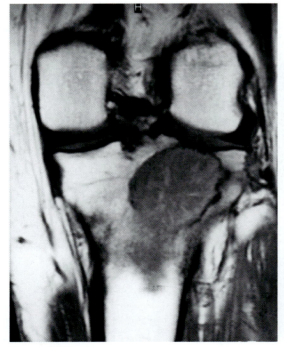

Figure 7-25   C

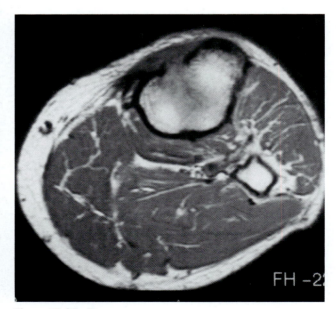

Figure 7-25   D

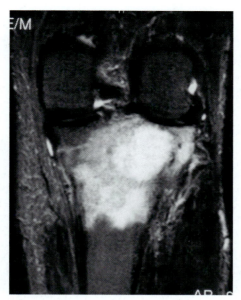

Figure 7-25 E

Findings: (**A, B**) Lateral and AP radiographs of the knee show a destructive process in the proximal tibia, with a larger, rounded proximal lesion and a smaller distal lesion. There may be vague rarefaction connecting these lesions, and there are some areas of surrounding sclerosis. The sclerosis does not completely surround the areas of destruction. No periosteal bone formation is present. There is no knee effusion. (**C**) Coronal T1-weighted MRI shows the proximal lesion extending to the tibial articular surface, with a partial rim of low-signal reactive bone. (**D**) Axial T1-weighted MRI through the more distal portion of the lesion shows a defect in the anterior tibial cortex, with well-localized soft tissue extension. (**E**) Coronal T2-weighted MRI shows bright signal within the proximal tibia. There is no involvement of the knee joint.

Differential Diagnosis: Infection, metastasis, lymphoma, adamantinoma, malignant transformation in Paget's disease, radiation, or osteonecrosis.

Diagnosis: Tuberculous osteomyelitis.

Discussion: Extensive bone destruction is present with minimal reactive bone formation. The appearance is more suggestive of infection than neoplasm because of the morphology of the destruction, but the lack of reactive bone formation would be unexpected for a pyogenic pathogen.

Tuberculous osteomyelitis not involving a joint is uncommon. On radiographs, advanced lesions such as this may mimic chronic pyogenic osteomyelitis, Brodie's abscess, tumor, or granulomatous lesions [36]. There are no particular imaging features that allow a conclusive radiologic diagnosis. Biopsy is mandatory to confirm the diagnosis. In one study, the prevalence of peripheral osteoarticular involvements in patients with known tuberculosis was 0.05%, with most of these cases involving the joint and the adjacent epiphyses [37]. Cases involving joints presented as destructive arthritis, whereas cases involving only bone had the appearance of lytic tumor.

Tuberculosis has undergone resurgence in recent years. Sites of predilection include the spine, hip, and knee. The mode of spread of mycobacterial infection to bone is hematogenous. Once settled in tissue, the host elicits an antigenic response, consisting of multinucleated giant cell and lymphocyte reaction. Caseating necrosis ensues, resulting in bony destruction and host reaction similar to pyogenic osteomyelitis. Marrow changes, as seen in the MRI, are similar to pyogenic infection, but the changes in tuberculosis often progress at a slower pace. Bursitis, as seen here, and tendinitis may be present. Phemister's triad in tuberculosis consists of juxtaarticular osteoporosis, peripheral erosions, and conspicuous lack of joint space alteration until late in the clinical course. When joint space obliteration does occur, it usually does so by fibrosis rather than bony ankylosis. Note the relative sparing of the cartilage space in this case. On radiographs, advanced tuberculous osteomyelitis may mimic chronic pyogenic osteomyelitis, Brodie's abscess, tumors, or other granulomatous lesions.

Clinical History: 24-year-old varsity football player.

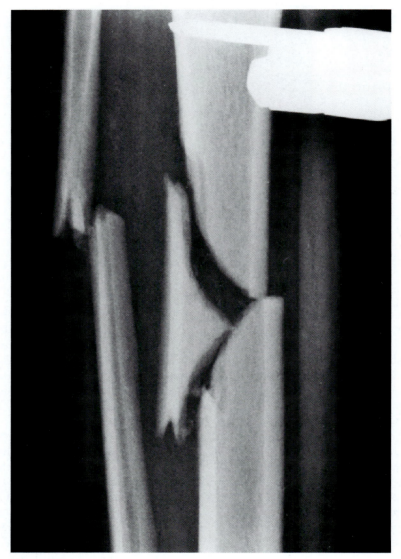

Figure 7-26

Findings: AP radiograph of the leg (detail). The patient has been visited by the orthopedic surgeon and placed in an external fixator. There is a comminuted fracture of the tibia.

Differential Diagnosis: None.

Diagnosis: Transverse fracture with butterfly fragment.

Discussion: Fractures caused by indirect loading result in injuries at a distance from the site of loading. They have fracture lines with predictable morphology, depending on the mode of loading. Bending results in tensile forces on the convex side of the bend, and compressive forces on the concave side of the bend. The tensile forces result in a transverse fracture, whereas the compressive forces result in symmetric oblique fractures and the butterfly fragment. Fractures of this morphology always result from loading in this manner, and the butterfly fragment will be on the concave side of the bend. Sometimes bending will result in a single oblique fracture on the concave side that connects with the transverse fracture, leaving a fracture line that resembles a hockey stick.

Clinical History: 29-year-old runner with knee pain.

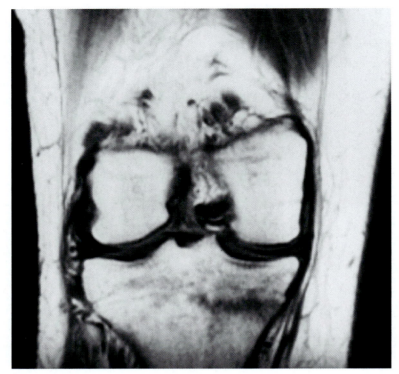

Figure 7-27   A

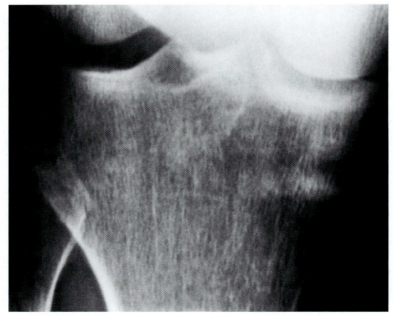

Figure 7-27   B

Findings: (A) Coronal T1-weighted MRI demonstrates a horizontally oriented linear band of low signal intensity in the proximal medial metaphysis. The radiographs at this time were normal. (B) Six weeks later, detail of AP radiograph demonstrates a linear band of increased sclerosis corresponding to the area of low signal on MRI.

Differential Diagnosis: None.

Diagnosis: Stress fracture.

Discussion: The linear band of decreased signal intensity within the tibial metaphysis is oriented perpendicular to the long axis, abuts the cortex, and is surrounded by an ill-defined area of decreased signal intensity that represents marrow edema. This constellation of findings is characteristic of a stress fracture. The clinical history and follow-up radiograph showing the sclerotic changes of healing confirms the diagnosis.

Stress fractures occur after repetitive, prolonged muscular activity that places more stress on an area of bone than usual. Bone responds by remodeling and strengthening itself to accommodate the additional stress, but there is a vulnerable period in which the bone is weakened by intracortical bone resorption in preparation for the formation of new bone. The term stress fracture encompasses both fatigue fractures and insufficiency fractures. Fatigue fractures, the type seen in athletes, are due to abnormal repetitive stresses exerted on normal bone (as in this case). Insufficiency fractures are due to normal stresses exerted on abnormal or insufficiently strong bone. For example, compression fractures of the spine in patients with senile osteoporosis are insufficiency fractures. The osteoporotic bone is no longer strong enough to withstand the normal compressive stress of the body weight.

The imaging features of stress fractures are usually straightforward: a linear band of increased density on radiography, linear decreased signal on T1-weighted or proton-density MRI, or a linear focus of radiotracer uptake. Characteristically, these linear abnormalities are oriented perpendicular to the long axis of the involved bone. Pathophysiologically, the findings are due to callus formation around trabecular microfractures. Earlier changes of stress reaction can be much more difficult to detect. Plain radiographs may be normal when the patient is first seen, or may show only very subtle resorptive changes within the cortex [38]. MRI and radionuclide examinations may show only amorphous areas of abnormality, although they often suggest the diagnosis long before it can be made by plain radiographs.

Fatigue fracture locations vary according to the specific type of physical activity. Runners are prone to develop them in the tibia. Military recruits are prone to develop them in the metatarsals and calcanei.

Clinical History: 2-year-old boy whose mother says he fell down while she was not watching.

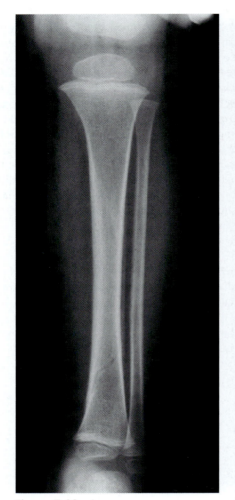

Figure 7-28   A

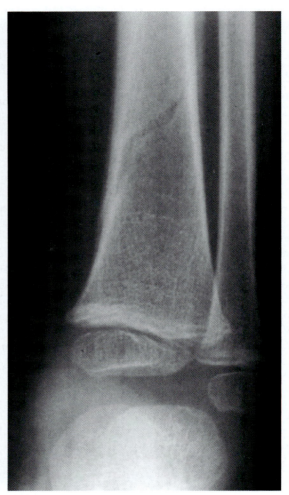

Figure 7-28   B

Findings: AP radiograph of the tibia (full and detail) shows a nondisplaced curved fracture of the distal tibial shaft.

Differential Diagnosis: Accidental fracture, inflicted trauma.

Diagnosis: Fracture, tibia (toddler's).

Discussion: There is a nondisplaced spiral-type fracture of the distal tibial metaphysis in this 2-year-old child. The age of the child and location of this fracture are typical of this stress-type injury. The repeated twisting falls of these young children as they are learning to walk result in this characteristic fracture.

Isolated spiral or oblique fractures of the tibial shaft are common injuries in ambulatory preschoolers (toddler's fracture). The fibula is usually intact. These injuries result from falls with torsion of the foot, and the traumatic episode is often innocuous or not witnessed. These fractures may be exceedingly subtle on radiographs because the low energy that produces the fracture is insufficient to displace it. The clinical presentation is often failure to bear weight, limping, or simply the appearance of pain when bearing weight. Follow-up examinations will show periosteal new bone, indicative of healing. Fractures from a similar mechanism may occur less frequently in the femur or metatarsals. Toddler's fractures must be distinguished from inflicted trauma in the battered child.

Clinical History: Three Army privates in basic training.

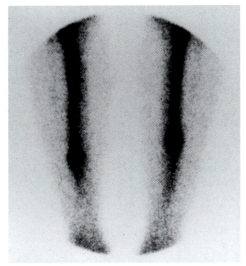

Figure 7-29   A

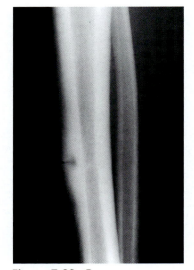

Figure 7-29   B

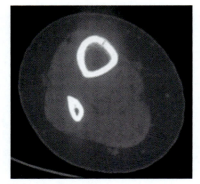

Figure 7-29   C

Findings: (A) Case 1. Radionuclide bone scan. Anterior camera view of both lower legs shows intense activity at the midshaft of both tibias, with a broad region of less focal and less intense activity along the proximal shafts. (B) Case 2. Lateral lower leg radiograph (detail). The anterior cortex of the tibia is markedly thickened. There is a transverse lucency extending from the periosteal surface partially through the cortex, with a poorly defined region of lucency around the deep margin of the lucency. (C) Case 3. Axial CT through the middle third of the tibial shaft shows a longitudinal lucent line through the anteromedial tibial cortex, with slight periosteal and endosteal reactive bone.

Differential Diagnosis: Stress fractures at different stages.

Diagnosis: Case 1: bilateral tibial stress fractures and stress remodeling. Case 2: anterior tibial stress fracture with nonunion. Case 3: longitudinal anterior tibial stress fracture.

Discussion: The radionuclide bone scan in Case 1 shows increased activity along both tibial shafts, which is consistent with stress remodeling. The more focal areas of activity correspond to stress fractures. The lateral radiograph of the lower leg in Case 2 shows the anterior tibial cortical thickening of stress remodeling, as well as the stress fracture. The lucency around the deep margin of the fracture line is indicative of nonunion. The CT in Case 3 shows a longitudinal fracture of the anteromedial tibial cortex involving the middle third of the shaft.

Stress fractures of the tibia are usually seen in athletic or military populations. It is estimated to occur in 20% of recruits and a favored location is the posterior, medial cortex of the proximal tibial diaphysis. The most contributory factor to this injury is related to tibial bending strength in the anterior to posterior direction [39]. Fractures involving the middle third of the tibia are much less common and pose problems with diagnosis as well as treatment. Usually these fractures are transverse, though on occasion they may be vertical, as in companion Case 3 [40]. Very often the initial radiographs show only thickening of the anterior cortex. Shin splints represent a milder condition in the same spectrum. An Aircast pneumatic brace may procure a quicker recovery and enable the patient to engage in athletic activities earlier [41].

Nonunion represents an uncommon complication, although anterior cortical midshaft tibial stress fractures are very prone to demonstrate this complication. In one series of athletes with these fractures, the overall time from initial symptoms to return to competition was 12.5 months [42]. If conservative therapy fails after a few months, then surgical treatment with resection of the fracture is advocated [43]. Intramedullary nailing may benefit patients with recurrent stress fractures, which are often seen in athletes and army recruits [44].

Clinical History: 10-year-old with knee trauma.

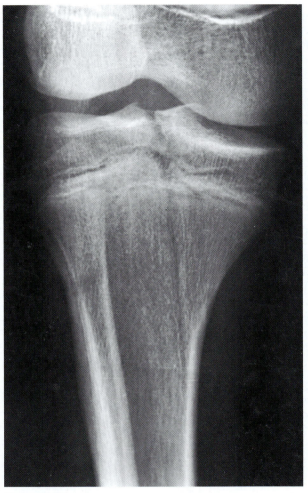

Figure 7-30

Findings: AP radiograph shows a vertical lucency originating in the notch region and extending to the metadiaphysis medial surface.

Differential Diagnosis: None.

Diagnosis: Salter type IV fracture.

Discussion: Fractures involving the growth plate (physis) of a long or short tubular bone are classified with the Salter-Harris system as type I, II, III, IV, or V.

- Type I fracture extends transversely through the plane of the physis.
- Type II fractures are the most common; they have a metaphyseal fracture fragment in addition to a physeal fracture.

- Type III fractures extend from the physis into the epiphysis.
- Type IV fractures have metaphyseal and epiphyseal involvement (as in this case).
- Type V fractures are due to axial loading; with an impaction crush injury of the physis.

The classification is important because it has prognostic significance. As one progresses from type I to type V there is a higher incidence of bad fracture outcome, with increased potential for growth disturbance or angular deformity. This is particularly true with lower extremity growth plate fractures.

Clinical History: 51-year-old man with nontender leg mass and foot drop.

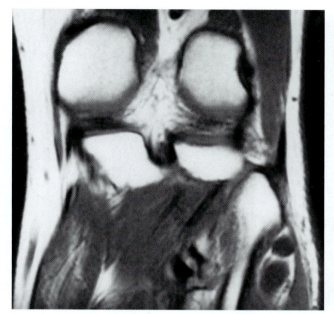
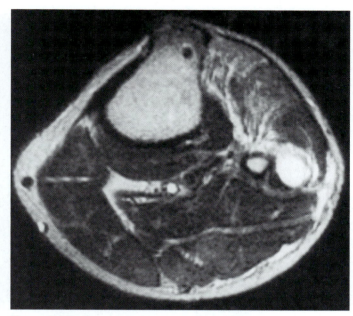

Figure 7-31   A   **Figure 7-31   B**

Findings: (**A**) Coronal T1-weighted MRI through the fibula shows lobulated mass lateral to the neck of the fibula with signal intensity similar to that of muscle, following the expected course of the peroneal nerve. The mass is separate from the bone. (**B**) Axial T2-weighted MRI shows high signal in the mass, lateral to the fibula. There is also atrophic change in the tibialis anterior muscle, consistent with peroneal nerve palsy. The lesion has no enhancement with intravenous gadolinium injection (not shown).

Differential Diagnosis: Peroneal nerve ganglion cyst, schwannoma, neurofibroma.

Diagnosis: Peroneal nerve ganglion cyst.

Discussion: The clinical history of mass and foot drop suggests a mass lesion causing a common peroneal nerve palsy. The findings on MRI are those of a cystic lesion. Peroneal nerve ganglion cysts probably arise from the synovial capsule of the proximal tibiofibular joint, and dissect along the sheath of the recurrent superior tibiofibular articular branch of the common peroneal nerve as they enlarge [45]. The lesions eventually reach the common peroneal nerve itself and lose their communication with the tibiofibular joint. Continued enlargement and cystic degeneration of the lesion results in signs and symptoms referable to mass effect on the common peroneal nerve. MRI is the most useful technique for demonstrating these lesions [46]. The differential diagnosis would include a nerve sheath tumor such as schwannoma or neurofibroma, but the absence of enhancement suggests a cystic lesion is far more likely. If imaging after gadolinium injection is delayed, the lesions may enhance because of gadolinium passage into the extracellular space.

Clinical History: 5-month-old boy with swollen, tender limbs.

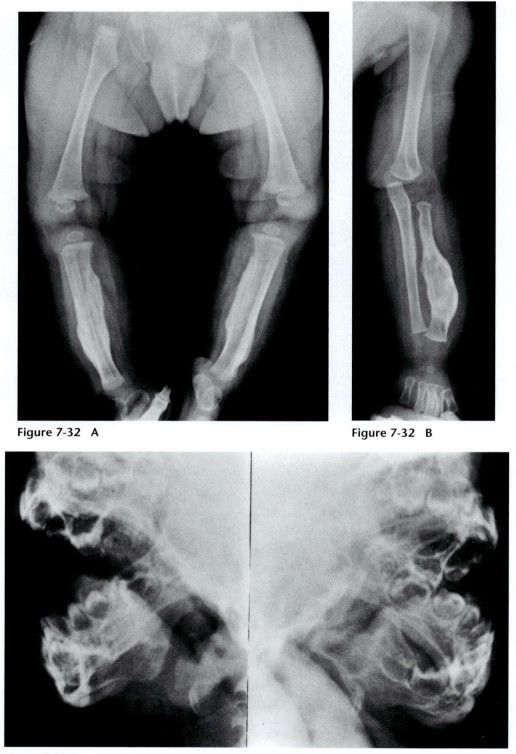

Figure 7-32   A

Figure 7-32   B

Figure 7-32   C

Findings: (A) AP radiograph of the lower limbs. Exuberant, solid periosteal bone formation is seen over the lower legs, with overlying soft tissue swelling. The periosteal bone partially obscures the underlying cortex. No fractures are present. (B) Radiograph of the upper limb shows similar solid periosteal bone along the radius. (C) Radiographs of the mandible show periosteal bone along the inferior margins.

Differential Diagnosis: Caffey's disease, hypervitaminosis A, long-term prostaglandin E administration, physiologic periostitis, infection, scurvy, battered child.

Diagnosis: Caffey's disease (infantile cortical hyperostosis).

Discussion: Caffey's disease, or infantile cortical hyperostosis, is a condition of unknown cause that is manifested by soft tissue swelling and new bone formation that begins adjacent to the cortex of ribs, long bones, and facial bones. The deposits of bone merge with the underlying bone and may cause marked thickening of the cortex. Involvement may be monostotic, but usually is polyostotic. Nearly all patients present before 5 months of age. Fever, hyperirritability, and soft tissue swelling, particularly over the mandible, are typical clinical features. The radiologic differential diagnosis in this age group includes conditions that have periostitis and hyperostosis. Rickets, scurvy, and battered child syndrome may have periostitis, hyperostosis, and subperiosteal elevation with subsequent ossification, but the absence of the additional specific features of these conditions should eliminate them as diagnostic possibilities. Hypervitaminosis A typically affects slightly older infants, and there is a predilection for metatarsal involvement and usually not facial or mandibular involvement. Long-term prostaglandin E administration for ductus-dependent cyanotic heart disease may be indistinguishable radiographically, but the clinical history should be definitive.

Clinical History: 35-year-old woman with foot drop.

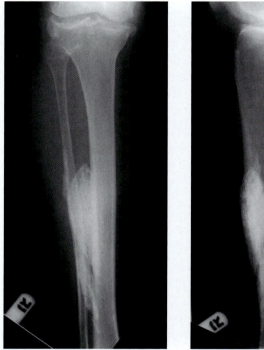

Figure 7-33   A   Figure 7-33   B

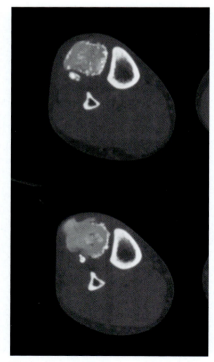

Figure 7-33   C

Findings: (A, B) AP and lateral plain radiographs show well-defined, dense sheets of calcification along the antero-lateral calf. (C) Axial CT shows the calcification is located in the anterior compartment of the leg. There is one main deposit of calcification and a few satellite lesions, all of which have well-defined sclerotic borders. The calcification is denser around the periphery of the lesion. There is no mass effect because the calcified lesion has replaced the musculature.

Differential Diagnosis: Calcific myonecrosis, myositis ossificans, tumoral calcinosis.

Diagnosis: Calcific myonecrosis.

Discussion: Peripheral calcifications in a lesion may be seen in myositis ossificans; however, these lesions demonstrate mature trabecular calcification as they evolve with sequential calcification from the periphery of the lesion to its center, and they typically do not demonstrate a fluid-filled central component. The changes illustrated in this case are more compatible with a diagnosis of calcific myonecrosis. Although dermatomyositis and polymyositis may demonstrate calcifications that are linear in nature, the calcifications typically are not isolated to a single muscle group.

Calcific myonecrosis is a posttraumatic lesion consisting of hematoma or cyst formation. Frequently there is a significant time lag between the insult and the presentation [47]. These lesions may demonstrate growth as well as other features simulating malignancy, and they may be confused for neoplastic processes such as soft tissue sarcomas. The radiologic manifestations consist of components of central liquefaction and calcification in a predominantly linear, peripheral distribution. It is this latter feature that facilitates its identification as a benign posttraumatic lesion in a similar spectrum to myositis ossificans, which also shows peripheral calcification. Adjacent bony erosion may be noted. On MRI, a heterogeneous intramuscular lesion may be demonstrated with only peripheral enhancement [48]. Imaging features help distinguish this from compartment syndrome, although an association may exist in some instances where calcific myonecrosis occurs as a result of the latter. Ischemia is another etiology for its occurrence [49].

Peripheral nerve damage may represent a common final pathway, since injury to the common peroneal nerve has been implicated in some instances. The superficial location of this nerve makes it more susceptible to injury, and it is the most commonly injured nerve in the lower extremity, with most documented cases of calcific myonecrosis occurring in a muscle innervated by this nerve [50]. Pathologically, these lesions consist of hypocellular fibrous tissue with hemosiderin-laden macrophages and cysts comprised of necrotic muscle tissue and hemorrhagic debris [51]. Recurrent hemorrhage within the lesion is probably responsible for its expansile nature. Surgical treatment carries a significant rate of complications, specifically from recalcitrant sinus tract formation and infection [52].

Clinical History: 18-year-old woman with multiple bone lesions.

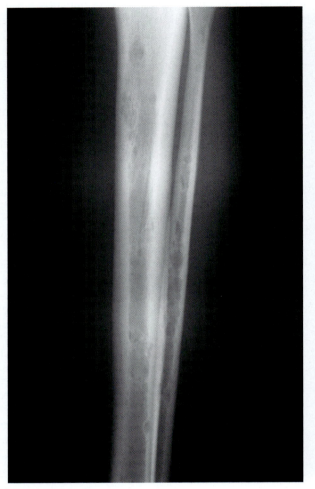

Figure 7-34 A

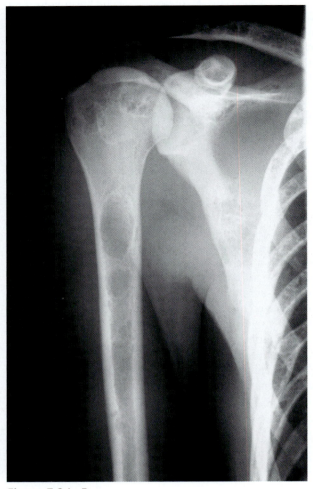

Figure 7-34 B

Findings: (A) Detail of AP radiograph of the lower leg shows confluent lobulated radiolucencies extending along the tibial and fibular shafts, with endosteal scalloping. There is no apparent cortical penetration or periosteal reactive bone. (B) AP radiograph of the humerus and shoulder shows similar radiolucent lesions in the shaft and head, clavicle, scapula, and ribs.

Differential Diagnosis: Cystic angiomatosis, metastases, lymphoma.

Diagnosis: Cystic lymphangiomatosis (cystic angiomatosis).

Discussion: Cystic lymphangiomatosis represents a proliferation of cystic spaces filled with lymphatic fluid. The lesions of cystic lymphangiomatosis do not differ histologically from cavernous or capillary hemangiomas, or from lymphangiomas, so these lesions are often referred to simply as cystic angiomatosis. Pathologically, cystic angiomas consist of numerous, dilated, cavernous, thin-walled vascular channels filling and sometimes eroding trabecular spaces. The radiologic appearance is solitary or multiple zones of rarefaction in the skeleton, typically involving more than one bone, not necessarily in a contiguous manner. Involvement of individual bones may include the epiphysis, metaphysis, or diaphysis. The margins tend to be well demarcated, without reactive bone formation and without mass effect. The differential diagnosis includes other solitary or multifocal bone lesions.

CASE 7-35

Clinical History: 18-year-old man with recurrent bone pain.

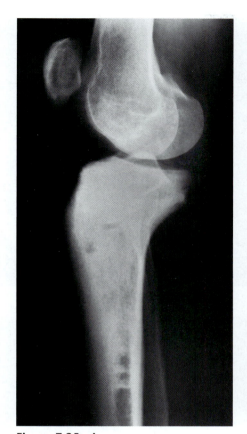

Figure 7-35   A

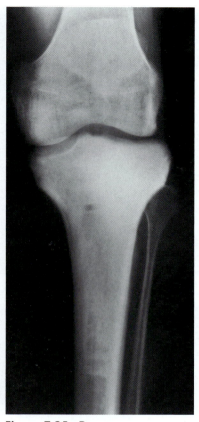

Figure 7-35   B

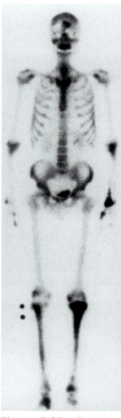

Figure 7-35   C

Findings: (A, B) Radiographs of the tibia show dense sclerosis obliterating the trabecular bone pattern and medullary space. The area of involvement includes the proximal end of the tibia, extending nearly to the midshaft as well as the medial femoral condyle. The cortex is intact, without destruction, expansion, or periostitis. A bone biopsy tract is present in the metaphysis. Similarly dense sclerosis is present in the medial femoral condyle. (C) Whole-body radionuclide bone scan shows increased activity in the left distal radius and thumb, left distal femur, left proximal tibia, left distal tibia, right proximal tibia, and right foot.

Differential Diagnosis: Infection, radiation changes, lymphoma, osteosarcoma.

Diagnosis: Chronic recurrent multifocal osteomyelitis.

Discussion: The differential diagnosis of multiple dense bones includes congenital, neoplastic, inflammatory, and metabolic conditions. In this case, the distribution of the process is the major clue to the diagnosis. Chronic recurrent multifocal osteomyelitis [53,54] is a distinct clinical entity in which recurrent episodes of clinical inflammatory bone disease involve different bones at different times. Cultures are negative by definition; if positive, the condition would be subacute osteomyelitis. Biopsy specimens are sterile but show chronic inflammatory changes, with a predominance of lymphocytes in the inflammatory infiltrates. Although the condition does not respond specifically to antibiotics, because it has a benign, self-limited course, patients nonetheless improve when given antibiotics. The recommended treatment is nonsteroidal antiinflammatory drugs [55].

Clinical History: 35-year-old woman with proximal muscle weakness.

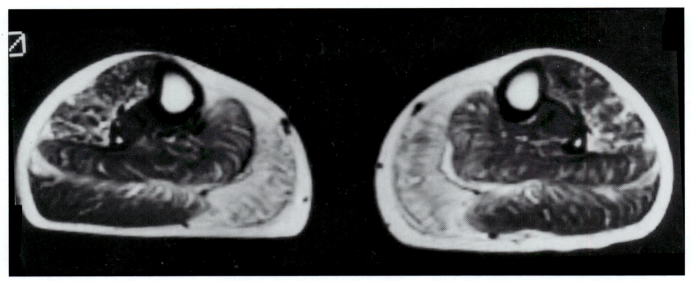

Figure 7-36   A

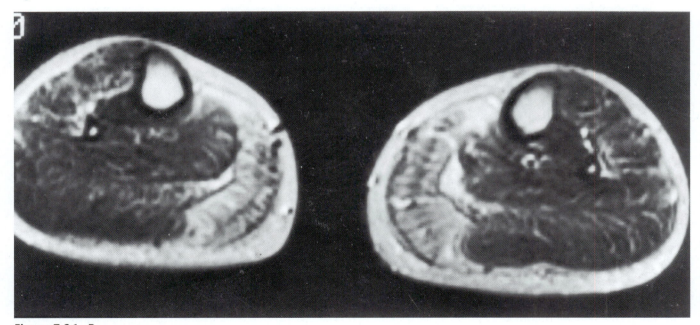

Figure 7-36   B

Findings: (A) Axial T1-weighted MRI shows bilaterally symmetric, abnormally high signal intensity in the gastrocnemius muscles. There is no mass effect or bony involvement. (B) Axial T2-weighted MRI also shows bilaterally symmetric, abnormally high signal intensity in the gastrocnemius muscles. Again, there is no mass effect.

Differential Diagnosis: Polymyositis, dermatomyositis, denervation or disuse atrophy, compartment syndrome, viral myositis, pyomyositis, rhabdomyolysis, lymphoma.

Diagnosis: Polymyositis.

Discussion: The symmetric involvement suggests a systemic disease, and the lack of mass effect would make lymphoma and pyomyositis much less likely than the other possibilities, but the diagnosis cannot be made without consideration of the clinical setting. Polymyositis and dermatomyositis are diseases of striated muscle characterized by diffuse, nonsuppurative inflammation and degeneration. Dermatomyositis has specific skin changes that are absent in polymyositis.

Polymyositis typically affects women between the ages of 20 and 40. It may begin with a flu-like illness and then progresses to increasing symmetric muscle weakness, initially prominent in the thighs. Skin changes (40% to 60%) and arthralgias or arthritis (20% to 50%) are variable. The disease may have many systemic manifestations, including cardiac, pulmonary, renal, ocular, neurologic, and gastroenteric symptoms. There is an association between polymyositis and the development of malignancy, but it is not as strong as the association between dermatomyositis and malignancy.

The first radiographic manifestation is that of subcutaneous fat and muscle edema [56,57]. This may resolve or progress to fibrosis or fatty replacement, with or without soft tissue calcification. The calcification classically outlines the fascial planes of muscles, but it may also be located in the subcutaneous tissue. CT may initially show muscle edema, and subsequently fatty replacement and calcification. On MRI, two types of muscle changes have been described. The earliest manifestation is inflammation of the muscle, which shows increased signal intensity on T2-weighted images and isointensity on T1-weighted images. Subsequently, fatty replacement may occur, and this manifestation shows increased signal intensity on both T1-weighted and T2-weighted MRI, as in this case. The hyperintensity of the muscle seen on T2-weighted or inversion recovery sequences appears to correlate with the clinical symptoms, and it may be more specific than laboratory parameters. Additionally, MRI has been shown to be cost effective in determining the site for diagnostic biopsy [58].

Clinical History: 59-year-old diabetic man with right lower extremity cellulitis and worsening sepsis, and companion case.

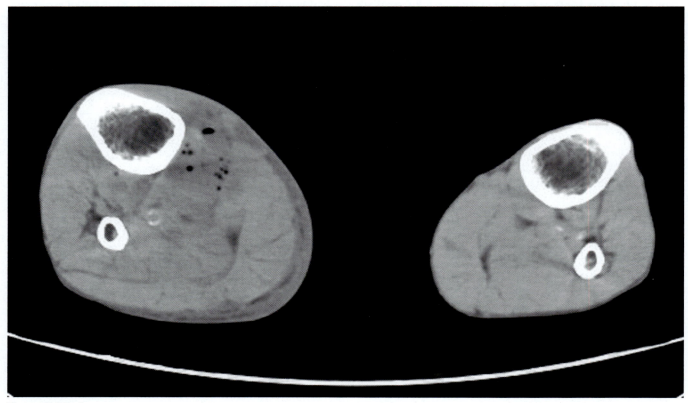

Figure 7-37 A

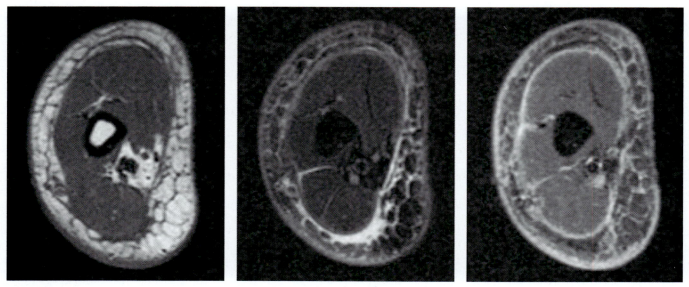

Figure 7-37 B

Findings: (A) CT through both lower legs shows marked swelling on the right side. A collection of gas bubbles and a region of low attenuation involves the flexor digitorum longus, tibialis posterior, and soleus muscles. The subcutaneous tissues are edematous. The bones appear uninvolved. Atherosclerosis is present. (B) Companion case. Axial T1-weighted, T2-weighted fat suppressed and enhanced T1-weighted fat suppressed sequences through the upper arm in another patient with the same disease show thickened, enhancing fascial planes.

Differential Diagnosis: Cellulitis, pyomyositis, necrotizing fasciitis, clostridial myonecrosis.

Diagnosis: Necrotizing fasciitis with abscess formation and cellulitis. The companion case is also necrotizing fasciitis and cellulitis, but without abscess formation.

Discussion: Necrotizing fasciitis is a severe infection involving deep fascial planes that often does not have a known causative factor or portal of entry for bacteria. Most patients have underlying conditions such as diabetes, alcoholism, or remote site of infection. These infections may progress rapidly, so rapid diagnosis and treatment is important for patient survival. The lower extremity is most commonly involved, but the process may also begin in the perineum, body wall, spine, or upper extremity. CT characteristics of necrotizing fasciitis include asymmetric fascial thickening and fat stranding, gas tracking along fascial planes, and abscesses [59]. MRI findings include thickening, high signal on T2-weighted or short tau inversion recovery (STIR) sequences, and enhancement of the deep fascia [60]. Fluid collections, abscesses, and gas may also be present. However, findings on CT or MRI may not be present in all cases. Because the results of imaging may be nonspecific or inconclusive, correlation with clinical factors is crucial. Treatment of necrotizing fasciitis generally includes surgical debridement, and the morbidity and mortality may be significant.

Clinical History: 62-year-old immunosuppressed man with painful calf swelling

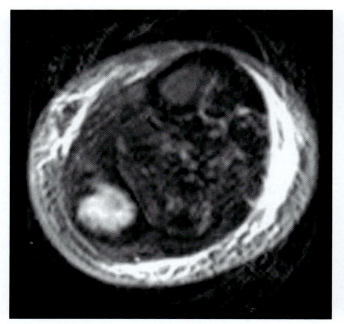

Figure 7-38   A

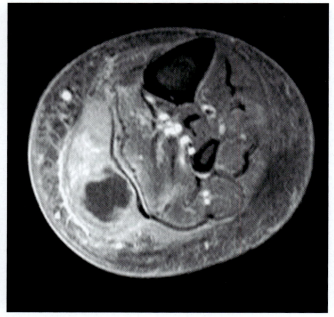

Figure 7-38   B

Findings: (**A**) Axial T2-weighted, fat-suppressed MRI shows heterogeneous high signal within a focal mass in the soleus muscle. Extensive subcutaneous edema is present. The bones are not involved. (**B**) Axial T1-weighted, fat-suppressed, post-gadolinium MRI shows enhancement in the soleus muscle and its surrounding fascia. The high-signal collection demonstrated on T2-weighted MRI does not enhance, nor does the anterior subcutaneous edema.

Differential Diagnosis: Pyomyositis with abscess, soft tissue sarcoma with necrosis or hemorrhage, muscle tear with hematoma.

Diagnosis: Pyomyositis with abscess.

Discussion: The inflammatory changes in the subcutaneous tissue and fascia would be very unusual features for a neoplasm or muscle tear. Pyomyositis, or pyogenic infection, is unusual outside of the tropics except in the setting of immunosuppression, either by drugs or the acquired immunodeficiency virus. In this case, cultures grew *Streptococci*.

Deep musculoskeletal infections are uncommon because muscle and bone are typically not exposed to pathogens in the environment, unlike the lung or gastrointestinal tract. Spontaneous infections typically follow an episode of mild trauma; presumably, there is a focus of hematoma or localized tissue necrosis that then becomes seeded hematogenously from another site. Entire muscles or muscle groups may become involved because they do not contain physical barriers to longitudinal spread of infection. Treatment is by surgical debridement and systemic antibiotics.

SOURCES AND READINGS

1. Rauch F, Glorieux FH. Osteogenesis imperfecta. *Lancet.* 2004;363: 1377–1385.

2. Therrell BL Jr, Berenbaum SA, Manter-Kapanke V, et al. Results of screening 1.9 million Texas newborns for 21-hydroxylase-deficient congenital adrenal hyperplasia. *Pediatrics.* 1998;10:583–590.

3. Cattaneo R, Villa A, Catagni M, Tentori L. Limb lengthening in achondroplasia by Ilizarov's method. *Int Orthop.* 1988;12:172–179.

4. De Bastiani G, Aldegheri R, Renzi-Brivio L, Trivella G. Limb lengthening by callus distraction (callotasis). *J Pediatr Orthop.* 1987;7:129–134.

5. Aldegheri R, Renzi-Brivio L, Agostini S. The callotasis method of limb lengthening. *Clin Orthop.* 1989;241:137–145.

6. Stoker DJ. Osteopetrosis. *Semin Musculoskelet Radiol.* 2002;6:299–305.

7. Synder M, Vera J, Harcke HT, Bowen JR. Magnetic resonance imaging of the growth plate in late-onset tibia vara. *Int Orthop.* 2003;27:217–222.

8. Iwasawa T, Inaba Y, Nishimura G, Aida N, Kameshita K, Matsubara S. MR findings of bowlegs in toddlers. *Pediatr Radiol.* 1999;29:826–834.

9. Cheema JI, Grissom LE, Harcke HT. Radiographic characteristics of lower-extremity bowing in children. *Radiographics.* 2003;23:871–880.

10. Lemyre E, Azouz EM, Teebi AS, Glanc P, Chen MF. Bone dysplasia series. Achondroplasia, hypochondroplasia and thanatophoric dysplasia: review and update. *Can Assoc Radiol J.* 1999;50:185–197.

11. Moore TE, King AR, Travis RC, Allen BC. Post-traumatic cysts and cyst-like lesions of bone. *Skeletal Radiol.* 1989;18:93–97.

12. Hensel KS, Harpstrite JK. Maisonneuve fracture associated with a bimalleolar ankle fracture-dislocation: a case report. *J Orthop Trauma.* 2002;16:525–528.

13. Babis GC, Papagelopoulos PJ, Tsarouchas J, Zoubos AB, Korres DS, Nikiforidis P. Operative treatment for Maisonneuve fracture of the proximal fibula. *Orthopedics.* 2000;23:687–690.

14. Unni KK. *Dahlin's Bone Tumors: General Aspects and Data on 11,087 Cases.* 5th ed. Philadelphia: Lippincott-Raven Publishers; 1996:333–342.

15. Murphey MD, Fairbairn KJ, Parman LM, Baxter KG, Parsa MB, Smith WS. Musculoskeletal angiomatous lesions: radiologic-pathologic correlation. *Radiographics.* 1995;15:893–917.

16. Hudson TM. Radiologic-Pathologic Correlation of Musculoskeletal Lesions. Baltimore: Williams & Wilkins; 1987:79–85.

17. Unni KK. *Dahlin's Bone Tumors: General Aspects and Data on 11,087 Cases.* 5th ed. Philadelphia: Lippincott-Raven Publishers; 1996:172–175.

18. Schajowicz F, McGuire MH, Santini Araujo E, Muscolo DL, Gitelis S. Osteosarcomas arising on the surfaces of long bones. *J Bone Joint Surg Am.* 1988;70-A:555–564.

19. Vanel D, Picci P, De Paolis M, Mercuri M. Radiological study of 12 high-grade surface osteosarcomas. *Skeletal Radiol.* 2001;30:667–671.

20. Campanacci M. Osteofibrous dysplasia of long bones: a new clinical entity. *Ital J Orthop Trauma.* 1976;2:221–237.

21. Alguacil-Garcia A, Alonso A, Pettigrew NM. Osteofibrous dysplasia of the tibia and fibula and adamantinoma. A case report. *Am J Clin Pathol.* 1984;82:420–424.

22. Hazelbag HM, Van den Broeck LJ, Fleuren GJ, et al. Distribution of extracellular matrix components in adamantinoma of the long bones suggesting fibrous-to-epithelial transformation. *Hum Pathol.* 1997;28:183–188.

23. Hazelbag HM, Werrels JW, Mollenomgers P, et al. Cytogenetic analysis of adamantinoma of long bones: further indications for a common histogenesis with osteofibrous dysplasia. *Cancer Genet Cytogenet.* 1997;97:5–11.

24. Bridge JA, Dembrinski A, De Boer J, et al. Clonal chromosomal disorders in osteofibrous dysplasia. Implications for histopathogenesis and its relationship with adamantinoma. *Cancer.* 1994;73:1746–1752.

25. Blackwell JB, McCarthy SW, Xipell JM, et al. Osteofibrous dysplasia of the tibia and fibula. *Pathology.* 1988;20:227–233.

26. Bloem JL, van der Heul RO, Schuttevaer HM, et al. Fibrous dysplasia versus adamantinoma of the tibia: differentiation based on discriminant analysis of clinical and plain film findings. *AJR Am J Roentgenol.* 1991;156:1017–1023.

27. Dominguez R, Saucedo J, Fenstermacher M. MRI findings in osteofibrous dysplasia. *Magn Reson Imaging.* 1989;7:567–570.

28. Nakashima Y, Yamamuro T, Fujiwara Y, et al. Osteofibrous dysplasia. A study of 12 cases. *Cancer.* 1983;52:909–914.

29. Ray D, Cohle SD, Lamb P. Spontaneous clostridial myonecrosis. *J Forensic Sci.* 1992;37:1428–1432.

30. Miguelez M, Aguado JM. Recurrent episodes of spontaneous clostridial myonecrosis related to colorectal carcinoma. *Clin Infect Dis.* 1996;22:582–583.

31. De Bastiani G, Aldegheri R, Renzi-Brivio L, Trivella G. Limb lengthening by callus distraction (callotasis). *J Pediatr Orthop.* 1987;7:129–134.

32. Nordkild P, Crone P. Spontaneous clostridial myonecrosis. A collective review and report of a case. *Ann Chirurg Gynaecol.* 1986;75:274–279.

33. Stephen MB. Gas gangrene: potential for hyperbaric oxygen therapy. *Postgrad Med.* 1996;99:217–224.

34. Tiegs RD. Paget's disease of bone: indications for treatment and goals of therapy. *Clin Ther.* 1997;19:1309–1329.

35. Renier JC, Leroy E, Audran M. The initial site of bone lesions in Paget's disease. A review of two hundred cases. *Rev Rhum Engl Ed.* 1996;63:823–829.

36. Vohra R, Kang HS, Dogra S, Saggar RR, Sharma R. Tuberculous osteomyelitis. *J Bone Joint Surg Br.* 1997;79:562–566.

37. Hugosson C, Nyman RS, Brismar J, Larsson SG, Lindahl S, Lundstet C. Imaging of tuberculosis. V. Peripheral osteoarticular and soft-tissue tuberculosis. *Acta Radiol.* 1996;37:512–516.

38. Mulligan ME. The "gray cortex": an early sign of stress fracture. *Skeletal Radiol.* 1995;24:201–203.

39. Milgrom C, Giladi M, Simkin A, et al. An analysis of biomechanical mechanism of tibial stress fractures among Israeli infantry recruits. A prospective study. *Clin Orthop.* 1998;231:216–221.

40. Jeske JM, Lomasney LM, Demos TC, Vade A, Bielski RJ. Longitudinal tibial stress fracture. *Orthopedics.* 1996;19:263–270.

41. Swensen EJ Jr, DeHaven KE, Sebastianelli WJ, et al. The effect of pneumatic leg brace on return to play in athletes with tibial stress fractures. *Am J Sports Med.* 1997;25:322–328.

42. Rettig AC, Shelbourne KD, McCarroll JR, Bisesi M, Watts J. The natural history and treatment of delayed union stress fractures of the anterior cortex of the tibia. *Am J Sports Med.* 1988;16:250–255.

43. Mabit C, Pecout C. Non-union of a midshaft anterior tibial stress fracture: a frequent complication. *Knee Surg Sports Traumatol Arthrosc.* 1994;2:60–61.

44. Chang PS, Harris RM. Intramedullary nailing for chronic tibial stress fractures. A review of 5 cases. *Am J Sports Med.* 1996;24:688–692.

45. Stack RE, Bianco AJ, MacCarty CS. Compression of the common peroneal nerve by ganglion cysts. *J Bone Joint Surg Am.* 1965;47-A:773–778.

46. Coakley FV, Finlay DB, Harper WM, Allen MJ. Direct and indirect MRI findings in ganglion cysts of the common peroneal nerve. *Clin Radiol.* 1995;50:168–169.

47. Mentzel T, Goodlad JR, Smith MA, et al. Ancient hematoma: a unifying concept for a post-traumatic lesion mimicking an aggressive soft tissue neoplasm. *Mod Pathol.* 1997;10:334–340.

48. Ryre KN, Bae DK, Park YK, et al. Calcific tenosynovitis associated with calcific myonecrosis of the leg: imaging features. *Skeletal Radiol.* 1996;25:273–275.

49. Broder MS, Worrell RV, Shafi NQ. Cystic degeneration and calcification following ischemic paralysis of the leg. *Clin Orthop.* 1977;122:193–195.

50. Janzen DL, Connell DG, Vaisler BJ. Calcific myonecrosis of the calf manifesting as an enlarging soft tissue mass: imaging features. *AJR Am J Roentgenol.* 1993;160:1072–1074.

51. O'Keefe RJ, O'Connell JX, Temple HT, et al. Calcific myonecrosis. A late sequela to compartment syndrome of the leg. *Clin Orthop.* 1995;318:205–213.

52. Malisano LP, Hunter GA. Liquefaction and calcification of a chronic compartment syndrome of the lower limb. *J Orthop Trauma.* 1992;6:245–247.

53. Bjorksten B, Boquist L. Histopathological aspects of recurrent multifocal osteomyelitis. *J Bone Joint Surg Br.* 1980;62-B:376–380.

54. Gamble JG, Rinsky LA. Chronic recurrent multifocal osteomyelitis: a distinct clinical entity. *J Pediatr Orthop.* 1986;6:579–584.

55. Chun CS. Chronic recurrent multifocal osteomyelitis of the spine and mandible: case report and review of the literature. *Pediatrics.* 2004;113:380–384.

56. Fujitake J, Ishikawa Y, Fujii H, Nishimura K, Hayakawa K, Tatsuoka Y. Magnetic resonance imaging of skeletal muscles in the polymyositis. *Muscle Nerve.* 1997;20:1463–1466.

57. Schweitzer ME, Fort J. Cost-effectiveness of MR imaging in evaluating polymyositis. *AJR Am J Roentgenol.* 1995;165:1469–1471.

58. Schweitzer ME, Fort J. Cost-effectiveness of MR imaging in evaluating polymyositis. *AJR Am J Roentgenol.* 1995;165:1469–1471.

59. Wysoki MG, Santora TA, Shah RM, Friedman AC. Necrotizing fasciitis: CT characteristics. *Radiology.* 1997;203:859–863.

60. Schmid MR, Kossmann T, Duewell S. Differentiation of necrotizing fasciitis and cellulitis using MR imaging. *AJR Am J Roentgenol.* 1988;170:615–620.

CHAPTER EIGHT
ANKLE AND FOOT

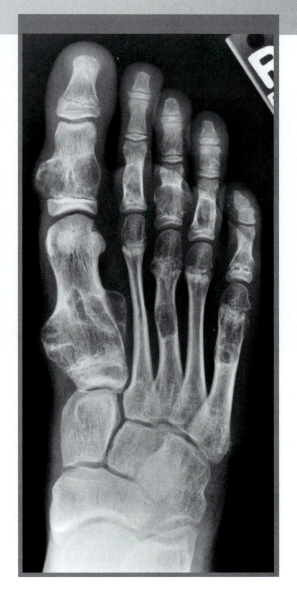

Clinical History: 71-year-old woman with chronic foot pain.

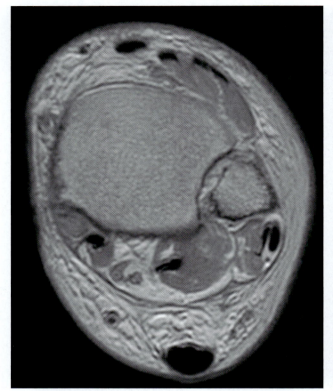

Figure 8-1 A

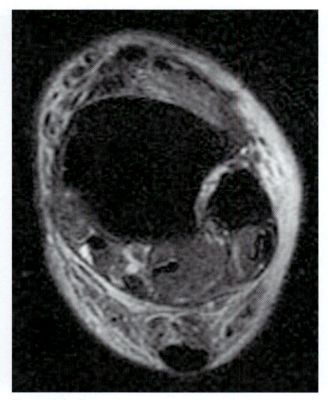

Figure 8-1 B

Findings: (A) Axial proton density and (B) T2-weighted, fat-suppressed magnetic resonance images (MRI) of the ankle shows a thickened posterior tibial tendon. There is increased T2-weighted signal within the tendon. Mild subcutaneous edema in the lateral ankle is an incidental finding.

Differential Diagnosis: None.

Diagnosis: Posterior tibial tendon (PTT) tear.

Discussion: The PTT is the largest and thickest of the three medial flexor tendons. The tendon courses under the medial malleolus and attaches to the medial navicular bone, the three cuneiforms, and the bases of the first to fourth metatarsals. Most PTT tears occur at the level of the medial malleolus. This tendon is one of the primary arch supporters for the foot. Tears of this tendon can cause flatfoot deformity and significant chronic pain and osteoarthritis [1]. Sinus tarsi syndrome has been described in association with PTT tear [2].

CASE 8-2

Clinical History: 9-year-old girl with ankle injury.

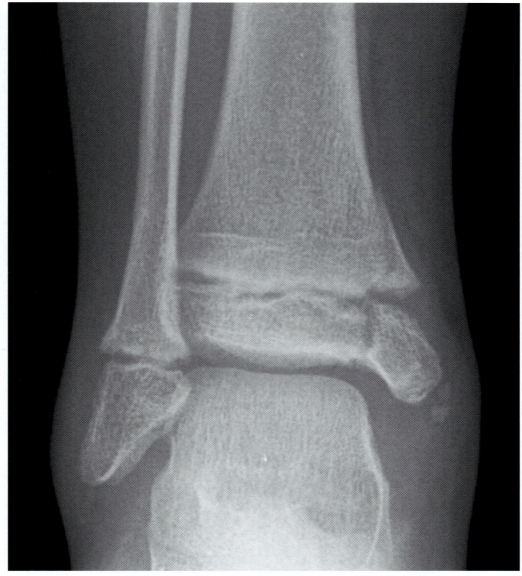

Figure 8-2

Findings: AP ankle radiograph shows an intraarticular fracture plane extending vertically through the medial aspect of the tibia, passing through the epiphysis, growth plate, and metaphysis, and separating the medial malleolus from the remainder of the tibia.

Differential Diagnosis: None.

Diagnosis: Salter type IV fracture, medial malleolus.

Discussion: Salter type IV fractures pass through the metaphysis, growth plate, and epiphysis. In this case, a vertical fracture in the sagittal plane can be seen passing through these three structures. These fractures require accurate open reduction and internal fixation (ORIF), because misalignment of the principal fragments would allow a bone bridge to form across the growth plate [3]. Such a bone bridge would tether the growth plate on one side and result in a progressive varus deformity as the open, lateral portion of the growth plate continued to lengthen the bone. The potential for deformity is greater in young children, who have a longer remaining growth period. The risk of complications is high if the fracture has more than 2 mm of displacement. A Salter type I or type II fracture of the fibula may be associated with this injury.

Clinical History: 15-year-old boy with football injury.

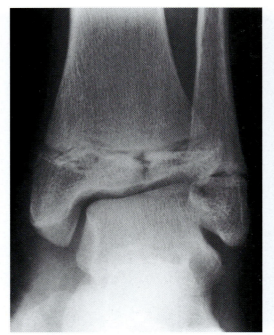

Figure 8-3   A

Figure 8-3   B

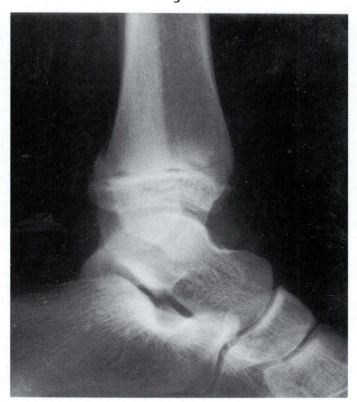

Figure 8-3   C

Findings: Anteroposterior (AP), mortise, and lateral radiographs demonstrate a vertical fracture through the epiphysis that runs from anterior to posterior, and an oblique fracture through the posterior distal tibial metaphysis. The medial malleolus is intact, as is the lateral metaphysis. The central part of the distal tibial growth plate is closed, the most medial portion of the growth plate is open, and the lateral portion is abnormally widened.

Differential Diagnosis: Salter type II fracture, Salter type III fracture, Salter type IV fracture, juvenile Tillaux fracture, triplane fracture.

Diagnosis: Triplane fracture.

Discussion: The radiographs show fractures of the distal tibia that appear to involve the growth plate. One fracture component extends through the metaphysis in the oblique coronal plane, and one fracture extends through the epiphysis in the sagittal plane. Because the fracture through the growth plate that connects the metaphyseal and epiphyseal fractures is in the axial plane, the components of this fracture occur in three different planes, defining the diagnosis of a triplane fracture. The triplane fracture has elements of Salter type II and type III fractures, and because it crosses the epiphysis, growth plate, and metaphysis, it can also be considered a Salter type IV fracture. The juvenile Tillaux fracture, in comparison, is a fracture in which the anterolateral aspect of the tibia epiphysis is avulsed by tension from the anterior tibiofibular ligaments during external rotation of the foot; the juvenile Tillaux fracture can be classified as a Salter type III fracture.

Triplane fractures only occur when physeal closure of the distal tibia is incomplete [4,5]. The distal tibial growth plate begins to close centrally, then medially, and finally laterally. Plantar flexion and external rotation are believed to be the mechanisms of injury in the triplane fracture, in which the lateral fragment of tibia that includes a portion of the epiphysis and metaphysis is avulsed by tension on the tibiofibular ligaments. Fracture of the fibula may accompany these injuries. When the separated epiphysis has two fragments, one of which has a portion of posterior tibial metaphysis attached to it and the other comprises a fragment of the medial epiphysis, then a three-part triplane fracture is produced. Three-part fractures are usually more severe than two-part fractures, since there is greater displacement of the epiphyseal fragments. ORIF is used more frequently for three-part injuries.

The mean age at the time of fracture is about 15 years in boys and 13 years in girls, with a range from about 12 to 17 years in boys and 10 to 15 years in girls. Triplane fractures comprise 15% and 7% of ankle fractures in boys and girls under the age of 18 years, respectively, but the proportion would be much higher in the age range in which these fractures occur. If an epiphyseal gap of 3 mm or greater remains after ORIF, there is a greater risk of premature physeal closure [6].

Clinical History: 4-year-old boy who refuses to walk.

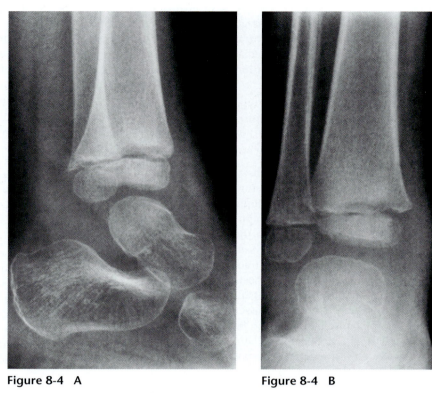

Figure 8-4   A

Figure 8-4   B

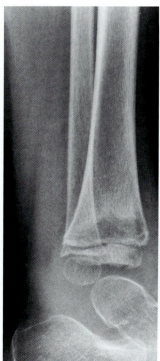

Figure 8-4   C

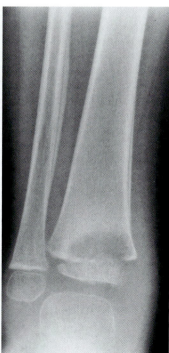

Figure 8-4   D

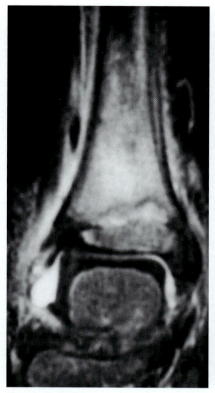

Figure 8-4   E

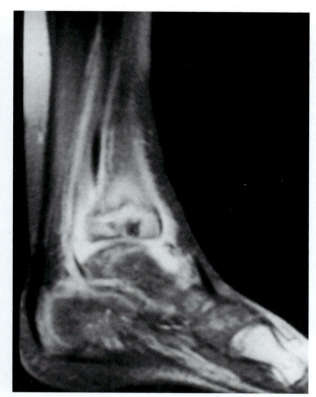

Figure 8-4   F

Findings: (**A, B**) Lateral and AP radiographs taken 2 weeks after initial presentation demonstrate a faint oval lucency of the distal tibial metaphyses with surrounding sclerosis. Soft tissue swelling is noted. Initial radiographs taken 2 weeks earlier were normal (not shown). (**C, D**) Radiographs taken 6 weeks after presentation show that the lucency has grown larger and more defined. Periosteal reaction extends up the shafts of the tibia and fibula. The soft tissue swelling is marked. (**E, F**) T2-weighted MRI taken 6 weeks after presentation demonstrates a focal area of increased signal in the distal tibial metaphysis, adjacent to but not crossing the growth plate, corresponding to the lucency noted on plain film. An ankle effusion and soft tissue edema is evident.

Differential   Diagnosis: Growth   plate   fracture;   osteomyelitis caused by pyogenic, granulomatous, or fungal organism; malignant tumor such as osteosarcoma, lymphoma, or Ewing's sarcoma.

Diagnosis: Atypical mycobacterium osteomyelitis.

Discussion: A growth plate fracture of the tibia in an otherwise healthy child should be healed at 6 weeks, although at 2-week follow-up, Salter type I fracture might show widening of the growth plate and sclerosis on the metaphyseal side. The asymmetry of the widening and sclerosis would be unusual for trauma. The enlarging lucency in the metaphysis suggests a destructive process such as osteomyelitis or

tumor. The location at the distal metaphysis is appropriate for hematogenous osteomyelitis, but the modesty of the reactive bone and the lack of involvement of the physis and epiphysis at the end of 6 weeks would be uncharacteristic of pyogenic osteomyelitis. The small size of the lesion would be distinctly unusual for a primary malignant bone tumor such as osteosarcoma, lymphoma, or Ewing's sarcoma, although the metaphyseal sclerosis could represent neoplastic bone. The diagnosis in this case was confirmed at open biopsy. The lucency consisted of a fluid-filled cystic space, and cultures of the fluid were positive.

Nontuberculous mycobacterial musculoskeletal infections may take the form of tenosynovitis, synovitis, or osteomyelitis [7]. The spectrum of pathologic findings includes virtually no inflammation, mild-to-severe nonspecific chronic infection, granulomas without necrosis, and caseating epithelioid granulomas indistinguishable from tuberculosis. These pathologic changes explain the blandness of the imaging features in this case. Multiple lesions in the metaphyses and diaphyses, sinus tracts, and osteoporosis are other features of atypical mycobacterial infections. Joint space narrowing, as in tuberculosis, is a late finding. Delays in the diagnosis of atypical mycobacterial osteomyelitis are common, and the disease may be multifocal. These infections occur in both immunocompromised as well as immunocompetent individuals [8].

Clinical History: 29-year-old man with lower leg swelling.

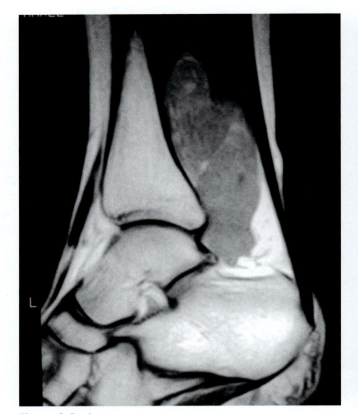

Figure 8-5   A

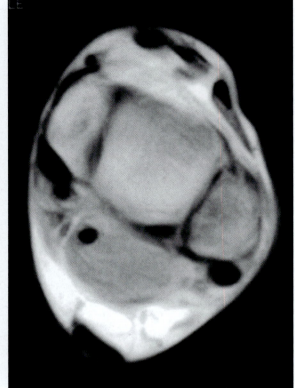

Figure 8-5   B

Findings: (A) Sagittal T1-weighted MRI shows a mass in the distal soleus muscle, extending inferiorly along the deep aspect of the Achilles tendon and abutting the posterior aspect of the tibia and ankle. The mass has a lobular contour and heterogeneous intermediate signal intensity. (B) Axial T1-weighted MRI at the level of the ankle joint shows the lesion in the posterior soft tissues, adjacent to the joint and surrounding the tendon of the flexor hallucis longus. The underlying bone is normal.

Differential Diagnosis: Soft tissue sarcoma, extraskeletal Ewing's sarcoma, lymphoma, benign soft tissue tumor, myotendinous injury, myositis ossificans, hematoma.

Diagnosis: Extraskeletal primitive neuroectodermal tumor (PNET).

Discussion: The finding of a large, lobulated, soft tissue mass in the deep tissues of the extremity of an adult is always cause for concern. There are no specific features on imaging that lead to the diagnosis in this case, but myotendinous injury, hematoma, and myositis ossificans are possibilities that should have a suggestive history (lacking in this case). The age of the patient is less than the peak incidence for a mesenchymal soft tissue sarcoma. A biopsy is necessary for diagnosis.

PNET is a sarcoma of neuroectodermal origin. It appears closely related to Ewing's sarcoma in histogenesis [9], with an appearance on light microscopy that may be indistinguishable (small, round, blue cells). Although both Ewing's sarcoma and PNET may be primary to bone or soft tissue, Ewing's sarcoma is much more likely to occur in bone, whereas PNET has an equal incidence in bone and soft tissue. Most patients with PNET are between 10 and 30 years old, with the most common soft tissue sites being the paravertebral region, the chest wall (called in this circumstance an Askin tumor), the retroperitoneum, and the lower extremities. Soft tissue PNETs present as rapidly enlarging soft tissue masses. Findings on imaging are nonspecific, and PNET is indistinguishable from Ewing's sarcoma on imaging [10]. The margins of the tumor may be well defined, as in this case, and sometimes encapsulated, or they may appear infiltrative. Areas of hemorrhage may be present, and contrast enhancement on MRI is typically intense. The treatment of PNET is chemotherapy and surgical resection, sometimes with radiation therapy as well. The prognosis for patients with PNET is less favorable than for patients with Ewing's sarcoma [11].

Clinical History: 34-year-old woman with foot pain.

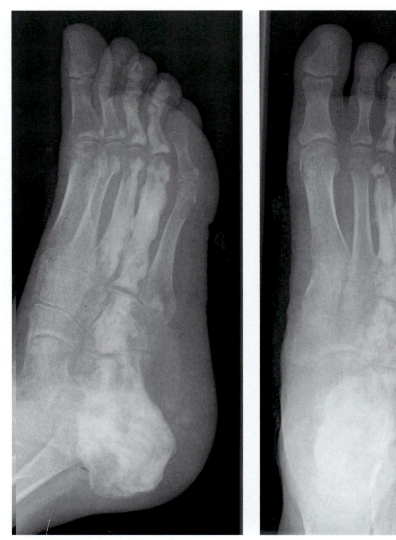

Figure 8-6   A

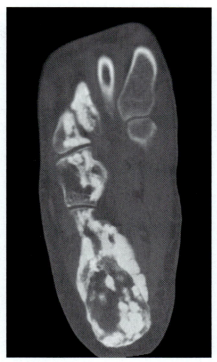

Figure 8-6   B

Findings: (A) Oblique and AP radiographs of the foot demonstrate wavy, dense sclerosis beginning in the calcaneus, involving the cuboid, and extending through the third and fourth metatarsals and toes. (B) Long axis computed tomography (CT) shows the sclerosis involving the cortex and medullary canal. There is no soft tissue mass or bone destruction.

Differential Diagnosis: Melorheostosis, trauma, chronic osteomyelitis, osteosarcomatosis.

Diagnosis: Melorheostosis.

Discussion: Melorheostosis is a disorder of unknown cause that can present at any age. The most common appearance is cortical hyperostosis that can be likened to dripping candle wax. Involvement is usually limited to a single extremity and is often along a sclerotomal distribution [12], in this case L5. When the soft tissues are involved, muscle and tendon contractures can lead to skeletal deformities such as scoliosis and growth disturbances. Most patients are asymptomatic, but this condition can painful [13]. Diseases associated with melorheostosis include osteopoikilosis, osteopathia striata, neurofibromatosis, and tuberous sclerosis. Treatment is most often surgical, to correct deformities and remove soft tissue masses [14].

Clinical History: 8-year-old boy with ankle pain.

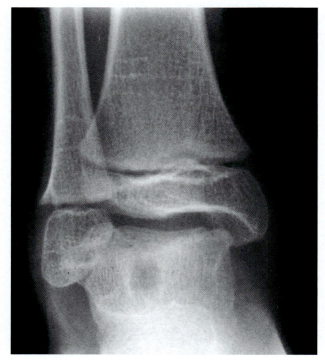

Figure 8-7   A

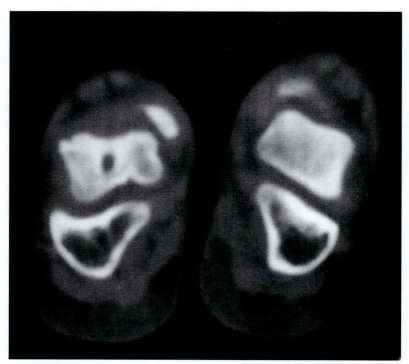

Figure 8-7   B

Findings: (A) AP radiograph of the ankle shows epiphyseal overgrowth, flattening of the talar dome, sclerosis, and cystic changes. A 1-cm lucency with sclerotic borders is noted in the medullary space of the talus. (B) CT of both ankles demonstrates a well-defined ovoid lucent lesion in the right talus with surrounding sclerosis. The lesion has soft tissue attenuation within. Articular irregularity is present at the dome of the talus, and the talus appears mildly contracted in size compared with the contralateral asymptomatic side. Soft tissue density within the ankle joint may represent fluid or synovial hypertrophy.

Differential Diagnosis: Hemophilia, juvenile idiopathic arthritis, septic arthritis, sickle cell disease.

Diagnosis: Hemophiliac pseudotumor.

Discussion: Abnormality of the articular surface of bone associated with synovial hypertrophy in a pediatric patient can be seen in juvenile idiopathic arthritis, hemophilia, and the rheumatoid-negative spondyloarthropathies. The cystic lesion is remote from the subarticular bone, which would be unusual for a subchondral cyst in the arthritic conditions mentioned, but could represent a pseudotumor from intraosseous hemorrhage in hemophilia.

Intraosseous bleeding and the subsequent inflammatory reaction that clears the hemorrhage may create radiolucent defects in bone, called pseudotumors. Repeated bleeding into a pseudotumor may cause it to recur and enlarge, simulating malignancy. Osteonecrosis or osteomyelitis in the setting of sickle cell disease involving the talus may have a similar appearance to this case. Septic arthritis may also result in osteomyelitis and osteonecrosis. Radiographic manifestations in hemophilia may be strikingly similar to certain arthritic conditions, particularly juvenile idiopathic arthritis. Because the pathomechanical basis for these findings differs (intraarticular hemorrhage with secondary inflammation versus chronic inflammation without hemorrhage), features specific for hemorrhage should be sought when attempting to distinguish between these diagnoses. The obvious differential point is the presence of a hemorrhagic effusion, which can be ascertained on MRI, but other differentiating features include localized periosteal reaction due to subperiosteal hemorrhage, and pseudotumor due to intraosseous hemorrhage.

Soft tissue hemorrhage may result in a soft tissue pseudotumor, which can cause pressure erosions and scalloping on the adjacent bone with or without exuberant periosteal reaction, again simulating neoplasm. Most pseudotumors arise near the large bones of the proximal skeleton in adults, but in younger patients, before skeletal maturity, they tend to occur distal to the wrist or ankle. Distal pseudotumors usually respond well to conservative management, whereas resection is often the treatment of choice for proximal pseudotumors [15]. Large proximal pseudotumors may lead to life-threatening hemorrhage. Emergent surgical treatment carries a significant intraoperative mortality.

Clinical History: 10-year-old boy with ankle pain.

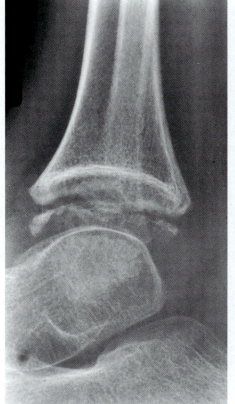
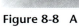

Figure 8-8   A

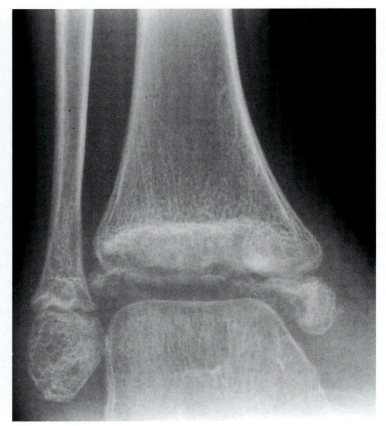

Figure 8-8   B

Findings: (A, B) Lateral and mortise radiographs of the ankle show disordered mineralization in the distal tibial epiphysis. The epiphysis is ossifying from multiple centers. There is a dense horizontal line of sclerosis across the distal tibial metaphysis. The ossification patterns in the medial and lateral malleoli are also disordered.

Differential Diagnosis: Osteonecrosis, epiphyseal dysplasia, trauma, osteomyelitis.

Diagnosis: Osteonecrosis in sickle cell disease.

Discussion: The appearance of the epiphysis with multiple centers of ossification is that of revascularized osteonecrosis. In this case, the patient was known to have sickle cell disease, and the clinical question was the cause of his ankle pain. Sickle cell disease is caused by an inherited structural defect in hemoglobin that leads to red cell dysfunction. The radiologic features of sickle cell disease in bone are the result of bone marrow hyperplasia, vascular occlusion, and osteomyelitis [16]. Hyperplasia of the bone marrow expands the marrow space. Vascular occlusion results in osteonecrosis. Any portion of any bone may be infarcted; frequent sites include the medullary space of long bones, growing epiphyses, and the hands. Involvement of growing epiphyses leads to growth disturbances. If the femoral head is involved, the pathophysiologic events and sequelae are indistinguishable from those of Legg-Calvé-Perthes disease. A growth disturbance in the vertebral body leads to development of H-shaped vertebrae. Localized infarctions of bone with repair or dystrophic calcification result in focal areas of bony sclerosis scattered about the skeleton.

Patients with sickle cell disease have a high incidence of osteomyelitis. Unlike hematogenous osteomyelitis in other situations, the infection in sickle cell disease is most frequent at the diaphysis of the long bones, where the oxygen tension is lowest. In approximately 50% of cases, *Salmonella* species or mixed flora are the causative organisms (their presence is exceedingly unusual under any other circumstance); the remaining cases are usually caused by *Staphylococcus* species. Chronicity and recurrence are common. Osteomyelitis may be difficult to differentiate from infarction on both clinical and radiologic grounds [17,18]; either one can be a complication of the other. The radiographic signs of osteomyelitis would superimpose on whatever preexisting bone changes existed from the sickle cell disease.

Clinical History: 32-year-old woman with chronic swelling and ankle pain.

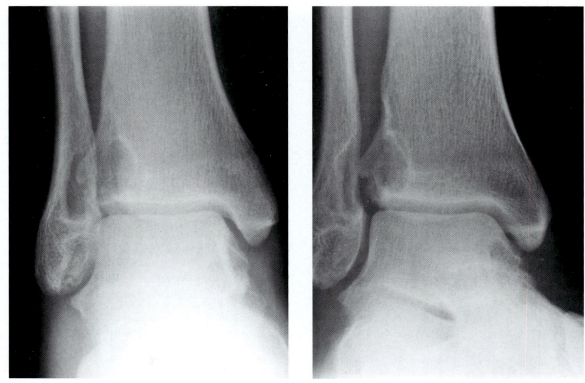

Figure 8-9   A

Figure 8-9   B

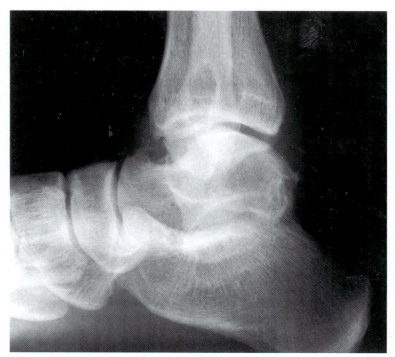

Figure 8-9   C

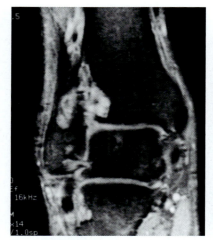

Figure 8-9   D

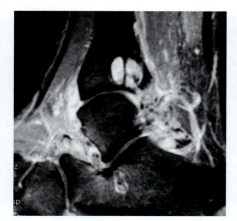

Figure 8-9   E

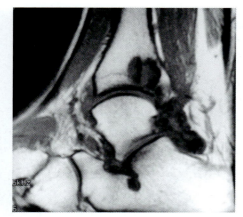

Figure 8-9   F

Findings: (A, B) AP and mortise radiographs of the ankle demonstrate erosive changes in the tibia and fibula. The erosions are shallow and have sclerotic margins. The cartilage space is preserved. The distribution of abnormality suggests a primary synovial process rather than a multifocal bone process. (C) Lateral radiograph shows erosive changes of the talus along the anterior superior aspect as well as the posterior aspect, indicating a diffuse process. (D–F) Coronal fat-saturated T2-weighted MRI, sagittal fat-saturated T2-weighted MRI, and sagittal T1-weighted MRI demonstrates profuse synovial hypertrophy and associated lesions in the subcortical bone, some of which appear to be communicating with the joint. There are low-signal-intensity foci within the hypertrophied synovium and within the intraosseous lesions.

Differential Diagnosis: Pigmented villonodular synovitis (PVNS), synovial osteochondromatosis, amyloid arthropathy, tuberculosis, synovial hemangiomatosis.

Diagnosis: PVNS.

Discussion: All of the entities in the differential diagnosis can demonstrate synovial hypertrophy and bony erosions. The lack of calcifications on the radiographs makes synovial osteochondromatosis much less likely. The low-MR-signal-intensity foci within the synovium and bone on T2-weighted images may be seen with PVNS or amyloidosis, but the monoarticular nature of the process favors PVNS over amyloidosis. These low-signal foci would not be expected with tuberculosis or hemangiomatosis.

PVNS is believed to be a benign neoplasm of the synovium. It is typically a monoarticular process that has a predilection for the large joints of the lower extremity, especially the knee [19]; however, any synovial joint may be involved. Radiographic findings include joint effusion, juxtaarticular erosions, and relative sparing of the cartilage space. In later stages, secondary osteoarthritis may be seen. Ankylosis is not a feature. The synovial masses generally do not calcify or ossify in PVNS, an important point of differentiation from synovial osteochondromatosis [20]. On MRI, PVNS demonstrates foci of low signal intensity on all pulse sequences due to widespread hemosiderin deposits from repeated episodes of intraarticular hemorrhage. These hemosiderin deposits also give the synovium a pigmented appearance at gross inspection. Amyloidosis may show a similar pattern of low-signal foci on MRI, but amyloidosis is most often a systemic, multiarticular process that is related to long-term hemodialysis [21].

PVNS is treated by synovectomy, but because complete surgical removal is difficult, recurrence rates may be as high as 50%. Development of malignancy in the setting of PVNS is an extremely rare event. Cases of malignant PVNS have been reported in patients with previously documented and treated benign PVNS, as well as in patients with PVNS and malignancy at initial presentation [22,23].

Clinical History: 63-year-old man with newly diagnosed prostate cancer.

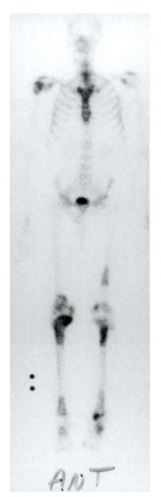

Figure 8-10   A

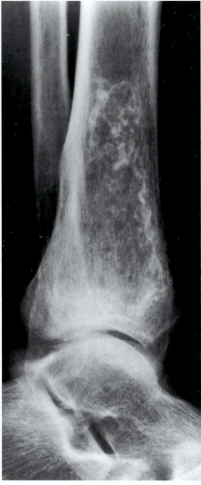

Figure 8-10   B

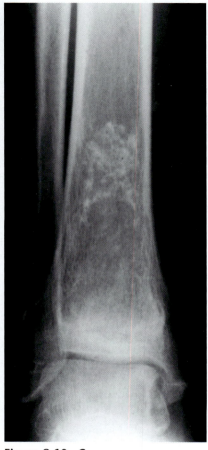

Figure 8-10   C

Findings: (A) Whole-body radionuclide bone scan demonstrates increased uptake in several locations, with particular involvement of the ends of the bones (bilaterally in the tibias, distal femurs, right proximal humerus, tali, and left distal femoral shaft). The sites of involvement are relatively large. The axial skeleton appears spared. (B, C) Two radiographic views of the distal right tibia demonstrate a lesion with a lacy calcified matrix and a sclerotic serpiginous rind. There is no cortical expansion or penetration.

Differential Diagnosis: Metastases, enchondroma, marrow infarction (osteonecrosis).

Diagnosis: Marrow infarction.

Discussion: Metastases typically involve the axial skeleton more than the appendicular skeleton. Lesions in the ankle and feet are unusual. Metastases also tend to be focal and discrete. Enchondroma and marrow infarcts can demonstrate radionuclide accumulation on bone scans. Accumulation in enchondromas is a reflection of reactive bone formation and enchondral ossification. Accumulation in infarcts is a reflection of repair and remodeling after revascularization. During the ischemic phase of marrow infarction, the bone scan may be cold or normal. Enchondroma and marrow infarction may have a similar radiographic appearance. The serpiginous rind of calcification and the location at the end of the bone is more suggestive of marrow infarction than enchondroma, and the multifocal involvement is more common in marrow infarction than in enchondroma.

There are multiple potential causes for marrow infarction, including exogenous steroids, alcoholism, sickle cell disease, trauma, Gaucher's disease, and pancreatitis. Abnormal fat metabolism in alcoholism and pancreatitis is believed to cause osteonecrosis by fat embolism. On MRI, medullary infarcts are usually multiple and have a diagnostic appearance. They have an irregular, serpiginous, sharply defined, low-signal border on T1-weighted and proton-density images, which often has high signal on T2-weighted images. This appearance corresponds to the margin of revascularization and remodeling. Contemporaneous radiographs are often normal, but the infarcted marrow may eventually calcify. This dystrophic calcification in infarcts may resemble the mineralized matrix of an endosteal cartilage tumor.

Clinical History: 35-year-old man felt pop and sharp pain while playing basketball.

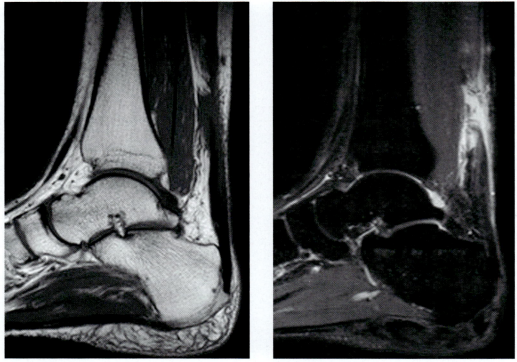

Figure 8-11   A   Figure 8-11   B

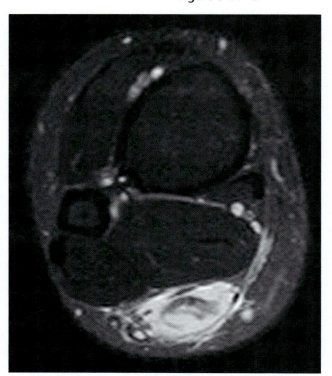

Figure 8-11   C

Findings: (A) Sagittal T1-weighted MRI shows loss of the normally black signal intensity of the Achilles tendon between the soleus muscle belly and the calcaneal insertion. (B, C) Sagittal inversion recovery and axial T2-weighted, fat-suppressed MRI shows discontinuity of the Achilles tendon approximately 5 cm proximal to the calcaneal attachment. The retracted margins of the tendon at the tear are thickened. Fluid (T2-weighted hyperintensity) is present through and around the tear.

Differential Diagnosis: Achilles tendinitis, Achilles tendon rupture.

Diagnosis: Achilles tendon rupture.

Discussion: The Achilles tendon is the primary plantar flexor of the foot and represents the confluence of the soleus and gastrocnemius tendons. Approximately 15 cm long in the average adult male, the Achilles tendon inserts on the calcaneus 1.5 cm below the superior margin of the posterior calcaneus. It is the largest and strongest tendon in the human body, with tensile strength similar to steel. The Achilles tendon is the only tendon in the ankle not invested in a synovial sheath. It derives its blood supply from the surrounding paratenon, adjacent muscular branches, and calcaneal insertion. Consequently, the portion of the tendon with the most tenuous blood supply is approximately 3 or 4 cm proximal to the calcaneal insertion.

Because of the great strength of the normal tendon, spontaneous or activity-related Achilles tendon tears do not occur without some underlying pathology. Rupture of the tendon can be considered to be the end point of tendinosis, a spectrum of disorders ranging from inflammation of the paratenon to partial tear and finally to complete rupture. Patients with underlying conditions, such as hyperparathyroidism, rheumatoid arthritis, renal failure, pseudohypoparathyroidism, pseudopseudohypoparathyroidism, and corticosteroid treatment, are predisposed to Achilles tendinosis and rupture, but the majority of patients who present with ruptures of the tendon have developed tendinosis while participating in sports-related activities [24]. Patients tend to be adults who participate in strenuous exercises on a limited, intermittent basis. Men are affected more than women by a ratio of approximately 3:1, and the mean age at injury in one large series was 41 years old [25].

Although ruptures can occur without warning, preexisting degenerative changes in the tendon can be documented on histologic examination, if sought. Rupture is more common on the left than the right. Evaluation of disease can be performed with either MRI or sonography. On MRI, the normal Achilles tendon is hypointense on all imaging sequences and flattened in morphology. Partial tears appear as high-signal intratendinous collections within a thickened tendon. Complete acute ruptures appear as a discontinuity that is typically filled with fluid or granulation tissue. Chronic tendinitis appears as diffuse thickening without the increase in signal intensity [26].

Clinical History: 22-year-old amateur rugby player with right ankle injury 3 weeks ago.

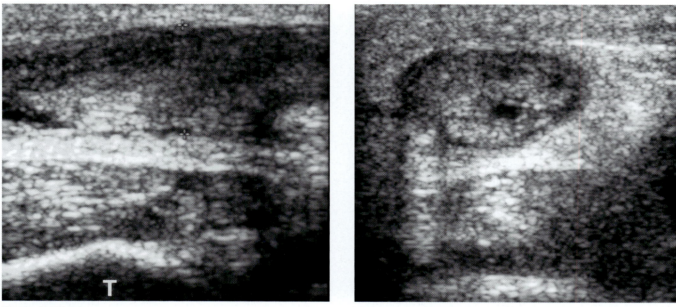

Figure 8-12   A

Figure 8-12   B

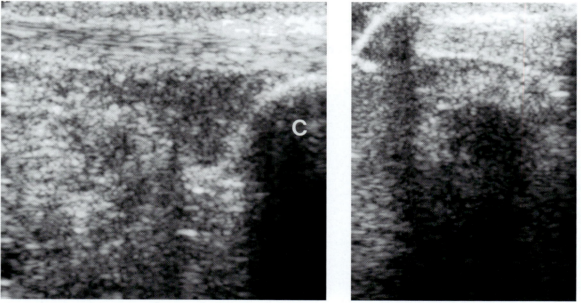

Figure 8-12   C

Figure 8-12   D

Findings: Right Achilles tendon. (A) Sonography of the Achilles tendon in the longitudinal plane, with the transducer placed on the posterior aspect of the heel cord, shows marked echogenic thickening of the entire tendon. The thickness of the tendon in the AP direction is 13 mm. No focal discontinuity of the tendon is demonstrated (T = tibia). (B) Sonography in the transverse plane shows the enlarged, ovoid cross-section of the Achilles tendon. A discrete hypoechoic region is present within the substance of the tendon. (C, D) Left Achilles tendon. Sonography of the uninjured contralateral Achilles tendon shows normal-thickness tendon in the longitudinal plane with slightly hypoechoic, organized, fibrillar texture. In the transverse plane, the tendon has a c-shaped cross-section (C = calcaneus).

Differential Diagnosis: Rupture of the Achilles tendon (partial or complete), tendinosis, hypercholesterolemia, postsurgical scar.

Diagnosis: Partial rupture of the Achilles tendon.

Discussion: The Achilles tendon is particularly amenable to diagnostic sonography because of its superficial location, large size, and simple anatomy. The normal Achilles tendon is a flat structure with an organized, slightly hypointense fibrillar structure. Thickness of the normal Achilles tendon increases with age and height [27]. Tendinosis is indicated by thickening of the tendon, with increased sagittal diameter and sometimes focal hypoechoic regions [28,29].

Tendon rupture is diagnosed when the fibers of an enlarged tendon are interrupted by fluid, fat, or hemorrhage that fills the gap between the ends of the tear. Real-time imaging while plantar and dorsiflexing the foot can be a valuable tool in distinguishing an incomplete from a complete tear. Complete tears typically occur 3 cm proximal to the insertion on the calcaneus. Treatment options include casting or operative repair. Most surgeons favor open repair in individuals interested in continuing athletic endeavors, as the re-tear rate is lower in this population. One study found a correlation between recovery time and the Achilles tendon's appearance on sonography in a population of patients with achillodynia, and suggested its use as a prognostic tool [30]. Common postsurgical findings after Achilles tendon repair include hypoechoic areas within the tendon, inhomogeneous echogenicity, and loss of the fibrillar structure. These morphologic changes were not correlated with the clinical outcome of the repair [31].

Clinical History: 26-year-old woman with skin problems.

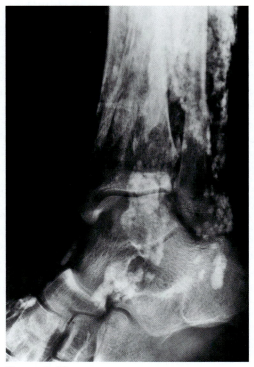

Figure 8-13

Findings: Oblique ankle radiograph. There is amorphous dense soft tissue calcification, distributed in vertical sheets. No underlying osseous abnormality is identified. No joint disease is present.

Differential Diagnosis: Dermatomyositis, systemic lupus erythematosus (SLE), scleroderma, hypervitaminosis D, hyperparathyroidism, pseudohypoparathyroidism, pseudopseudohypoparathyroidism, parasitic infection.

Diagnosis: Dermatomyositis.

Discussion: Extensive soft tissue calcification is present, some of which is subcutaneous, but some appears to be intramuscular and possibly intratendinous. The calcifications are amorphous in character, without defined internal structure. Numerous disorders can be associated with soft tissue calcifications, including dermatomyositis, SLE, scleroderma, hypervitaminosis D, hyperparathyroidism, pseudohypoparathyroidism, pseudopseudohypoparathyroidism, and parasitic infection.

Dermatomyositis is an idiopathic disorder with non-infectious inflammation of the skin and skeletal muscle. Polymyositis involves muscle alone. Multiple types of the disease have been described based on the clinical presentation, and a clinical form associated with underlying malignancy has been described. Regardless of subtype, nearly all patients experience muscle weakness, usually proximal. Skin rashes and arthralgias are common clinical findings and may be the presenting symptoms. Involvement of cardiac, pulmonary, renal, neurologic, and gastrointestinal tissues will alter the presentation. Laboratory tests reveal elevation of creatine kinase during active inflammation, and electromyographic alterations can be detected. Soft tissue findings tend to be more common and severe in children than adults. Soft tissue swelling may be appreciated by dedicated soft tissue films in areas of complaint, but soft tissue calcifications represent the most dramatic radiographic finding. Distinct patterns of soft tissue calcification have been described, the most common of which are linear, sheet-like calcification in the interfascial planes. Reticular and rounded calcifications may be seen in the subcutaneous tissues, and deep rounded calcifications are common. In childhood disease, spontaneous remission of soft tissue calcifications has been reported with the onset of puberty. Joint changes on radiographs are rare and usually limited to soft tissue swelling. Distal tuft resorption may be seen in association with soft tissue calcification, which may be confused with scleroderma.

MRI is a useful method for evaluating the extent and activity of disease. Actively involved muscle tends to demonstrate increased signal on T2-weighted images; inversion recovery or fat-suppressed, T2-weighted images are the most sensitive method for displaying these changes [32]. Antimyosin scintigraphy may be even more sensitive than MRI for detecting active disease [33]. Identification of active disease is useful for directing biopsy.

CASE 8-14

Clinical History: 73-year-old woman with persistent lateral foot pain after twisting her ankle.

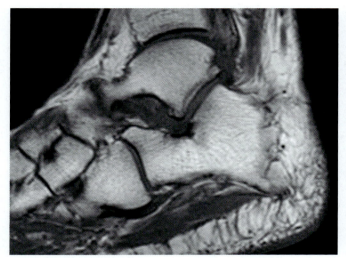

Figure 8-14 A

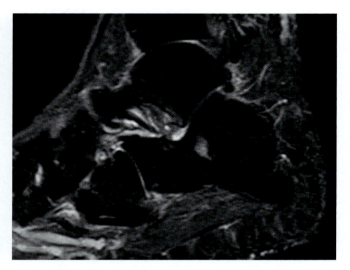

Figure 8-14 B

Findings: (A, B) Sagittal T1-weighted and inversion recovery MRI of the hindfoot shows edema and resultant loss of the normal fat signal within the sinus tarsi region.

Differential Diagnosis: None.

Diagnosis: Sinus tarsi syndrome.

Discussion: The sinus tarsi is the space between the talar neck and distal calcaneus. This space contains ligaments, neurovascular structures, and fat. In a severe ankle inversion injury, inflammation or hemorrhage in this region may produce chronic pain. The ligaments within the sinus tarsi may also be torn, producing a sensation of instability. MRI can demonstrate ligamentous tears within the sinus tarsi—usually the cervical ligament or interosseous talocalcaneal ligament [34][35]—as well as edema or fibrosis within the surrounding fat. Sinus tarsi syndrome may also occur due to flatfoot deformities and inflammatory arthropathies [36]. Treatment is usually conservative. An arthroscopic subtalar joint synovectomy is an effective treatment when conservative measures fail [37].

CASE 8-15

Clinical History: 47-year-old alcoholic with chronic ankle pain but no history of trauma.

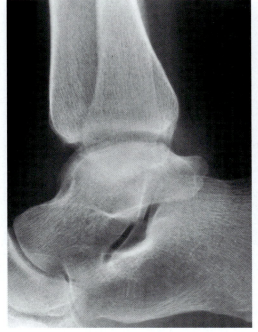

Figure 8-15 A

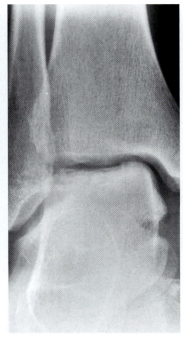

Figure 8-15 B

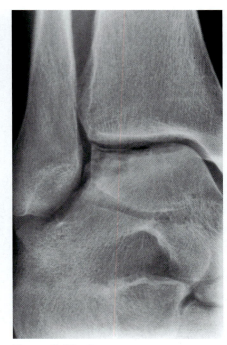

Figure 8-15 C

Findings: (A–C) Lateral, AP, and mortise radiographs of the right ankle show subchondral lucency, subchondral sclerosis, and flattening of the talar dome.

Differential Diagnosis: Osteochondral fracture, osteonecrosis, osteoarthritis, neuropathic osteoarthropathy.

Diagnosis: Osteonecrosis.

Discussion: The radiographic findings of linear subchondral lucency, subchondral sclerosis, and collapse of the articular surface are diagnostic of osteonecrosis (avascular necrosis) involving an articular surface. Note the preservation of joint space and normal appearance of the tibial plafond, indicating that the disease process is primary to the talus rather than the joint itself. The opposing joint surface is typically normal in osteonecrosis until late in the disease, when manifestations of secondary degenerative joint disease may be seen. Once revascularization of the necrotic bone has become reestablished, attempts at repair by creeping substitution result in sclerosis as new viable bone is apposed to necrotic bone. Sclerosis represents the earliest radiographic manifestation of osteonecrosis. Resorption of bone may re-

sult in a loss of mechanical strength, sometimes leading to subchondral fracture. Subchondral fracture may be evident as linear subchondral lucency—the crescent sign—and it is a highly specific sign of osteonecrosis. The subchondral fracture may even contain nitrogen gas formed in the joint during traction. Continued application of forces across the joint with associated attempts at repair leads to collapse of the articular surface, as in this case. The joint surface may then fragment, and resulting joint incongruity eventually leads to the development of osteoarthritis.

Atraumatic osteonecrosis of the talar dome has numerous causes, including alcoholism, SLE, sickle cell disease, excessive corticosteroids (endogenous or exogenous), pancreatitis, dysbarism, and marrow packing disorders such as Gaucher's disease. Some cases have no apparent cause, but the majority of patients with atraumatic osteonecrosis of the talus have osteonecrosis elsewhere, especially the femoral head, and approximately half have bilateral involvement of the tali [38]. Atraumatic osteonecrosis is relatively uncommon, with most cases of osteonecrosis being related to fractures of the talar neck [39].

CASE 8-16

Clinical History: 26-year-old man in a motorcycle accident.

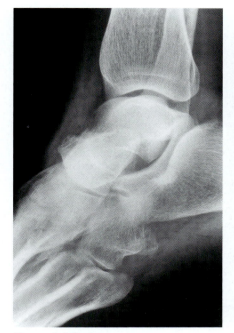

Figure 8-16   A

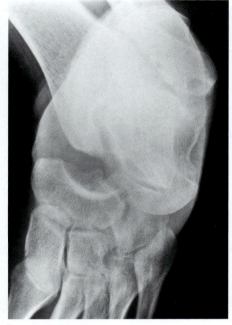

Figure 8-16   B

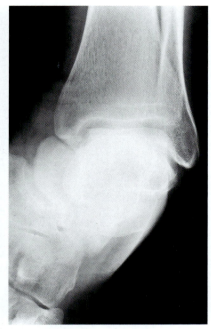

Figure 8-16   C

Findings: (A) Lateral radiograph of the foot. The talus remains within the ankle mortise, but the relationship of the posterior facets of the talus and calcaneus is abnormally widened and oriented. Easy to overlook, the head of the talus overlaps the navicular, rather than articulating with it. (B) Oblique and AP radiographs of the ankle and foot. The entire midfoot has dislocated medially and inferiorly. Most obvious are the naked articular surfaces of the distal aspect of the talus and the proximal aspect of the navicular.

Differential Diagnosis: None.

Diagnosis: Subtalar dislocation.

Discussion: Simultaneous dislocation of the talocalcaneal and talonavicular joints is referred to as subtalar dislocation. Of the ligamentous supports about the talus, the talonavicular and talocalcaneal ligaments and capsules are weaker than the calcaneonavicular ligaments and capsule and the ankle ligaments, so the entire midfoot and calcaneus may dislocate as a single unit [40]. Most of these injuries represent high-energy trauma, such as that sustained in motorcycle accidents or falls from a height, but relatively minor stumbling trauma may also cause this injury. Approximately 90% of subtalar dislocations are closed. In approximately 80% of cases, the foot dislocates medial to the talus. Severe open subtalar dislocations occur in major trauma [41], typically motorcycle accidents. Associated injuries include injuries of the tibial nerve, ruptures of the posterior tibial tendon, lacerations of the posterior tibial artery, and articular fractures of the subtalar joint, talonavicular joint, and talar dome. The outcome is often poor, and the risk of osteonecrosis of the talus is significant.

Clinical History: 18-year-old adolescent boy with painful flatfoot deformity.

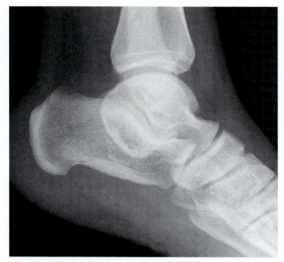

Figure 8-17   A

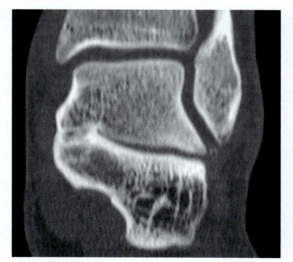

Figure 8-17   B

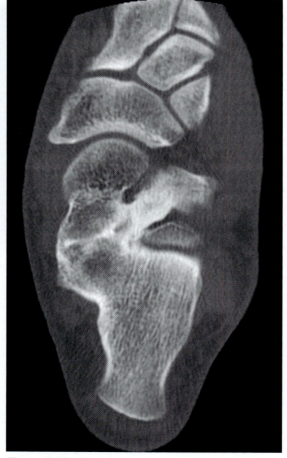

Figure 8-17   C

Findings: (A) Lateral radiograph of the foot shows talocalcaneal coalition, "absent middle facet" sign, and C-sign. The posterior facet of the subtalar joint can be seen. (B) Coronal CT shows a bony coalition between the talus and calcaneus at the sustentaculum tali; the posterior facet is visible and not bridged. (C) Axial CT shows the bony coalition between the calcaneus and the talus.

Differential Diagnosis: Tarsal coalition, surgical fusion.

Diagnosis: Tarsal coalition.

Discussion: A tarsal coalition is an abnormal bony or fibrous articulation between two tarsal bones. The condition is congenital and appears to result from lack of segmentation rather than fusion of a fully developed joint [42]. Tarsal coalitions are found most commonly as isolated deformities, but they may occur in association with other ipsilateral limb deformities as well as generalized syndromes. Heritable cases of apparently autosomal dominance have been described. Most symptomatic cases are either coalitions between the calcaneus and the navicular (calcaneonavicular), or between the calcaneus and the talus (talocalcaneal). These coalitions may be bilateral in approximately 50% of cases.

A talocalcaneal coalition prevents the rotational and gliding motions at the subtalar joint that normally occur during walking, resulting in a painful flatfoot deformity. The coalition may be fibrous, cartilaginous, or osseous. Typically, the coalition is cartilaginous but becomes ossified as the skeleton matures; with ossification comes rigidity and the onset of symptoms. With calcaneonavicular coalitions, the loss of subtalar motion is partial, and the pain is generally confined to the region of the coalition itself.

Special views and conventional or computed tomography may be necessary to identify the presence and the precise site of coalition. An indirect sign of a coalition between the calcaneus and the talus is talar beaking. A talar beak is a bony spur from the anterior superior aspect of the talus consequent to limited subtalar motion, hypoplasia of the head of the talus, and dorsal subluxation of the navicular bone. A talar beak may occur in any condition that causes abnormal talonavicular motion. The C-sign may be evident on lateral views when a middle facet coalition is present. The dome of the talus forms the top of the C, the coalition forms the middle, and the sustentaculum forms the bottom. The middle facet of the subtalar joint should be visible in normal patients. Thus, when the middle facet is absent, a coalition should be suspected [43]. Coalitions between other adjacent tarsal bones are rare and generally asymptomatic.

Clinical History: 1-month-old male infant with foot deformity.

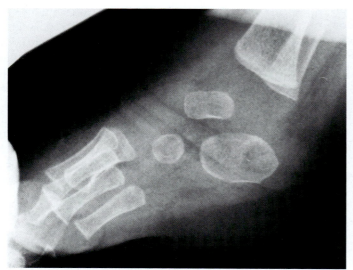

Figure 8-18 A

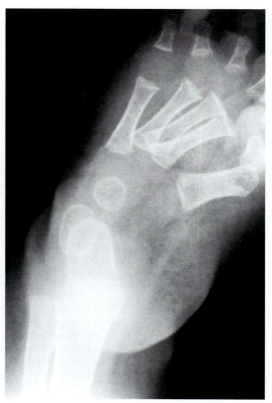

Figure 8-18 B

Findings: (A) Lateral radiograph of the foot shows that the long axes of the talus and calcaneus are nearly parallel. The longitudinal arch is abnormally high. (B) AP radiograph of the foot shows an abnormally narrow talocalcaneal angle, with severe adduction and supination of the forefoot.

Differential Diagnosis: Clubfoot, vertical talus, metatarsus adductus, skewfoot.

Diagnosis: Classic clubfoot (talipes equinovarus).

Discussion: Radiographic criteria for the diagnosis of certain congenital foot deformities in infancy are based on lateral and AP views obtained while weight-bearing, or with dorsiflexion stress simulating weight-bearing. In the normal foot, until the age of about 2 years, the long axis of the talus and the long axis of the calcaneus form an angle (talocalcaneal angle) that is about 40 degrees on both lateral and AP radiographs. If one considers the talus to be fixed in the ankle mortise, then abnormal varus (medial) alignment of the calcaneus relative to the talus will reduce the talocalcaneal angle in the AP projection, and abnormal valgus (lateral) alignment will increase it. Because of the geometric and

ligamentous linkage between the talus and the calcaneus, the changes in the talocalcaneal angles will be approximately equal on both AP and lateral radiographs. Thus, on AP and lateral radiographs, a small talocalcaneal angle (close to parallel, perhaps 10 degrees or less) is called hindfoot varus, and a large talocalcaneal angle (perhaps 70 degrees or more) is called hindfoot valgus.

Talipes equinovarus, or classic clubfoot, is a common congenital abnormality with an incidence of 1 per 1,000 live births. The condition is bilateral in about half the cases, and is three-times more common in boys than in girls. When unilateral, it is usually the left foot that is abnormal. The deformity is believed to be caused by a combination of intrauterine and genetic factors. Clubfoot may also occur in association with arthrogryposis, meningomyelocele, and other neuromuscular and genetic syndromes. The key radiologic finding is hindfoot varus (decreased talocalcaneal angle) combined with forefoot plantar flexion and supination. Depending on the severity and rigidity of the deformity, clubfoot may be treated by serial manipulation and casting, or surgical release of the soft tissues and realignment of the foot.

CASE 8-19

Clinical History: Infant with family history of foot deformities.

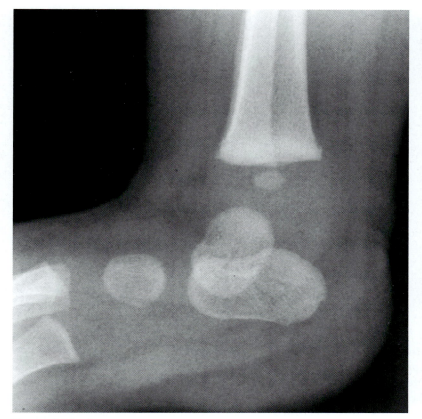

Figure 8-19 A

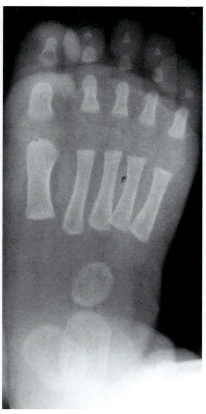

Figure 8-19 B

Findings: (A) Lateral radiograph of the foot shows an increased angle between the long axes of the talus and calcaneus (talocalcaneal angle). (B) AP radiograph of the foot shows an increased talocalcaneal angle. The forefoot is pronated.

Differential Diagnosis: Clubfoot, vertical talus, metatarsus adductus, skewfoot.

Diagnosis: Congenital vertical talus.

Discussion: Congenital vertical talus is an unusual deformity characterized by hindfoot valgus (increased talocalcaneal angle) and dorsal dislocation of the navicular on the talus [44]. The navicular adapts to its abnormal position by becoming wedge shaped, and the forefoot is pronated as a consequence. The plantar arch will be flattened and, in severe cases, a rocker-bottom deformity (convex plantar surface of the foot) may result. The anterior and middle facets of the subtalar joint may be absent or replaced by fibrous tissue. Approximately half of the cases of congenital vertical talus occur in isolation; the remainder occurs in association with neurofibromatosis, arthrogryposis, meningomyelocele, or other central nervous system or genetic syndromes. Acquired vertical talus may occur in association with conditions such as cerebral palsy, poliomyelitis, and spinal muscular atrophy. Overcorrection of a classic clubfoot may create a vertical talus.

Clinical History: Infant with foot deformity.

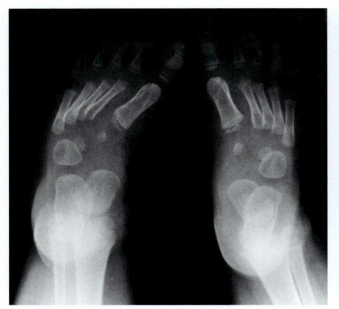

Figure 8-20   A

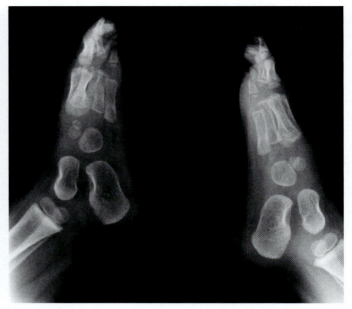

Figure 8-20   B

Findings: (A, B) AP and lateral radiographs demonstrate that the forefoot is adducted in varus, more pronounced on the left. There is an overall convex lateral border of the foot soft tissues, and a concave medial border. The hindfoot and midfoot is normal.

Differential Diagnosis: Talipes equinovarus, skewfoot, metatarsus adductus.

Diagnosis: Metatarsus adductus.

Discussion: Metatarsus adductus is a congenital deformity characterized by medial deviation of the forefoot, without abnormality of the hindfoot [45]. It is the most common congenital foot deformity, with an incidence 10 times greater than classic clubfoot. The condition is bilateral in most cases, and it is thought to result from intrauterine positioning. Two-thirds of these deformities are detected at birth, and the remainder becomes noticeable during the first year of life.

The cause of the deformity has not been elucidated, but there is a hereditary component, as 25% of affected infants have a first-degree relative with similar findings. In the majority of cases, the deformity is flexible and resolves without treatment.

Metatarsus adductus can be recognized on radiographs by the marked medial deviation of the metatarsals with a normally aligned hindfoot. On weight-bearing radiographs or simulated weight-bearing radiographs in infants, a line drawn along the longitudinal axis of the calcaneus (calcaneal axial line) should extend through the base of the fourth metatarsal on an AP projection. If the forefoot is angulated medial to this line, it is adducted. An adducted forefoot occurring in combination with hindfoot valgus is called skewfoot, a different and unusual deformity that frequently requires surgical correction.

CASE 8-21

Clinical History: 54-year-old woman with podiatric problems.

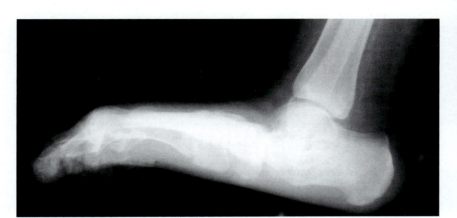

Figure 8-21   A

Figure 8-21   B

Findings: (**A**) Lateral radiograph of the foot shows an extreme flatfoot deformity. There are no hypertrophic bony changes, bone fragments, or dislocation. Extensive vascular calcification is present. (**B**) AP radiograph of the foot shows the flatfoot deformity with pronation of the forefoot and valgus deviation of the toes. The bones are osteopenic, but erosive changes are absent.

Differential Diagnosis: Heritable connective tissue dysplasia (such as Ehlers-Danlos syndrome, Marfan's syndrome), SLE, arthrogryposis, congenital vertical talus, diabetic neuropathy, rheumatoid arthritis, stroke.

Diagnosis: Systemic Lupus Erythematosus (SLE).

Discussion: A severe flatfoot deformity in association with extensive vascular calcification is a common association in diabetic neuropathy, but the bony changes of neuropathic arthropathy are absent from this case. Congenital vertical talus also results in a severe flatfoot deformity but, in older patients, degenerative arthritis dominates the clinical picture. Ehlers-Danlos syndrome and arthrogryposis are conditions in which infants present with joint laxity, whereas adults present with contractures. The absence of erosive changes eliminates rheumatoid arthritis as a consideration, although the osteoporosis and alignment deformities would otherwise be suggestive. The presence of severe vascular disease in combination with atrophy suggests stroke as a possibility.

Abnormalities of the hand can be found in about half of the patients with SLE, but abnormalities of the foot are found in about two-thirds [46]. The severity of the changes is related to the duration of disease. Nearly all patients with nonerosive deforming arthropathy of the hands (Jaccoud's type of arthropathy) will also have passively correctable joint deformities of the foot [47]. Such deformities include hallux valgus, subluxation of the lesser metatarsophalangeal (MTP) joints, and widening of the forefoot. Erosive or cystic changes of bone and cartilage are typically not seen in SLE, and neither are hypertrophic changes such as subchondral sclerosis, osteophyte formation, or asymmetric joint space narrowing. Vascular disease in SLE generally involves the microvascular circulation, but macrovascular occlusive disease occurs occasionally and is presumably related to immune complex-mediated endothelial damage [48]. Extensive vascular disease below the inguinal ligament in SLE has a poor prognosis, often resulting in treatment by amputation.

Clinical History: 37-year-old woman with foot pain.

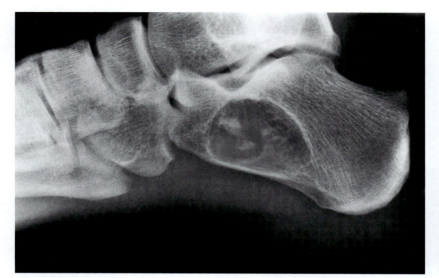

Figure 8-22   A

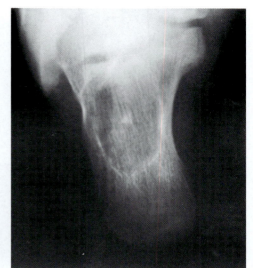

Figure 8-22   B

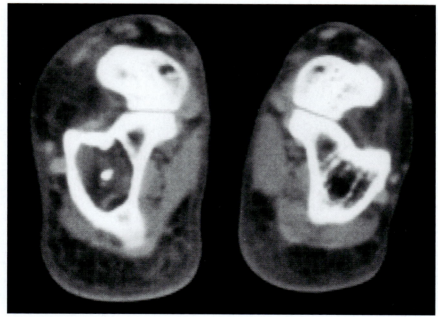

Figure 8-22   C

Findings: (A, B) Lateral and Harris View radiographs of the calcaneus demonstrate a geographic medullary lesion with sclerotic borders and lucent center. Dystrophic calcification is contained centrally. (C) Coronal CT demonstrates that part of the lesion has low attenuation coefficients consistent with fat.

Differential Diagnosis: Cyst, lipoma, giant cell tumor, eosinophilic granuloma.

Diagnosis: Intraosseous lipoma.

Discussion: Unicameral bone cyst, aneurysmal bone cyst, giant cell tumor, lipoma, and eosinophilic granuloma may produce a lucent, well-defined lesion in the calcaneus. The anterior calcaneus is a particularly good site for unicameral bone cyst and intraosseous lipoma. A few foci of calcifications are typical for the intraosseous lipoma, and correspond to areas of dystrophic calcification. Fat attenuation on the CT further supports this diagnosis. The other diagnostic possibilities would not be fat containing. Soft tissue lipomas are more common than their osseous counterparts. Most cases of intraosseous lipomas are found in the long bones, and 15% are seen in the calcaneus [49]. They classically have a lucent appearance, with a thin sclerotic border and nonaggressive features. Central dystrophic calcification is a cardinal feature of lipoma in the calcaneus, and a fatty constituent may be identified on MRI or CT. The histologic picture is mature adipose tissue mixed with a few degenerated bone trabeculae.

Clinical History: 55-year-old woman unable to continue a new, aggressive exercise program because of heel pain.

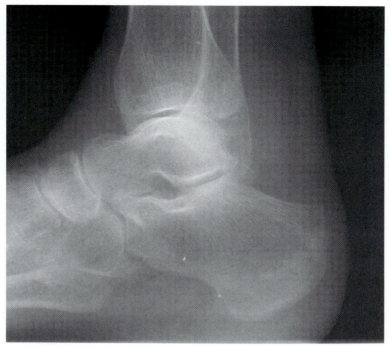

Figure 8-23   A

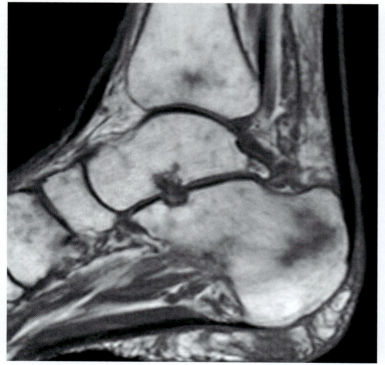

Figure 8-23   B

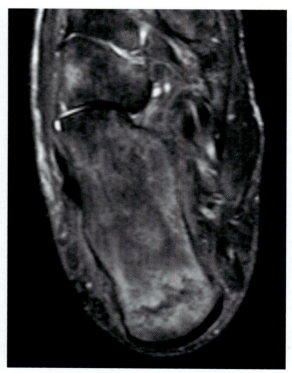

Figure 8-23   C

Findings: (A) Lateral radiograph of the calcaneus shows an irregular band of sclerosis in the tuberosity, oriented perpendicular to the major weight-bearing trabeculae. The margins of the sclerosis are somewhat fluffy. (B) Sagittal T1-weighted MRI shows a region of dark, curvilinear signal in the posterior calcaneus. (C) Axial T2-weighted, fat-suppressed MRI shows the dark linear signal surrounded by edema.

Differential Diagnosis: Traumatic fractures, fatigue fractures, pathologic fractures.

Diagnosis: Calcaneal fatigue fracture.

Discussion: The linear morphology and fluffy character of the sclerosis is characteristic of healing fatigue fracture. The history suggests that the lesion is related to locomotor activity. The lack of mass or bone destruction eliminates possibilities such as blastic metastases or lymphoma.

Stress fractures may be divided into fatigue fractures, where normal bone fractures in response to abnormal loads, and insufficiency fractures, where abnormal bone fractures in response to normal loads. Fractures through focal lesions such as tumors are called pathologic fractures. Stress fractures through trabecular bone are similar to stress fractures through tubular bones, except that the individual weight-bearing trabeculae produce calcified endosteal callus. In aggregate, these form the fluffy densities visible on radiographs. Unlike traumatic fractures, the cortex is typically intact. As these fractures heal, the sclerosis remodels and ultimately disappears. The appearance and evolution of stress fractures is not related to the site or the character of the inciting stress. Although the tibia was the most commonly affected bone by stress fractures in one study of military recruits, the posterior calcaneal tuberosity was the most commonly affected site [50].

Clinical History: 25-year-old woman with polyarticular arthritis.

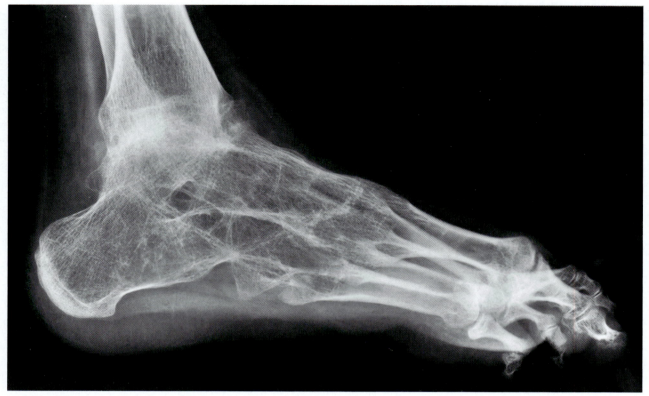

Figure 8-24

Findings: Lateral radiograph of the foot demonstrates fusion of the ankle, hindfoot, midfoot, and MTP joints. Diffuse osteopenia is noted.

Differential Diagnosis: Juvenile idiopathic arthritis, sequelae of trauma or infection, corrected clubfoot.

Diagnosis: Juvenile idiopathic arthritis.

Discussion: The ankylosis of nearly the entire ankle and foot with osteopenia and remodeled bone suggests juvenile idiopathic arthritis as the underlying cause. Trauma, infection, and surgery are other situations where fusion of the foot may occur. Juvenile idiopathic arthritis [51], formerly known as juvenile chronic arthritis or juvenile rheumatoid arthritis, is a designation that includes seronegative juvenile-onset rheumatoid arthritis (Still's disease), juvenile onset of seropositive adult-type rheumatoid arthritis, and the seronegative spondyloarthropathies. The radiologic findings in juvenile idiopathic arthritis reflect the effect of a chronic inflammatory arthritis on a growing skeleton, and are generally not specific for a particular clinical entity. The radiographic findings include soft tissue swelling, osteoporosis, periostitis, erosions, ankylosis, and growth disturbances. The earlier the age of onset, the more severe the findings. Not all findings are likely to be present together, but combinations of these findings should point to the diagnosis. The disease may remit in adulthood, but permanent muscle wasting, growth deformities, loss of function from ankylosis, and secondary osteoarthritis are common sequelae. MRI and ultrasound is becoming more important in the evaluation and monitoring of patients with this disease [52].

Clinical History: 45-year-old man with heel pain, and a companion case.

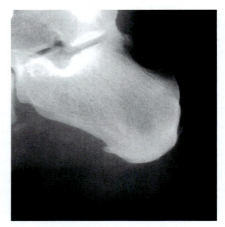

Figure 8-25   A

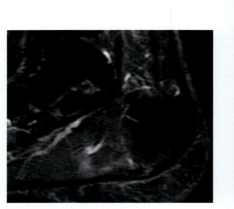

Figure 8-25   B

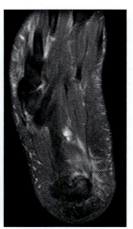

Figure 8-25   C

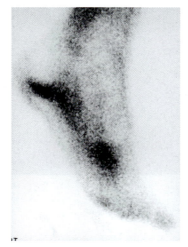

Figure 8-25   D

Findings: (**A**) Lateral radiograph shows loss of the normal sharp tissue-fat plane at the plantar aspect of the attachment of the plantar aponeurosis to the calcaneus. (**B, C**) Companion case. Sagittal inversion recovery and axial T2-weighted, fat-suppressed MRI shows thickening and increased signal of the attachment of the plantar aponeurosis. There is mild edema in the adjacent subcutaneous fat and calcaneal bone marrow. (**D**) Lateral camera image of blood pool portion of three-phase radionuclide bone scan shows increased activity at the calcaneal attachment of the plantar aponeurosis.

Differential Diagnosis: Plantar fasciitis, plantar fibromatosis, rupture of the plantar fascia, subcalcaneal bursitis, calcaneal stress fracture, spondyloarthropathy, rheumatoid arthritis.

Diagnosis: Plantar fasciitis.

Discussion: The plantar aponeurosis is a strong band of connective tissue that originates at the calcaneus and extends distally to coalesce with the ligaments that attach to the toes. Plantar fasciitis is an inflammatory process involving the plantar aponeurosis, typically at its origin. Plantar fasciitis can occur with repetitive microtrauma and is a somewhat common cause of heel pain in runners [53]. Approximately 7% of injuries in distance runners are related to plantar fasciitis. The plantar fascia stretches during the first half of the stance phase of walking or running, storing potential energy. Approximately 90% of this energy is returned as it recoils like a spring during the push-off. Peak stress as high as 3 times body weight occurs at the time of midstance, when most of the weight-bearing forces have been transferred from the hindfoot to the ball of the foot.

The most common presenting symptom of plantar fasciitis is pain, especially on rising in the morning. Tenderness may be found along the course of the plantar fascia or at its origin on the medial aspect of the calcaneal tuberosity. Radiographs may be normal or may show swelling and loss of fat-tissue planes along the plantar aponeurosis. Radionuclide studies most often show increased activity along the plantar fascia on early images, with focal accumulation of radiotracer at the inferior aspect of the calcaneus on delayed static images [54]. MRI shows signal intensity changes at the proximal aspect of the calcaneus [55]. Plantar fasciitis may also be a feature of rheumatoid arthritis and the seronegative spondyloarthropathies [56].

Clinical History: 41-year-old woman with painful mass on plantar aspect of foot.

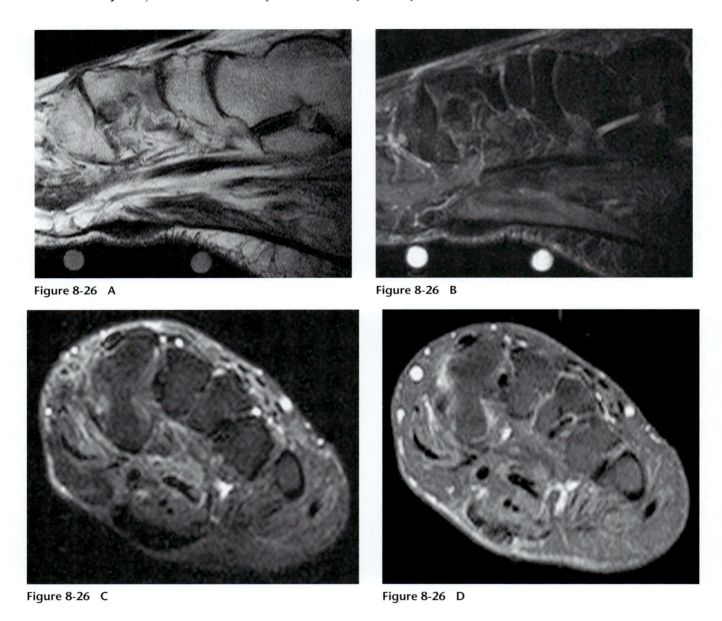

Figure 8-26   A

Figure 8-26   B

Figure 8-26   C

Figure 8-26   D

Findings: (A–C) Sagittal T1-weighted and sagittal inversion recovery, and coronal T2-weighted, fat-suppressed MRI shows a low-signal, lobulated mass in the subcutaneous tissues of the foot under the longitudinal arch. The mass involves the plantar aponeurosis and abuts the underlying musculature. (D) T1-weighted, gadolinium-enhanced, fat-suppressed MRI shows heterogeneous enhancement.

Differential Diagnosis: Soft tissue sarcoma, foreign body granuloma, fibromatosis, metastasis, giant cell tumor of tendon sheath, abscess.

Diagnosis: Plantar fibromatosis.

Discussion: The fibromatoses encompass a group of lesions that demonstrate fibrous proliferation and may be locally aggressive, but do not possess metastatic potential. Broad subdivisions include superficial and deep fibromatoses. The superficial variety has a predilection for the lower extremity. Common varieties of this class of lesions include palmar fibromatosis, plantar fibromatosis, and nodular fasciitis. They differ from keloids and cicatricial fibromatosis in that they possess a greater cellular constituent in their matrix, specifically myofibroblasts [57]. On MRI, these lesions classically demonstrate decreased signal intensity on all pulse sequences, although a relatively more cellular lesion (with a higher cell to collagen ratio than typically present) may confer a higher signal intensity on T2-weighted pulse sequences [58,59]. Variability in the MRI appearance of these lesions on T1-weighted, T2-weighted, and proton-density-weighted pulse sequences may be related to the relative preponderance of the various constituents seen in the lesion, which include collagen, spindle cells, and mucopolysaccharides.

Plantar fibromatosis is a slow growing, unencapsulated, nodular lesion that most frequently occurs in the plantar aponeurosis. Patients are typically adults who present with one or more firm, fixed, painless subcutaneous nodules in the plantar aspect of the foot. The MRI features commonly noted in plantar fibromatoses include an infiltrative margin, isointensity to muscle on T1-weighted MRI, and hyperintensity to muscle on T2-weighted images [60]. The lesions are well defined superficially against the normal adjacent subcutaneous fat, but may be inseparable from the underlying muscle. Enhancement patterns are variable, but profuse enhancement after contrast was seen in 60% of cases of plantar fibromatosis in one study on MRI [61].

Clinical History: 47-year-old woman with heel pain and swelling.

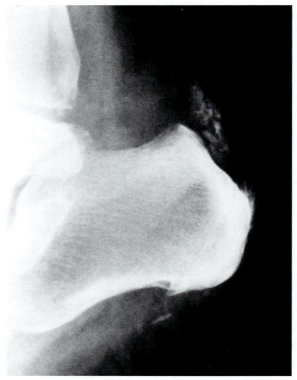

Figure 8-27

Findings: Lateral radiograph of calcaneus shows soft tissue calcification posterior to the calcaneus but anterior to the Achilles tendon, in the location of the retrocalcaneal bursa. No erosions of the underlying bone are present.

Differential Diagnosis: Hydroxyapatite deposition disease, gouty arthritis, pyrophosphate arthropathy, spondyloarthropathy, synovial osteochondromatosis.

Diagnosis: Hydroxyapatite deposition disease (calcific retrocalcaneal bursitis).

Discussion: Hydroxyapatite deposition disease is a heterogeneous group of conditions that have in common the abnormal presence of amorphous hydroxyapatite (basic calcium phosphate) crystals in the soft tissues. Ion contaminants such as carbonate, magnesium, fluoride, and chloride will be present within the crystals. Probably the result of multiple causes, there may be more than one mechanism of deposition. The radiologic manifestations of hydroxyapatite deposition disease are similar to other crystal-associated conditions [62]: asymptomatic deposits, acute crystal-induced synovitis, and chronic destructive arthropathy.

Hydroxyapatite deposition disease typically involves the periarticular soft tissues, tendons, ligaments, bursae, and joint capsules rather than the articular cartilage and sub-chondral bone. Deposits of hydroxyapatite in the soft tissues appear on radiographs as dense, homogeneous, sharply marginated, and amorphous calcifications. They may have linear, angular, or round shapes and, unlike chondrocalcinosis, the calcifications do not conform to hyaline or fibrocartilage structures.

Recurrent episodes of calcific tendinitis or calcific bursitis are commonly associated with hydroxyapatite deposits. Most patients are adults in their 50s or 60s and present with acute pain, swelling, and tenderness. Symptoms respond rapidly to nonsteroidal anti-inflammatory agents. When the retrocalcaneal bursa is involved, the Achilles tendon is usually the site of hydroxyapatite deposits. Tendons may go on to atrophy and rupture, but it is unclear whether the deposits initially caused the local tissue damage, or whether preexisting tissue damage allowed the deposits to accumulate. The process is usually monoarticular, but multiple joints may be involved at the same time or successively. Other common sites of involvement include the supraspinatus tendon, the long head of the biceps tendon, the extensor tendons of the wrist, the myotendinous attachments along the linea aspera (thigh adductors) and at the medial border of the proximal tibia (pes anserinus), the olecranon bursa, the trochanteric bursa, and the ischial bursa.

Clinical History: 26-year-old man with heel pain and swelling.

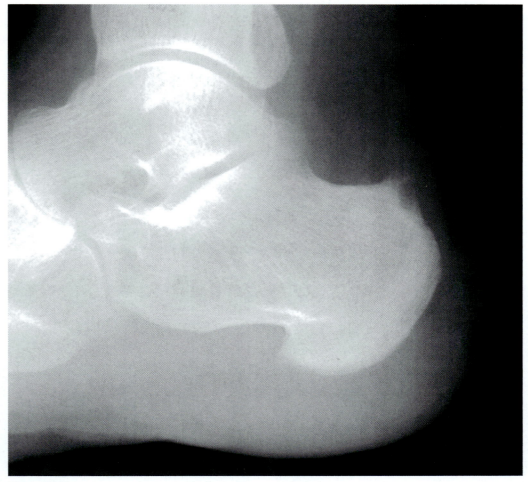

Figure 8-28

Findings: Lateral radiograph of the calcaneus shows effusion in the retrocalcaneal bursa. Fluffy periostitis is present at the origin of the plantar aponeurosis on the plantar aspect of the calcaneus.

Differential Diagnosis: Reiter's disease, psoriatic arthritis, ankylosing spondylitis, rheumatoid arthritis, plantar fasciitis.

Diagnosis: Reiter's disease.

Discussion: The calcaneus is a characteristic site of radiographic abnormalities in Reiter's disease. The prevalence of radiographic abnormalities involving the calcaneus among patients with Reiter's disease is 25% to 50%. The calcaneus may be the only site or the predominant site of findings, and correlative symptoms are frequently present. Bilateral changes are common. At the posterior aspect of the calcaneus, retrocalcaneal bursitis and Achilles tendinitis results in thickening of the soft tissues and poorly defined erosions of the adjacent calcaneus. Unlike psoriatic arthritis or ankylosing spondylitis, enthesophytes at the Achilles tendon insertion are rare in Reiter's disease. On the plantar surface of the calcaneus, erosions, hyperostosis, and enthesophytes may be present. Initially, the enthesophytes are poorly defined and fuzzy in outline, but they often become better defined as they mature, and may become indistinguishable from the common plantar calcaneal spurs seen in normal patients. The presence or absence of radiologic evidence of enthesopathy correlates poorly with the presence or absence of clinical symptoms [63]. Although both osteoporosis and erosions may be seen in Reiter's disease, the associated bony proliferative changes help to distinguish it from rheumatoid arthritis.

Clinical History: 71-year-old diabetic man with foot problems.

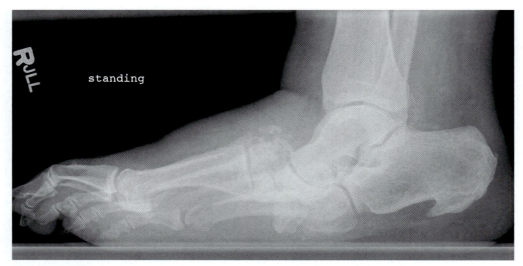

Figure 8-29   A

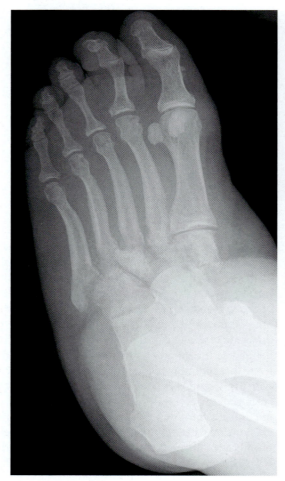

Figure 8-29   B

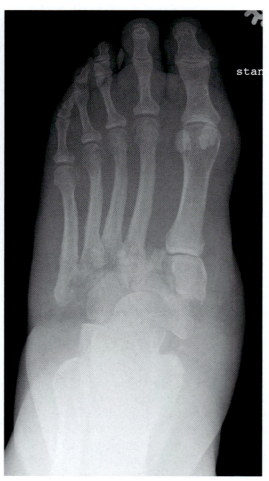

Figure 8-29   C

Findings: (A) Standing lateral radiograph of the foot shows over-riding of the metatarsals over the midfoot, with fragmentation and soft tissue swelling. The midfoot points into the plantar soft tissues, resulting in a rocker-bottom deformity. There is a plantar calcaneal spur. (B, C) Oblique and AP radiographs demonstrate fragmentation at the Lisfranc joint with subluxation of the lesser metatarsals.

Differential Diagnosis: Neuropathic osteoarthropathy, infection, trauma.

Diagnosis: Neuropathic osteoarthropathy.

Discussion: Neuropathic joints (also called Charcot joints) have lost proprioception and deep pain sensation. With continued use of the joint, relaxation and hypotonia of the supporting structures lead to malalignment and recurrent injury. Rapidly progressive erosion of the articular cartilage, reactive subchondral sclerosis, fractures, and fragmentation of the subchondral bone results in a disorganized joint. The presence of joint debris induces synovitis and chronic effusion. The damage and derangement may occur over a period of days to weeks, with relatively little symptomatology. Both lower motor neuron (peripheral) and upper motor neuron (central) lesions may result in neuropathic osteoarthropathy.

Diabetic neuropathy is the most common lower motor neuron lesion causing neuropathic osteoarthropathy. Other causes include alcoholism, tuberculosis, amyloidosis, leprosy, peripheral nerve trauma, steroids, and congenital indifference to pain. Syringomyelia is the most common upper motor neuron lesion. Other causes include meningomyelocele, trauma, multiple sclerosis, tabes dorsalis (syphilis), and cord compression. Neuropathic osteoarthropathy occurs in 0.1% of all diabetics and in 5% of those with diabetic neuropathy. Diabetic peripheral neuropathy causes loss of pain sensation and proprioception, leading to exceptional wear and tear without patient awareness of injury. The most frequent site of involvement is the foot (80%), especially the tarsometatarsal, intertarsal, and MTP joints; involvement may be unilateral or bilateral. Tarsometatarsal fracture-dislocation (Lisfranc fracture-dislocation) may occur spontaneously or with minimal trauma. Extensive sclerosis, osteophytosis, fractures, bony fragmentation, subluxation, dislocation, bony debris, effusion, and subchondral cysts are common findings. Chronic osteomyelitis is also relatively common in the diabetic foot, and the possible combination of neuropathic osteoarthropathy with infection can pose a diagnostic dilemma. MRI with gadolinium enhancement may be helpful in this circumstance.

Clinical History: Acute pain and swelling in foot.

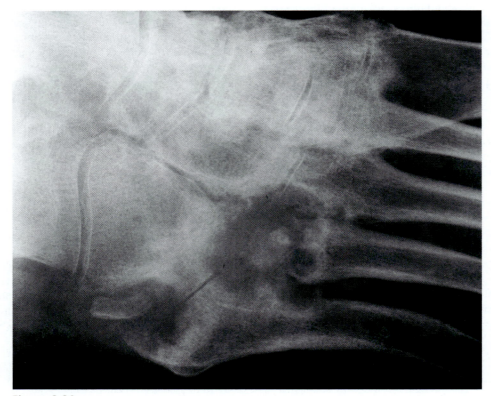

Figure 8-30

Findings: AP detail radiograph of the foot demonstrates erosions of the third, fourth, and fifth MTP joints, with sclerotic margins. Increased density is noted in the center of the erosions.

Differential Diagnosis: Osteoarthritis, rheumatoid arthritis, tophaceous gout, psoriatic arthritis, ankylosing spondylitis.

Diagnosis: Tophaceous gout.

Discussion: The well-defined nature of the erosions indicates the process is indolent. The lack of fusiform soft tissue swelling, uniform joint space loss, or juxtaarticular osteoporosis allows exclusion of an inflammatory arthropathy. These findings, particularly in this distribution, represent gouty arthropathy. Gout represents deposition of urate crystals into soft tissues, and patients are typically hyperuricemic. Hyperuricemia can be due to excessive production of uric acid, decreased renal clearance of uric acid, or a combination of the two. The majority of cases of gout are idiopathic, without known secondary disease to account for elevated levels of serum uric acid. Males are more frequently affected than females (20:1), and patients tend to be 40 to 50 years old at the onset of disease.

The disease most frequently manifests in the lower extremities, with 75% to 90% of patients having involvement of the first MTP joint. The first interphalangeal (IP), tarsometatarsal, ankle, and knee joints are frequently involved. Upper extremity involvement is common, particularly in the hands and elbows. In the past, 50% to 60% of patients would subsequently develop arthropathy, but this percentage has been decreased by pharmaceutical intervention. Patients typically do not have radiographically apparent arthropathy accompanying the initial onset of disease, and intermittent symptoms are usually present for years before findings become apparent. Lumpy, bumpy, soft tissue swelling may be seen due to tophaceous deposits, which are typically over extensor surfaces. Mineralization is usually preserved. Erosions tend to occur at the margins of joints or in a paraarticular distribution. The erosions of gout are typically well marginated and may demonstrate sclerotic borders. Despite erosive changes that may be extensive, the joint space is preserved until late in the disease, and lack of joint space narrowing is one of the most helpful clues to distinguish this erosive arthropathy from other erosive disorders. Tophaceous deposits may extend under the periosteum and produce overhanging edges at the margins of erosions, which is a helpful differentiating feature.

CASE 8-31

Clinical History: 15-year-old male basketball player.

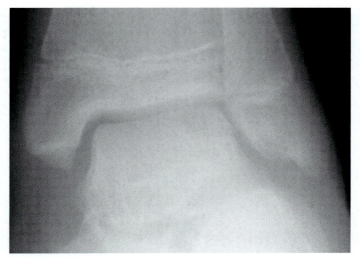

Figure 8-31 A

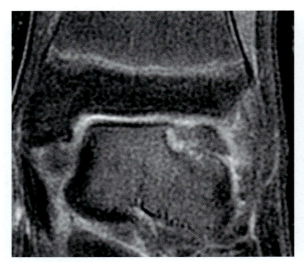

Figure 8-31 B

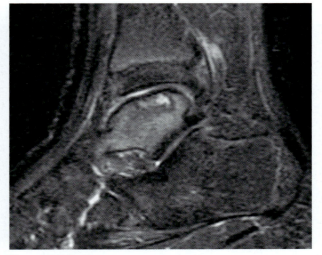

Figure 8-31 C

Findings: (A) Oblique radiograph demonstrates a crescentic lucency at the lateral aspect of the talar dome. (B, C) Coronal T2-weighted, fat-suppressed and sagittal inversion-recovery MRI shows an osteochondral injury to the lateral talar dome with fluid tracking beneath the fragment.

Differential Diagnosis: Osteochondral lesion, arthritis, fracture.

Diagnosis: Osteochondral lesion of the talus.

Discussion: Osteochondral lesions of the talar dome, formerly referred to as osteochondritis dissecans, are focal injuries to the cartilage and subchondral bone that typically occur secondary to trauma. It is controversial whether the osteochondral injury occurs at the time of the traumatic event, or whether it is the consequence of resultant instability [64]. In some cases, there is no history of trauma. On radiographs, there is a focal lucency in the anterolateral or posteromedial talar dome. MRI best demonstrates injury to the overlying cartilage and can identify fluid beneath the bone fragment, suggesting fragment instability. Treatment is initially conservative, with immobilization and then physical therapy. Surgical intervention consists of arthroscopic loose body removal, debridement, and drilling of the osteochondral lesion [65].

Clinical History: Monoarticular arthritis.

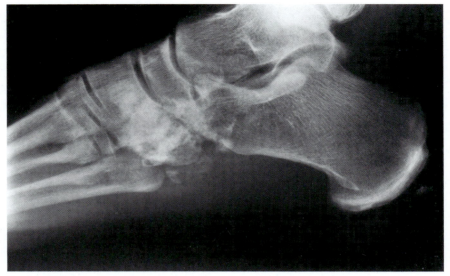

Figure 8-32   A

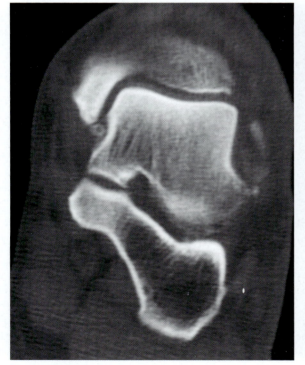

Figure 8-32   B

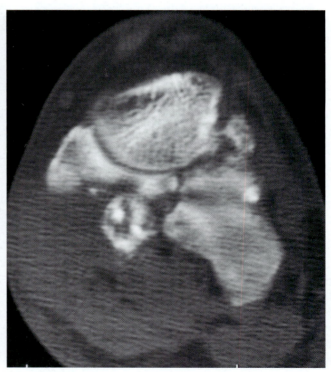

Figure 8-32   C

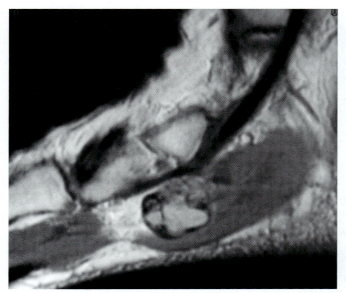

Figure 8-32 D

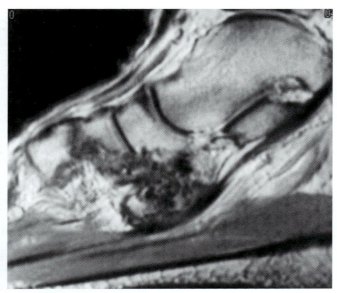

Figure 8-32 E

Findings: (A) Lateral radiograph demonstrates multiple ossific fragments projecting over the cuboid. (**B, C**) Coronal CT demonstrates secondary osseous erosion and well-defined, corticated ossific fragments. One is interposed between the medial malleolus and talus. (**D, E**) Sagittal T1-weighted MRI demonstrates osseous erosion of the talonavicular articulation and cuneiforms by the masses that are heterogeneous on all pulse sequences, but some focal hyperintense signal on T1 is seen, which suggests mature ossification with contained fatty elements.

Differential Diagnosis: PVNS, synovial chondromatosis, hemangiomatosis.

Diagnosis: Synovial osteochondromatosis.

Discussion: The complex anatomy of the foot makes diagnosis from the conventional radiograph difficult, since it is impossible to characterize the calcification and its relationship to underlying bone. CT was very helpful in this case, revealing multiple rounded osteochondral fragments within the talocalcaneal navicular joints. Erosive changes are not associated with joint space narrowing, osteoporosis, or dissolution of the joint. The MRI examination with low signal on both T1-weighted and T2-weighted images puts PVNS in the differential, but the osteocartilaginous loose bodies shown on CT are very unusual in PVNS. Hemangiomatosis in the soft tissues with pheboliths could account for the calcifications and erosions, but the cross-sectional images are inconsistent. Synovial chondromatosis is the best diagnosis, given the radiologic findings.

Synovial chondromatosis is a self-limiting metaplasia of the synovium that presents as a monoarticular arthropathy or, in unusual cases, within a tendon sheath of the hand or foot. This disease is 2 to 4 times more common in men and tends to present in middle-aged patients who have complaints of swelling, stiffness, and pain. The knee is the most commonly involved joint, followed by the elbow, hip, and shoulder; however, any joint may be involved.

Not all cases of synovial chondromatosis (33%) have radiographically identifiable osteocartilaginous loose bodies. The loose bodies of this disease tend to be small, numerous, and uniform in size, as opposed to the large, scattered, osteocartilaginous densities that may accompany osteoarthritis or osteochondritis dissecans. Although degenerative changes may be a late manifestation of synovial chondromatosis, the loose bodies in extent and number are more prominent than the osteoarthritic changes, and there is relative preservation of the joint space, since the patients tend to present early in the course of the disease. Erosions are appreciated more commonly in tight joints than capacious articulations such as the knee.

CT is very helpful in complex areas of anatomy, such as the temporomandibular and intervertebral joints, in characterizing the extent of erosions and confirming the extraosseous nature of densities seen on conventional radiography. MRI is also very helpful in determining the extent of disease, and the multiplanar capabilities of this technique are particularly helpful in this regard. The most common appearance on MRI is that of an intraarticular process that is intermediate on T1-weighted images and bright on T2-weighted images, with focal areas of low signal on both sequences from ossification. Areas of increased signal on T1-weighted images within ossific loose bodies corresponding to fat may be appreciated [66].

Clinical History: Medial foot mass for 10 years.

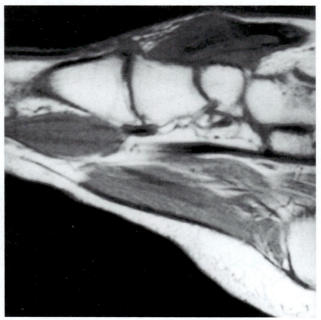

Figure 8-33   A

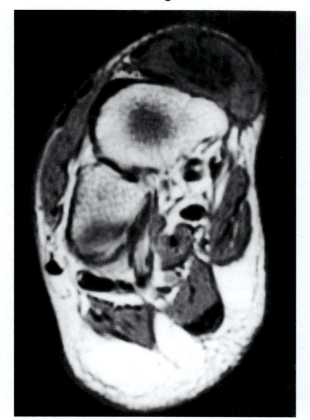

Figure 8-33   B

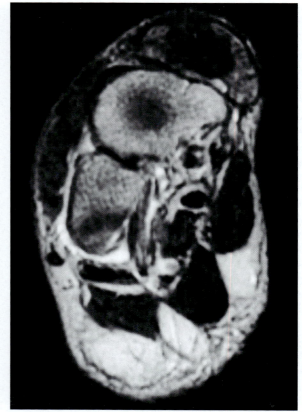

Figure 8-33   C

Findings: (A) Sagittal T1-weighted MRI demonstrates a low-signal-intensity, well-defined mass medial and dorsal to the foot. The extensor hallucis longus tendon is incorporated into the mass. (B, C) Axial T1-weighted images, without and with contrast, demonstrate minimal enhancement of the well-defined mass.

Differential Diagnosis: Giant cell tumor of tendon sheath, synovial sarcoma, synovial chondromatosis, unusual infection such as *Mycobacterium marianum*.

Diagnosis: Giant cell tumor of the tendon sheath.

Discussion: Soft tissue masses around the ankle joint are uncommon. The neurovascular bundle is not involved, making the diagnosis of peripheral nerve sheath tumor unlikely. The lack of direct tendon involvement makes the diagnosis of clear cell sarcoma unlikely. The diagnosis of synovial sarcoma must be considered with a soft tissue mass around the ankle. However, the mass appears to arise in the flexor hallucis tendon sheath, and the most likely diagnoses include processes that might arise from the tenosynovial sheath, such as giant cell tumor of the tendon sheath, synovial chondromatosis, and an unusual infection such as *Mycobacterium marianum*. The lack of inflammatory changes in the surrounding soft tissues makes tuberculosis unlikely, and the lack of calcifications within the mass lowers the likelihood but does not exclude the diagnosis of tenosynovial chondromatosis.

The most likely diagnosis, given the radiologic findings, is giant cell tumor of the tendon sheath, which is a benign synovial proliferative disorder, histologically indistinguishable from PVNS, that involves a joint. Giant cell tumor of the tendon sheath occurs most commonly in patients in their 30s through 50s, and presents more frequently in females than males with an approximate 2:1 ratio. This lesion most frequently presents in the hand, with only 5% to 15% of cases occurring in the foot, most typically in the first and second rays. In approximately 15% to 21% of cases, pressure erosion of adjacent bone can be seen, and bone may even be invaded, though rarely. Intralesional calcifications may be seen in 6% of cases, which makes radiologic distinction between giant cell tumor of tendon sheath and tenosynovial chondromatosis difficult. The mass appearance is typically nonspecific on T1-weighted images, and usually demonstrates intermediate signal. The diagnosis is usually considered based on T2-weighted images, which often reveal regions of intermediate to low signal. The relatively low signal on T2-weighted images is likely due to hemosiderin seen pathologically within these lesions. The MRI appearance varies, likely due to varying degrees of hemosiderin deposition. Moderate to intense enhancement is seen after contrast administration [67]. On ultrasound, these lesions are homogenously hypoechoic and have detectable internal blood flow [68].

Clinical History: 47-year-old man with trauma from motor vehicle crash.

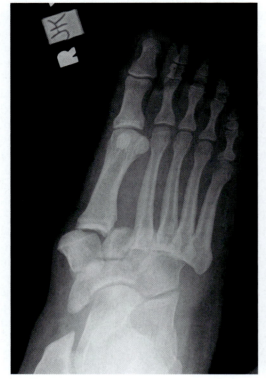

Figure 8-34 A

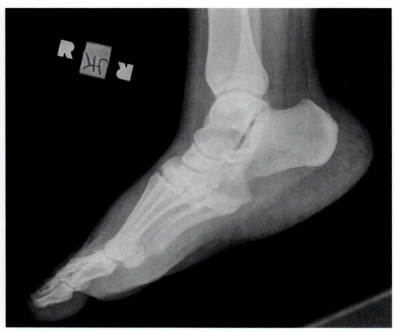

Figure 8-34 B

Findings: AP and lateral radiographs of the foot show fracture-dislocations of the tarsometatarsal joints. The first metatarsal has been separated from the metatarsals of the lesser toes and is displaced dorsally and medially relative to the first cuneiform. The first cuneiform has been dislocated medially. The metatarsals of the lesser toes have dislocated dorsally and laterally as a group

Differential Diagnosis: None.

Diagnosis: Lisfranc fracture-dislocation, divergent type.

Discussion: Lisfranc fracture-dislocation refers to any fracture-dislocation involving multiple tarsometatarsal articulations. Abduction forces cause a lateral shift of the forefoot relative to the midfoot, frequently accompanied by fracture at the base of the second metatarsal and cuboid. Misalignment of the second metatarsal relative to the second cuneiform is a prerequisite for the diagnosis. The bases of the second through fifth metatarsals are connected by ligaments. Although there is a ligament connecting the second metatarsal to the medial cuneiform, and a ligament connecting the medial cuneiform to the first metatarsal, there is no ligament joining the first and second metatarsals at their bases. When all of the metatarsals are dislocated laterally together, the injury may be called homolateral. When the first metatarsal is separated from the metatarsals of the lesser toes, the injury may be called divergent. Although the findings in this case are gross, if the metatarsals spontaneously relocate after the injury the findings may be very subtle and shown only by CT [69] or MRI. Stress views may be helpful in equivocal cases.

CASE 8-35

Clinical History: 74-year-old woman with foot pain.

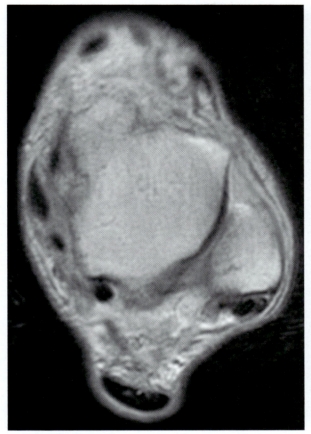

Figure 8-35 A

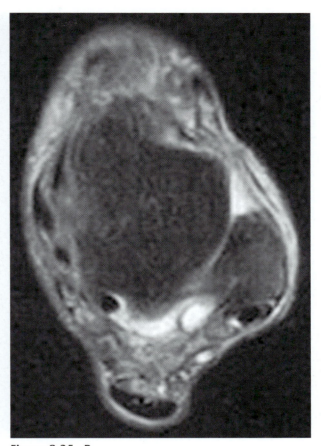

Figure 8-35 B

Findings: Axial proton-density (**A**) and T2-weighted, fat-suppressed (**B**) MRI through the ankle demonstrates three tendons located posterior to the lateral malleolus. A small ankle effusion is present.

Differential Diagnosis: None.

Diagnosis: Peroneus brevis tendon split tear.

Discussion: The peroneus longus and brevis tendons are located on the posterior lateral aspect of the ankle and are major everters of the foot, with the peroneus brevis being more effective [70]. The brevis attaches to the base of the fifth metatarsal. The longus has a broad-based insertion on the plantar surface of the base of the first metatarsal and medial cuneiform. Complete and partial tears can be seen in both of these tendons. Longitudinal split tears occur within the peroneus brevis during dorsiflexion when the brevis tendon is wedged between the lateral malleolus and peroneus longus tendon. When the peroneus brevis tendon splits, the peroneus longus tendon is partially surrounded by the two main peroneus brevis bundles [71]. Longitudinal peroneus brevis split tears are a clinically under-appreciated cause of lateral ankle pain [72].

Clinical History: 12-year-old girl with anemia.

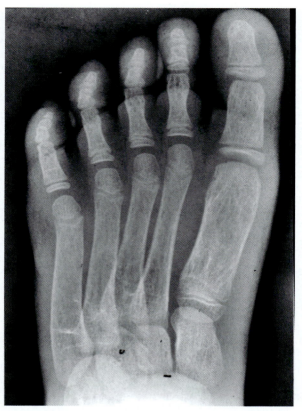

Figure 8-36

Findings: AP radiograph of foot. The marrow spaces are enlarged, causing the bones to have thin, scalloped cortices without much medullary structure. The shape of the long bones lacks the normal constriction of the diaphyses and gentle flaring of the metaphyses. Osteopenia is present.

Differential Diagnosis: Hemoglobinopathy, Gaucher's disease, leukemia, Pyle's disease, fibrous dysplasia.

Diagnosis: Thalassemia.

Discussion: Thalassemia comprises a group of disorders caused by inherited abnormalities of globin production that lead to ineffective hematopoiesis and anemia. The defect is in the synthesis of one of the globin chains. There are many types of thalassemia distinguished on the basis of the specific globin chain affected and the particular defect present. Limb deformities and metaphyseal abnormalities are common skeletal manifestations of thalassemia. Marrow expansion of the metaphysis and limb deformities occur more frequently in females and more often with earlier institution of desferrioxamine therapy [73]. Other skeletal manifestations may include widening of the diploic space, a hair-on-end pattern in the skull, and diminished pneumatization of the paranasal sinuses. Osteoporosis may predominate in adult-hood, and this may occur predominantly on the basis of marrow hyperplasia [74]. Ischemic necrosis and infection of bone and soft tissue, in addition to growth disturbances, are potential complications of hemoglobinopathies in general [75]. Undertubulation is nonspecific and may be seen in multiple conditions. Widening of the marrow spaces with osteopenia is a hallmark feature of marrow replacement processes. In the younger patient, this raises the possibility of hemoglobinopathies.

In thalassemia, β-chain synthesis is defective and α-chain synthesis predominates. The extraneous α-globin chain production causes intracellular precipitation of this compound, which in turn causes hemolysis, derangement of erythropoiesis, and enlargement of the marrow spaces. Treatment, such as hypertransfusion, may diminish hyperactive erythropoiesis and thereby decrease the degree of marrow expansion. Complications of this are best appreciated on MRI and include iron overload. Iron deposition in several organs may be seen, and this may impart low signal intensity to the bone marrow [76]. Additional chelation therapy may limit the degree of iron deposition, which may appear less prominent in the peripheral skeleton [77].

Clinical History: 23-year-old man with chronic foot swelling.

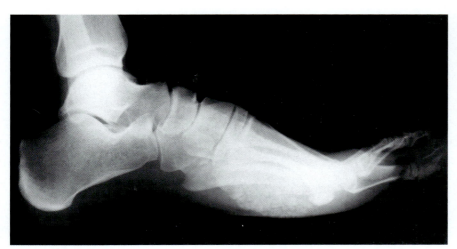

Figure 8-37   A

Figure 8-37   B

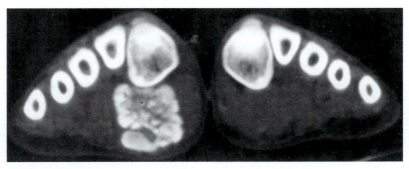

Figure 8-37   C

Findings: (A, B) Lateral and oblique radiographs of the foot show amorphous calcification in the plantar soft tissues. No changes in the bone are present. (C) Axial CT (bone windows) shows calcifications with occasional fluid levels in the plantar soft tissues.

Differential Diagnosis: Tumoral calcinosis, synovial osteochondromatosis, hydroxyapatite deposition disease, foreign body granulomas, osteosarcoma.

Diagnosis: Idiopathic tumoral calcinosis.

Discussion: Idiopathic tumoral calcinosis is an uncommon disorder characterized by accumulations of calcium hydroxyapatite crystals in the periarticular soft tissues with granulomatous reaction [78]. An inborn error in phosphorus metabolism is thought to be the cause of these nonneoplastic lesions. About one-third of reported cases are familial. The masses tend to grow slowly over many years to large size; symptoms may be caused by their physical bulk. Most are discovered in the first or second decade of life. These accumulations are comprised of multiple globules of calcification separated by radiolucent bands. Fluid levels are usually present but may not be evident, except on CT. The lesions are frequently found in the normal location of bursae. Fibrous septa may create a chicken-wire pattern of lucencies between the calcific densities. Smooth erosions of the bone surfaces adjacent to the lesions may be found. The treatment is surgical, but local recurrences are not uncommon.

Clinical History: 29-year-old amateur runner with foot pain.

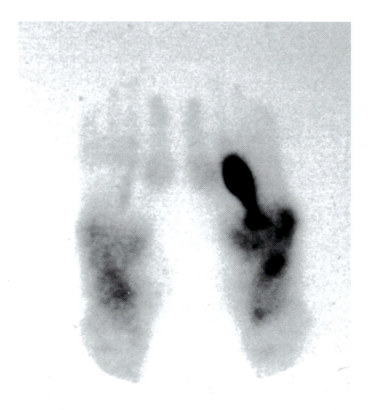

Figure 8-38 A

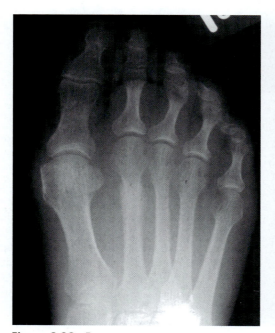

Figure 8-38 B

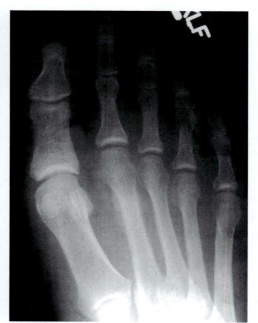

Figure 8-38 C

Findings: (A) Camera view of radionuclide bone scan shows intense activity in the second metatarsal. (B, C) Radiographs of the foot show fluffy, fusiform periosteal callus surrounding the distal shaft of the second metatarsal. No fracture line is evident.

Differential Diagnosis: None.

Diagnosis: Metatarsal stress fracture.

Discussion: On radiographs, stress fractures of long bones are evident as thin radiolucent lines that involve only a portion of the cortex, and are therefore incomplete fractures. By the time most cortical stress fractures are visible on plain film, callus is usually present. Sometimes the callus is visible, but the fracture line itself cannot be demonstrated. A lucent line that is completely surrounded by sclerotic bone represents a stress fracture with nonunion. On radionuclide bone scan, the accelerated remodeling may be apparent as a diffuse but patchy increase in tracer accumulation. Stress fractures are focal hot spots. On MRI, stress fractures may show extensive endosteal and periosteal edema and evidence of bone healing. An actual fracture line is frequently not seen. The bone scan and MRI is far more sensitive than plain films for detecting stress reaction and stress fractures. Periosteal new bone formation and endosteal thickening in the absence of a demonstrable fracture line usually represents stress reaction, which is a healing process that occurs in the presence of microfractures. This process may be demonstrable by radionuclide bone scan if plain films are unrevealing. The condition is also called traumatic periostitis. The most common fatigue fractures in the forefoot occur at the shaft or neck of the second or third metatarsals [79].

Clinical History: 22-year-old woman with foot pain.

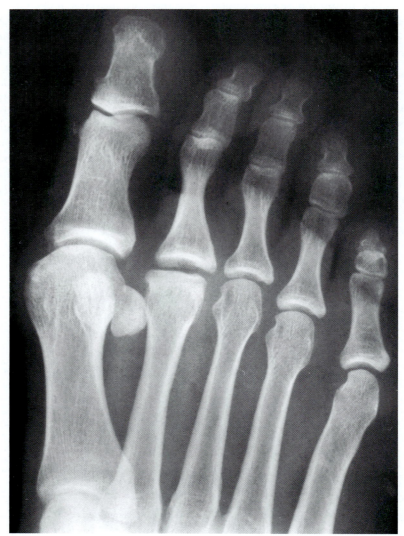

Figure 8-39

Findings: AP radiograph of the foot (detail of toes). The head of the second metatarsal is broad, flat, and dense. A corresponding adaptive change has occurred in the proximal end of the proximal phalanx.

Differential Diagnosis: Posttraumatic osteoarthritis, postinflammatory osteoarthritis, Freiberg's infraction.

Diagnosis: Freiberg's infraction.

Discussion: The bones of the second MTP joint are dysplastic, suggesting a pathologic process involving the joint that occurred during skeletal growth. Both trauma and infection could involve a metatarsal joint and cause enough damage to result in secondary osteoarthritis. The dysplastic changes suggest an abnormality of growth rather than direct injury, and the relative preservation of the cartilage space would be inconsistent with arthritis as the primary disease. Freiberg's infraction is an osteochondrosis of the second metatarsal head that occurs in the second decade while the epiphysis is still present. Of unknown etiology, it is believed to represent osteonecrosis, revascularization, subchondral collapse, and remodeling of the second metatarsal head. Chronic repetitive trauma leading to osteochondral injury and osteonecrosis has been suggested as the underlying cause [80]. Secondary degenerative arthritis occurs in early adulthood. The initial presentation is pain and tenderness over the metatarsal head, which typically resolves within a year or two. Chronic pain suggests the onset of secondary degenerative change. The condition is much more common in females.

Clinical History: 22-year-old woman with chronic foot swelling.

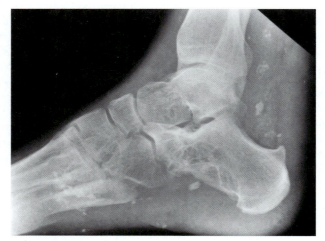

Figure 8-40   A

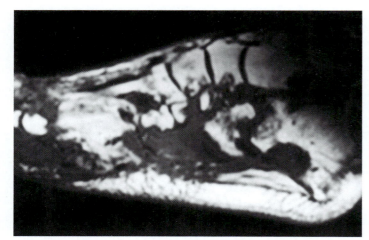

Figure 8-40   B

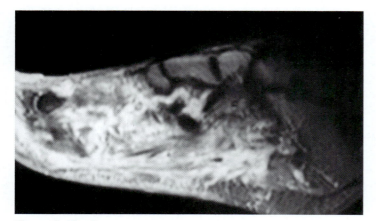

Figure 8-40   C

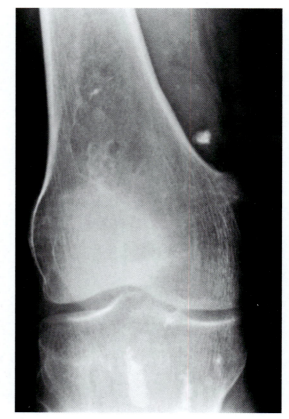

Figure 8-40   D

Findings: (A) Lateral radiograph. Multiple soft tissue calcifications are noted, most of which are round or linear. There is an erosion of the undersurface of the calcaneus and subtalar joint as well as the cuneiforms at their articulations with the metatarsals, with reinforcement of the existing trabecular pattern. (B, C) Sagittal T1-weighted MRI without and with contrast demonstrates predominantly T1 hypointensity, with an area of T1 hyperintensity at the metatarsal bases and marked enhancement of the soft tissue mass. (D) AP radiograph of the knee demonstrates additional soft tissue calcifications. A distal femoral central lucent lesion with scalloped borders and chondroid calcification is noted.

Differential Diagnosis: Ollier's disease, Maffucci's syndrome, idiopathic tumoral calcinosis, synovial osteochondromatosis.

Diagnosis: Maffucci's syndrome.

Discussion: The differential diagnosis of the foot includes entities that have soft tissue calcification. When the calcifications are recognized as phleboliths and the femoral lesion is recognized as an enchondroma, the diagnosis of Maffucci's syndrome should be considered. MRI confirms the presence of hemangiomas in the foot and, if necessary, could confirm the presence of the enchondroma in the femur.

Maffucci's syndrome is a mesodermal dysplasia consisting of multiple enchondromas and soft tissue hemangiomas. Maffucci's syndrome is much less common than multiple enchondromatosis (Ollier's disease), which itself is rather uncommon. The hemangiomatosis may be localized or extensive, and may occur anywhere in the skin or subcutaneous tissues. Malignant transformation of the bone lesions to chondrosarcoma has been recognized to occur in 20% of cases, based on retrospective reviews of the literature [81], but the lifetime risk of chondrosarcoma in these patients is probably much higher. The soft tissue hemangiomas are frequently found in close proximity to the bony lesions, and they may undergo malignant transformation, although with much less frequency [82].

Clinical History: 46-year-old woman with polyarticular arthritis.

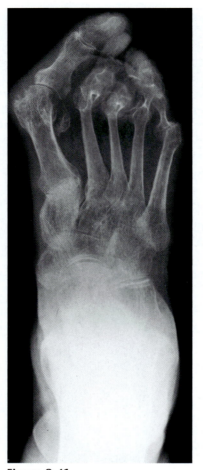

Figure 8-41

Findings: AP radiograph of the forefoot. There is diffuse osteopenia. Severe hallux valgus and metatarsus primus varus is present, and there are large erosions at the first metatarsal head. Marginal erosions are seen along the medial aspect of the IP joint of the great toe, at the MTP joints of the lesser toes, and at the lateral sesamoid. The erosions appear to have a thin sclerotic border. A cock-up toe deformity with overriding is present at the third toe. The cartilage spaces of the MTP joints of the lesser toes are difficult to see because of the alignment abnormalities, but diffuse narrowing is evident at the second toe. There is a relative lack of hypertrophic bone.

Differential Diagnosis: Rheumatoid arthritis, tophaceous gout, psoriatic arthritis, osteoarthritis.

Diagnosis: Rheumatoid arthritis.

Discussion: The symptoms of rheumatoid arthritis in the hand may also be found in the forefoot, including juxtaarticular and chronic osteoporosis, marginal erosions, subchondral cysts, and diffuse joint space narrowing. The MTP joints tend to be the site of greatest involvement. The relative lack of hypertrophic bone formation, such as osteophytes and subchondral sclerosis, eliminates osteoarthritis and neuropathic osteoarthropathy as possibilities. The erosions are marginal, involving the bare area of the bone that is not covered by cartilage, and is therefore directly exposed to the inflammatory pannus. Inflammatory erosions tend to have poorly defined margins, and the sclerotic rim seen in this case is indicative of healing and lack of acute disease activity. The presence of this sclerotic rim raises the question of tophaceous gout, but the distribution of disease would be unusual for gout. Furthermore, the erosions in gout represent a combination of bone loss and bone reaction, and the overhanging edges characteristic of this process are absent. Erosions in rheumatoid arthritis represent pure bone loss. Psoriatic arthritis may have an appearance that overlaps with the appearance of rheumatoid arthritis, but severe erosions in psoriatic arthritis are often more central and intraarticular rather than marginal. Periostitis would also be a distinguishing feature that is frequently present in psoriatic arthritis, but usually absent from rheumatoid arthritis.

Clinical History: 11-year-old girl.

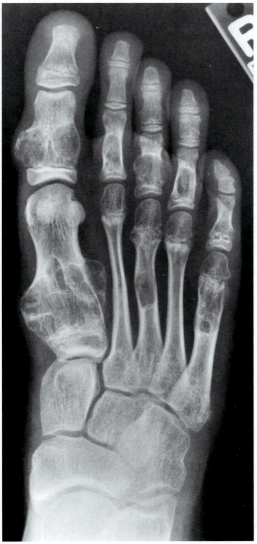

Figure 8-42

Findings: AP radiograph of the foot shows multiple lesions deforming the foot. Many of the larger lesions are expansile, with thinned but intact overlying cortex. Some lesions have mineralized matrix with punctate calcifications. The second metatarsal has remodeled around the adjacent large lesion in the first metatarsal.

Differential Diagnosis: None.

Diagnosis: Multiple enchondromatosis (Ollier's disease).

Discussion: Multiple enchondromatosis (Ollier's disease) is a nonfamilial, nonheritable, diffuse growth abnormality in which the tubular bones may be bowed and shortened to a variable extent and filled with multiple enchondromas. The severity of involvement may range from a few lesions with mild deformities to countless ones with severe deformities. The lesions often become stable at puberty, but their growth may continue throughout the patient's lifetime. The individual lesions are radiologically and histologically identical to solitary enchondromas, but patients with multiple enchondromatosis may have as high as a 30% to 50% risk of developing chondrosarcoma in their lifetime. A lesion that becomes painful in the absence of pathologic fracture should trigger consideration of possible malignancy.

Clinical History: 37-year-old man with enlarging foot mass. There was no history of fracture.

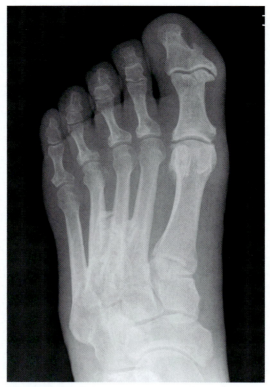

Figure 8-43   A

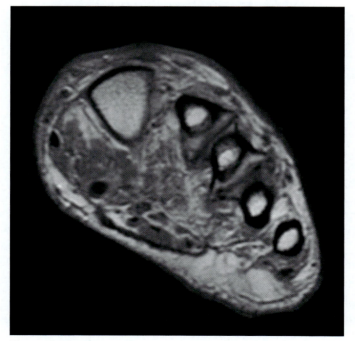

Figure 8-43   B

Findings: (A) AP view of the foot shows an ossific lesion involving the shafts of the second, third, and fourth metatarsals. Incidental degenerative changes are seen at the great toe. (B) MRI through the short axis of the foot shows that the ossific lesion arises from the cortex of both the second, third, and fourth metatarsal shafts, and has the form of mature, reactive periosteal bone formation. There are broad pseudoarticulations. The original cortices and marrow spaces of the involved metatarsals are still delineated.

Differential Diagnosis: Fracture, florid reactive periostitis, bizarre parosteal osteochondromatous proliferation (BPOP), acquired osteochondroma (Turret exostosis).

Diagnosis: BPOP (Nora's lesion).

Discussion: The conventional radiograph shows a lesion comprised of mature bone overlying the metatarsal shafts, which appear otherwise intact. The maturity of the bone indicates the lesion is indolent, but it is difficult to tell how the process is related to the underlying metatarsals. The MRI shows that the lesions have no medullary continuity with the underlying metatarsals, eliminating the diagnosis of osteochondroma. Parosteal osteosarcoma presents as an ossific mass arising from the surface of bone, but involvement of multiple bones would be exceedingly rare, and the mass consists entirely of mature bone without soft tissue component or destruction. This leaves a category of lesions known as reactive lesions of the bone surface, which commonly occur in the hands and feet. Included in this category are florid reactive periostitis, BPOP, and acquired osteochondroma (Turret exostosis). Radiographically, these lesions may be indistinguishable from one another. Pathologic distinction is based on the amount and character of reactive spindle cells, cartilage, and bone formation.

These lesions are related to myositis ossificans and are thought to occur as a result of trauma. Patients are typically 20 to 40 years old. The middle and proximal phalanges of the hand are most commonly affected. The chief radiologic differential is osteochondroma, which is not surprising, since these lesions often have a metaplastic cartilage cap. The lack of cortical and medullary continuity on cross-sectional imaging excludes the diagnosis, as mentioned earlier. BPOP pathologically consists of prominent bone and cartilage formation with atypical cells in both cell lines, leaving the pathologist vulnerable to the erroneous microscopic diagnosis of malignancy if the radiographic appearance is not considered [83,84,85]. BPOP is a benign disease with low likelihood of recurrence after resection. CT is also an excellent method of examining diseases that involve the cortex and extensive mineralization, and in these situations, CT may be preferable to MRI.

Clinical History: 45-year-old woman with painful feet.

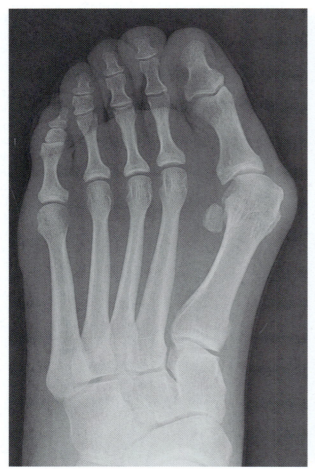

Figure 8-44   A

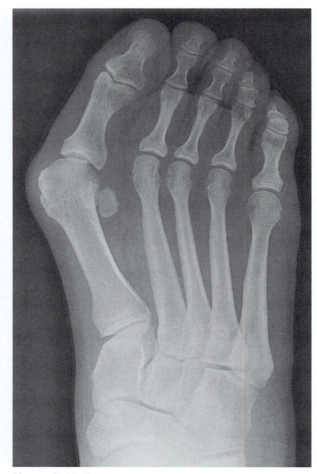

Figure 8-44   B

Findings: (A, B) AP and oblique radiographs of the left foot show lateral deviation of the great toe and medial deviation of the first metatarsal. The articular surface of each first metatarsal head is 50% uncovered. The lateral sesamoid is subluxated laterally from beneath the first metatarsal head. The great toe is slightly rotated externally along its long axis. Soft tissue prominence is present over the medial aspect of the first metatarsal head.

Differential Diagnosis: Hallux valgus, gout, rheumatoid arthritis, SLE.

Diagnosis: Hallux valgus.

Discussion: The presence of a soft tissue lump at the first MTP joint suggests tophaceous gout, but the absence of erosions would be inconsistent. The lateral deviation of the great toe and the medial deviation of the first metatarsal (hallux valgus, metatarsus primus varus) define hallux valgus, also called bunion deformity. The soft tissue lump represents a distended bursa covering the medial prominence of the metatarsal head. Osteoarthritis is commonly associated with hallux valgus, but it is a secondary feature. Hallux valgus is also a common feature of rheumatoid arthritis, but in this case there are no other findings to suggest that diagnosis.

Foot problems are common in the United States and other well-heeled societies; perhaps 12% of Americans, most of them women, have had an operation on the foot. As many as 80% of adult American women experience pain while wearing shoes, and the prevalence of hallux valgus is approximately 50% [86]. Shoes that are too tight in the forefoot have been implicated as a principal cause of hallux valgus [87]. Familial factors are also important, particularly in children and adolescents [88].

The first MTP joint has a strong plantar capsule and sesamoid mechanism, and a thin dorsal capsule. The extensor hallucis longus and brevis tendons pass through a hood mechanism over the dorsal aspect of the first MTP joint to insert on the toes. The two heads of the flexor hallucis brevis incorporate sesamoid bones and have separate shallow grooves in which to run. The abductor hallucis inserts on the plantar medial aspect of the proximal phalanx, and the adductor hallucis anchors the sesamoid mechanism and inserts on the plantar lateral aspect of the proximal phalanx. As the great toe deviates laterally and the first metatarsal deviates medially (the causal relationship between these two processes is incompletely understood), the first MTP joint subluxates laterally. The first metatarsal head slides medially off the sesamoids, which are tethered by the adductor hallucis, and secondary degenerative changes occur at the sesamoid articulations as they are pulled out of their grooves. The abductor hallucis tendon displaces to the plantar aspect, pronating the proximal phalanx, and the flexor and extensor tendons act as a bowstring to worsen the deformity. In advanced cases, the great toe may deviate so far that it crosses underneath the second toe.

The severity of a bunion deformity may be assessed by the degree of great toe deviation, the angle between the first and second metatarsals, and the amount of lateral subluxation of the sesamoids. These measurements should be made on weight-bearing radiographs. When surgical treatment is called for, a wide variety of operations are possible, consisting generally of combinations of osteotomies to realign the bones, and soft tissue repairs to maintain the reduction [89]. Other common foot deformities that occur in the lesser toes include the claw toe (extension at the MTP joint, flexion at the proximal IP [PIP] and distal IP [DIP] joints), the hammer toe (extension at the MTP joint, flexion at the PIP joint, hyperextension at the DIP joint), and the mallet toe (isolated flexion at the DIP joint). As if these problems were not enough, women's high-heeled shoes have been implicated in the development of medial and patellofemoral compartment osteoarthritis of the knee [90].

Clinical History: 59-year-old woman with pain.

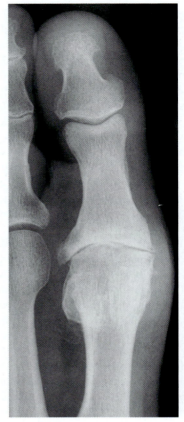

Figure 8-45 A

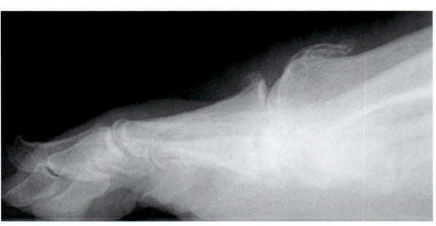

Figure 8-45 B

Findings: Radiographs of the great toe show asymmetric cartilage space narrowing, subchondral sclerosis, and prominent osteophytes at the first MTP joint. Alignment of the great toe and first ray is normal.

Differential Diagnosis: None.

Diagnosis: Hallux rigidus (hallux limitus).

Discussion: Hallux rigidus is characterized by restriction of motion at the first MTP joint. The condition is also called hallux limitus, because the range of motion is very limited. This limitation in motion is usually in the dorsal direction and is most commonly associated with a mechanical block caused by periarticular osteophytes [91]. These osteophytes tend to form a horseshoe-shaped collar of hypertrophic bone around the medial, dorsal, and lateral aspects of the first metatarsal following the articular margin, often with match-

ing bony hypertrophy of the proximal phalanx. The condition follows the natural history of osteoarthritis and has a prevalence of about 2% in individuals older than 50. Various conditions may result in hallux rigidus, including generalized, idiopathic osteoarthritis, posttraumatic osteoarthritis, metabolic disorders such as crystal arthropathies, and congenital disorders such as a long first ray or abnormal gait. Most patients present with chronic pain, but fracture of an osteophyte or presence of a new loose body may result in an acute exacerbation. Mechanical symptoms from impingement of the dorsal bony hypertrophy on shoes may occur, and impingement of the dorsal digital nerve as it passes over the bony hypertrophy may cause burning pain or paresthesias. Females are affected twice as often as males, and most symptomatic patients are in the adolescent or elderly age groups.

Clinical History: 47-year-old woman with severe foot problems and skin rash.

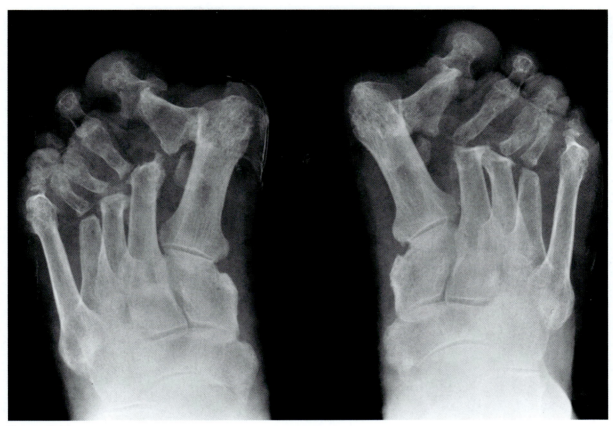

Figure 8-46

Findings: AP radiograph of both feet shows severe bilateral abnormalities. Both feet show marked valgus deviation of the great and lesser toes, with lateral subluxations that are most prominent at the great toe MTP joints. The ends of the bones of the MTP joints have been eroded, particularly at the second through fourth toes, with a suggestion of pencil-in-cup deformity at several sites. Erosions and subluxations are present at the IP joints of the great toes. Bone mineralization is normal or perhaps slightly decreased, and soft tissue swelling is relatively modest compared with the severity of the forefoot joint changes. The intertarsal joints are nearly intact, but proliferative bone is present along the medial aspects of the navicular and medial cuneiform bones.

Differential Diagnosis: Rheumatoid arthritis, psoriatic arthritis, Reiter's disease, ankylosing spondylitis, neuropathic osteoarthropathy, trauma.

Diagnosis: Psoriatic arthritis (arthritis mutilans).

Discussion: The severity of the joint changes fits the descriptive term arthritis mutilans. Although in many cases it is difficult, and perhaps not important, to determine the underlying pathophysiology, the exercise is worthwhile because the diagnostic reasoning is similar in early, subtle disease. There is obvious bilateral, symmetric polyarticular disease. The central, intraarticular erosions suggest a spondyloarthropathy as the underlying disease rather than rheumatoid arthritis, because the erosions in rheumatoid arthritis tend to occur at the margins of the joint. Erosions in rheumatoid arthritis are unlikely to assume a pencil-in-cup morphology. Radiographic changes in Reiter's disease are typically rather mild, and proliferative rather than erosive changes predominate. The severity of these changes would be unusual for ankylosing spondylitis. Neuropathic osteoarthropathy and posttraumatic osteoarthritis may involve the feet bilaterally, but there is very little reactive bone formation and there is a complete lack of osseous debris.

Clinical History: 48-year-old man with foot problems.

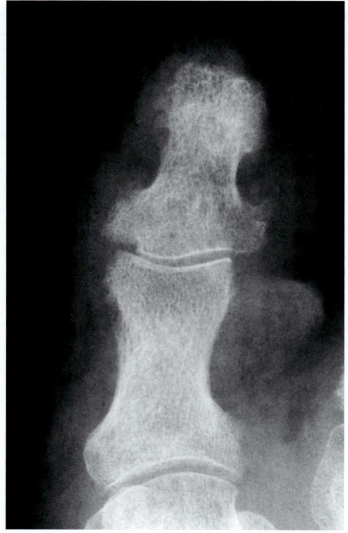

Figure 8-47

Findings: AP radiograph of the great toe. The articular ends of the IP joint have been eroded. Bone mineral density is maintained, and there is marked periosteal reaction about the joints.

Differential Diagnosis: Psoriatic arthritis, Reiter's disease, ankylosing spondylitis, rheumatoid arthritis, septic arthritis, resection arthroplasty.

Diagnosis: Psoriatic arthritis.

Discussion: Severe erosions of the IP joint suggest an inflammatory process, but one that has not progressed to ankylosis. The periosteal new bone formation is fluffy (the morphology associated with periostitis), rather than linear (the morphology that would be associated with infection). The lack of osteoporosis argues against rheumatoid arthritis, but osteoporosis in the feet of rheumatoid patients is often less striking than osteoporosis in the hands and upper limbs. Foot surgery actually has a greater prevalence among adults in the United States than inflammatory arthritis, so postsurgical change is always a consideration when a joint is missing. The age of the patient is more suggestive of psoriatic arthritis than Reiter's disease.

Clinical History: 22-year-old college football player.

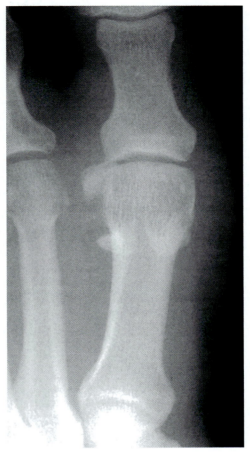

Figure 8-48

Findings: AP radiograph of the forefoot with attention to the first MTP joint shows transverse fractures of the medial (tibial) and lateral (fibular) sesamoids. The fracture fragments are distracted by several millimeters.

Differential Diagnosis: None.

Diagnosis: Sesamoid fracture (turf toe).

Discussion: Traumatic fractures of the sesamoid bones of the great toe may occur with dorsal dislocation of the first MTP joint. The medial and lateral heads of the flexor hallucis brevis attach to the medial and lateral sesamoid bones, respectively, which then attach to the proximal plantar aspect of the proximal phalanx of the great toe through the plantar capsule. Dorsal dislocation of the great toe at the MTP joint produces severe tensile loading of the sesamoid mechanism and is the basis for these distracted transverse fractures. Alternatively, the plantar capsule may rupture distal to the sesamoids. These injuries are typically sustained when force is applied to the dorsiflexed great toe in activities such as football, motor vehicle accidents, equestrian stirrup injuries, and falls from heights. The term "turf toe" refers to the higher frequency of these injuries in football players who play on artificial turf as opposed to grass [92].

Stress fractures of the sesamoids are more common injuries than traumatic fractures, and they occur in various athletic activities, including dance and distance running. Because the flexor hallucis brevis tends to distract the fragments, nonunion is a common complication. Although resection of the sesamoid fragments is the most common operative treatment for such nonunions, bone grafting may be successful [93]. Stress fractures occur more commonly in the medial sesamoid [94], whereas traumatic fractures occur more commonly in the lateral sesamoid. Sesamoid fractures may be distinguished radiographically from bipartite sesamoids by the absence of rounded contours and circumferential cortical margins. MRI can differentiate between nondisplaced sesamoid fractures and other causes of sesamoid pain including sesamoiditis, osteonecrosis, osteomyelitis, arthritis, and bursitis [95].

SOURCES AND READINGS

1. Churchill RS, Sferra JJ. Posterior tibial tendon insufficiency. Its diagnosis, management, and treatment. *Am J Orthop.* 1998;27:339–347.

2. Anderson MW, Kaplan PA, Dussault RG, Hurwitz S. Association of posterior tibial tendon abnormalities with abnormal signal intensity in the sinus tarsi on MR imaging. *Skeletal Radiol.* 2000;29:514–519.

3. Crawford AH. Ankle fractures in children. *Instr Course Lect.* 1995;44:317–324.

4. Karrholm J. The triplane fracture: four years of follow-up of 21 cases and review of the literature. *J Pediatr Orthop B.* 1997;6:91–102.

5. El-Karef E, Sadek HI, Nairn DS, Aldam CH, Allen PW. Triplane fracture of the distal tibia. *Injury.* 2000;31:729–736.

6. Barmada A, Gaynor T, Mubarak SJ. Premature physeal closure following distal tibia physeal fractures: a new radiographic predictor. *J Pediatr Orthop.* 2003;23:733–739.

7. Marchevsky AM, Damsker B, Green S, Tepper S. The clinicopathological spectrum of non-tuberculous mycobacterial osteoarticular infections. *J Bone Joint Surg Am.* 1985;67:925–929.

8. Hirsch R, Miller SM, Kazi S, Cate TR, Reveille JD. Human immunodeficiency virus-associated atypical mycobacterial skeletal infections. *Semin Arthritis Rheum.* 1996;25:347–356.

9. Granowetter L, West DC. The Ewing's sarcoma family of tumours: Ewing's sarcoma and peripheral primitive neuralectodermal tumor of bone and soft tissue. *Cancer Treat Res.* 1997;92:253–308.

10. Kransdorf MJ, Murphey MD. *Imaging of Soft Tissue Tumors.* Philadelphia: Saunders; 1997:264–269.

11. Kimber C, Michalski A, Spitz L, Pierro A. Primitive neuralectodermal tumours: anatomic location, extent of surgery, and outcome. *J Pediatr Surg.* 1998;33:39–41.

12. Levine SM, Lambiase RE, Petchprapa CN. Cortical lesions of the tibia: characteristic appearances at conventional radiography. *Radiographics.* 2003;23:157–177.

13. Rhys R, Davies AM, Mangham DC, Grimer RJ. Sclerotome distribution of melorheostosis and multicentric fibromatosis. *Skeletal Radiol.* 1998;27:633–636.

14. Donath J, Poor G, Kiss C, Fornet B, Genant H. Atypical form of active melorheostosis and its treatment with bisphosphonate. *Skeletal Radiol.* 2002;31(12):709–713.

15. Rodriguez-Merchan EC. Management of the orthopaedic complications of haemophilia. *J Bone Joint Surg Br.* 1998;80:191–196.

16. Smith JA. Bone disorders in sickle cell disease. *Hematol Oncol Clin North Am.* 1996;10:1345–1356.

17. Rifai A, Nyman R. Scintigraphy and ultrasonography in differentiating osteomyelitis from bone infarction in sickle cell disease. *Acta Radiol.* 1997;38:139–143.

18. Sadat-Ali M, al-Umran K, al-Habdan I, al-Mulhim F. Ultrasonography: can it differentiate between vasoocclusive crisis and acute osteomyelitis in sickle cell disease? *J Pediatr Orthop.* 1998;18:552–554.

19. Al-Nakshabandi NA, Ryan AG, Choudur H, et al. Pigmented villonodular synovitis. *Clin Radiol.* 2004;59:414–420.

20. Baker ND, Klein JD, Weidner N, Weissman BN, Brick GW. Pigmented villonodular synovitis containing coarse calcifications. *AJR Am J Roentgenol.* 1989;153:1228–1230.

21. Cobby MJ, Adler RS, Swartz R, Martel W. Dialysis-related amyloid arthropathy: MRI findings in 4 patients. *AJR Am J Roentgenol.* 1991;157:1023–1027.

22. Kalil RK, Unni KK. Malignancy in pigmented villonodular synovitis. *Skeletal Radiol.* 1998;27:392–395.

23. Bertoni F, Unni KK, Beabout JW, Simm FH. Malignant giant cell tumor of the tendon sheaths and joints (malignant pigmented villonodular synovitis). *Am J Surg Pathol.* 1997;21:153–163.

24. Newnham DM, Douglas JG, Legge JS, Friend JA. Achilles tendon rupture: an underrated complication of corticosteroid treatment. *Thorax.* 1991;46:853–854.

25. Levi N. The incidence of Achilles tendon rupture in Copenhagen. *Injury.* 1997;28:311–313.

26. Tuite MJ. MR imaging of the tendons of the foot and ankle. *Semin Musculoskelet Radiol.* 2002;6:119–131.

27. Koivunen-Niemela T, Parkkola K. Anatomy of the Achilles tendon (tendo calcaneus) with respect to tendon thickness measurements. *Surg Radiol Anat.* 1995;17:263–268.

28. Kainberger FM, Engel A, Barton P, Huebsch P, Neuhold A, Salomonowitz E. Injury of the Achilles tendon: diagnosis with sonography. *AJR Am J Roentgenol.* 1990;115:1031–1036.

29. Astrom M, Gentz CF, Nilsson P, Rausing A, Sjoberg S, Westlin N. Imaging in chronic Achilles tendinopathy: a comparison of ultrasonography, magnetic resonance imaging and surgical findings in 27 histologically verified cases. *Skeletal Radiol.* 1996;25:615–620.

30. Archambault JM, Wiley JP, Bray RC, Verhoef M, Wiseman DA, Elliott PD. Can sonography predict the outcome in patients with achillodynia? *J Clin Ultrasound.* 1998;26:335–339.

31. Rupp S, Templehof S, Fritsch E. Ultrasound of the Achilles tendon after surgical repair: morphology and function. *Br J Radiol.* 1995;68:454–458.

32. Maillard SM, Jones R, Owens C, et al. Quantitative assessment of MRI T2 relaxation time of thigh muscles in juvenile dermatomyositis. *Rheumatology (Oxford).* 2004;43:603–608.

33. Lofberg M, Liewendahl K, Lamminen A, Korhola O, Somer H. Antimyosin scintigraphy compared with magnetic resonance imaging in inflammatory myopathies. *Arch Neurol.* 1998;55:987–993.

34. Lektrakul N, Chung CB, Lai Ym, et al. Tarsal sinus: arthrographic, MR imaging, MR arthrographic, and pathologic findings in cadavers and retrospective study data in patients with sinus tarsi syndrome. *Radiology.* 2001;219:802–810.

35. Lektrakul N, Chung CB, Lai Ym, et al. Tarsal sinus: arthrographic, MR imaging, MR arthrographic, and pathologic findings in cadavers and retrospective study data in patients with sinus tarsi syndrome. *Radiology.* 2001;219:802–810.

36. Rosenberg ZS, Beltran J, Bencardino JT. From the RSNA Refresher Courses. Radiological Society of North America. MR imaging of the ankle and foot. *Radiographics.* 2000;20(Spec No):S153–S179.

37. Oloff LM, Schulhofer SD, Bocko AP. Subtalar joint arthroscopy for sinus tarsi syndrome: a review of 29 cases. *J Foot Ankle Surg.* 2001;40:152–157.

38. Delanois RE, Mont MA, Yoon TR, Mizell M, Hungerford DS. Atraumatic osteonecrosis of the talus. *J Bone Joint Surg Am.* 1998;80:529–536.

39. Inokuchi S, Ogawa K, Usami N, Hashimoto T. Long-term follow up of talus fractures. *Orthopedics.* 1996;19:477–481.

40. Bohay DR, Manoli A II. Subtalar joint dislocations. *Foot Ankle Int.* 1995;16:803–808.

41. Goldner JL, Poletti SC, Gates HS III, Richardson WJ. Severe open subtalar dislocations: long-term results. *J Bone Joint Surg Am.* 1995;77:1075–1079.

42. Drennan JC. Tarsal coalitions. *Instr Course Lect.* 1996;45:323–329.

43. Liu PT, Roberts CC, Chivers FS, et al. "Absent middle facet": a sign on unenhanced radiography of subtalar joint coalition. *AJR Am J Roentgenol.* 2003;181:1565–1572.

44. Drennan JC. Congenital vertical talus. *Instr Course Lect.* 1996;45:315–322.

45. Greene WB. Metatarsus adductus and skewfoot. *Instr Course Lect.* 1994;43:161–177.

46. Reilly PA, Evison G, McHugh NJ, Maddison PJ. Arthropathy of hands and feet in systemic lupus erythematosus. *J Rheumatol.* 1990;17:777–784.

47. Mizuntani W, Quismorio FP Jr. Lupus foot: deforming arthropathy of the feet in systemic lupus erythematosus. *J Rheumatol.* 1984;11:80–82.

48. Calamia KT, Balabanova M. Vasculitis in systemic lupus erythematosis. *Clin Dermatol.* 2004;22:148–156.

49. Gonzalez JV, Stuck RM, Streit N. Intraosseous lipoma of the calcaneus: a clinicopathologic study of three cases. *J Foot Ankle Surg.* 1997;36:306–310.

50. Greaney RB, Gerber FH, Laughlin RL, et al. Distribution and natural history of stress fractures in U.S. Marine recruits. *Radiology*. 1983;146:339–346.

51. Cohen PA, Job-Deslandre CH, Lalande G, Adamsbaum C. Overview of the radiology of juvenile idiopathic arthritis (JIA). *Eur J Radiol*. 2000;33:94–101.

52. Johnson K, Gardner-Medwin J. Childhood arthritis: classification and radiology. *Clin Radiol*. 2002;57(1):47–58.

53. DeMaio M, Paine R, Mangine RE, Drez D Jr. Plantar fasciitis. *Orthopedics*. 1993;16:1153–1163.

54. Ozdemir H, Ozdemir A, Soyucu Y, Urguden M. The role of bone scintigraphy in determining the etiology of heel pain. *Ann Nucl Med*. 2002;16:395–401.

55. Morrison WB. Magnetic resonance imaging of sports injuries of the ankle. *Top Magn Reson Imaging*. 2003;14:179–197.

56. Gerster JC, Vischer TL, Bennani A, Fallet GH. The painful heel. Comparative study in rheumatoid arthritis, ankylosing spondylitis, Reiter's syndrome, and generalized osteoarthrosis. *Ann Rheum Dis*. 1977;36:343–348.

57. Kiryu H, Tsuneyoshi M, Enjoji M. Myofibroblasts in fibromatoses. An electron microscopic study. *Acta Pathol Jpn*. 1985;35:533–547.

58. Sundaram M, McGuire MH, Schajowicz F. Soft tissue masses: histologic basis for decreased signal intensity (short T2) on T2-weighted MR images. *AJR Am J Roentgenol*. 1987;148:1247–1250.

59. Yacoe ME, Bergman AG, Ladd AL, Helman BH. Dupuytren's contracture: MR imaging findings and correlation between MR signal intensity and cellularity of lesions. *AJR Am J Roentgenol*. 1993;160:813–817.

60. Pasternack WA, Davison GA. Plantar fibromatosis: staging by magnetic resonance imaging. *J Foot Ankle Surg*. 1993;32:390–396.

61. Morrison WB, Schweitzer ME, Wapner KL, Lackman RD. Plantar fibromatosis: a benign aggressive neoplasm with a characteristic appearance on MR images. *Radiology*. 1994;193:841–845.

62. Hayes CW, Conway WF. Calcium hydroxyapatite deposition disease. *Radiographics*. 1990;10:1031–1048.

63. Secundini R, Scheines EJ, Gusis SE, Riopedre AM, Citera G, Maldonado Cocco JA. Clinico-radiological correlation of enthesitis in seronegative spondyloarthropathies (SNSA). *Clin Rheumatol*. 1997;16:129–132.

64. Takao M, Ochi M, Uchio Y, Naito K, Kono T, Oae K. Osteochondral lesions of the talar dome associated with trauma. *Arthroscopy*. 2003;19:1061–1067.

65. Barnes CJ, Ferkel RD. Arthroscopic debridement and drilling of osteochondral lesions of the talus. *Foot Ankle Clin*. 2003;8:243–257.

66. Kramer J, Recht M, Deely DM, et al. MR appearance of idiopathic synovial osteochondromatosis. *JCAT*. 1993;17:772–776.

67. Kitagawa Y, Ito H, Amano Y, Sawaizumi T, Takeuchi T. MR imaging for preoperative diagnosis and assessment of local tumor extent on localized giant cell tumor of tendon sheath. *Skeletal Radiol*. 2003;32:633–638.

68. Middleton WD, Patel V, Teefey SA, Boyer MI. Giant cell tumors of the tendon sheath: analysis of sonographic findings. *AJR Am J Roentgenol*. 2004;183:337–339.

69. Goiney RC, Connell DG, Nichols DM. CT evaluation of tarsometatarsal fracture-dislocation injuries. *AJR Am J Roentgenol*. 1985;144:985–990.

70. Otis JC, Deland JT, Lee S, Gordon J. Peroneus brevis is a more effective evertor than peroneus longus. *Foot Ankle Int*. 2004;25:242–246.

71. Rosenberg ZS, Beltran J, Cheung YY, Colon E, Herraiz F. MR features of longitudinal tears of the peroneus brevis tendon. *AJR Am J Roentgenol*. 1997;168:141–147.

72. Dombek MF, Lamm BM, Saltrick K, Mendicino RW, Catanzariti AR. Peroneal tendon tears: a retrospective review. *J Foot Ankle Surg*. 2003;42:250–258.

73. Williams BA, Morris LL, Toogood IR, Penfold JL, Foster BK. Limb deformity and metaphyseal abnormalities in thalassemia major. *Am J Pediatr Hematol Oncol*. 1992;14:197–201.

74. Giuzio E, Bria M, Bisconte MG, et al. Skeletal changes in thalassemia major. *Ital J Orthop Traumatol*. 1991;17:269–275.

75. Johanson NA. Musculoskeletal problems in hemoglobinopathies. *Orthop Clin North Am*. 1990;21:191–198.

76. Brasch RC, Wesbey GE, Gooding CA, Koerper MA. MRI of transfusional hemosiderosis complicating thalassemia major. *Radiology*. 1984;150:767–771.

77. Levin TL, Sheth SS, Ruzal-Shapiro C, Abramson S, Piomelli S, Berdon WE. MRI marrow observations in thalassemia: the effects of primary disease, transfusional treatment, and chelation. *Pediatr Radiol*. 1995;25:607–613.

78. Steinbach LS, Johnston JO, Tepper EF, Honda GD, Martel W. Tumoral calcinosis: radiologic-pathologic correlation. *Skeletal Radiol*. 1995;24:573–578.

79. Eisele SA, Sammarco GJ. Fatigue fractures of the foot and ankle in the athlete. *Instr Course Lect*. 1993;42:175–183.

80. Brower AC. The osteochondroses. *Orthop Clin North Am*. 1983;14:99–117.

81. Sun TC, Swee RG, Shives TC, Uni KK. Chondrosarcoma in Maffucci's syndrome. *J Bone Joint Surg Am*. 1985;67:1214–1219.

82. Lewis RJ, Ketcham AS. Maffucci syndrome: functional and neoplastic significance. Case report and review of the literature. *J Bone Joint Surg Am*. 1973;55:1465–1479.

83. Nora EF, Dahlin DC, Beabout JW. Bizarre parosteal osteochondromatous proliferations of the hands and feet. *Am J Surg Pathol*. 1983;7:245–250.

84. Bandiera S, Bacchini P, Bertoni F. Bizarre parosteal osteochondromatous proliferation of bone. *Skeletal Radiol*. 1998;27:154–156.

85. Meneses MF, Unni KK, Swee RG. Bizarre parosteal osteochondromatous proliferation of bone (Nora's lesion). *Am J Surg Pathol*. 1993;17:691–697.

86. Thompson GH. Bunions and deformities of the toes in children and adolescents. *Instr Course Lect*. 1994;45:355–367.

87. Coughlin MJ, Thompson FM. The high price of high-fashion footwear. *Instr Course Lect*. 1995;44:371–377.

88. Frey CC. Trends in women's shoewear. *Instr Course Lect*. 1995;44:385–387.

89. Coughlin MJ. Hallux valgus. *J Bone Joint Surg Am*. 1996;78:932–966.

90. Kerrigan DC, Todd MK, Riley PO. Knee osteoarthritis and high-heeled shoes. *Lancet*. 1998;351:1399–1401.

91. Shereff MJ, Baumhauer JF. Hallux rigidus and osteoarthrosis of the first metatarsophalangeal joint. *J Bone Joint Surg Am*. 1998;80:898–908.

92. Rodeo SA, O'Brien S, Warren RF, Barnes R, Wickiewicz TL, Dillingham MF. Turf-toe: an analysis of metatarsophalangeal joint sprains in professional football players. *Am J Sports Med*. 1990;18:280–285.

93. Richardson EG. Hallucal sesamoid pain: causes and surgical treatment. *J Am Acad Orthop Surg*. 1999;7:270–278.

94. Biedert R, Hintermann B. Stress fractures of the medial great toe sesamoids in athletes. *Foot Ankle Int*. 2003;24:137–141.

95. Karasick D, Schweitzer ME. Disorders of the hallux sesamoid complex: MR features. *Skeletal Radiol*. 1998;27:411–418.

APPENDIX: COMPUTED TOMOGRAPHY CASES

APPENDIX: MAGNETIC RESONANCE IMAGING CASES

HAND AND WRIST

ELBOW, ARM, AND SHOULDER

SPINE

PELVIS

PROXIMAL FEMUR AND THIGH

KNEE

LOWER LEG

ANKLE AND FOOT

APPENDIX: CASE LISTING BY PATHOPHYSIOLOGY

TRAUMA

MALIGNANT AND AGGRESSIVE TUMORS

Osteosarcoma

Chondrosarcoma

Primary Marrow Cell Tumors

Small Cell Sarcomas

Soft Tissue Sarcoma

Miscellaneous

BENIGN LESIONS

Benign Bone Forming Lesions

Benign Cartilage Lesions

Benign Fibrous Lesions

Benign Cystic Lesions

Miscellaneous Benign Bone Lesions

Benign Soft Tissue Lesions

METASTATIC TUMORS

Metastases

Hematologic Malignancies Involving Bone Secondarily

INFLAMMATORY ARTHRITIS

Rheumatoid Arthritis

Connective Tissue Disease

Spondyloarthropathy

Juvenile Idiopathic Arthritis (Juvenile Chronic Arthritis)

NON-INFLAMMATORY JOINT DISEASE

Osteoarthritis

Neuropathic Arthropathy

Crystal-Associated Diseases

Miscellaneous Joint Conditions

Toxic Conditions

INFECTION

Osteomyelitis

Joint Infections

Spine Infections

Miscellaneous Infections

MISCELLANEOUS

Osteonecrosis

Marrow and Storage Diseases

Hematologic Diseases

Miscellaneous Conditions

POSTSURGICAL IMAGING